ANTONY

OXFORD MEDICAL PUBLICATIONS

Primary Surgery

Volume Two Trauma

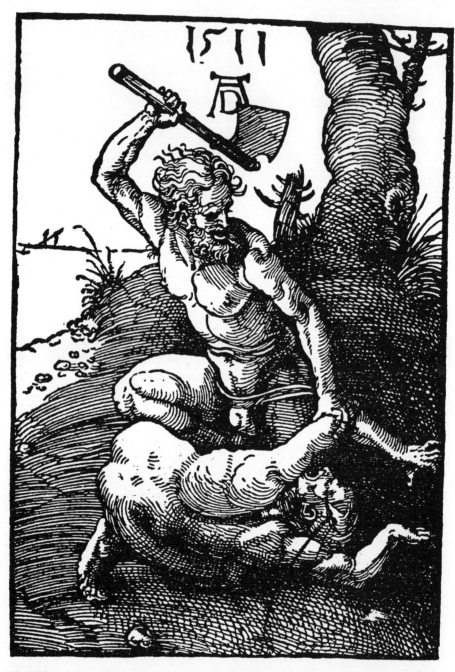

The Bible's earliest reference to trauma, and an expression of man's innate violence which will be the cause of so many of the injuries you have to treat. Cain is slaying Abel as Albrecht Dürer imagined them. Had Cain desisted at this point, as we are told he did not (Genesis iv:8), Abel might have required the control of arterial bleeding (**3.2, 55.1**), a wound toilet (**54.1**), the care of an open head wound (**63.6**) and treatment for a fracture of the vault of his skull (**63.7**).

Primary Surgery

Volume Two
Trauma

NELSON AWORI, MB ChB (East Africa), FRCS (ED.), DRCOG (Lond),
Professor of Urology, Chief Transplant Surgeon, Kenyatta National Hospital, Chairman Dept. of Surgery University of Nairobi.

JAMES CAIRNS OGDS (Zambia), OBE, MB BChir (Cantab), FRCS (Eng),
Director, St Francis Hospital Katete, Zambia.

GERALD HANKINS FRCS (Eng),
Honorary Surgeon, The Shanta Bahwan Hospital, Kathmandu, Nepal.

JOSIAH W. HIADZI DTM (Hamburg), FA Chir (Hamburg), FWACS,
Professor of Surgery and Head of Department, University of Science and Technology, and Komfo Anokye Teaching Hospital, Kumasi Ghana.

JOHN H. JAMES MBChB (St Andrews), FRCS (Ed),
Consultant Plastic Surgeon, Shotley Bridge Hospital, Co. Durham; formerly Consultant Leprosy and Plastic Surgeon, The African Medical Research and Education Foundation (AMREF), Nairobi, Kenya.

SAMIRAN NUNDY MB BChir (Cantab), FRCS (Eng),
Associate Professor at the All India Institute of Medical Sciences, New Delhi, India.

GERISHOM M. SANDE MBChB (East Africa), MMed (Nairobi),
Consultant Neurosurgeon and Head of the Section of Neurosurgery, Kenyatta National Hospital Nairobi, Kenya.

JOHN E. STEWART MD (Harvard); ABOS, 1951; AAOS, 1959;
Clinical Professor Emeritus (Orth), University of Washington School of Medicine; Orthopaedic Consultant, Harborview Trauma Centre, Seattle; formerly Senior Orthopaedic Consultant, Kilimanjaro Christian Medical Centre; Consultant, Rotary International Program Against Polio, Malawi.

Sir MICHAEL WOOD CBE, MBBS, FRCS (Eng)
Director, 'AMREF' The African Medical Research and Education Foundation, Nairobi, Kenya

Edited by
MAURICE KING MD (Cantab), FRCP (Eng), MFCM,
Senior Lecturer in Community Medicine in the University of Leeds; Lately Staff Member with the German Agency for Technical Cooperation (GTZ) in Nyeri Kenya.

PETER C. BEWES MB BChir (Cantab), FRCS (Eng),
Consultant Surgeon to The Birmingham Accident Hospital; formerly Honorary Surgeon to the Kilimanjaro Christian Medical Centre, Tanzania.

Illustrated by DEREK ATHERTON and IVANSON KAYAI

This low-priced edition was funded by the Wellcome Trust.

OXFORD DELHI KUALA LUMPUR
OXFORD UNIVERSITY PRESS

Oxford University Press, Walton Street, Oxford OX2 6DP
Oxford New York Toronto
Delhi Bombay Calcutta Madras Karachi
Kuala Lumpur Singapore Hong Kong Tokyo
Nairobi Dar es Salaam Cape Town
Melbourne Auckland Madrid
and associated companies in
Berlin Ibadan

Oxford is a trade mark of Oxford University Press

Published in the United States
by Oxford University Press Inc., New York

© GTZ 1987

First published 1987
Reprinted 1993 (with corrections)

British Library Cataloguing in Publication Data
King, Maurice
Trauma.—(Primary surgery; v. 2)—
(Oxford medical publications)
1. Wounds and injuries—Treatment
I. Title   II. Series   III. Series
617'.21   RD93
ISBN 0-19-261598-X (Low Priced Edn)
ISBN 0-19-261599-8 (Pbk)

Library of Congress Cataloging in Publication Data
Trauma.
(Primary surgery; v. 2) (Oxford medical publications)
Includes index.
1. Wounds and injuries. I. Awori, Nelson.
II. King, Maurice H. (Maurice Henry)   III. Series.
IV. Series: Oxford medical publications.   [DNLM:
1. Wounds and Injuries.   WO 100 P952 v.2]
RD31.P848   vol. 2   617 s   86-12815
[RD93]   [617'.1]
ISBN 0-19-261598-X (Low Priced Edition)
ISBN 0-19-261599-8 (pbk)

Printed in Great Britain by
Wm Clowes Ltd.,
Beccles, Suffolk

Foreword

The production of this manual on Trauma was
sponsored by the German Federal Ministry for Economic
Cooperation within the scope of the Technical Cooperation
Agreement with the Republic of Kenya, under project
number 78.2048.3-01.100. It was compiled by Maurice King
in close collaboration with Kenyan and other experts.

The manual contains the collective views of an international
group of experts. The methods and techniques described
correspond to the state of the art with regard to their
feasibility in rural hospitals where sophisticated technical
equipment may not be available. The manual cannot,
however, replace personal instruction by a qualified expert.
Neither the editor nor the publisher may be held responsible for any damage resulting from the application of the
described methods. Any liability in this respect is excluded.

Dr. R Korte, GTZ
Department of Health,
Nutrition and population Activities.
German Agency for Technical Cooperation
Postfach 5180D
6236 ESCHBORN
West Germany

Contents

50 Introduction

50.1 A system of traumatology

Trauma is so universal that the Declaration of Alma Ata included the care of the common injuries as an an essential part of Primary Care. This manual, the second in the series, describes how you as a non—specialist doctor can prevent much of the death and disability that are the result of trauma—for every patient who dies, at least two are permanently disabled, most of them at or near the most productive period of their working lives.

Here are the injured patients you will see:—

(1) A few patients whose injuries threaten their lives, and who may die at various intervals after the accident: (a) Patients who die immediately, within minutes, from lacerations of the brain, brain stem, or spinal cord. Most of these patients present at the mortuary, and account for about half of those who eventually die. (b) Patients who die within a few hours of the accident from bleeding into the skull, thorax, or abdomen, or from multiple lesser injuries. (c) Patients who die days or weeks later from infection or multiple organ failure. There is little you can do for patients in groups (a) or (c); those in group (b) are your main challenge, because you can usually save them using quite simple technology—if you apply it soon enough—within four hours of the accident and if possible much sooner. This needs rapid transport and rapid surgery.

(2) Some patients who need admitting to hospital, but are in no danger of death. You will probably find that about half the beds in your hospital will be surgical and about half the patients in them will have been injured.

(3) Some patients with quite severe injuries whom you can treat as out—patients.

(4) Very many patients with only minor injuries. Although the injuries may look trivial, many of these patients are wage earners and want to be back at work quickly. If you don't treat them carefully, complications may keep them away from work for weeks.

We have classified the methods of treatment that injured patients need into the three levels shown in Fig. 50-1. Like most classifications it is only a working compromise.

Level One, the care of a severely injured patient as a whole. When you first see a severely injured patient start with Section 51.3 and approach him systematically.

Level Two, the general methods. Some of these apply anywhere in the body and are those for shock (53.2), burns (58.1), split skin grafting (57.5), plastercraft (70.6), skin traction (70.10), skeletal traction (70.11), and amputations (56.1). Other general methods, such as opening and closing the abdomen, and making a colostomy, are described in Book One.

The general methods for particular regions of the body are those for injuries of a patient's eyes (60.1), his face (61.1), his maxillofacial region (62.1), his lower jaw (62.7), his head (63.1), his spine (64.1), his chest (65.1), his abdomen (66.1), his lower urinary tract (68.1), and his hands (75.1).

Level Three, specific methods and specific injuries, form most of the book, and assume a knowledge of the methods in Level Two. For example, the methods for each particular amputation describe only the details peculiar to each site, and assume that you know the general method.

If a patient is seriously ill with many injuries, you may need to work through all three levels. But if he only has a minor injury, such as a subungual haematoma (75.5), you can work at Level Three only. You are unlikely to forget Level One, but you may forget to refer to the general methods in Level Two. For example, don't treat a severe finger injury without following the 'General method for a hand injury' (75.1).

USE THE METHODS AT ALL THREE LEVELS

After first aid at the scene of the accident, we describe the care of an injured patient as a whole, the care of his airway, and the management of shock. Then come wounds, and with them artery, nerve, and tendon injuries. This is followed by

THE STRUCTURE OF THIS BOOK

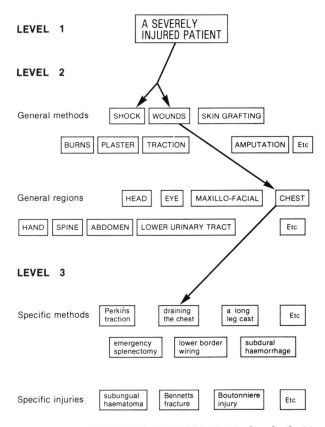

Fig. 50-1 THE STRUCTURE OF THIS BOOK is in three levels: (1) The care of a severely injured patient. (2) The general methods for the body as a whole and for partricular regions. (3) Specific methods and specific injuries. The patient shown here with the arrows was severely injured, so he needed the methods in Section 51.3 for a severe injury, and also those for airway obstruction (52.1), shock (53.2), a chest injury (65.1), and an intercostal drain (65.2).

methods for skin grafting and for the burns they are mostly used to treat. After a brief discussion of radiation injuries, the rest of the book is arranged anatomically, starting at a patient's head and working down his trunk. Then come general methods for his limbs (plaster, traction, and amputations), followed by specific injuries of his arms and then his legs, the more proximal ones first.

DIDIER (34) said that he had been hit on the scrotum by a bag of coffee. His scrotum was large and swollen and a quantity of bloody fluid was aspirated from it. Two days later he started vomiting and complained of abdominal pain. He had not passed flatus or a stool since admission. A strangulated inguinal hernia was diagnosed and 50 cm of necrotic gut was removed at laparotomy, after which he recovered uneventfully. LESSON Patients quite often ascribe the onset of their condition to some quite coincidental trauma.

50.2 Preventing trauma

Trauma—the tearing apart, burning, crushing, maiming, lacerating, and irradiating of the human frame is potentially one of the most preventable of mankind's afflictions. Injuries are the result of accidents or of violence, either personal, communal, or international. Almost all of them could be prevented, so what we say now about the absolute importance of prevention, applies to all injuries in later pages. Common prudence would prevent most of the injuries described here.

Road accidents are a major cause of death and disability in the developing world, so that measures to prevent them are urgent. Among other things, this means: (1) Seat belts for all front and, if possible, back seat passengers also. (2) The absolute rule that nobody should ever drive after having taken any alcohol whatsoever, not even a single drink. (3) The strict enforcement of traffic regulations and the separation, where possible, of motorized traffic from pedestrians. (4) In many developing countries better driving instruction and more strictly examined driving tests are an urgent need. Most of us are much more likely to die early from trauma than from anything else, so the personal precautions in this list apply particularly to ourselves.

Accidents with agricultural machines are often gravely mutilating, especially in rural communities using such machines for the first time. Proper precautions would prevent many injuries, so would elementary preventive measures in factories. Very often the same hazard causes the same injury in a succession of patients, so always ask how an injury was caused. If it was caused by something that might injure someone else, do your best to see that the danger is removed.

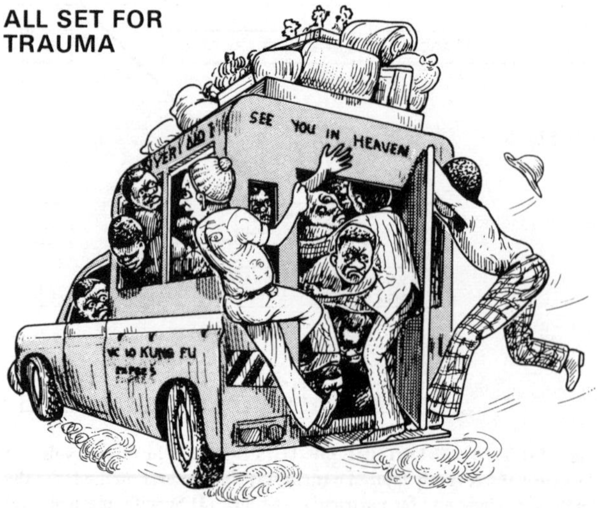

Many injuries, particularly burns to children, happen at home, and these too can be prevented by simple precautions.

In many societies social disintegration is causing increasing violence. As the result, many of the injuries you see will be due to fists, teeth, bottles, knives, sticks, and bullets, many of them inflicted under the influence of drink.

No form of trauma is in such desperate need of prevention as the 'megatrauma' from a nuclear holocaust. Many thoughtful people are now asking not if it will occur, but *when* it will occur. Preventing it is so important that it is considered separately in Chapter 59.

LIFTING AN INJURED PATIENT

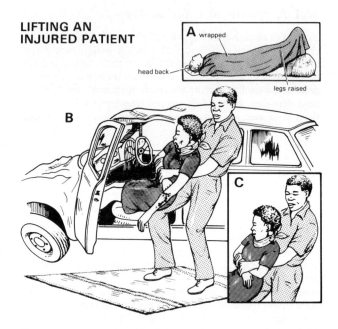

Fig. 50-3 LIFTING AN INJURED PATIENT. When a shocked patient is waiting for transport, lie him as in A,—horizontal, his legs raised, and his head tilted backwards. Wrap him up for warmth, but don't overheat him. B, lift him onto your thighs, kneel, and then slide him onto a blanket or a stretcher. If his arm is injured let it hang free. C, if both his arms are normal, lock your arms under both of his. These passers-by have no headboard to slide behind him and steady his cervical spine. *Adapted from Hans Pacy with kind permission.*

ALL SET FOR TRAUMA

Fig. 50-2 ALL SET FOR TRAUMA, especially head injuries (63.1), crush injuries of the chest (65.6), and fractures of the pelvis (76.2), femur (78.4), and tibia and fibula (81.1). *Adapted from a Kenyan newspaper.*

50.3 At the scene of the accident

A severe accident kills some patients instantly. Other patients die shortly afterwards from causes that could have been prevented, if they had been properly treated immediately after the accident. It is the purpose of first aid to prevent this unnecessary death and disability *before the patient ever reaches hospital*. The first people to help are usually the public passing by, so that the average knowledge of first aid in the community as a whole should be high. Try to do all you can to increase it, and particularly to teach the police first aid.

If possible, send a nurse or medical assistant with the ambulance. You will probably be unable to keep one on permanent standby, so put your most intelligent and interested driver in charge of the ambulance and teach him the first aid described below. Interest him by letting him see how you care for injured patients in the theatre. His tasks include the care of a patient's airway, and transport in the recovery position. An ambulance driver should also be able to immobilize the joints on either side of a fracture until a patient reaches hospital, so as to minimize pain, bleeding, shock, and further damage to the tissues.

EXTRACTING A TRAPPED PATIENT

A

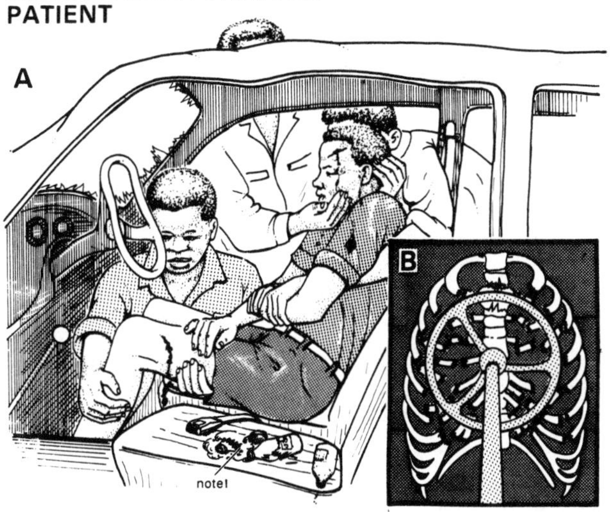

Fig. 50-4 EXTRACTING A TRAPPED PATIENT. One man uses the grip shown in the previous figure, another stabilizes the patient's neck and keeps his airway clear, while a third eases his legs out. B, shows what the steering wheel has done to his chest. *After Hans Pacy with kind permission.*

THE MINIMUM REQUIREMENTS FOR AN AMBULANCE

THE AMBULANCE BOX The contents of this should include a self inflating (AMBU) bag, face masks, oral airways, firm pads of sterile dressings, slings, crepe bandages, a head-board, a sucker, and Thomas splints or padded fracture boards. Pillows are also useful for splinting.

If you can send a suitably competent nurse or medical assistant with the ambulance, include bottles of a plasma expander or 0.9% saline, drip sets, and intravenous cannulae.

If you are called to the scene of an accident yourself, take a laryngoscope, an intubation set, a self-inflating bag, and a non–rebreathing valve.

IF YOU ARE FIRST AT THE SCENE OF AN ACCIDENT, you may be in command, so your first duty is to supervise. Warn other traffic by displaying a red triangle, or hazard warning lights, or other lights, or by any other means. Extinguish lighted cigarettes or other fire hazards and ask drivers to switch off their engines. Get uninjured people out of vehicles onto a place of safety, then remove the casualties.

THE MINIMUM FIRST AID Here are some of the things to teach your ambulance driver.

He should be able to: (1) Clear the patient's airway by holding his jaw forward and removing blood, vomit, and foreign bodies from his mouth. (2) Insert an oropharyngeal airway. (3) Use a sucker. (4) *Place the patient in the recovery position for transport back to hospital.* Not doing this is a common critical mistake. (5) Lift and carry a patient appropriately, particularly if he is suspected of having a spinal injury, as in Fig. 64-4. (6) Fit a temporary cervical collar. (7) Control bleeding by raising a wounded limb, by applying local pressure to a wound, and by pressing on the pressure points. (8) Ventilate a patient with a self–inflating bag. (9) Close an open chest wound. (10) Give external cardiac massage and mouth–to–mouth ventilation. (11) Treat shock by putting a patient into the legs–up position.

CAUTION ! (1) Transporting an unconscious accident victim on his back without proper attention to his airway is a major cause of unnecessary death. (2) The use of a tourniquet (55.1) is likely to do more harm than good.

FIRST AID FOR FRACTURES

Spine Move the patient with great care as in Section 64.3. If necessary, move him on a board or a door, or strap him to a plank.

Pelvis Tie three triangular bandages firmly round the patient's pelvis, put pads between his legs and tie them together.

Arm (1) Put his arm in a sling and bandage it firmly to his body. Or, (2) tie his arm to a splint which reaches to his axilla.

Fractures above the knee Put the patient's leg in a well padded Thomas splint. Take especial care to pad the neck of his fibula to prevent paralysis of his common peroneal nerve. If necessary, pad his leg well and hold it in place in a Thomas splint with a few plaster bandages.

Lower leg fractures If no Thomas splint is available, pad a piece of wood or bamboo, or even a palm branch, and tie this to the patient's injured leg, or bandage his injured leg to his normal one.

Other sections describe the first aid for obstruction of a patient's upper airway (52.1), burns (58.1), tension pneumothorax (65.5), and flail chest (65.6).

51 The severely injured patient

51.1 Caring for a severely injured patient

A severely injured patient can be a very gruesome sight—so don't panic! There will be much to do, so call for a nurse, a medical assistant, or an anaesthetist to help you. Two people can often work on the same patient simultaneously. First, preserve the patient's life, particularly by restoring his airway and restoring his blood volume. *More injured patients lose their lives unnecessarily from respiratory obstruction than from any other cause.* After you have done this, take the patient's history from anyone who was present at the accident. Extend this by quickly questioning the patient himself. Later, you can take a more complete history and examine him more thoroughly.

You will have to act quickly; no two injuries are quite the same, so vary the usual sequence of history taking and examina-tion. Train yourself to recognizse the urgent situations quickly while they are still treatable, especially rupture of a patient's spleen or liver, or an extradural haematoma.

MORE LIVES ARE LOST FROM FAILING TO CARE FOR THE AIRWAY THAN FROM ANY OTHER CAUSE

Many mistakes are caused by not examining a patient carefully. His peripheral injuries are unlikely to kill him even if you do miss them, but you can easily overlook serious central ones, especially injuries to his chest and abdomen. You will not miss bone sticking out of his trouser leg, but you can easily miss

AN ACCIDENT RECEPTION AREA

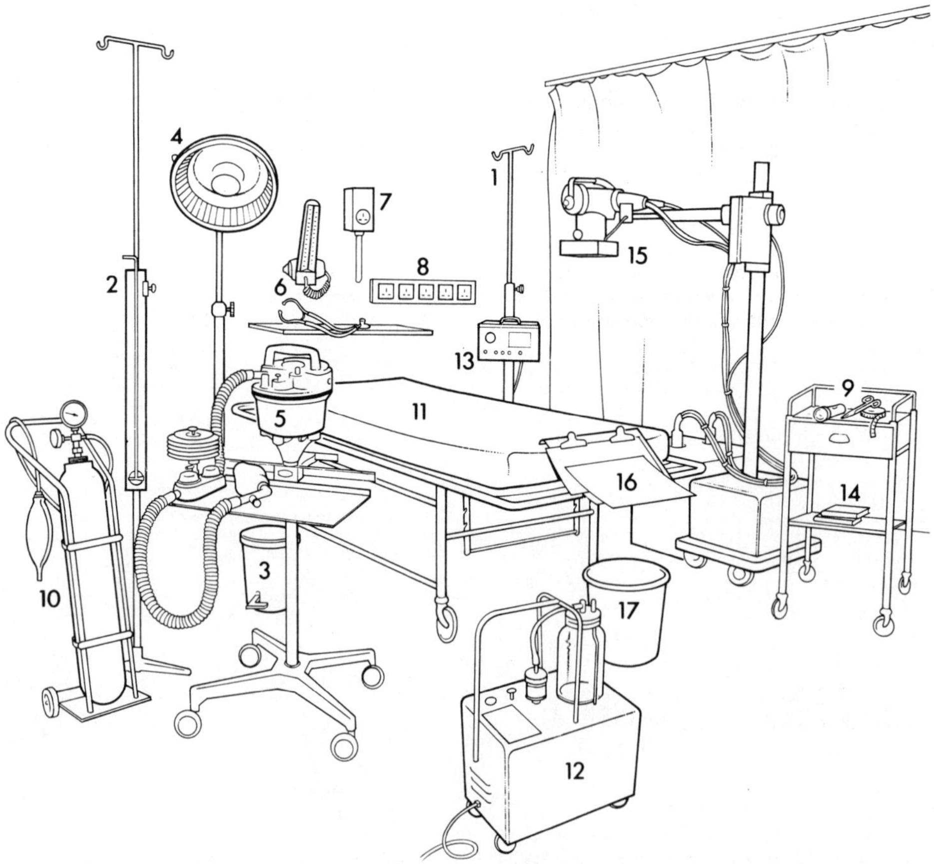

Fig. 51-1 AN ACCIDENT RECEPTION AREA. You may not be able to provide all these things, but try to provide most of them. The best place to take a severely injured patient may be your intensive care unit. (1) Drip–stand, (2) central venous pressure set, (3) sluice bin, (4) mobile lamp, (5) a completely equipped anaesthetic machine (and a ventilator if you have one), (6) sphygmomanometer and stethoscope, (7) large plug for X-ray machine, (8) several power points, (9) tape measure, torch, and scissors, (10) oxygen cylinder and flow meter with rebreathing bag, (11) special bed or tipping trolley, (12) sucker, (13) blood warming bath, (14) admission books, (15) X-ray machine, (16) charts, (17) bin for clothes. You will also need an ophthalmoscope and an auriscope, a labelling pen, urine test strips, drip sets, intravenous fluids and cannulae, and a chest drain set (65.2).

blood in his thoracic cavity or a slowly developing haemoperitoneum.

You will need enough space to work in and the right equipment. Figure 51-1 shows the ideal set–up. Try to have as much of this equipment as you can immediately available. You are unlikely to have a special accident treatment area, so the best place to take an injured patient may be the simple intensive care unit described in Section 19.1 of *Primary Anaesthesia* or the theatre.

There are no hard and fast rules as to what should be first aid at the scene of an accident and what is only possible in hospital. Many of the procedures which follow are practical in both situations. When a patient has arrived in hospital, don't let him wait around. If he needs a laparotomy for an abdominal injury, he should be *on the operating table within an hour of admission.*

• *TROLLEY, resuscitation, tiltable at the head and foot, with a radio–translucent surface, a device to hold cassettes underneath, holders for an oxygen cylinder and a drip attachment, also a wire basket for the patient's clothes and his property.* You will find this very useful. In spite of its detailed specifications, it is really quite simple.

THE CARE OF A SEVERELY INJURED PATIENT

ORDER OF PRIORITIES This is a summary of what follows— *be systematic and examine the patient in an orderly way.* (1) Clear his airway and maintain it. (2) Deal with any obvious chest injury. (3) Control any external haemorrhage. (4) Assess his circulatory state and correct it. (5) Note his level of consciousness and assess injury to his head (including testing his reflexes and examining his pupils). (6) Examine his abdomen and pelvis; look for fractures of his pelvis. Look for signs of internal bleeding. Note the state of his bladder. (7) Look for wounds and fractures of of his limbs. (8) Look for signs of injury to his spine.

IF THE PATIENT IS IS TRAPPED IN A VEHICLE, cut away the parts trapping him with great care. Move him carefully as in Section 64.3 to avoid injury to his spine. Keep him lying flat.

IS HE ALIVE ? Ask your ambulance driver to call you and let you see a seriously injured patient in the ambulance before he is moved. If he is not obviously alive, feel his carotid pulse, and listen for heart sounds with a stethoscope. If these are absent, and there is any evidence that they have only stopped in the last few minutes, attempt cardiopulmonary resuscitation as in A 3.5. Your task will be easier if you have three helpers, one to perform mouth–to–mouth ventilation, another to perform external cardiac massage, and a third to fetch help.

A PATIENT IN THE RECOVERY POSITION

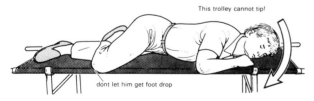

Fig. 51-2 A PATIENT IN THE RECOVERY POSITION. Lie him on his side with his thorax at 45° to the horizonal. You can support his chest with a pillow, but don't let it interfere with his breathing. His head is extended to provide a free airway. His uppermost arm is flexed in front of his trunk with his hand under his jaw to provide additional support. His lower arm is behind his back. To prevent him rolling over, you can flex his upper or his under leg, depending on his injury, while the other leg remains extended. He will be more stable with his under leg flexed. If he is on a stretcher for any length of time, don't let it press on his common peroneal nerve and cause foot drop. *From the Field Surgery Pocket Book with the kind permission of Guy Blackburn.*

If the patient is unconscious, can you rouse him by pressing one of his supraorbital notches firmly with your nail?

IMMEDIATE LIFE-SAVING PROCEDURES

CHECK THE PATIENT'S AIRWAY This is a summary of the methods in Chapter 52. You may need any of the methods in Fig. 52-1. (1) Clear any vomit or foreign bodies from the patient's mouth. Sweep your finger deeply into his mouth and pharynx. Suck out his pharynx. (2) Move his head and neck into the position in which he breathes best (A 4.2). (3) Make sure that his head is slightly dependent so that blood and secretions can drain. Unless particular injuries make it impractical, he will probably be best in the recovery position, if he is not already in it. (4) Insert an oropharyngeal airway if he is unconscious and will tolerate it.

If the patient is sufficiently unconscious after a head injury for you to insert a tracheal tube, insert one. As soon as his level of consciousness improves, he will make spontaneous efforts to remove it.

If his airway is obstructed and intubation is impossible, as with a severe maxillary injury in an adult, you can do a cricothyroid puncture with a needle, or a tracheostomy. In a child you will have to do a tracheostomy.

SOME LIFESAVING MEASURES

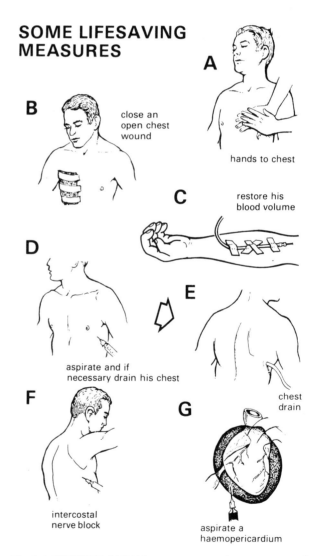

Fig. 51-3 SOME LIFE–SAVING MEASURES. A, if a patient has a flail chest, put your hands on it to control it. B, close an open chest wound. C, after severe bleeding, restore the blood volume. D, and E, if a patient has had a chest injury, aspirate his pleural cavity, and if necessary insert an underwater seal drain. F, after a severe chest injury an intercostal nerve block may greatly help breathing. F, if a patient has a haemopericardium, aspirate it. *After Naclerio, with the kind permission of Grune and Stratton.*

If he is not breathing adequately after the above measures, either ventilate him with a self inflating bag (A 10.3), or mouth–to–mouth (A 3.5). Give him oxygen. Think of the possibility of a pneumothorax (65.5) or a flail chest (65.6). Feel for deviation of his trachea, and for the position of his apex beat.

CONTROL SEVERE EXTERNAL BLEEDING Do this as in Section 55.1. You will probably find firm pressure on the wound most useful.

If a knife, dagger, arrow, or spear is still in the patient's body, leave it there until he reaches the theatre. If you remove it he may bleed severely.

APPLY URGENT MEASURES FOR SEVERE CHEST IN-JURIES A patient may need treatment for an open chest wound (65.7), a tension pneumothorax (65.5), a haemothorax (65.4), or a flail chest (65.6).

TREAT HYPOVOLAEMIC SHOCK Assess this by the methods in Section 53.2. If a patient is severely shocked, can you feel a pulse? Record its rate and his blood pressure. Set up an intravenous line by one of the methods in A 15.2. If he is in severe hypovolaemic shock and you are sufficiently skilled, the best method is to use a large bore catheter threaded into the great vessels of his upper trunk by the methods in A 19.2. Start by giving him a litre of Ringer's lactate or 0.9% saline.

If he is severely shocked and you are sufficiently skilled, set up a CVP (central venous pressure) line, as in A 19.2. This requires the insertion of a fairly wide bore catheter into a central vein or into his superior vena cava.

Continue the treatment of shock as in Section 53.2.

CAUTION ! Take blood for cross matching. If possible, take the sample before the patient's veins collapse, and before you give him a colloid such as dextran, which may interfere with cross matching. At the same time take blood for measuring his haemoglobin or haematocrit.

THE HISTORY OF A SEVERE INJURY

Take a brief history now and complete it later. Exactly what happened at the accident? First question any witnesses, then the patient himself. How did his body have to withstand the trauma of the accident? If you can find this out, you will know better what injuries to expect. For example, if he was hit by a car, expect 3 injuries, one from the bonnet, one from the bumper and another from the road.

If he is conscious ask him where his pain is? Does he have abdominal pain? This is always important (66.1). Has he passed urine since the accident? (68.1)

Don't forget his ordinary medical history. Perhaps he has a history of mental illness, or is taking drugs, such as insulin, steroids, or anticonvulsants.

IS THE PATIENT UNCONSCIOUS AFTER A SEVERE INJURY?

How does he respond when you press his supraorbital margin firmly with your thumb nail?

IS HE PARALYSED ?

Paralysis is easily missed, so don't forget a quick test to exclude quadriplegia, paraplegia, or a brachial plexus injury.

If he is conscious, ask him to move his arms and legs. If his legs are working, he has no serious spinal cord injury. Or, pinch one of his legs, and see if he complains.

If he is unconscious, check his pattern of breathing.

The following things suggest a spinal injury: (1) An accident in which there was violent movement of his neck, especially if he also has head or face wounds. (2) Severe occipital, shoulder, or arm pain. (3) Weakness or numbness in his arms or legs.

Don't move him until you have evaluated his injury. You cannot immediately exclude an injury to his spinal cord, so assume he has one and move him lying flat and without flexing or extending his spine as in Section 64.3.

Cervical cord injuries can come on insidiously, so don't allow him to stand or sit up.

THE PRELIMINARY EXAMINATION OF A SEVERELY INJURED PATIENT

Clean the blood from his face, and note if it is coming from his nose or ears. If necessary, cut away his blood stained clothing. His history and immediate signs and symptoms will tell you what to expect, so look elsewhere for the detailed history and examination of his major injuries, such as those to his head (63.1), spine (64.3), thorax (65.1), abdomen (66.1), and pelvis (76.1).

LOOK FOR FRACTURES Feel his limbs gently through his clothes. If there seems to be an injury underneath, you may have to cut them away along the seams. Compress his chest from front to back to test for fractured ribs (65.1).

On each side, feel the whole length of all his subcutaneous bones, the margins of his orbits, his clavicles, his olecranons, the subcutaneous borders of his ulnae, his patellae, and his tibiae.

CAUTION ! (1) Don't forget to look for blood at the tip of his urethra (68.1). (2) Observe and record all bruises. If these bear the imprint of his clothing, the injury underneath them is likely to be severe. (3) Carefully turn him onto his side and examine his back. Deformity and bruising here may indicate an injured spine (64.6). (4) If he has any limb injuries, make sure that he has no injured tendons (55.11), nerves (55.8), or vessels (55.2) in his wrists, fingers, ankles, or feet.

WOUNDS Remove any large pieces of clothing or foreign bodies which come away easily. Cover any wounds or open fractures and do the rest of the exploration in the theatre (54.1).

PERIPHERAL CIRCULATION Check the peripheral pulses of all his four limbs, especially the circulation peripheral to any limb injuries, particularly if he has supracondylar fractures of his humerus or femur. If a limb is cold and blue, a peripheral pulse is absent, or the capillary return to his nail beds is slow, you may need to reduce a fracture or dislocation urgently.

CAUTION ! A delay of only 4 hours in restoring the circulation to a limb can cause muscle necrosis (70.4).

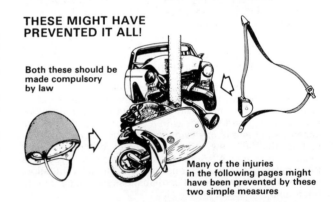

THESE MIGHT HAVE PREVENTED IT ALL!

Both these should be made compulsory by law

Many of the injuries in the following pages might have been prevented by these two simple measures

Fig. 51-4 THESE MIGHT HAVE PREVENTED HIS MOST SERIOUS INJURIES. Seat belts prevent most severe maxillofacial injuries and chest injuries. A crash helmet will usually prevent a head injury, but not a fracture of the cervical spine, so when you remove one, do so carefully, as in Fig. 64-1.

DRUGS Restore a patient's respiration and circulation before you give him an analgesic. If you expect internal injuries, avoid morphine until you have planned a course of action. If he has severe multiple injuries, pain is not so much of a problem.

If a patient is merely restless, this probably indicates progressive bleeding rather than severe pain. He probably does not need morphine.

If he is in pain, give him small doses of intravenous morphine or pethidine. See also Section A 8.7. Dilute 10 mg of morphine in 10 ml of saline and give him fractions of 1 ml at a time intravenously until you have relieved his pain.

CAUTION ! (1) Don't give him an *intramuscular* narcotic until you have excluded head and abdominal injuries, because they will confuse the diagnosis. You can give him *small* intravenous doses before you are certain of his diagnosis. If he has a head injury, he only needs morphine if he is conscious and has other injuries. (2) If he has a severe injury, such as a dislocated hip, he needs morphine—analgesic tablets are not enough!

OXYGEN If a patient has a severe abdominal or chest injury, or a low haemoglobin, give him oxygen. Otherwise it is unlikely to be useful.

X-RAYS IN SEVERE INJURIES

Defer these until you have resuscitated the patient. If films are scarce, don't X-ray the obvious. Where possible, try to do all X-rays in one trip. Wheel him to the theatre on a trolley with a radio–translucent top, so that he can be X-rayed on it with the minimum of movement. Splint limb fractures before he goes. This will minimize blood loss, and make positioning easier.

Take a chest X-ray and a supine view of the patient's abdomen. Where possible, take the chest X-ray in the erect position. But beware—this is dangerous if he is shocked.

If he is critically injured, X-ray only his major lesions initially. If you suspect a foreign body, X-ray the wound. If he has multiple injuries and needs an anaesthetic, X-ray him to exclude pneumothoraces, which would make anaesthesia dangerous.

CAUTION ! If you suspect a chest injury, but cannot confirm it clinically, X-ray him again in 48 hours. Lack of clinical signs does not exclude a haemothorax or pneumothorax of considerable size.

Before treating any peripheral fracture, make quite sure he has no proximal dislocation. If in doubt, X-ray him.

If you suspect an injury to his cervical spine, accompany him to the X-ray department yourself to supervise the way he is moved.

RECORDS IN SEVERE INJURIES

Complete these, record even negative findings, and make a management plan for the patient. If his consciousness is impaired, start a head injury chart. Prescribe all drugs and fluids. If there are many casualties, use Fig. 51-8.

ALLERGIES If possible, ask if he is allergic to any drugs, particularly antibiotics.

TETANUS PROPHYLAXIS Don't forget this, see Section 54.11.

SOME SEVERE INJURIES

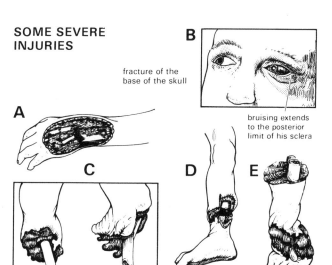

fracture of the
base of the skull

bruising extends
to the posterior
limit of his sclera

Fig. 51-5 SOME SEVERE INJURIES. A, a severe injury of the back of the hand exposing its extensor tendons. This patient would probably benefit from the groin flap in Section 75.27. B, fracture of the base of the skull (63.1). C, amputations of both legs. This is the patient JACK whose legs were torn off by a farm machine (54.3). D, a severe open fracture of the lower leg (81.12). E, another traumatic amputation of the lower leg.

THE LATER EXAMINATION OF A SEVERELY INJURED PATIENT

Examine him again later after you have attended to his more obvious injuries. As he recovers, expect to find more injuries. Although you may have saved his life from a severe head injury, a finger fracture which you missed may trouble him ever after. A brachial plexus injury (71.3) is easily missed at the time of the accident.

CHILDREN WITH SEVERE INJURIES

A severely injured child is in special danger, particularly from thoracic injuries, because: (1) His blood volume is small, with the result that a correspondingly small loss can be fatal. So replace any blood he loses, even if it is only a little. (2) His air passages are small and are easily blocked.

FLUIDS FOR SEVERE INJURIES

If a patient is shocked, he will probably be thirsty. Don't give him any fluids by mouth, including tea, even in minor injuries, because he may need a general anaesthetic. But, if you don't have enough intravenous fluids, and he is not going to be operated on for some hours, an oral electrolyte fluid (58.5) can be life–saving, especially if you have many casualties to treat at the same time. Prevent a patient's relatives from giving him food or fluids when they should not.

NASOGASTRIC TUBE A patient's stomach may be full and he may regurgitate its contents. So if he is drowsy or unconscious, or has severe injuries to his chest or abdomen, pass a nasogastric tube. This does not remove the risk of vomiting, perhaps with fatal results, but it does reduce its probability.

FEEDING A SEVERELY INJURED PATIENT

Intense catabolism occurs some days after a severe injury. This is proportional to its severity, is worse if the injury is infected, and is especially important in severe burns, so see Section 58.11.

ANAESTHESIA FOR A SEVERELY INJURED PATIENT

A patient may have been injured soon after his last meal. His stomach will empty very slowly. So, if he needs an anaesthetic, be safe, and use local anaesthesia when you can. If you have to give him a general anaesthetic, take the necessary precautions for anaesthetizing a patient with a full stomach (A 16.5).

If you are operating on a patient with multiple injuries, take the opportunity to insert traction tongs or Steinmann pins while he is in the theatre. Where possible, try to care for all his injuries at the same time.

REFERRING A SEVERELY INJURED PATIENT

(1) Never refer or evacuate a patient with an insecure airway—secure it first. (2) Even if a patient is not shocked, he must have a secure intravenous line—travel often causes shock in an injured patient.

GENERAL METHODS FOR PARTICULAR REGIONS

Read on for the general methods for injuries of a patient's: eyes (60.1), face (61.1), maxillofacial region (62.1), head (63.1), spine (64.1), chest (65.1), abdomen (66.1), kidneys (67.1), urinary tract, (68.1) or hand (75.1). Refer also to methods for specific injuries.

If a patient has lost consciousness after an injury, care for him as a head injury.

If he is severely injured, dead, or dying, talk to the relatives yourself, don't leave this task to the nurses. If possible, give them the opportunity to talk to him.

SEVERE INJURIES ARE OFTEN MISSED

51.4 Monitoring an injured patient

You have now done all you can for an injured patient for the moment, but there may be more to do at any time, so assess him thoroughly at *definite intervals of time* to observe any changes in his condition, because changes will then be more obvious. Change is gradual, and you are more likely to observe it if you retain a mental picture of him at one moment and then return 15 minutes or half an hour later. You may perhaps observe a change of 10 points in his pulse, increasing pallor, or the onset of sweating. These last two cannot easily be measured and charted, yet they often preceed a catastrophic fall in his blood pressure. If you have even a simple intensive care unit, this is the place for him while he is seriously ill, before and after his operation (19.1).

MONITORING A SEVERELY INJURED PATIENT

Record the patient's pulse and his blood pressure and, when necessary, his CVP (A 19.2)—if you are skilled enough to be able to insert a central venous line. When necessary, record his state of consciousness with a head injury chart (63.2), his fluids with a fluid balance chart (A 15-5), and his abdominal girth (66-2).

Make sure that the nurses who make these charts know that their role is life-saving.

CAUTION ! Watch him carefully for the development of a silent pneumothorax. Percuss his lungs daily. Reduced vocal resonance is a useful sign of a haemothorax.

A DOUBLE INJURY

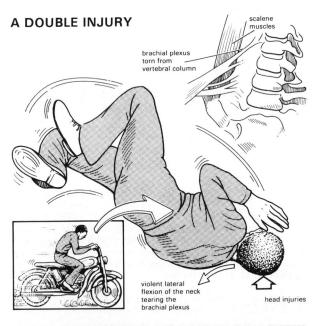

Fig. 51-6 A DOUBLE INJURY—HEAD AND BRACHIAL PLEXUS. This patient has been thrown from his motor cycle, injuring his head and his brachial plexus. He might also easily fracture both his upper and lower arms and his legs, and have internal injuries, especially a ruptured spleen. *From an unknown source.*

51.5 Some particularly difficult combined injuries

Although a patient can have almost any combination of injuries, there are some pairs of injuries in which one of the pair is often missed. If you find the more obvious injury of the pair, look for the other one.

A head injury and an injury of the patient's cervical spine. The same force can easily produce both these injuries. The patient may be unconscious from his head injury and so unable to complain of pain in his neck. Later, he may recover from his head injury only to find himself quadriplegic, or with a severe injury

to his brachial plexus. So, if a patient has a head injury, suspect that he may have a neck injury also.

A neck injury and obstruction to a patient's upper respiratory tract. This can be the result of a severe injury to his lower jaw. Support his head and neck continuously in a neutral position, until you have seen AP (anteroposterior) and lateral X-rays of his cervical spine. Hyperextending his neck to look at his larynx, or to intubate him, may damage his cervical spine seriously. Careful nasotracheal intubation or a temporary laryngotomy is safer.

An abdominal injury combined with any other severe injury, particularly a head injury. A severe injury elsewhere may distract your attention from a patient's abdomen. If he is unconscious he may be unable to complain of abdominal pain. Examine him carefully, review him frequently, and, if necessary, use the special methods in Section 66.1.

A chest injury and an abdominal injury. This is a common and difficult combination. Both the surgery and the anaesthesia for a thoracotomy are too difficult to be described here. If you cannot do one, at least be sure to: (1) insert a chest drain with an underwater seal before you operate, and (2) intubate the patient.

Multiple injuries and a haemothorax. A haemothorax would not be so deadly if it were not so easily missed. It may not be noticeable on the initial X-ray, especially in an AP film, but blood may accumulate slowly and silently over several days after the initial X-ray. So if a patient has multiple injuries, watch for a haemothorax over a week or more.

Other common combinations. (1) A chest injury and an injury to a patient's thoracic spine. (2) A fracture of his femur and a dislocation of his hip on the same side (77.4). (3) A fracture of his pelvis with a rupture of his urethra, and less often his diaphragm. (4) A pelvic fracture, a lumbar fracture, and paraplegia.

RAM (28) was one of several casualties brought in about 10 p.m. after a road accident. It had been a difficult night, and there had already been an emergency Caesarean section that evening. He did not look particularly ill and his blood pressure was normal, but surgical emphysema was observed over his left chest. Another patient had a severe malleolar fracture so RAM was second on the list. By 2 a.m. he was severely shocked, and was thought to have an abdominal injury. The anaesthetic assistant gave him ketamine and intermittent suxamethonium, but was unable to intubate him. His ruptured spleen was successfully removed, and a rupture in his diaphragm repaired, but he died just before the equipment for a chest drain could be assembled. LESSONS (1) If a patient has a chest injury, it usually takes precedence over that to his abdomen. (2) If you cannot do a thoracotomy at least drain his chest using an underwater seal. (3) A sterile chest drain set must always be instantly available (65.2).

ONE CAUSE OF MASS CASUALTIES

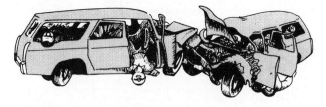

Fig. 51-7 ONE CAUSE OF MASS CASUALTIES. Fourteen people died in this crash on the Kaduna—Zaria road. Several others were seriously injured. Better driving instruction and stricter driving examinations might have prevented it.

51.6 Mass casualties

Sooner or later, ten casulties, or fifty, or even a hundred or more will arrive in your hospital after a bus accident, a fire or some civil disturbance. What are you going to do? The first principle is to approach the problem calmly and thoughtfully, avoiding undue hurry. The second is to have a *practical* plan prepared and know what it is. With luck, you will have warning of the disaster. More often, your first awareness of it will be the sudden arrival of many patients. The first half hour will be the worst, and if this goes smoothly, the rest of the plan probably will too.

Your first requirement will be space. One way to obtain it is to evacuate a ward, and, if necessary, to remove the beds. There will be room for more patients if you put mattresses for them in rows on the floor.

The most surgically experienced person should 'triage' (grade) the casualties. First, separate the living from the dead. Then grade the living into three groups. Priority One patients have life threatening injuries, such as penetrating wounds of the chest or abdomen, head injuries, or hypovolaemic shock. These are the patients whose lives you might save and who need an immediate operation. Priority Two patients have such severe injuries that they are likely to die anyway. Priority Three patients have only minor injuries and will probably recover, even if treatment is delayed. Operate on them last.

The decisions as to what to do with each patient should be made by the triage officer. It is the task of the non—surgeons to set up drips and take blood, etc. In a big disaster, and if you have enough staff, divide them into two shifts, each of which works for 12 hours, and then has 12 hours rest. There will be plenty to do, so make sure that everyone has some useful task and does it.

A MASS CASUALTY FORM

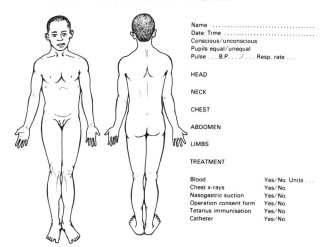

Name ....
Date: Time ....
Conscious/unconscious
Pupils equal/unequal
Pulse ... B.P. .../... Resp. rate ...

HEAD

NECK

CHEST

ABDOMEN

LIMBS

TREATMENT

Blood	Yes/No. Units ...
Chest x-rays	Yes/No.
Nasogastric suction	Yes/No.
Operation consent form	Yes/No.
Tetanus immunisation	Yes/No.
Catheter	Yes/No.

Fig. 51-8 A MASS CASUALTY RECORD FORM. Mark the position of the patient's injuries on the chart. *Kindly contributed by John Jellis.*

THERE MUST BE A DISASTER PLAN

MASS CASUALTIES

We assume that you are the senior triage officer. Your task is to direct other people, not to become involved in the care of particular patients yourself.

As soon as you learn of the disaster, order the present shift to stay on duty, and summon the shift which is off duty. Send immediately for whatever supplies and help you think you will need.

EMERGENCY EQUIPMENT FOR MASS CASUALTIES

You will need quantities of intravenous fluids, drip sets and dressings, and a supply of 1.5 mm×40 mm intravenous needles that you can quickly boil up and use to set up drips. Have these ready.

THE ADMINISTRATION OF MASS CASUALTIES

Clear a ward, designate it as 'the mass casualty area', and choose a nearby room for minor operations under local anaesthesia. Warn all departments, such as the laboratory and the X-ray department, to prepare for action. Get the sterilizers ready, assemble and sterilize the general sets and minor suture sets.

TRIAGE AND RECORDS

Triage the patients and allocate them to particular doctors, or, if necessary, medical assistants or nurses. Ask a clerk to stick lables on each patient's forehead indicating his category, and to make out a record sheet for each patient, like that in Fig. 51-8. This is reproduced again larger on an endpaper, so that you can photocopy it. If a patient's name is not known, give his label and his form a number.

Staff who have been allocated patients can then start examining and treating them, concentrating entirely on their own patients. Their first task should be to attend to airways and set up drips. Go round looking for seriously ill patients who have been missed in the first triage. These are usually the silent ones; the fit ones will probably be shouting for attention. Visit each staff member in charge of patients to find out what he has discovered, and record your instructions.

Meanwhile, the next most surgically competent person goes to the theatre and waits for the first patient to be sent to him by the triage officer.

After treatment, return all patients to the mass casualty area, so that they are all together. Put a doctor directly responsible to you in charge of them.

RELATIVES

should be kept separately somewhere else. Put someone with good public relations ability in charge of them to reassure them, and to answer their questions as best he can. Only in exceptional circumstances allow them near the patients. Ask them to donate blood.

PARTICULAR INJURIES

Where necessary, secure each patient's airway (52.1), control bleeding (55.1), seal any open chest wounds (65.7), and set up drips. Only an occasional patient will have severe facial injuries and need an emergency tracheostomy. For the others, an oropharyngeal airway will be enough. Some will need nasogastric suction and some catherization (68.1). Undress all casualties, and don't forget to look at all their backs.

OPERATION

Decide which are the urgent operations and do these first; many fractures, for example, can wait a few days. When you operate, be radical, try to do everything necessary at one operation, because there may be no chance to do another. Do radical excisions, and, where necessary, guillotine amputations.

Your assistants can go down the rows of patients in the ward sewing up minor wounds and dressing them.

TETANUS

Don't forget tetanus prophylaxis (54.12). It is tragic to work hard to save lives, only to lose them weeks later quite unnecessarily from tetanus. Some days later, if you are worried about tetanus, ask patients to open their mouths as you go round the wards. Those who have difficulty doing so may have it.

DIFFICULTIES WITH MASS CASUALTIES

If INTRAVENOUS FLUIDS AND DRESSINGS are scarce, try to save as many patients as possible with a good chance of survival. Treat those whose lives might be saved with 3 litres before those who need 15 litres.

Provided there are no contraindications, such as an abdominal injury or intestinal obstruction, you can give burns patients an oral salt and sodium bicarbonate solution, such as Moyer's solution (NaCl 4 g, NaHCO$_3$ 1.5 g in water to a litre) or (NaCl 5 g, NaHCO$_3$ 4 g, in water to a litre). These solutions are adequate for adults with burns of up to 15%. They have been used to treat burns of up to 30% successfully.

If you run out of dressings, use any clean cloth you have.

52 The airway

52.1 The general method for airway obstruction

If a patient survives his original injury, the next hazard that he has to overcome is obstruction to his airway. Making sure that he can breathe must thus be your your first priority. He is in particular danger if: (1) He is unconscious from a head injury (63.1) which depresses his cough reflex and causes him to lose control of his tongue and jaw. (2) His face, mouth, mandible, or neck has been injured (62.1). (3) His face or his respiratory tract has been burnt (58.27). (4) Rarely, his larynx or trachea may be injured (52.4).

The most important single measure in preventing airway obstruction is to make sure that a patient is transported in the recovery position (51-2). After this, the next methods are those which are also used to prevent obstruction during anaesthesia. These are described in Section 4.2 of Primary Anaesthesia, *and are shown in Fig. 52-1. Most of them are quick, and if one does not succeed, try the next one rapidly. The earlier ones are almost always enough. If they fail, and a patient is conscious or partly conscious, try 'awake intubation'. This is safe, it will not unduly distress him, and it is not practised as often as it should be. Laryngotomy and tracheostomy are rarely needed, but, when a patient does need them, he needs them urgently to save his life. You should find yourself intubating patients frequently, but doing a laryngotomy or tracheostomy only rarely. They are difficult to manage.*

NEVER REFER A PATIENT WITH AN INSECURE AIRWAY

THE GENERAL METHOD FOR AIRWAY OBSTRUCTION

DIAGNOSIS Try to diagnose that a patient's airway is obstructed early. Watch for noisy breathing, restlessness and confusion, cyanosis of his mucous membranes (often a difficult sign to detect), sweating and hypertension (caused by carbon dioxide retention), a fast pulse (later becoming slow as his myocardium fails), forceful movements of his chest wall, and intercostal and subcostal indrawing.

If he makes wet bubbling sounds, there is fluid in his respiratory tract, which needs removing.

If he has inspiratory stridor, his larynx is probably obstructed.

If he has to-and-fro stridor, his trachea is probably obstructed.

CAUTION ! Airway obstruction can be completely silent.

PREVENTION Make sure that the ambulance men transport him in the recovery position (A, Fig. 52-1).

THE TREATMENT OF AIRWAY OBSTRUCTION

Extend the patient's neck and draw his jaw forwards (B, Fig. 52-1). Remove pieces of vomit or foreign bodies from his pharynx with your finger (C). Insert an oropharyngeal airway (D).

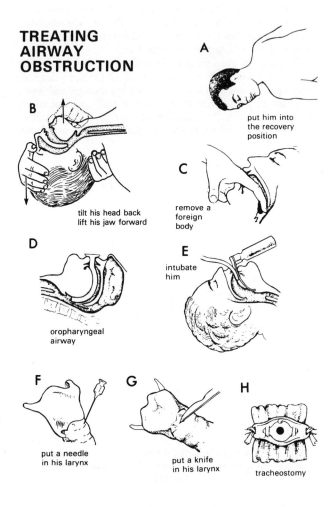

TREATING AIRWAY OBSTRUCTION

A put him into the recovery position

B tilt his head back lift his jaw forward

C remove a foreign body

D oropharyngeal airway

E intubate him

F put a needle in his larynx

G put a knife in his larynx

H tracheostomy

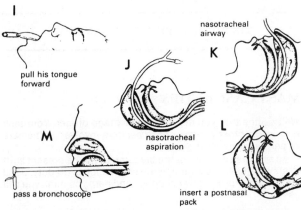

I pull his tongue forward

J nasotracheal aspiration

K nasotracheal airway

L insert a postnasal pack

M pass a bronchoscope

Fig. 52-1 METHODS FOR AIRWAY OBSTRUCTION. Try the earlier and easier methods first. *After Naclerio, by kind permission of Grune and Stratton*

If he is noisy, restless, and is struggling for breath, you can intubate him while he is still awake or partly conscious as described below (E).

If he is unconscious, you can intubate him as if he were anaesthetized (A 13.2).

CAUTION ! (1) If you suspect that a patient has a spinal injury, extending his neck to pass a tracheal tube may injure his spinal cord if you are not careful. Fortunately, most cervical spine injuries are flexion ones, and the little extension or even the neutral position required for intubation is not dangerous—provided you remember to avoid too much extension. (2) Nasotracheal intubation is more difficult, and there will not be a cuff on the tube.

If intubation fails or is impractical, do a laryngotomy with a needle (F), or a knife (G), or do a tracheostomy (H). Unfortunately, a temporary laryngotomy is difficult to manage.

If a patient has a maxillofacial injury (62.1), you may need to pull his tongue forward with forceps or a stitch (I), or pass a nasotracheal catheter (J), or give him a nasotracheal airway (K), or apply a postnasal pack (L). Sometimes he may need bronchoscopic aspiration (M).

THE AWAKE INTUBATION OF A SEVERELY INJURED PATIENT

SEDATION If a patient is conscious, give him an opioid, intravenously or intramuscularly. The intravenous morphine that he may already have had may be enough. If he is moribund, no sedation is necessary.

METHOD If possible, and especially if a patient is not fully conscious or is a child, try to intubate him without using a local anaesthetic. This will take some minutes to act, and will delay the return of his protective reflexes.

If necessary, draw 5 ml of 4% lignocaine into a syringe and needle. Ask him to open his mouth and spray 1 to 1.5 ml of solution onto and over the back of his tongue.

Ask him to close his eyes and breathe deeply. Reassure him, and then gently introduce a well lubricated laryngoscope over his tongue until you see the tip of his epiglottis. Then spray a further 1 to 1.5 ml of solution onto it.

When you see his vocal cords, spray the remaining 2 to 3 ml into his upper larynx and between his cords.

When his cords are widely abducted, pass the tracheal tube into his trachea and inflate the cuff. He will cough a little, but he will soon tolerate the tube. With his airway isolated, you can, if necessary, induce him intravenously.

CAUTION! Don't let a patient's tracheal tube remain in place for more than 48 hours with the cuff inflated. Deflate the cuff as soon as is safe, or it will ulcerate his tracheal mucosa. Tracheal tubes vary, and you can leave some in longer than others. Even if you have been successful in intubating him, he may still need a tracheostomy later.

IF YOU CANNOT INTUBATE, DO A LARYNGOTOMY
DON'T LET A TRACHEAL TUBE STAY IN PLACE
MORE THAN 48 HOURS

52.2 Laryngotomy and tracheostomy

If a patient's respiration is obstructed and you cannot relieve it by simpler methods or by intubation, you may *occasionally* have to open his respiratory tract below the obstruction. You can enter it through his cricothyroid membrane, or his trachea.

As a useful emergency method, you can pass two or more large (1.5 mm) short needles through his cricothyroid membrane, whatever age he is. In an adult (but not in a child) you have the additional possibility of opening his cricothyroid membrane (laryngotomy) with a sharp knife. If necessary, you can do this in 30 seconds or less—*it may be so urgent that you do not have time to sterilize the knife.* As an emergency procedure in an adult this is simpler and safer than the other alternative, which is an

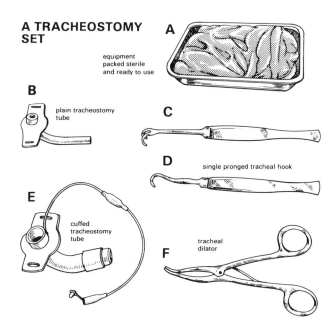

Fig. 52-2 A TRACHEOSTOMY SET. Always have this ready and sterile. You may need it in a hurry.

emergency tracheostomy. Permanent impairment of the patient's voice or airway is unusual after a laryngotomy. But it is a temporary procedure only, so he will need a formal tracheostomy later.

If possible *anticipate* the need for an emergency tracheostomy and do it as an elective procedure under local anaesthesia, ketamine, or tracheal anaesthesia. It will: (1) Provide immediate relief for a patient's upper airway obstruction. (2) Reduce his dead space by 100 ml and nearly double his alveolar ventilation. (3) Provide an opening through which you can suck out secretions. (4) Provide him with an airway that can be continued indefinitely.

But, a tracheostomy will also: (1) Greatly diminish the effectiveness of his cough reflex. (2) Short circuit the humidifying effect of his upper respiratory tract, and so dry his tracheal mucosa and make his bronchial secretions more viscid. (3) Make infection of his lower respiratory tract much more likely, so careful aseptic procedures are essential. (4) Occasionally cause severe bleeding. (5) Carry the risk of tracheal stenosis later, especially in a child.

Intubation is almost always possible, so that tracheostomy is only very rarely necessary. Only do it if: (1) Intubation fails or is unsatisfactory, and there is no other way of maintaining an injured patient's airway. Or, (2) intubation has to be prolonged for more than 48 hours. If his tracheostomy proves to be unnecessary later, you can close it. If it was necessary, you have saved his life. Even so, a tracheostomy has serious risks, especially when nursing care is poor. Here are two patients whose lives it saved.

OMARI (36) was crushed by some heavy scaffolding in a sugar works. He was dyspnoeic with paradoxical movement on the left side of his chest, which had no breath sounds and diminished vocal resonance. It was resonant anteriorly, and dull at the base posteriorly. His trachea and apex beat were shifted to the right. X-rays confirmed the diagnosis of multiple fractured ribs with a flail chest and a left haemopneumothorax.

A chest drain connected to an underwater seal was inserted in his left midaxilla, and he was given oxygen. Much air and a litre of blood flowed into the drain bottle, but he remained distressed and cyanosed. His chest was too painful to allow him to cough. Secretions began to accumulate, so he was bronchoscoped and copious sputum sucked out. Unfortunately, bronchoscopy was too traumatic to be repeated. Further X-rays showed diffuse mottling throughout both his lung fields. A tracheostomy was done, and his trachea was repeatedly aspirated, after which his general condition improved and his cyanosis disappeared. Eight days later his tracheostomy tube was removed and 3 weeks after discharge, he returned to work.

HAMID heard a lion chasing his cows. He went out with his spear, but the lion leapt at him, biting his throat, and penetrating his larynx. He arrived in hospital at the point of death, with blood bubbling from his mouth. It obscured his oedematous distorted larynx, so that intubation was impossible. A tracheostomy was done with some difficulty under local anaesthesia. He immediately began to breathe normally. Much blood was sucked from his trachea, and blood stopped coming from his mouth. He recovered completely.

You will need tracheostomy equipment in a hurry, so have a set ready sterilized in the theatre. You will need it for other indications, besides trauma, and particularly for respiratory infections in children. Here is the equipment for it.

• *DILATOR, tracheal, extra small for children, one only.* Use this to dilate the trachea before inserting a tracheostomy tube.

• *TUBE, tracheostomy, plain, uncuffed, reusable, with 15 mm termination, 15 Ch one, 18 Ch one, 21 Ch two, 24 Ch three, 27 Ch four, 30 Ch three, 36 Ch one, 42 Ch one, one carton of 15 assorted tubes only.* Traditionally a silver tracheostomy tube was used with an inner tube and obturator. Plastic ones are equally good, but they must be firm enough to hold their shape in the trachea.

• *TUBE, tracheostomy, standard, cuffed and reusable complete with obturator and one way valve, 24 Ch two, 27 Ch two, 30 Ch two, 36 Ch two, 39 Ch one, 42 Ch one, one carton of 10 assorted tubes only.*

• *RETRACTOR, tracheostomy, single, sharp hook, blunt, one only.*

• *RETRACTOR, tracheostomy, double hook, blunt, two only.* If you don't have one of these, use a Langenbeck retractor instead.

LARYNGOTOMY AND TRACHEOSTOMY

EMERGENCY LARYNGOTOMY

INDICATIONS Any of those given below for a formal tracheostomy when the patient is in immediate danger of death, and there is no time to do a formal tracheostomy.

METHOD Put anything under the patient's shoulders that will extend his neck, and make his larynx more prominent.

Find the prominence of his thyroid cartilage in the midline, and follow it downwards to the prominence of his cricoid cartilage, as in A, Fig. 52-3. Feel these on your own throat now.

Use your finger nail to mark the depression formed by his cricothyroid membrane in the midline between his thyroid and cricoid cartilages.

You can now insert needles or a knife.

USING NEEDLES (patients of any age) Insert 2 or more short wide bore (1.6 mm or larger) needles through the patient's cricothyroid membrane (B). Give him oxygen through one of them if necessary. Or, use a disposable needle and cannula ('Medicut') and leave it in place.

USING A KNIFE (patients over 10 years only) Make a vertical midline incision over the patient's thyroid and cricoid cartilages (C). Retract the subcutaneous tissues between your fingers. Spread the wound apart until you can see his cricothyroid membrane.

Insert the first 2 cm of the tip of a solid bladed knife horizontally through the patient's cricothyroid membrane as near his cricoid cartilage as you can (D). This will avoid his cricothyroid arteries which run across the membrane superiorly.

CAUTION ! Stand clear as you cut, you may be showered with droplets of blood and secretions as he coughs through his tracheostomy wound.

Widen the opening in his cricothyroid membrane. Put the handle of the scalpel into it horizontally, and turn it through 90° (E). If you don't have a tracheostomy tube, put any convenient tube into the hole.

Do an elective tracheostomy as soon as you can. If you delay it, perichondritis, stenosis, and subglottic oedema may follow.

EMERGENCY TRACHEOSTOMY

INDICATIONS Children and desperate emergencies only. A formal tracheostomy after intubation is safer.

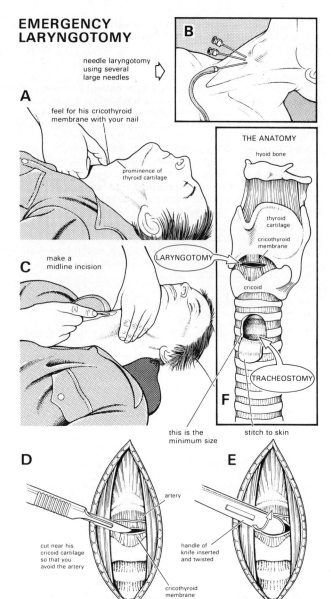

EMERGENCY LARYNGOTOMY

needle laryngotomy using several large needles

A — feel for his cricothyroid membrane with your nail

prominence of thyroid cartilage

THE ANATOMY
hyoid bone
thyroid cartilage
cricothyroid membrane
cricoid

C — make a midline incision

LARYNGOTOMY

TRACHEOSTOMY

this is the minimum size

stitch to skin

D — cut near his cricoid cartilage so that you avoid the artery

cricothyroid membrane

artery

E — handle of knife inserted and twisted

Fig. 52-3 EMERGENCY LARYNGOTOMY. You may need to do this for any of the indications for a formal tracheostomy when the patient is in immediate danger of death, and there is no time to do one. *With the kind permission of Peter London.*

METHOD There will not be time to make a flap, so make a vertical cut just above the patient's suprasternal notch. Make room underneath his skin with any convenient blunt instrument.

Neglect bleeding for the time being, unless it makes finding his trachea difficult. Leave his first and second rings and cut his third and fourth. There will be less chance of a stricture here. Turn the knife sideways. He will cough profusely. Insert a tracheostomy tube and stitch it to his skin.

FORMAL TRACHEOSTOMY

INDICATIONS The main indications in trauma are: (1) When intubation fails or is unsatisfactory, and there is no other way of maintaining an injured patient's airway. (2) When intubation has to be prolonged for more than 48 hours. Acute respiratory infection in children is the most common overall indication.

Intubation which has failed or is impossible in a patient with:
(1) Severe cyanosis who is dying of respiratory obstruction. (2) Severe jaw injuries. (3) Severe laryngeal injuries. (4) Severe burns of the face.

Severe chest injuries in which a patient with a flail chest or lung contusion is becoming increasingly cyanosed and has failed to respond to the insertion of a chest drain for a thorax or pneumothorax.

Severe head injuries in which a patient is in deep coma and has already had burr holes and treatment for cerebral oedema. He has been intubated and hyperventilated with a ventilator. He is now beginning to run the risk of complications from his tracheal tube. Oral and bronchoscopic suction are proving inadequate.

Also: (1) Respiratory obstruction due to a diphtheritic membrane or some other respiratory infection, especially in a child. (2) The need for prolonged ventilation. (3) Massive secretions needing frequent bronchoscopy. (4) Poliomyelitis, with respiratory paralysis. (5) Respiratory obstruction following thyroidectomy.

EQUIPMENT A sucker and catheter. A tracheal retractor or hook. A suitable tracheal tube, as listed above. The inner tube should be 3 mm longer than the outer one, so that secretions remain inside it. If you aim to prevent secretions accumulating, or to provide continuous anaesthesia with positive pressure ventilation, use a cuffed tube with a long curve, so that it makes an adequate airtight seal. Choose it carefully. *Don't use too small a tube.* If it is too long, it may reach to a patient's carina and block one of his bronchi. An incorrectly fitting tube may erode an artery and cause severe bleeding.

ANAESTHESIA (1) Intravenous ketamine. (2) Give the patient a general anaesthetic and pass a tracheal tube. (3) Infiltrate his tissues with a local anaesthetic solution (A 5.4). Local anaesthesia on a struggling patient is difficult; if you use it, find some sturdy helpers. Before any tracheostomy, warn the patient that he may not be able to talk immediately after the operation.

OPENING THE TRACHEA If you are inexperienced, make a 5 cm vertical incision starting just below the patient's cricoid cartilage, as in A, Fig. 52-4. When you have had successes, make a transverse incision 5 cm long 2 cm below the border of his cricoid cartilage. Cut through the patient's subcutaneous fat, and his cervical fascia (C).

CAUTION! (1) From now on use blunt dissection. Use it to raise short flaps and expose his anterior jugular vein and the underlying muscles.

Use blunt dissection to define and separate the fibrous median raphe between his right and left sternohyoid muscles. His sternothyroid muscles lie slightly deeper, find them and retract them laterally. You will now see the isthmus of his thyroid gland and part of his trachea. They vary considerably.

If the isthmus of his thyroid is small, there is no need to divide it.

If the isthmus of his thyroid is large and interferes with your approach to his trachea, divide it. Make a small horizontal incision through his pre-tracheal fascia over the lower border of his cricoid cartilage. Put a small haemostat into the incision and feel behind his thyroid isthmus and its fibrous attachment to the front of his trachea (D). When you have found the plane of cleavage, use blunt dissection to separate the isthmus from the trachea. Put a large haemostat on each side of the isthmus, and cut it. Later, oversew the cut surfaces or tie them (E).

Put sutures into the skin edges ready to close the wound round the tube later.

Insert a tracheal hook below his cricoid cartilage and pull his trachea forwards and upwards (not illustrated). Have a sucker and a catheter ready.

CAUTION ! Control all bleeding before you open the patient's trachea. Cut the membrane below its second or third ring transversely, and keep the sucker near the opening. Then stand clear. If there is blood in his trachea, he will cough it everywhere.

Turn a flap (F) containing his second tracheal ring downwards and insert the tube. The flap will act as a guide to direct the tube into his trachea and will make changing it easier. A flap largely eliminates the great danger of a tracheostomy, which is inability to replace the tube quickly when it has come out accidently. When the tube is safely in place, stitch the flap to his skin.

CAUTION ! (1) Don't disturb his first tracheal ring. (2) Don't remove any trachea. (3) Don't incise more than 40% of the circumference of his trachea, or severe stenosis may follow.

Inject 2 ml of lignocaine into the stoma in his trachea; he will tolerate the tube more easily with his mucosa anaesthetized.

INSERTING AND FIXING THE TUBE

With the obturator in the tube, place the tube in the patient's trachea (G). You will find this easier if you use the tracheal dilator (H). Remove the obturator, and replace it by the inner tube.

The tube must not slip out, so stitch it and tie it in two places: (1) On either side of the tube pass a silk suture through a bite of skin and tie it through the slots on the outer tracheal tube. (2) Tie the tube in place with tapes round the patient's neck. Tie it with his head well flexed, or the tapes may become slack when he sits up in bed with his head forward.

Pack vaseline gauze round the tube, and bring the edges of the skin incision together with sutures. Leave a little space round the tube, to minimize the danger of subcutaneous emphysema.

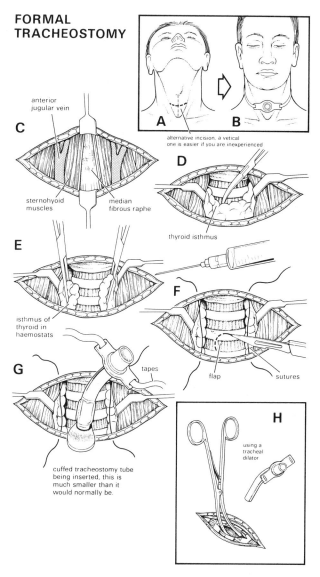

FORMAL TRACHEOSTOMY

Fig. 52-4 A FORMAL TRACHEOSTOMY. A, the choice of incisions. B, the tube finally in place. C, incising the patient's skin and pre-tracheal fascia. D, passing a haemostat behind the isthmus of his thyroid. E, clamping his cut thyroid. F, cutting the flap in his second tracheal ring. G, inserting the tracheal tube; this has been drawn much smaller for convenience. H, using a tracheal dilator. *With the kind permission of Peter London.*

13

CAUTION ! (1) Don't stitch his skin too lightly or too loosely round the tube. Surgical emphysema can be caused by: (a) closing his skin too tightly round the tube (causing him to drive air out into his tissues when he coughs round a partly blocked tube), or (b) closing it too loosely, enabling him to draw air into his tissues when he makes a panic inspiration through a blocked tube. (2) To avoid emphysema, *don't let the tube become blocked.* (3) If you use a cuffed tube, avoid too short a cuff or too high a pressure inside it. (4) Deflate the cuff 4 hourly for 15 minutes to reduce the risk of his tracheal mucosa necrosing.

THE POSTOPERATIVE CARE OF A TRACHEOSTOMY

Keep the patient in a steam room to prevent crusts forming in the tube. If necessary use a steam kettle or squirt a fine spray of saline into the tube every 15 minutes. Suck out secretions with a soft sterile catheter. Suck them out only as you withdraw it. Avoid prolonged or too frequent suction.

CAUTION ! Suck out his trachea aseptically. This is no less important than catheterizing his bladder aseptically. Use a fresh, sterile catheter each time. Remove and clean the *inner* tube every 4 hours during the first few days.

If viscid secretions have formed, loosen them by injecting 3 ml of sterile saline solution and then aspirate.

If the tube easily slips out, change it for one with a better shape. If necessary, take a soft tissue lateral X-ray of the patient's neck, to show how the tube is lying in his trachea.

CAUTION ! (1) Try not to change the outer tube before the fourth postoperative day. If you take it out too soon, it may be difficult to replace. Check the tension of the tapes regularly. (2) Minimize the risk of infection by sucking out his trachea regularly under careful aseptic precautions.

Later, insert a smaller tube and tell the patient to try to breathe and speak with his finger over the hole. As soon as he can do this easily, remove the tube.

DIFFICULTIES WITH A TRACHEOSTOMY

If there is FIERCE BLEEDING while you are inserting a tracheostomy tube the blood may be coming from: (1) The veins of the patient's anterior jugular system. (2) The isthmus of his thyroid. (3) The wall of his trachea. If blood enters his trachea round the tracheostomy tube, immediately insert a cuffed tube. Then open the wound and tie any bleeding vessels. Next time make a vertical incision.

If the patient's tracheostomy TUBE SLIPS OUT, you may have: (1) Made the tracheostomy in the wrong place. (2) Used the wrong shape of tube. (3) Failed to adjust the tapes round his neck. (4) Not stitched the outer tube's flanges to his skin.

If the INNER TUBE BLOCKS, change it frequently, humidify the air he breathes, and suck regularly.

If his TRACHEA BECOMES STENOSED, it has probably done so because you opened it below the level of the second tracheal ring.

If he CANNOT TOLERATE THE REMOVAL OF THE TUBE, the reason may be psychogenic. If he is an adult, gradually reduce its size, then cork it for progressively longer periods before removing it.

52.3 Injuries of the larynx and trachea

Injuries to a patient's nose (62.4) and mouth (62.1) are discussed elsewhere. Injuries to his larynx and trachea are rare and difficult. His main danger is the aspiration of blood into his lungs and surgical emphysema (65.10). Try to pass a cuffed tube beyond the wound, either through his nose or mouth, or through the wound itself. A tube will also reduce the danger of emphysema.

53 Shock

53.1 Four kinds of shock

There are several kinds of shock, but the final mechanism in all of them is a fall in a patient's cardiac output which reduces the supply of blood to his brain, kidneys, gut, liver, lungs, and muscles. His brain is the most sensitive of these organs.

Hypovolaemic shock is our main concern here. A patient's blood volume can fall because of: (1) Sudden bleeding, either external or internal. (2) The slow loss of plasma from his circulation due to burns or peritonitis. (3) The loss of extracellular fluid as the result of vomiting, diarrhoea, intestinal obstruction or fistulae. In theory, the treatment of all these kinds of shock is straightforward—restore his blood volume with balanced electrolyte solutions or whole blood as appropriate. Section 14.3 of *Primary Anaesthesia* describes the treatment of surgical dehydration.

Vasovagal shock or neurogenic shock is the result of a strong sensory or emotional stimulus which causes widespread vasodilation and bradycardia. Trauma, either severe or trivial, is one such stimulus. The patient may yawn, feel hot, sweat, and then lose consciousness. He breathes with slow deep sighs, he becomes cold and pale, his blood pressure falls, and he has a slow pulse. If he lowers his head or lies down, he rapidly recovers.

Vasovagal attacks are common and normally harmless, but they can be important because: (1) Their symptoms can be added to those of hypovolaemic shock and make a patient seem worse than he really is. The critical sign is his pulse. *If this is slow, suspect that there is a strong vasovagal component to his symptoms.* (2) If vasovagal shock is added to hypovolaemia, he may collapse suddenly during the induction of anaesthesia. (3) Vasovagal shock can complicate such procedures as the manipulation of fractures. (4) If he remains seated upright during a vasovagal attack, his brain becomes anoxic and he may die.

Septic shock is caused by bacteria releasing endotoxins which cause circulatory collapse, especially when antibiotics kill them in large numbers in a patient's circulation when he is septicaemic. Although this might logically be considered in Volume One, with the surgery of sepsis, it is more conveniently included here.

Cardiogenic shock has many medical causes, the most important one being cardiac infarction. There are also two important surgical causes—bruising of the heart and cardiac tamponade (65.9), due to blood in the pericardial cavity. This is rare but it is important because you can treat it. Don't transfuse a patient if he is in cardiogenic shock, unless there are other reasons for doing so. More fluid in his circulation can weaken myocardial contractility and add to the work of his heart.

There are difficulties in diagnosing and managing hypovolaemic shock: (1) Diagnosing internal bleeding may not be easy, so (a) remember the possibility of an ectopic pregnancy, and (b) don't forget that shock developing after trauma may be due to bleeding into a patient's peritoneal cavity or behind it, into his pleural cavities (65.4), or into the muscles round fractures, particularly those of his pelvis or femur. He can die from bleeding into any of these places, without any blood appearing on the surface. (2) Shock is not the only cause of reduced consciousness in an injured patient—he may be drunk, drugged, concussed, hypoxic or hypoglycaemic; he may also be suffering from a head injury. Sometimes he is unconscious for more than one of these reasons—the combination of a head injury and abdominal bleeding is common. Finally, (3) don't diagnose an infarct without some positive evidence for it, such as precordial pain and no signs of any other cause of shock.

53.2 Hypovolaemic shock after an injury

A patient in hypovolaemic shock is intensely pale with cold extremities. The first signs to suggest that insufficient blood is reaching his brain are drowsiness and withdrawal from his environment, although he can be deceptively alert and euphoric. As shock deepens he becomes agitated, delirious, and finally comatose. His pulse is rapid, and his blood pressure low. When you pinch one of his nails, its bed empties of blood and takes a long time to fill up. His breathing is fast and rapid. He is thirsty and acidotic, and he passes little urine.

He has two main ways of compensating for the blood he loses: (1) He immediately constricts the vessels in his skin and gut. About 75% of the blood is in the veins, so venous constriction is particularly effective. (2) Later, he slowly absorbs the extracellular fluid from his tissues, with the result that his skin loses its elasticity, and his eyes sink into their sockets. Although this maintains his blood volume, it dilutes his remaining red cells, so that his haemoglobin falls and he becomes anaemic over several days.

Both these mechanisms have their limits. A normal adult's blood volume is 80 ml/kg or about 5.5 litres. Whether he goes into shock, or not, depends on how much blood he loses. If he loses 10% of it (500 ml) he is unlikely to show signs of shock, but if he loses 20% of it (a litre) he almost certainly will. Provided he loses less than a third of his blood volume (2 litres), he can usually maintain his blood pressure above 100 mm. If he loses half of it (about 3 litres) for more than a few minutes, he dies. So a shocked adult needs a transfusion of *at least a litre, and if he is severely shocked he may need 3 litres.* If he continues to bleed, he may need much more. A child has a smaller blood volume, so that a given loss is proportionately more serious in him.

BEWARE OF A CHILD'S SMALL BLOOD VOLUME

When you try to decide how shocked a patient is, remember that: (1) His condition is never static. From moment to moment he will be getting better or worse. (2) Shock usually develops slowly over several hours, although it can develop rapidly. (3) A single sign may not be reliable, so use several. (4) His symptoms may be out of proportion to the volume of blood he has lost. A small loss may occasionally cause severe shock and vice versa. (5) A falling blood pressure is an unreliable sign, and occurs late. For example, the blood pressure of a child or young adult may not fall at all, until it finally falls catastrophically, when he has lost a third or more of his blood volume. Try to restore the blood volume *before* this happens. *A rising pulse rate is an*

THE BLOOD VOLUME IN CHILDREN

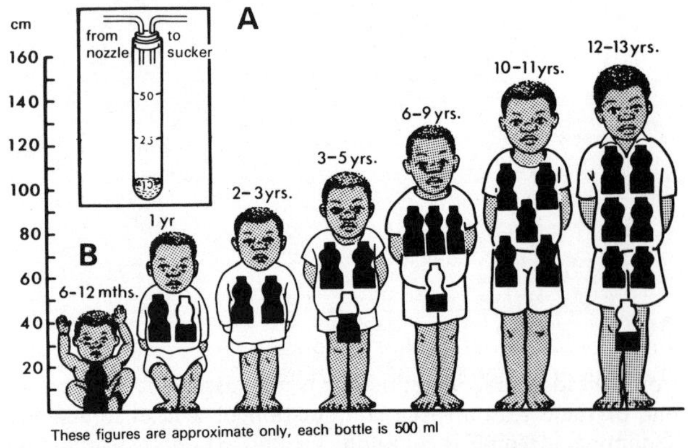

Fig. 53-1 THE BLOOD VOLUME IN CHILDREN. A, when you operate on a child, put a graduated test tube in your suction line. B, the loss of even a little blood can cause severe shock in a small child. Each one of these bottles contains 500 ml. *After Brenda Vaughan.*

earlier and more reliable sign than a falling blood pressure. But even the pulse may not rise until late, particularly if the patient is old. A good pulse volume, a warm pink skin (if he is Caucasian), well filled veins, and a good urine output, are better signs of an adequate blood volume than a normal blood pressure. If a patient's systolic blood pressure falls below 100 mm after an injury, he needs an infusion. If it falls below 80 mm he needs it urgently.

IN HYPOVOLAEMIA THE BLOOD PRESSURE MAY FALL LATE

Electrolyte solutions are useful replacements for lost blood. If a patient can only maintain his cardiac output, he can meet the oxygen demands of his tissues even if his haemoglobin falls as low as 8 g/dl. He is only likely to need a blood transfusion if: (1) He has lost 1000 ml of blood or more. Or, (2) his haemoglobin later falls below 10 g.

If an adult is in severe hypovolaemic shock, give him a large volume (2 to 3 litres) of an electrolyte solution fast, preferably Ringer's lactate, but if necessary 0.9% saline, or glucose saline. Then assess his needs by evaluating his clinical response. Unfortunately, these solutions will leave his circulation in an hour or two. Colloids like dextran stay in it longer; you can give him dextran 70 in 0.9% saline to replace up to 30% of his blood volume, or up to about 2 litres if he is an adult. Giving more may damage his kidneys.

If possible, try to stop him bleeding, then restore his blood volume, and then operate on him. If he is bleeding externally, this it should not be difficult (55.1). If he is bleeding internally, *resuscitate him as best you can, and then operate.* He will probably need a laparotomy. He will not die from anaemia while you do this, but he may die from hypovolaemia. His blood pressure should be over 80 mm before surgery starts. Ideally, it should have remained over 100 mm for at least 20 minutes. But, if he does not respond to resuscitation, an immediate laparotomy is his only hope. For example, if he has ruptured his spleen, try to get your hand on his splenic pedicle as soon as you can—bold action may save his life. You are like a person who is trying to fill a bath without first putting in the plug. Somehow, you will have to put in the plug.

Restoring a patient's blood pressure is not a sufficient aim in itself. A good pulse volume, warm extremities, and a systolic pressure of only 70 mm, are better than a normal systolic pressure, cold extremities, and a rapid pulse. *The surest way to know if you have given a patient enough fluid is to put a catheter in his bladder, and to monitor his urine output.*

The common mistake is to underestimate the volume of blood that a patient has lost, and so to give him *too little fluid too slowly.* You are unlikely to give a young healthy person too much fluid before you realize that his circulation is normal. But in an old hypertensive or cardiac patient, be more cautious. You can precipitate cardiac failure before you have corrected his hypovolaemia. Ideally, such a patient needs a CVP monitor (A 19.2).

Anaesthesia is dangerous if a patient is severely shocked (16.7), because he is only maintaining his blood pressure by severe vasconstriction; a general anaesthetic abolishes this, so does subarachnoid (spinal) anaesthesia in the lower half of the body. If he is desperately ill, local infiltration anaesthesia may be best (A 5.4, A 6.7).

WHEN IN DOUBT INFUSE
OPERATE AS SOON AS A PATIENT IS FIT FOR SURGERY
THE COMMON MISTAKE IS NOT TO GIVE ENOUGH FLUID

GRADING SHOCK

			← Skin	→				
Degree of Shock	**Blood pressure**	**Pulse quality**	**Temperature**	**Colour**	**Circulation**	**Thirst**	**Urine output**	**Mental state**
None	Normal	Normal	Normal	Normal	Normal	Normal	Normal	Clear and distressed
Slight	To 20 per cent decrease	Normal	Cool	Pale	Definite slowing	Normal	Normal	Clear and distressed
Moderate	Decreased 20 per cent to 40 per cent	Definite decrease in volume	Cool	Pale	Definite slowing	Definite	Reduced	Clear and some apathy unless stimulated
Severe	Decreased 40 per cent to non recordable	Weak to imperceptible	Cold	Ashen to cyanotic (mottling)	Very sluggish	Severe	Oliguria	Apathetic to comatose; little distress except thirst

Fig. 53-2 GRADING HYPOVOLAEMIC SHOCK Don't rely on one sign only, use as many as you can. Measure the patient's blood pressure, and the rate and quality of his pulse; assess the colour of his skin; ask him if he is thirsty, assess his mental state. Later, his urine volume will be the best guide. *From the Field Surgery Pocket Book, with the kind permission of Guy Blackburn.*

HYPOVOLAEMIC SHOCK

This extends Section 51.3 on the care of a severely injured patient. You have diagnosed shock, and have already inserted an intravenous line.

MINIMIZING SHOCK These things make hypovolaemic shock worse, so try to avoid them: (1) Rough handling. (2) Prolonged or rough operating, including (a) the repeated vigorous manipulation of fractures, (b) the prolonged handling of gut through too small an incision, (c) too many operations on the day of the injury. (3) Ignoring intra–operative bleeding by failing to use warm packs, or to tie or clamp bleeding vessels. (4) Associated dehydration due to severe vomiting, diarrhoea, or sweating. (5) Warming a patient with hot water bottles or shock cradles. Warmth may overcome the vasoconstriction that he needs to maintain his circulation, so don't let a shocked patient get too warm. Instead, put a blanket over him to prevent him losing heat and actually getting cold.

SOME INJURIES DO NOT CAUSE SHOCK, so that if a patient has one of them and is shocked, suspect that it is not the cause of his shock and that he has some other injury also, probably an abdominal one. Injuries which do not by themselves cause shock include: (1) Any minor injury. (2) Head injuries. (3) Maxillofacial injuries.

IMMEDIATE TREATMENT Raise the patient's legs at right angles to his body. The blood in them will give him an autotransfusion and increase the venous return to his heart. Don't tilt him with his head down because: (1) It is uncomfortable. (2) It causes cererebral congestion, and (3) it impairs the movement of his diaphragm.

HOW SHOCKED IS HE ?

Don't rely on one sign only, use as many as you can. Apply the rules Fig. 53-2. Measure his blood pressure, and the rate and quality of his pulse; assess the colour of his skin; ask him if he is thirsty, assess his mental state. Later, his urine volume will be the best guide.

Feel the warmth and wetness of his forehead and hands. Are his hands or his nose cold? If his feet are cold, how far up his legs does the coldness go? If he is cold below the knee, he has lost 30% of his blood volume.

How full are his peripheral veins? Judge this from two signs: (1) Empty any convenient superficial vein by pressing it between two of your fingers. Remove your distal finger, and see how fast the empty vein fills up. (2) Look at the veins on the dorsum of his ankle. If they are invisible through a white skin, he is likely to be in hypovolaemic shock. This sign is less valuable in a dark one.

What is the capillary pressure in his nail beds? Press the blood out of one of them. How quickly does it fill up?

What is the pressure of his interstitial fluid? Look for: (1) sunken eyes, (2) loss of skin elasticity, (3) lowered eyeball tension, and (4) in severe cases, a Hippocratic facies. These are late signs.

If his respiration is shallow and rapid (air hunger), he is severely shocked.

If possible, and if you are sufficiently skilled, insert a central venous line (A 19.2) and measure his central venous pressure (CVP). This will be useful for monitoring treatment.

CAUTION ! (1) A falling blood pressure is a late sign of increasing shock. (2) Don't give him vasopressor drugs.

HOW MUCH BLOOD HAS HE LOST EXTERNALLY? A patient's history will be of some help. On the floor or on his clothes 100 ml of blood covers about a thousand square centimetres, or one square foot. A litre covers about a square metre (or square yard).

HOW MUCH BLOOD HAS HE LOST INTERNALLY? The volume of your fist is about 500 ml (one unit of blood or fluid). For each mass of soft tissue swelling equal to this, he needs a unit of replacement fluid. Fractures cause approximately the following blood loss. Upper limb fractures 1 unit. Tibia and fibula 2 units. Femur 1.5 units. Pelvis or multiple fractured ribs 2 to 6 units. For each rib fracture you can see on the X-ray, estimate 100 ml. If a fracture is open, add another 0.5 to 1 unit. A patient's abdomen or thorax can hold 3 litres of blood

or more. If he has multiple injuries he can thus lose much blood.

CAUTION ! (1) Lost blood need not reach the surface. (2) The loss of only a few hundred millilitres may be fatal in a small child, as in Fig. 53-1.

DOES THE SEVERITY OF HIS SHOCK MATCH THE VOLUME OF BLOOD HE HAS LOST? Perhaps the patient has a fractured forearm and a fractured femur with an average sized haematoma, yet a litre of blood does not resuscitate him. He probably lost more blood externally at the site of the accident, or he has lost it into his abdomen or chest.

If he has a fast pulse and a low blood pressure with only a small wound, suspect that he has some serious internal injury, or, if a day or two has passed since the accident, some massive infection or gas gangrene.

THE MANAGEMENT OF A PATIENT IN HYPOVOLAEMIC SHOCK

This follows on from Section 51.3. You have taken blood for cross matching, and set up at least one good intravenous line, by the methods in A 15.2. If the patient is bleeding externally, you have controlled it (55.1). He is receiving oxygen. His management during (A 4.4) and after the operation (A 4.5), or when burns (58.4) or dehydration (A 15.3) are causing his shock, are described elsewhere.

CATHETER Insert an indwelling catheter and attach it to a urine bag. Or, collect his urine in a 250 ml plastic measuring cylinder. If you suspect a urethral injury, insert the catheter suprapubically (68.1). An adequate urine output will be the

ESTIMATING BLOOD LOSS

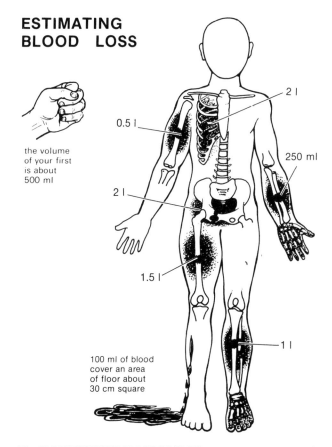

the volume of your first is about 500 ml

0.5 l

2 l

250 ml

2 l

1.5 l

1 l

100 ml of blood cover an area of floor about 30 cm square

Fig. 53-3 ESTIMATING BLOOD LOSS. When you examine an injured patient, try to estimate how much blood he has lost. The volume of your fist is about 500 ml (one unit of blood or fluid). For each mass of soft tissue swelling equal to this, he needs a unit of replacement fluid. For each rib fracture you can see on the X-ray, estimate 100 ml. If a fracture is open, add another 0.5 to 1 unit. A patient's abdomen or thorax can hold 3 litres of blood or more. If he has multiple injuries he can thus lose much blood. *After Hamilton Bailey, with the kind permission of Hugh Dudley.*

most useful indication that you have treated his hypovolaemic shock adequately. Examine the first urine from this catheter. Look especially for blood, and if possible culture it.

If, later, no urine appears in the bag, make sure: (1) that the catheter is not kinked, and (2) that the inlet spigot has been removed from the bag.

If the catheter only produces a little urine and some blood, suspect that he has a bladder or urethral injury (68.1).

HOW MUCH FLUID SHOULD YOU GIVE HIM AND HOW FAST?

A severely shocked patient must have an effective intravenous line (A 15.2), if necessary, from two drips. If possible, replace the volume of blood you calculate he has lost. In very severe hypovolaemia give him a litre in 5 minutes. If he is shocked enough to have air hunger and a blood pressure less than 60 mm, he will need 2 or 3 litres.

If he is reasonably young, transfuse him at the most rapid convenient rate until the signs of shock go.

If he is old, or hypertensive, or has vascular or coronary disease, give him repeated rapid transfusions of about 100 ml, watching his jugular venous pressure carefully between each transfusion. Do this until there are signs that his cardiac output is normal. A change in his JVP or CVP is more important than its absolute value. Listen to the bases of his lungs for crepitations.

BLOOD TRANSFUSION If you are fortunate enough to be able to give more than 4 units, warm them. The only safe way to do this is to fit two drips sets together and lead the coiled tubes through a water bath at 37°C measured with a thermometer. Too much cold blood may cause ventricular fibrilation. After you have given 12 units of blood, give him 5 ml of a 10% solution of calcium chloride, or 10 ml of a 10% solution of calcium gluconate for every 3 or 4 units of blood you transfuse.

FLUID BALANCE CHART Start this (A 15.5).

WHEN HAVE YOU GIVEN ENOUGH FLUID TO A SEVERELY SHOCKED PATIENT?

(1) Monitor his skin temperature. If you have transfused him adequately, his skin will become warm, dry, and pink (if he is Caucasion), instead of being cold, damp and white. His nail beds now fill up again after you have emptied them and his nose becomes warm. These signs may sometimes be delayed, even if transfusion is satisfactory. (2) A normal blood pressure is a good sign, but perfusion can be inadequate, even if it is normal. (3) An adult's urine flow should be *at least* 20 ml/hour, and preferably 30 to 60 ml (1 ml/kg hour). If you have transfused him adequately, it should reach this value very soon after the injury.

CAUTION! Watch for: (1) A rise in his jugular venous pressure. (2) Basal crepitations.

IF YOU ARE MONITORING A PATIENT'S CVP, when he is oligaemic, you can give him fluid safely and rapidly until it rises 12 cm of water.

If his CVP is over 15 cm, you are overtransfusing him, or he has a failing heart.

If his CVP rises, but his blood pressure and peripheral circulation do not improve, give him isoprenaline 0.5 to 10 micrograms/minute by intravenous infusion.

METABOLIC ACIDOSIS If a patient is severely shocked he will be acidotic. So give an adult 100 mmol of sodium bicarbonate, and another 50 mmol an hour or two later if necessary (A 15.1).

HOW WELL DOES THE PATIENT RESPOND TO TRANSFUSION? Shock from a fractured femur or a bleeding limb responds rapidly. If a patient's shock does not respond, suspect an abdominal or thoracic injury.

LATER MANAGEMENT For the care of hypovolaemia during and after the operation, see 'Primary Anaesthesia' 5.4 and 5.5.

DIFFICULTIES WITH HYPOVOLAEMIC SHOCK

If you are in DOUBT AS TO THE CAUSE OF A PATIENT'S SHOCK, and he is fit enough, prop him up with his legs horizontal and his trunk at 45°. His neck veins should not be visibly distended. If they are, his jugular venous pressure is raised. He probably has some medical condition, or a bruised heart, or cardiac tamponade, or overtransfusion. If you can see an upper level in the blood in his neck veins, estimate how many centimetres it is above his sternal angle.

If his BLOOD PRESSURE FAILS TO RISE: (1) You have probably failed to give him enough fluid. (2) He may have been in shock too long. (3) He may have acute adrenocorticosteroid lack due to previous steroid therapy. This will weaken the response of his adrenal cortex to stress. Or, he may have some other cause of adrenocortical insuffiency.

If his VENOUS PRESSURE AND HIS PULSE RATE RISE, he has BASAL CREPITATIONS, PERIORBITAL OEDEMA AND A HEADACHE, you have given him too much fluid. The more usual mistake is to give him too little. Slow down the infusion, give an adult 40 to 80 mg of frusemide intravenously. If his kidneys are working normally, he will then have a massive diuresis. If necessary repeat the frusemide after 6 hours.

A SHOCKED PATIENT MUST HAVE A CATHETER IN HIS BLADDER

53.3 Renal failure after an injury

If you don't transfuse a patient in severe hypovolaemic shock rapidly and adequately, he either dies immediately, or the cortices of his kidneys necrose so that his kidneys fail. Post traumatic renal failure is thus the major complication of hypovolaemic shock. Although a period of acute hypovolaemia can injure his lungs, his heart or his liver, it is its effect on his kidneys that is so marked and so preventable. The more severe his hypovolaemia and the longer it lasts, the more likely are his kidneys to stop working and shed their tubular cells. If they do, days or weeks may elapse before they start working again. During this time he can die from uraemia, potassium intoxication, or infection. Prevent these disasters by treating hypovolaemic shock quickly. In good units post traumatic renal failure has almost disappeared, but preventing it may require 50 units of blood. It can also complicate extensive burns, crush injuries, severe muscle wounds (especially if they are heavily infected), or transfusion reactions.

If a patient passes *no* urine, suspect that his catheter is kinked or blocked, or that his urinary tract is obstructed. If he passes less than 20 ml an hour (for a child, see Fig. 58-6), suspect that he has post traumatic renal failure. Before diagnosing it, consider these other possibilities:

(2) He may still be hypotensive due to hypovolaemia. If his blood pressure is still below 80mm, or his peripheral circulation is still severely constricted, his glomerular filtration rate will be low. If you correct his hypovolaemia and restore his blood pressure, his urine output may increase, *but only provided that hypotension has not lasted long enough to damage his kidneys.*

(2) He is showing the metabolic response to injury. If his urine output is low, look for signs of hypovolaemia and renal failure. If you have excluded these, his urine output may be low because of the 'metabolic response to trauma' due to increased antidiuretic hormone secretion. This may reduce his urine output for 8 to 36 hours. Don't rely on this diagnosis unless his condition is stable in other respects, his urine is chemically normal and its specific gravity is high. The practical consequence of this is that you should not infuse more fluid to increase his urine output if all other signs are satisfactory.

If you have excluded these two conditions, and a patient has passed less than 20 ml/hour of urine for 12 hours, he probably has acute post traumatic renal failure. Diagnose it early, before his blood urea starts to rise, by monitoring his urine output. His kidneys are probably failing if: (1) The specific gravity of his urine is less than 1016 in the absence of glycosuria or albuminuria, or (2) there is pigment or protein in his urine, whatever its specific gravity.

If he recovers, he will go through two phases:

(1) An oliguric phase during which his kidneys cannot correct for his water and electrolyte intake, so you will have to restrict these for him. While he is oliguric, one of his dangers is that too much potassium will enter his plasma from dead or dying tissues, so try to minimize this. Unfortunately, you cannot diagnose the earlier phases of hyperkalaemia clinically. Don't give him potassium containing solutions such as Darrow's solution or Ringer's lactate in this phase. It may be followed gradually or suddenly by the next one.

(2) A phase of diuresis, during which he may pass 6 to 9 litres of urine a day, regardless of his fluid intake. While this phase lasts, he is in danger of losing electrolytes. So replace them, and the water he loses. One difficulty is knowing when to stop giving him large volumes of fluid. If you go on giving them, he has to go on excreting them, so you won't know if he needs them or not!

POST TRAUMATIC RENAL FAILURE

If possible, refer the patient. If you cannot refer him, treat him like this.

THE OLIGURIC PHASE OF POST TRAUMATIC RENAL FAILURE

CORRECT THE CAUSE For example, correct any hypovolaemia, treat a burn, or severe muscle injury. Even if you can refer him, do this first.

CORRECT HIS INITIAL WATER AND ELECTROLYTE DEFICIT Chart the water and electrolytes he has lost and those he has been given. Correct his calculated water and electrolyte deficit before you start the period of fluid restriction.

RESTRICT HIS WATER AND ELECTROLYTES Give him his measured output of water, plus an estimate of his insensible loss. Give it as water by mouth, or intravenously as 5% dextrose. Don't give him any solutions containing electrolytes, except those necessary to replenish his losses, because he cannot excrete them.

His measured output is the total volume of his urine, and any vomit, or watery diarrhoea.

His insensible loss in a temperate climate will be about 500 ml, in the tropics it may be 1000 ml or more.

CAUTION ! (1) Don't include blood, plasma, or plasma substitutes in these estimates. (2) Don't allow his thirst to influence the volume of his intake. Watch that he does not over hydrate himself. (3) The dose of many antibiotics, especially gentamicin, needs to be modified in the presence of renal failure. (4) Don't give him diuretics.

WEIGH HIM If possible, do this daily. He should lose about 500 g daily after his initial fluid replacement. If he gains weight, he is retaining fluid and is being over hydrated.

MINIMIZE THE RISE OF HIS PLASMA POTASSIUM (1) Remove all dead and dying tissue with a really thorough wound toilet. (2) Avoid hypoxia. If he needs an anaesthetic, try to use local anaesthesia. (3) Don't give him potassium in any form. There is potassium in milk and orange juice, Darrows and Ringer's lactate, in soup and meat, and in many drugs. (4) Minimize catabolism with a high energy no protein diet.

HIGH ENERGY NO PROTEIN DIET If he has no nausea, gastric suction, or intestinal lesions, try to to give him at least 400 g of glucose or lactose, or, failing these, sucrose, daily by mouth or by nasogastric tube. This will give him 6.7 MJ (1,600 kcal).

OTHER MEASURES Give him 20 ml of 50% glucose with 10 units of soluble insulin into a large vein, preferably his vena cava, repeated 6 hourly (19.2).

THE DIURETIC PHASE OF POST TRAUMATIC RENAL FAILURE

Every 24 hours during this phase give him 1500 ml of fluid plus his urine output for the previous 24 hours. Give him a litre of 0.9% saline and a litre of 5% dextrose and the balance as half strength Darrow's solution. This contains 17 mmol/l of potassium. The normal potassium requirements are about 35 mmol/daily. He may need 6 to 10 litres of fluid a day.

If his urine specific gravity is still very low at 4 days, you are probably keeping his diuresis going by overinfusing him. Try cautiously reducing his fluid intake.

CAUTION ! Don't start protein feeding until he is passing at least 1500 ml of urine a day, and his blood urea is below 25 mmols (250 mg/dl). Starting it too early increases the danger of uraemic complications.

53.4 Septic shock

Although septic shock might be considered out of place in a system of traumatology, it is more conveniently discussed with other kinds of shock, than with the surgery of sepsis. This is the draining of pus from the many sites in which it can collect, and is described in Chapters 5 to 8 of Volume One.

Septic shock is a common cause of surgical death. Once it has developed, a patient has a 50% chance of death, even in a good unit. His outlook is better if he is young and his history is short. It is the result of the release of endotoxins from lysed bacteria, especially Gram negative bacilli, into his circulation. It is not the same as septicaemia caused by intact living bacteria. Provided the bacteria remain intact, a patient can be septicaemic without being shocked.

Septic shock usually starts suddenly. The drop in a patient's blood pressure may be castastrophic. He may be disoriented, confused, delirious, or comatose. He breathes rapidly. His blood pressure is low. He is always febrile, and his pulse is fast. A characteristic sign is a high rectal (or vaginal) temperature and

SEPTIC SHOCK

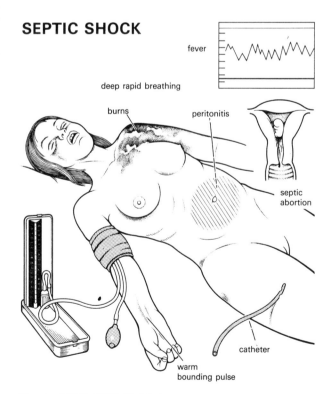

fever

deep rapid breathing

burns

peritonitis

septic abortion

catheter

warm bounding pulse

Fig. 53-4 SOME SITES OF INFECTION IN SEPTIC SHOCK. Septic shock usually starts suddenly. The drop in a patient's blood pressure may be castastrophic. He (or she) may be disoriented, confused, delirious, or comatose. A patient in septic shock breathes rapidly, his blood pressure is low, he is always febrile, and his pulse is fast. *Kindly contributed by Samiran Nundy.*

cold extremities. A patient in septic shock is acidotic and breathes deeply and rapidly. He may have diarrhoea and ileus simultaneously. He is usually jaundiced, is often anaemic, and passes little or no urine (a bad sign). He may develop DIC (disseminated intravascular coagulation), and bleed from a wound, from his nose, or his gut, or into his urine. His heart, lungs and kidneys may fail, causing pulmonary oedema and oliguria.

There are two kinds—'warm' and 'cold'; the cold may follow the warm: (1) In the less common, less lethal warm kind, typically caused by Gram positive cocci, the patient has warm, pink (if he is Caucasian) extremities, a large pulse pressure and a bounding pulse. (2) In the more common and even more dangerous cold kind, usually caused by Gram negative bacilli, he has cold and clammy extremities.

Suspect that a patient is in septic shock if he is already infected and suddenly becomes severely ill and hypotensive. The source of his infection can be peritonitis (6.2), septic abortion (16.3), infected burns (58.23), the transfusion of infected blood, pyaemia, or the instrumentation of an infected bladder (22.8). Or, his infection may be hidden, and make diagnosis difficult.

Treatment is urgent. The first consideration is to give him fluids, and to adjust the volumes you give to his urine output. Measuring his CVP is not useful, even if you can measure it, because he can develop pulmonary oedema when it is in the normal range.

SEPTIC SHOCK

Take blood cultures, and culture pus from any septic lesion.

OXYGEN Give the patient oxygen through a mask.

NURSING Tepid sponging will comfort him. Don't let him develop hyperpyrexia.

ANTIBIOTICS Give him large doses of not less than three bactericidal antibiotics, if possible intravenously, as a bolus injection. Choices include: (1) Benzyl penicillin 5-10 megaunits 4 hourly with chloramphenicol 1 g 6 hourly, or streptomycin 500 mg 6 hourly. (2) Gentamicin 2 to 5 mg/kg daily by intramuscular or slow intravenous injection in divided doses every 8 hours. In renal failure increase the interval between the doses. (3) Methicillin 1 g by intramuscular or slow intravenous injection 4 to 6 hourly. (4) Kanamycin 15 to 30 mg/kg daily by slow intravenous injection in divided doses

every 8 to 12 hours. (5) Cephaloridine 0.5 to 1 g every 8 to 12 hours by intramuscular or slow intravenous injection. The maximum dose is 6 g daily, or 4 g in patients over 50 or within 2 days of surgery. Give children 20 to 40 mg/kg daily in divided doses, to a maximum of 4 g. (3) Metronidazole for anaerobes. By mouth 400 mg 8 hourly. By rectum 1 g 8 hourly for 3 days then 1 g 12 hourly. Intravenously give 500 mg 8 hourly up to 7 days. Give a child 7.5 mg/kg 8 hourly by any route.

WHICH INTRAVENOUS FLUID? Be guided by his serum electrolytes. If you cannot measure these, give him 0.9% saline, 5% dextrose in 0.9% saline, Ringer's lactate, or Darrrow's solution. Hyponatraemia is common, so 5% dextrose alone is unsafe. He would probably also benefit from a colloid such as dextran.

HOW MUCH FLUID? He may need as much as 50 ml/kg/24hrs in addition to his normal daily water requirements in Fig. 58.6. An adult may need 6 litres in 24 hours. Be guided by his hourly urine output. Aim for a urine output of at least 30 ml/hr.

If he develops pulmonary oedema, give him frusemide 100 to 200 mg two or three times daily. If possible, watch his sodium and especially his potassium level and correct them.

If he develops into acute left ventricular failure, give him digoxin 0.5 mg, repeated as necessary. If an electrocardiogram is available, use it as a guide to therapy. If not, count his pulse and apex beat together. If he has a pulse deficit, you are over digitalizing him.

OTHER DRUGS *After* you have given him adequate fluids, consider giving him the following drugs, they are not so important as giving him adequate fluids.

Dopamine which will increase his cardiac output and tissue perfusion. Give him 1 to 4 micrograms/kg/min. To give this dissolve 4 mg in 500 ml of fluid.

Chlorpromazine which may relieve his peripheral vasoconstriction. If his extremities are cold and clammy give him chlorpromazine 0.5 mg/kg.

Steroids are of doubtful value. Give him dexamethazone 50 mg (or its equivalent) intravenously, and repeat this every 4 to 6 hours.

DRAIN PUS If you can drain the septic focus, do so. Timing is important: he must be fit enough to stand the procedure, so overcome shock first. Do the simplest possible operation. This will need courage because he will be very ill, and he may not survive it. It may however save his life. You may need to evacuate a septic abortion, drain a pelvic or subphrenic abscess, or re–explore his abdomen.

54 Wounds

54.1 Preventing infection—the wound toilet

A wound can heal in two ways. Either it can heal by first intention, quickly, with no sepsis, and with the minimum of scarring. Or, it can heal by second intention, slowly by granulation, perhaps with the discharge of pus, and eventually with much scarring. Unfortunately, when you see a wound you often will not know what it is going to do. If you sew it up immediately by primary suture, will it heal elegantly by first intention? Or will it break down and pour out pus?

Answering this question depends on understanding the timing of events as a wound heals after a major injury in a shocked patient. During the first few hours the body's first priority is to maintain the circulation to the patient's brain (53.1) at the expense of that to his less essential organs, including his skin and bones. Meanwhile, the bacteria which have entered his wound have their own time scale. What they do depends greatly on the nature of his wound, and on how much foreign material and dead tissue there is in it, especially dead muscle. Even if there is much debris and dead tissue and conditions favour them, they multiply little in the first 6 hours. From 6 to 12 hours they are beginning to multiply, but after 24 hours they are multiplying fast. If infection is going to occur, it will be established after 24 hours. By about the third day, the body's priorities will have changed, the blood supply to the patient's wound will have increased, and it will be in the ideal state for healing and resisting infection.

You will see the following kinds of wound, depending on the time since the injury, its severity (particularly the amount of dirt, dead tissue, and especially dead muscle present), and the patient's ability to overcome infection.

(1) A wound which presents within the first 6 hours. The challenge before you is to remove all damaged tissue and the dirt by toileting the wound *before the bacteria in it can start multiplying.* Even a few hours can be important, so don't delay.

(2) A wound presenting at any time with obvious systemic or local signs of infection. These signs don't start for 6 hours, and become more serious the longer the delay. Bacteria are now established in the dead tissue, and are passing into the lymphatics around the wound. If you do too vigorous a toilet, you may spread the infection further, so treat the wound as an infection. *Gently* remove any slough without disturbing the surrounding tissue, drain the wound, or pack it with dry gauze, or apply a hypochlorite ('Eusol') dressing, and give the patient an antibiotic. This is the delayed wound toilet described in Section 54.5. A day or two later, when you have controlled his infection, you may be able to complete the toilet of his infected wound.

(3) A wound which is more than 48 hours old, without systemic or local signs of infection. By this time the patient has overcome any bacteria that might have been present, so you can safely toilet his wound as vigorously as is necessary.

(4) A wound with much dead tissue in it, which presents between 6 and 48 hours after the injury without any obvious signs of infection. Deciding what to do can be difficult. Should you do a vigorous toilet, or should you merely drain it? The wisest course is to treat it as (2) above and do a gentle toilet, repeating this later if necessary.

Time is critical. If a patient has a severely contaminated wound, he needs a wound toilet, *immediately* he reaches hospital. Delay is inexcusable. Grossly contaminated wounds and crush injuries are acute emergencies. Every hour's delay makes his chances of an uncomplicated recovery less likely.

SEVERE WOUNDS ARE ACUTE EMERGENCIES

After you have toileted a wound, when should you close it? This mostly depends on the interaction of three factors: (1) How much dead tissue or debris there is inside it. (2) Where the wound is. You can close most wounds of a patient's face or hands by immediate primary suture. But in the shaded areas in Fig. 54-1 the risk of infection, and particularly gas gangrene makes immediate primary suture unwise, especially if a wound is heavily contaminated. (3) The time since the injury. You may be able to close a wound immediately if you have toileted it *within 6 hours of the injury,* before the bacteria in it have started to divide. But if there is much dead tissue or debris, you would be wiser to leave it for delayed primary suture. *If you are in any doubt, leave a wound open for delayed primary closure on the third day.* The patient will have overcome his infection, and his tissues will be in their most active healing state. His wound will heal by first, not second intention, just as it would do if you sutured it immediately, but it will heal much more certainly.

The common mistakes are: (1) Not to do an adequate wound toilet. (2) Not to leave a wound open for delayed primary closure. Neglect of these things delays wound healing, and may cause traumatic osteomyelitis, or the need for an amputation. There

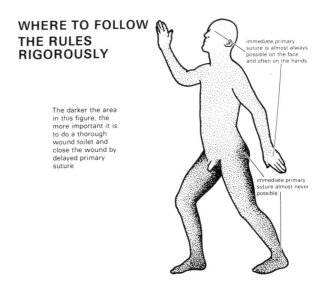

WHERE TO FOLLOW THE RULES RIGOROUSLY

immediate primary suture is almost always possible on the face and often on the hands

The darker the area in this figure, the more important it is to do a thorough wound toilet and close the wound by delayed primary suture

immediate primary suture almost never possible

Fig. 54-1 WHERE TO FOLLOW THE RULES RIGOROUSLY. The rules are: (1) do a thorough wound toilet, (2) close a wound by delayed primary suture whenever you are in any doubt. The darker the area in this figure, the more important these two rules are. *Kindly contributed by Peter Bewes.*

is seldom any indication for suturing any wound in the interval between 6 hours and the third day, with the possible exception of clean knife wounds

There are two parts to a wound toilet: (1) Do a social cleaning of the wound and the skin round it to wash away bacteria and foreign material. Use soap, a soft nail brush and plenty of water poured in, or saline. You may need many litres, a few spongefuls are not enough. (2) Do a surgical toilet with a scalpel to remove damaged tissue, so that the patient's inflammatory response can get to every part of it. If his wound is large and dirty, toileting it may take you an hour.

Adapt the way you toilet a wound to its severity and its site. Only the severest and most disadvantageously sited wounds in Fig. 54-1 need all the measures described below. At one extreme, a recent clean, incised, knife wound of the scalp needs a social toilet only, and no surgical toilet. At the other extreme you will need to remove much dead muscle from a grossly contaminated wound. Don't hesitate to use a nail brush; it is the best way to remove ingrained dirt, such as occurs when a limb has been dragged along a road.

If there is *any* contamination, a wound toilet is necessary. For example, if a patient treads on a nail, don't merely give him antibiotics and hope for the best. Instead, excise the puncture wound, curette the track, and leave it open.

You will need these methods: (1) The immediate wound toilet described below, for all wounds which present early, and for those which present late without infection. (2) Immediate primary suture, which can follow it if the indications are right (54.2). (3) Delayed primary closure or skin grafting at 3 days, which should be the rule for severe wounds (54.4), especially if they are contaminated or in dangerous areas. (4) A delayed wound toilet for infected wounds which present late (54.5). (5) Secondary closure, usually by skin grafting, for wounds which are starting to heal by granulation at 10 days (54.6). (6) A method for chronic wounds which are months or years old (54.7).

You cannot prevent bacteria entering a wound at the time of the injury, but you can prevent them entering a wound *in the hospital*. A common error is not to toilet and suture wounds in a sterile manner. So make sure you do this, and your staff do so too.

**ALL WOUNDS NEED A TOILET
MODIFY THE TOILET TO THE NEEDS OF THE
WOUND**

THE IMMEDIATE WOUND TOILET

Here is a general method for most wounds, large or small. Goto other sections for wounds of a patient's scalp (63.6), his face (61.1), or his hands (75.1).

ADMISSION Don't hesitate to admit a patient, even if he has quite a minor wound, especially if it is below his knee, in his buttock or his perineum, or on his abdomen or chest.

X-RAYS If he might have a foreign body or a fracture, X-ray his wound in two planes to locate it. Glass is usually radio–opaque.

INDICATIONS *All* wounds need some kind of toilet. The simplest toilet (applicable, say, to eyelid wounds) is dabbing on antiseptic after ordinary washing and exploring to remove obvious dirt. Most wounds need more than this, some very much more. The more the dead tissue, the more thorough must be your toilet.

CONTRAINDICATIONS The contraindications to a radical toilet are signs of established infection, such as a foul discharge, lymphangitis, lymphadenitis, or fever. You will not find them in wounds under 6 hours old, so with these wounds you can always do a radical toilet.

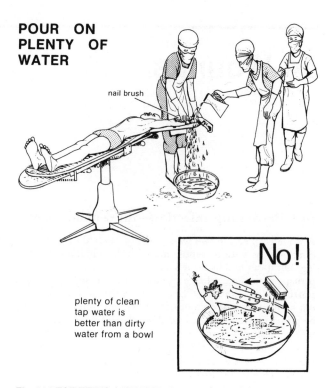

POUR ON PLENTY OF WATER

nail brush

No!

plenty of clean tap water is better than dirty water from a bowl

Fig. 54-2 TOILETING A WOUND. Pour on plenty of clean water when you toilet a wound. This patient has been anaesthetized with ketamine.
Kindly contributed by Peter Bewes

EQUIPMENT A minor operation set (4.11), two *fairly soft* nail brushes, two skin hooks, soft rubber tubing for a finger tourniquet, or a pneumatic tourniquet. Several litres of clean water, which need not be boiled. Saline is better; make it by adding two level teaspoonfuls of salt to a litre of water. Soap and aqueous chlorhexidine. You will need a good light. If you are in any doubt, use the main theatre.

TOURNIQUET A tourniquet may sometimes be useful, but don't use one routinely, because it makes distinguishing between living and dead tissue more difficult.

ANTIBIOTICS A thorough wound toilet is more important than any antibiotic. If a patient's wound is severe and particularly if it is heavily contaminated, give him a perioperative antibiotic, as in Section 2.7, before you start his surgical toilet.

ANAESTHESIA Don't hestitate to anaesthetize a patient, even if his wound is quite small. You cannot toilet it adequately if he is conscious.

If he might have injured his nerves and tendons, test them before you anaesthetize him—clinical tests while he is conscious are more reliable than poking about in his wound after he is anaesthetized.

If his wound is large, use regional or general anaesthesia. Ketamine is adequate.

If a patient's wound is small, you can do a nerve block, or you can use a fine needle to inject local anaesthetic solution from his wound into the surrounding tissues. This is particularly useful in children.

THE SOCIAL TOILET OF A WOUND

Do this in two stages before you drape a patient, first the surrounding skin, then the wound.

(1) Pack the patient's wound with a sterile swab to keep it dry while you clean the skin around it with tap water, ordinary soap, and a nail brush. Ask your assistant to pour on more tap water, until the patient's skin is very clean.

(2) Now remove the swab and clean the wound itself. If the dirt is ingrained, use a fresh soft boiled nail brush and gloved or scrubbed hands. You can use a nail brush in a wound. Push it into the dirty tissues of the wound with gentle rotating movements. Don't use vigorous side to side scrubbing

DIRECTIONS FOR EXTENDING WOUNDS

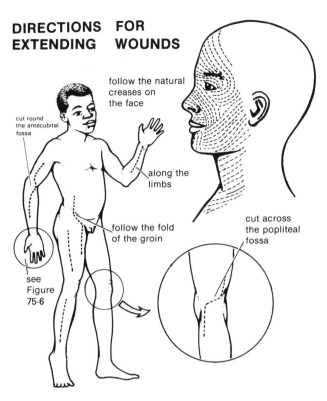

cut round the antecubital fossa

follow the natural creases on the face

along the limbs

follow the fold of the groin

cut across the popliteal fossa

see Figure 75-6

Fig. 54-3 DIRECTIONS FOR EXTENDING WOUNDS. Follow the crease lines in a patient's face (see also Fig. 61-3). Extend wounds in the length of limbs and don't cut across flexures.

movements. Put a basin under the wound, so that your assistant can pour clean water over it continually. Don't immerse it in a basin of water.

THE SURGICAL TOILET OF A WOUND

Paint the skin round the wound with cetrimide or chlorhexidine. Don't use iodine, because this will damage more tissue. Drape it.

CAUTION ! Treat the tissues kindly. Don't grab them with large artery forceps, or swab them violently; this injures them, and makes them less able to resist infection.

Use a scalpel and a pair of forceps to cut away all dirt and ingrained mud etc. Flush smaller foreign bodies out of the wound with sterile Ringer's lactate, saline, or sterile water in a 50 ml syringe, or an ear syringe. You may find pieces of wood, metal, gravel or clothing. *Explore* the patient's wound. Probing for foreign material is not enough. If necessary, open it widely to look into its depths.

If, for any reason, you have to leave a foreign body, such as deeply embedded bullet, tell the patient so.

Remove all clots and join up all cavities so that they drain readily.

EXTEND THE WOUND, if necessary, in the length of the limb. If you have to open up a flexure, make an S–shaped incision, as in Fig. 54-3. If nerves or vessels have been injured, extend his wound appropriately to reach them.

INJURED TISSUES IN A WOUND

Injured skin. Except on the patient's face cut away 3 mm of the skin margin round the wound, as in A, Fig. 54-4. Don't undermine the skin edges.

Injured fat readily necroses, so cut it back freely until you reach healthy yellow fat which is not bruised.

Injured muscle and fascia. Cut away all torn fascia and open up fascial planes (B). Put retractors in the wound so that you can see inside it. Cut away all dead muscle (C). Dead muscle looks darker and bluish, it does not bleed or ooze when you cut it, and it does not contract when you pinch it with forceps. Snip it away until you reach healthy muscle which

contracts and oozes where you cut it. Be radical, dead muscle is an ideal culture medium for clostridia. If you are in doubt as to whether muscle is alive or dead, cut it out! The patient has muscle to spare and will not miss it.

If there are loose pieces of bone which are not attached to periosteum or muscle, they are ischaemic and will die anyway. Remove them. Leave pieces which are still attached to periosteum. Don't scrape live muscle or periosteum from the surface of a bone, because the bone under it may die.

If his bone is exposed in the wound, there are several things you can do:—

If there is muscle nearby, use this to cover the exposed bone. This is usually easy with the femur, the radius or the ulna, because reduction (usually traction) will pull the bone back into the wound. Covering an exposed tibia is not so easy.

If the exposed area of bone is large, you can cover it with moist gauze. Apply sterile saline several times a day, and change the gauze daily. After several months the outer cortex of the bone will slough and you can graft the granulations under it.

If the exposed area is clean, you can graft it with split skin. If this later falls off to leave white dry bone, chisel it away until you reach red cancellous bone, as in Fig. 81-12. You can graft this immediately, but it is probably wise to wait 3 or 4 days for a bed of suitable granulations to form.

If tendons lie exposed see if they are covered by paratenon (the normal fine vascular covering of a tendon). A split skin graft will not take on naked white or dry tendons, but it will usually take if they are still covered by paratenon. If the extensor tendons of a patient's hand are exposed, and there is no such layer, and you cannot refer him, consider doing the groin flap in Section 75-27. If you can refer, him cover his tendons temporarily with split skin and vaseline gauze.

If nerves or vessels are exposed, try to cover them with adjacent tissue, or a simple flap, as in Section 57.11.

If you are not sure if tissue is alive or dead, it is alive if it bleeds or blanches on pressure. If you are still not sure, inspect the wound at 48 hours and remove more dead tissue if necessary. This is wiser than waiting for infection.

SURGICAL TOILET AND DELAYED SUTURE

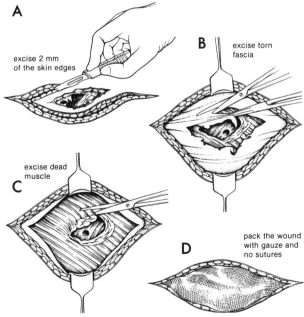

A

excise 2 mm of the skin edges

B

excise torn fascia

C

excise dead muscle

D

pack the wound with gauze and no sutures

Fig. 54-4 SURGICAL TOILET AND DELAYED SUTURE. A, the skin edges are being excised. B, torn fascia is being excised. C, dead muscle is being removed. D, the wound has been packed with gauze and is being left open for delayed primary suture. *After Farquharson, with kind permission*

SPECIAL STRUCTURES If clinical examination shows that a nerve has been injured, explore it and look at it. If one side is gaping, clean it carefully and suture the epineurium to approximate the ends accurately.

Look elsewhere for the treatment of cut tendons (55.11), cut nerves (55.9), torn arteries (55.6), open fractures (69.7), and open joint wounds (69.8).

RELIEVING TENSION IN THE WOUND If a patient's tissues show any tendency to burst out of his wound, open up his deep fascia longitudinally down the whole length of the muscle compartment involved. This will prevent the compartment syndrome (70.4), and is especially important in the forearm (73.7) and the lower leg (81.14); it may even hasten the union of a fracture.

CONTROLLING BLEEDING FROM A WOUND

If you are using a tourniquet, release it. If bleeding is very severe, see Section 55.1.

If you are not using a tourniquet, bleeding or oozing should start as you cut away dead tissue. If it does not, you have not yet reached viable tissues, so you are not cutting away enough. If the wound is extensive, pack one part of it while you clean another.

Most of the bleeding will probably have stopped by the time you have finished toileting the wound. If larger arteries spurt at you, tie them with silk or linen thread. Tie smaller vessels with fine monofilament. Avoid catgut, especially thick catgut, because it makes a good culture medium.

If necessary, control oozing with packs (3.1), leave them on for 10 or 20 minutes, and apply more if necessary.

SUTURES AND DRESSINGS If you have had to do an extensive wound toilet, the wound will *not* be suitable for immediate primary suture. So pack it with gauze, as in D Fig. 54-4 Aim for dryness and coolness. Loosely bandage the gauze in place, making sure the bandages do not restrict the circulation.

If the wound is in a limb, raise it (75-1, 81-1).

PREVENT TETANUS in all wounds, as in Section 54.11.

PREVENT GAS GANGRENE, when necessary, as in Section 54.13. If a patient has a severe muscle wound of his buttock, thigh, calf, axilla, or retroperitoneal tissues, give him penicillin 1.5 megaunits every 4 hours starting immediately after the injury. Or, give him tetracycline.

SPLINTS TO IMMOBILIZE THE LIMB If he has a severe wound of a limb, immobilize it. Skeletal traction is safest. Or, use a plaster back slab. If you use a circular cast, bivalve it immediately, a slit down one side is not enough to prevent swelling. Elevate it.

A SECOND SURGICAL TOILET If you see more dead tissue at the time of the delayed closure, toilet his wound again.

THE COMMON MISTAKE IS FOR A WOUND TOILET NOT TO BE THOROUGH ENOUGH

54.2 Immediate primary suture

This is the suture of a wound within six hours of the injury, but *it is only safe if the wound is clean, and if it contains no dead tissue.* All other wounds are best packed with gauze and left open to see what happens 3 days later (54.4).

When you suture any wound, aim to: (1) Close it at all points and in all planes. Suture it so as to obliterate dead spaces in which blood and exudate can collect as in B, and C, Fig. 54-5. If you allow them to collect, as in F, and G, in this figure, they may become infected, and when they finally organize they will cause a denser scar. (2) Cause as little trauma as you can by using sharp needles and fine sutures. Avoid heavy toothed forceps, blunt knives, and tissue forceps on the skin edges.

SUTURING A WOUND

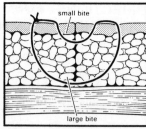

vertical mattress sutures will prevent inversion of the skin edges

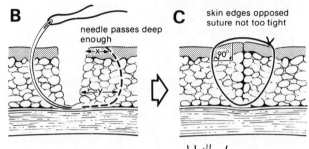

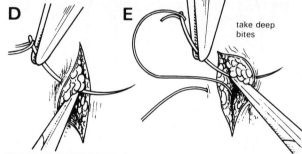

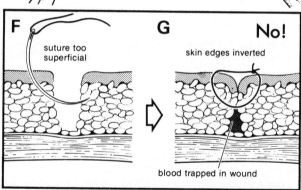

Fig. 54-5 SUTURING A WOUND. A, a vertical mattress suture is an excellent way of making sure that skin edges are everted. There is a small superficial bite and a large deeper one. B, and C, show a correctly placed suture. The dotted line in B, shows the path of the suture. If 'X' is smaller than 'Y', the skin edges will be everted. The suture should enter the skin at 90°. D, and E, the edges of the wound have been everted to get a good bite of tissue. F, and G, show how NOT to do it; the suture is too superficial and the skin edges are inverted. *From various sources, partly Hamilton Bailey with the kind permission of Hugh Dudley*

IMMEDIATE PRIMARY SUTURE

You have just toileted the wound as in Section 54.1, and have now to decide if it is suitable for immediate or delayed primary suture. For face wounds goto Section 61.1.

INDICATIONS (1) In most parts of the body, primary suture is only indicated if a wound: (a) is clean cut, as by a knife or broken glass, (b) is less than 6 hours old, (c) contains no doubtfully viable tissue, and (d) can be sutured without undue tension. (2) Most wounds of the head, face, and neck, and small clean wounds on the hands, arms, and scalp, are suitable for immediate primary closure for up to 24 hours because their blood supply is so good. (3) Close all wounds of the dura, and the pleural and peritoneal cavities, by immediate primary suture. If necessary, you can leave the tissues over them for delayed suture.

If all the other conditions apply, except that you cannot bring the skin edges together, you may be able to close the wound by primary skin grafting (57.5).

CONTRAINDICATIONS These are also mostly the indications for *delayed* primary suture. They are: (1) Wounds more than 6 hours old, or with dirty or damaged tissue. (2) All severe wounds, crush injuries, gunshot wounds and bites, either human or animal. (3) Any wound in which immediate or delayed primary split skin grafting might be a better way of providing skin cover, for example degloving injuries. (4) Wounds in severely shocked patients whose peripheral circulation is so poor as to seriously weaken wound repair (5) *All open fractures (69.7)*. (6) Most open joint wounds (69.8). (7) Wounds in anyone who is about to be sent on a long journey. (8) Lack of antibiotics, so that you have nothing to give a patient if his wound does become infected. (9) *ALL war wounds*, especially all missile wounds.

METHODS FOR IMMEDIATE PRIMARY SUTURE

Before you start to close a wound, be sure to control bleeding adequately. Failure to do this is a common cause of infection, necrosis, and breakdown. Close the patient's skin and deep tissues with *interrupted* monofilament sutures.

If a wound is shallow and the cosmetic result is important, you may be able to use subcuticular sutures as in I, and J, Fig. 61-2.

If the cosmetic result is not important, use deep interrupted sutures, as in in B, and C, Fig. 54-5. Insert them at 90° to his skin. Put them across the wound, close to the skin edges, so that if they do interrupt the blood supply, they do so in as little skin as possible.

If the wound is deeper, or fat is friable, use interrupted vertical mattress sutures as in A, Fig. 54-5. The large bite closes spaces deep in the wounds, and the small one prevents inversion of the skin edges.

Don't drain the wound; if you expect much discharge, close it by delayed primary suture.

CAUTION ! (1) Don't make the sutures too tight, or put them too close. Exudate should be able to escape from between them. (2) Close all dead spaces.

If you cannot bring the skin edges together, you may be able to undercut them. The level at which you do this is important: (1) In the face, undercut just deep to the dermis (61.1). (2) In the scalp, undercut between the galea and the pericranium. (3) If more than minimal undercutting is necessary in the limbs, do it between the superficial and deep fascia. If you cannot easily bring the skin edges together, graft the wound.

CAUTION ! (1) Undercutting more than 1 cm has its dangers, especially haematoma formation. Split skin grafting may be safer. If you fear infection, mesh it (57.5). (2) Always leave some fat under the skin. If you undermine it too superficially, it will necrose.

POSTOPERATIVE CARE Leave skin sutures in from 4 to 14 days, depending on the thickness and blood supply of the patient's skin. Four days will be enough on the neck or scalp. Ten to 14 days may be necessary on the lower leg, feet, and toes. Remove them earlier if there is increasing pain, pyrexia or pus.

DIFFICULTIES WITH A SUTURED WOUND

If a patient's WOUND BLEEDS WITHIN 24 HOURS (reactionary haemorrhage), a ligature has slipped, or a clot has become dislodged. Bleeding is sudden, and may be massive. Prevent it by tying careful double ligatures on larger vessels.

If his WOUND BLEEDS AFTER 24 HOURS (secondary haemorrhage), sepsis has probably eroded a blood vessel. There may be a small warning bleed before a large vessel bursts. Prevent it by preventing sepsis (2.3).

The treatment for both kinds of haemorrhage is the same. Try to control bleeding with large pressure dressings, such as laparotomy pads. If this fails, take the patient to the theatre, open his wound gently, and tie the vessel. If you cannot find the source of the bleeding, pack it, and remove the pack in

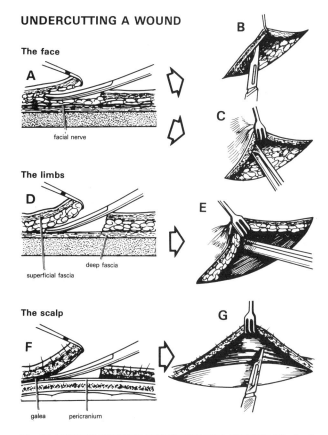

UNDERCUTTING A WOUND

The face

The limbs

The scalp

Fig. 54-6 UNDERCUTTING THE EDGES OF A WOUND. The levels at which you should do this vary with the wound. A, undermining the face superficial to the branches of the facial nerve, using either a scalpel (B), or scissors (C). D, and E, undercutting the skin of the limbs between the superficial and deep fascia. F, and G, undercutting the scalp between the galea and the pericranium. *After Ian McGregor with kind permission.*

the theatre 3 days later. If local pressure fails to control the bleeding, you may very rarely need to tie the vessel proximally (3.3 etc.).

If his WOUND FAILS TO HEAL, or leaves a sinus, think first of a foreign body. If this might be a possibility explore it.

54.3 Some bitter lessons from early suture

Here are two cases where the indications for primary suture were not observed.

IBRAHIM (6 years) was admitted in severe shock with a gross open fracture of his tibia and a bad laceration of his anus. His wound was carefully toileted, and his leg amputated below his knee. The stump was closed by primary suture and drained. His anus was treated by wound toilet, and a proximal defunctioning colostomy was done. He was given antibiotics, but his amputation stump became so badly infected that his leg had later to be amputated above his knee.

MUSTAFA (46 years) had a minor fracture of his fibula, and a wound over the medial side of his ankle, away from the fracture. A wound toilet was done and the wound was stitched, as the doctor who was caring for him said 'to convert a compound fracture into a simple one'. He was then transferred to another hospital and was given antibiotics. Nevertheless, sepsis had spread within his ankle joint so severely that its ligaments sloughed, it fell open and the surrounding bone necrosed. He required five more operations, including sequestrectomy, drainage, and skin grafts. Finally, he was left with an ankylosed ankle.

What were the mistakes ? Both patients had a social toilet and a surgical toilet. The most probable mistake was to suture their wounds too early. The boy would probably not have lost his knee if his original amputation stump had been closed by delayed primary or secondary suture. Sutures inevitably damage the blood supply a little, and kill some tissue, which may tip the delicate balance towards the spread of infection. Both wounds should have been left open, and only closed when they showed signs of healing. Here, by contrast, are some patients whose wounds were left open.

KAMAU (35 years) had a bad injury to his right hand. He was treated in another hospital but discharged himself when he was told 'when the suppuration is over we will amputate your hand'. His hand was indeed seriously injured, with its palm torn open. It was toileted under a tourniquet and bleeding controlled with packs. His wound was then left wide open under a gauze pack. Within 6 days it was granulating well and was ready for grafting. The grafts took and he is now using his hand normally.

NJOROGE (25 years) was a bus driver with a severely torn forearm. Lacerated tendons, crushed muscle, bruised torn fat, and damaged ischaemic skin lay ingrained with mud in the depths of his dirty ragged wound. All damaged tissue was cut away, and even some of his tendons, until only healthy bleeding muscle, viable skin, and fat were left in his wound. Packs took 20 minutes to control bleeding, but only a few small arteries needed tying. His wound was left widely open under a gauze dressing, and it, too, was ready for grafting in 6 days. All the grafts took and he is now driving his bus.

JACK (51 years) was standing in cattle manure and slurry when he had his legs torn off by a farm machine. Manure was deeply ingrained in what was left of his calf muscles. A social toilet was done using about 15 litres of water. This was followed by a thorough surgical toilet, and below knee amputations, using long flaps and delayed primary suture. Both knee joints were saved and he is now walking on bilateral below knee prostheses.

Although these are only a few cases, they are examples of a very effective way of managing wounds. A patient usually needs no antibiotics, if he does need one, penicillin is usually enough. If you are in any doubt how to close a wound, wait to see what happens. *Delay in closing it will not lengthen a patient's stay in hospital, but an unwise decision to close it immediately may cause disaster.*

IF YOU ARE IN DOUBT, DON'T CLOSE A WOUND IMMEDIATELY

54.4 Delayed primary suture (dps)

This is the most widely useful way of closing a wound. It means closing a wound between the 3rd and the 7th day, usually on the 3rd day. It does not mean waiting for about 10 days until granulations have formed. That is secondary suture.

In nature all wounds heal by granulation, so that immediate primary suture is a recent human invention. Delayed primary suture is thus closer to the conditions under which human tissue evolved. Also, it makes good use of a universally available chemical which is lethal to the anaerobes causing gas gangrene—the oxygen of the air. The main way in which wound care in most hospitals needs changing is: *(1) more emphasis on a really adequate wound toilet, and (2) much less on immediate primary closure.* Many tragedies, including osteomyelitis and death, result from treatment which is perfect in every way, except that the wound was sutured immediately, when delayed closure would have been wiser. *The temptation is great because a wound looks so much tidier when it is neatly sewn up!* Unfortunately, dirt, dead tissue and bacteria may all be hidden under a beautifully sutured wound. If a patient arrives in your ward with his wound sutured, and you are not sure about the adequacy of the toilet, or the correctness of immediate primary suture, reopen his wound and look at it. If necessary, leave it open and suture it later.

DELAYED PRIMARY SUTURE

INDICATIONS These are mostly the contraindications to immediate primary suture given in Section 54.2.

You toileted the patient's wound as in Section 54.1, and have decided on delayed primary suture. You have now brought him back to the theatre 3 days later to look at his wound.

If there are no signs of infection, close it by the same methods as for immediate primary suture. Disturb it as little

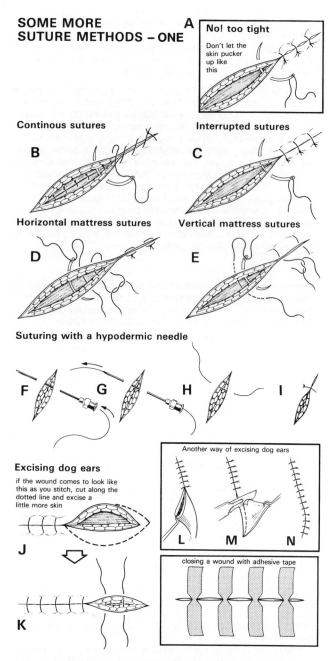

SOME MORE SUTURE METHODS – ONE

A **No! too tight**
Don't let the skin pucker up like this

Continous sutures

B

Interrupted sutures

C

Horizontal mattress sutures

D

Vertical mattress sutures

E

Suturing with a hypodermic needle

F   G   H   I

Excising dog ears
if the wound comes to look like this as you stitch, cut along the dotted line and excise a little more skin

J

K

Another way of excising dog ears

L   M   N

closing a wound with adhesive tape

Fig. 54-7 MORE SUTURE METHODS—ONE. A, sutures pulled too tight—never draw them as tight as this. B, horizontal continuous sutures. C, interrupted sutures. D, horizontal mattress sutures. E, vertical mattress sutures. F, to I, suturing with a hypodermic needle. J, and K, and L, M, and N, removing dog ears. *Kindly contributed by Peter Bewes.*

as possible, irrigate it with saline to remove blood clot. Excise any necrotic tissue. Clean its edges, but don't freshen them. If necessary, undercut them (54-6). Bring them together with interrupted monofilament sutures. Apply a pressure dressing and, if necessary, splint his limb as before.

CAUTION ! (1) Control all bleeding. Use packs and avoid ligatures if you can. A haematoma will ruin the chance of success. (2) Don't close the wound under tension.

If there are signs of infection, leave the wound open for secondary suture (54.6), or a secondary skin graft.

If you have had to excise any necrotic tissue, delay suture for two more days.

If you cannot bring the edges together, consider grafting. If the gap is more than 6 to 8 cm you will probably have to graft it. If the wound is on a patient's forearm, hand, or calf, you will have to graft much smaller areas.

POSTOPERATIVE CARE If the wound is superficial, leave it for 10 to 12 days. If it is large and deep, inspect it in the theatre after 5 days. Remove the stitches at 10 to 12 days and start exercises.

54.5 Delayed wound toilet

If a patient presents eight hours or more after the injury with a wound which is already infected, a vigorous wound toilet might spread the organisms further, so you will have to do a more gentle one. Infected operation wounds are described elsewhere (2.8).

SECONDARY WOUND TOILET

INDICATIONS Infected wounds 8 hours or more after the injury.

METHOD If any stitches have already been placed in the patient's wound, remove them and lay it open. If necessary relieve tension by splitting the fascia. If pus is present, culture it.

If the edges of the wound are acutely inflamed, or there is lymphangitis, lymphadenitis, or fever, give the patient an antibiotic, and make sure you toilet his wound under antibiotic cover, or you may spread the infection and cause septicaemia. If he has none of these signs, antibiotics are unlikely to be helpful. Remove all necrotic tissue; open up any pockets of pus; remove any infected blood clot, dead bone or foreign bodies.

Be cautious and try not to open up tissue planes at a distance from the edges of his wound. *This is especially important if you have no adequate antibiotic.*

Eliminate any dead spaces, and provide dependent drainage. Pack the wound with dry gauze or apply a hypochlorite ('Eusol') dressing.

You will probably be able to close the wound some days later by delayed primary suture or by grafting. Immobilize the patient's wound, and elevate his limb (81-1, 75-1).

DIFFICULTIES WITH AN INFECTED WOUND

If a patient's WOUND IS LARGE, and continues to discharge for many days, check his haemoglobin, transfuse him if necessary, and give him a high protein diet.

If his INFECTED, STINKING, DISCHARGING WOUND IS DIFFICULT TO MANAGE, try: (1) Soaking it in a bucket or a bath. (2) Immobilizing it in plaster gutter or splint. Lay it widely open and pack it with gauze. If the wound is not too big, and you need to immobilize a fracture, cover it with a complete cast, and cut a window in it. Make sure the dressings compress it firmly to stop it herniating.

54.6 Secondary suture

If the closure of a wound is delayed beyond 10 days, granulation tissue will grow over it. You will have to close it by secondary suture, rather than by delayed primary suture, although there is no sharp dividing line between these two methods. By now its edges will be indurated and and will be less easy to bring together, so you are more likely to have to graft it. It will also have a growing epithelial edge with an inadequate blood supply. You will need to excise this ingrowing edge, and you may have to prepare the granulations before you can graft them (57.3).

SECONDARY SUTURE

A wound is probably ready for secondary suture when its granulations are favourable by the criteria in Section 57.3. If they are unsuitable, prepare them by the methods in that section.

Apply a tourniquet, where possible. Excise the new epithelium at the edge of the wound, undercut its edges, and gently scrape the granulation tissue off the surface of the wound. Release the tourniquet, and control bleeding.

If you can bring the edges together without too much tension, suture them with a few interrupted sutures. Make sure the sutures go underneath the granulation tissue, not through it.

If you cannot bring the skin edges together, graft the bare area. If sepsis is not completely controlled, be sure to mesh the graft. This is the most usual situation.

54.7 Chronically infected wounds

A chronically infected wound may be months or years old, and so scarred that you cannot bring its edges together by suture. The fibrous tissue at its base may be so dense that you have to excise it first. A chronic tropical ulcer (Chapter 29) is an extreme example of a wound of this kind.

CHRONIC WOUNDS

Don't forget: (1) Neurological causes for chronic ulcers, particularly leprosy (test for anaesthesia and feel for thickened nerves). (2) In Uganda, Buruli ulcer.

WOUND TOILET Give the patient a bath, clean his wound well with soap and water and shave the skin round it. Examine it to find out exactly which structures are involved. If there are extensive sloughs or any sequestra, do a thorough wound toilet (54.1).

If the granulations are unfavourable, prepare them, as in Section 57.3 before you then graft them. Change the dressings at least every day, taking care to avoid cross infection. Change them twice daily in the few days before grafting.

Pad the wound and bandage it. A plaster back slab may make the patient more comfortable.

If scar tissue has had time to develop (3 weeks or more), excise it and the subcutaneous layers until you have exposed healthy fascial planes. Wait 3 days for new granulations to form and then graft. You can graft immediately, but the graft will be more likely to take if you wait a few days. A large infective wound will cause the patient to lose much weight. So feed him up (58.12).

CAUTION ! (1) If he is anaemic, treat him. (2) Have you considered the possibility that his ulcer might be tuberculous? These ulcers are often multiple, and there may be a sinus. Antituberculous drugs cure tuberculous ulcers rapidly.

IF AN ULCER DOES NOT HEAL THINK OF TB

54.8 Wounds which leave flaps

The simplest wound to leave a flap is a 'V' – shaped laceration. The apex of the 'V' is likely to necrose, so try to replace it without stitching, and warn the patient that healing may be delayed. If a stitch does seem necessary, use the apical stitch in Fig. 54-8.

With larger flaps, you can do three things: (1) You can replace a flap. (2) You can excise and discard it. (3) You can excise it and use it to make a graft. When you treat a wound with a flap you have two decisions to make. Firstly, should you keep the flap? Secondly, what should you do with the fat under it?

Replace a flap if: (1) Its edges bleed. (2) It becomes pale when you press its base and pink again when you let it go. (3) Its base is wider than its length. And, (4) the wound under it is clean. Otherwise, excise it. If you decide to keep it, hold it in place with adhesive strapping rather than sutures.

Fat impedes the diffusion of nutrients from the surface of a wound to the overlying skin of a flap. So trim off any obvious lumps of fat from under a flap as in Fig. 54-9. If a flap is very

MORE SUTURE METHODS – TWO

Inserting an apical stitch

make these apical stitches whenever you suture a jagged cut

A

B

pass the suture through the apex close to the skin edge

if you fail to insert an apical stitch a piece of skin sticks out

C No!

No!

Removing a suture

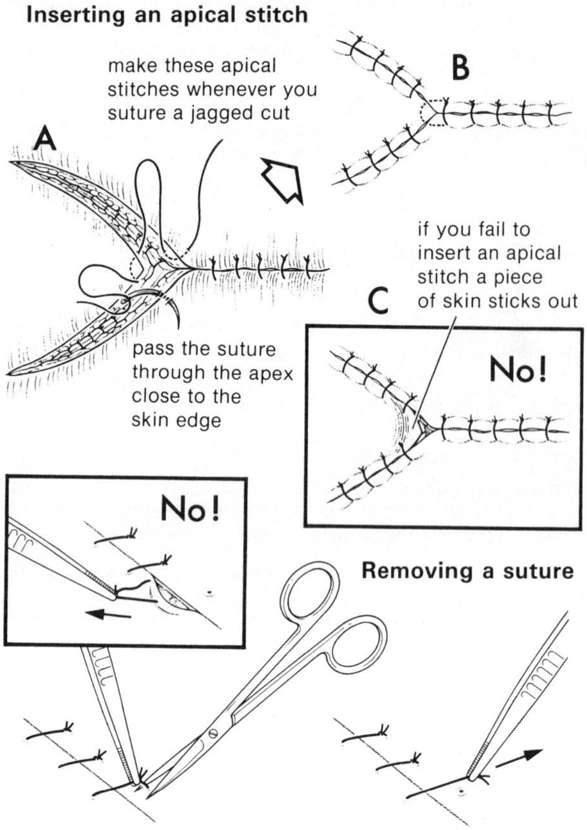

Fig. 54-8 MORE SUTURE METHODS—TWO. A, and B, you can suture the smallest flaps with an apical stitch. C, and D, make sure your nurses know how to remove sutures correctly, or they may open the wound as they do so. Pull out a suture so that a wound tends to close rather than to open. *Partly after Hamilton Bailey with the kind permission of Hugh Dudley.*

TRIMING THE FAT OFF A FLAP

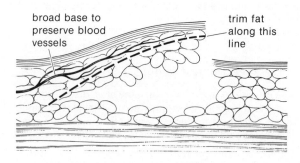

broad base to preserve blood vessels

trim fat along this line

Fig. 54-9 TRIMMING THE EXCESS FAT OFF A FLAP will help it to unite better. Preserve the full thickness of its base, which contains its blood vessels.

AVULSION INJURIES

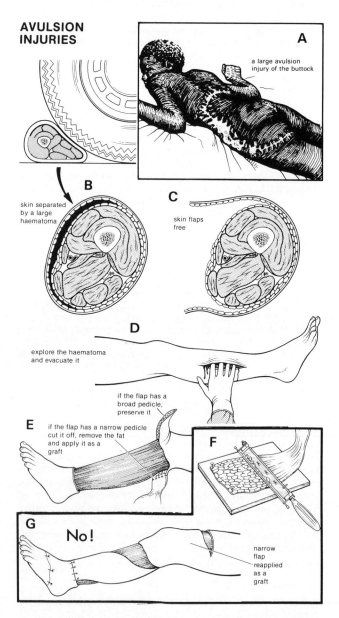

a large avulsion injury of the buttock

A

skin separated by a large haematoma

B

skin flaps free

C

explore the haematoma and evacuate it

D

if the flap has a broad pedicle, preserve it

if the flap has a narrow pedicle cut it off, remove the fat and apply it as a graft

E

F

G No!

narrow flap reapplied as a graft

Fig. 54-10 DEGLOVING INJURIES can detach a flap completely as in E, or cause a closed injury as in B. Don't try to reapply flaps as in F, and G. Instead, remove them and graft the raw areas 3 to 5 days later. *From various sources, partly with the kind permission of Peter London.*

---

thick, trim it so that it has a thinner margin and a thicker base which preserves its blood vessels. Make sure that: (1) the patient does not lie on it, and (2) it is uppermost, if it is very thick, so that gravity keeps it in place.

54.9 Degloving or avulsion injuries

These are extreme versions of the injury in the previous section. If a vehicle runs over a patient's limb, it may tear large flaps of skin from the tissues under them. If his skin is hanging loose, as in A, or C, in Fig. 54-10, the diagnosis is obvious, but if it is merely separated from the tissues underneath by a haematoma, as in B, the diagnosis is not so easy. To begin with his skin may look quite normal, and only necrose later. If you are in any doubt, feel it carefully, to make sure it is attatched to the tissues underneath, and look at it again 48 hours later.

If you suture a large piece of degloved skin back in place, it will die, so manage the patient as described below.

DAMAYANTI (34 years) had a motor accident in which a large part of her buttock was avulsed, as in A, Fig. 54-10. Fortunately, it had a broad base and did not necrose. She was nursed in the position shown with the flap uppermost. While she lay like this for many weeks, both her arms developed such severe contractures that she was later unable to move them. LESSONS (1) Nurse the patient in a position which will allow gravity to hold a flap in place. (2) Any limb held in an abnormal position for any length of time is liable to develop contractures. So, unless there is some very good reason for not doing so, put all immobilized limbs through their full range of movements each day.

DEGLOVING INJURIES

If the patient has no skin wound, aspirate the haematoma. Or, incise it, and explore it, to see how much undermining there is, as in B, C, and D, Fig. 54-10. Turn back the skin flaps, and excise or replace them as described below.

If the patient has an open skin wound, excise any grossly damaged skin.

If a flap has a base which is broader than its length, preserve it, trim the fat underneath it as in Fig. 54-9, and reapply it immediately as in E, Fig. 54-10.

If a piece of skin is free, or has a base which is too narrow to let it survive as a flap, excise all the degloved skin and fat and manage the patient's raw wound as described below.

If raw surfaces remain uncovered, take split skin grafts (57.5). Apply them immediately, if the base is favourable (as with muscle). If it is unfavourable, take the grafts, store them (57.8), and cover the wound with dry dressings. At 3 to 5 days when granulations are forming, remove the dressings, and any dead tissue, and apply the stored graft.

CAUTION ! (1) If there is a tyre mark on the patient's skin, he will certainly have a degloving injury under it. (2) Never replace any flap of skin which is longer than its base.

54.10 Missile wounds

Missile wounds, which were only seen by army surgeons in the past, are now common in many of the district hospitals of the developing world. If a patient reaches you alive, you will probably be able to save him, provided his heart or his major blood vessels or his large gut have not been injured. The most important steps are a thorough wound toilet and delayed primary closure.

The higher the velocity of a missile, the greater the damage it does. A low velocity missile, as from a pistol, drills only a narrow track, with little damage around it. A high velocity missile from a modern high velocity rifle, causes an explosion in the tissues with extensive cavitation. Small entry and exit wounds may conceal gross damage inside.

Try to visualize the structures that a missile may have passed through. This is difficult because it may take a very remarkable path, as in Fig. 54-11. If there is no exit wound, look for the missile inside the patient by taking X-rays in two planes.

The wounds from standard rifle bullets are least likely to be infected, because firing will have sterilized them and they do not cause much tissue destruction. Both 'home made', unsterile low velocity missiles, and high velocity missiles causing bursting injuries, are more likely to result in severe infected wounds. Antibiotics have the same rather uncertain role that they have in other wounds (54.1).

de Wind C M, 'Management of missile injuries in a peripheral hospital. Tropical Doctor 1984;14:157-159

MISSILE WOUNDS

See elsewhere for missile wounds of a patient's head (63.6), and his abdomen (66.2).

Resuscitate and anaesthetize him. Leave any existing dressings on until you reach the theatre. Excise the entry and exit wounds, and remove all devitalised tissue.

If the entry and exit wounds are small and there is not much tenderness in between, it is probably a low velocity injury. You will probably be able to toilet it and save the patient's limb. There is likely to be only a narrow track; cleaning it of all visible debris may be enough. If the track is superficial, unroof it by joining the entry and exit wounds. If it runs more deeply, you may be able to flush it through with saline.

If the exit wound is large, the patient's limb grossly swollen, his bone much fragmented and he is severely shocked, he has probably been injured by a high velocity missile. You you may have to remove much blood clot, dead muscle, and many bone fragments. Prepare for major surgery. Occasionally, you may have to amputate his limb.

MISSILE WOUNDS

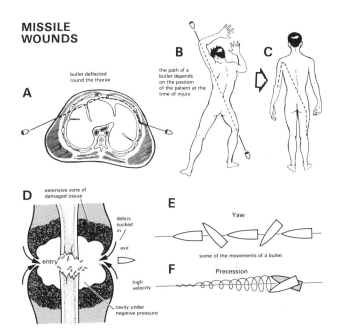

Fig. 54-11 MISSILE WOUNDS may take a curious path. The missile may be deflected by bone (A), or take a path that depends on the position of the patient at the time of the injury, as in B, and C. D, shows a high velocity missile creating a cavity surrounded by damaged tissue and causing a partial vacuum which sucks in debris. E, and F, show some of the complex movements that can increase the damage that a missile does as it goes through a patient *A, B, and C, after Naclerio, by permission of Grune and Stratton. D, E, and F, from the Field Surgery Pocket Book with the kind permission of Guy Blackburn.*

Control all bleeding, leave the wound open (except for face wounds which can be closed immediately), and cover it with gauze.

After 3 to 6 days, bring the patient back to the theatre and inspect his wound under general or local anaesthesia. If it looks clean and there are no signs of infection, close it by delayed primary suture. If if is not clean and there is dead tissue present, do a further wound toilet.

CAUTION ! (1) Don't forget tetanus prophylaxis. (2) If you are going to refer a patient, do the necessary early treatment first—reduce a fracture, drain his chest, or explore his abdomen. (3) If removing a missile is going to be more dangerous than leaving it in, leave it. There are many asymptomatic missile carriers.

DIFFICULTIES WITH MISSILE INJURIES

If a patient's BONE HAS BEEN COMMINUTED by the missile, toilet the wound as above, and then leave it unsutured and dressed inide a cast without a window. Consider sending him home. Remove the cast at 4 to 6 weeks. You will probably find a clean healing wound filled with granulation tissue, and a fracture that is uniting clinically and radiologically as it should.

If his THORAX is involved, a thoracotomy may not be necessary, and you will probably not be able to do one anyway. Drain a haemothorax or haemopneumothorax (65.4 and 65.5). The lung is remarkably resistant to missile injuries.

54.11 Preventing surgical tetanus

The prevention of surgical tetanus depends on: (1) A thorough wound toilet (54.1). (2) The active immunization of everyone in childhood. Further methods at the time of the injury are: (3) Passive immunization to give immediate cover. (4) Active immunization with tetanus toxoid. (5) Antibiotics, usually penicillin, to limit the multiplication of *Clostridium tetani*. Vary your regime according to the patient's immune state and the nature of his injury by following the methods below.

Toxoid is cheap, widely available, and seldom causes reactions. When they do occur, they are unlikely to be serious, so there is no need to test for sensitivity. The disadvantage of tetanus toxoid is that it does not provide immediate cover. If a non–immune patient has a high risk wound, you can either give him human tetanus immune globulin (HTIG) which is expensive and scarce, but has few side effects, or horse antitetanus serum, which is cheaper, and more widely available, but is more likely to cause serious hypersensitivity.

In practice, passive immunization is much less valuable than the other methods of prevention, and one experienced contributor advised us to leave it out entirely. In a busy hospital, where most patients do not know if they have been immunized or not, you will need a simple regime, *so give 0.5 ml of tetanus toxoid to ALL patients with any wound, however small.* If you wish, you can combine this with passive immunization of the most dangerous cases only.

The prevention of tetanus is one of the targets of WHO's global EPI program. As more children are immunized and populations become increasingly immune, it should become rarer.

AZIZ (26 years) fell drunk from a second floor verandah and dug both his forearm bones into the earth. His wound was closed by primary suture without a wound toilet. 5 days later he developed tetanus and died. At post mortem a quantity of earth was found in his wounds. LESSON The critical step in preventing tetanus is a thorough wound toilet.

PREVENTING SURGICAL TETANUS

RISKS **The risk of tetanus is small** in a clean cut, minimally contaminated wound. But it can occasionally follow even a trivial one.

The risk of tetanus is great in burns, deep puncture wounds, injuries of the leg, thigh, buttocks, or axilla; in heavily contaminated wounds, especially crush injuries, and in wounds where there is much injured muscle, especially if they occurred on cultivated land, or if dung has been applied to the wound.

WOUND TOILET Toilet the patient's wound thoroughly and leave it open.

WHAT TO DO TO PREVENT TETANUS

If you are sure the patient has had adequate tetanus toxoid previously, there are the following possibilities. (Adequate means two injections of toxoid, one of which must have been given during the previous 5 years).
If the risk is small, no further prophylaxis is necessary.
If the risk is great or doubtful, give him a booster dose of toxoid, and antitetanus immunoglobulin or serum (optional), and a megaunit of penicillin.
If he has not had adequate tetanus toxoid previously, assess the risks.
If the risk of tetanus is small, one dose of toxoid is enough.
If the risk is large or doubtful, give him toxoid, and a megaunit of penicillin, and antitetanus immunoglobulin, or serum. Continue penicillin for five days, or until his wound has healed. If his wound occurred more than 6 hours previously, his need for passive immunization is greater. Give him further doses of tetanus toxoid after 6 to 8 weeks and 4 to 6 months to complete his course.

IMMUNIZATION Immunize a patient on the indications given above. Give the antitoxin and the toxoid with different syringes in different sites.
Passive immunization If possible, give the patient antitetanus immune globulin of human origin (HTIG) ('Humotet') 500 units intramuscularly. If you don't have this, give him horse antitetanus serum 1500 units intramuscularly.
CAUTION ! If you use antitetanus serum, test him for sensitivity. Inject 0.1 ml subcutaneously into his skin. Wait one hour. If there is any redness or any symptoms, he is allergic and should not have any more.

Active immunization Give an adult tetanus toxoid, 0.5 ml, intramuscularly. One dose gives little immunity, a second dose 6 to 8 weeks later gives more, a third dose 4 to 6 months later produces a high level of immunity. Give him another dose 5 years later, and every 10 to 15 years thereafter.

DIFFICULTIES IN PREVENTING TETANUS
If the REGIME ABOVE IS IMPRACTICAL, give all patients with any wound tetanus toxoid. If the risk of tetanus is high, give them prophylactic penicillin also.

GIVE TETANUS TOXOID TO ALL PATIENTS WITH WOUNDS

TETANUS

A preventable surgical tragedy!

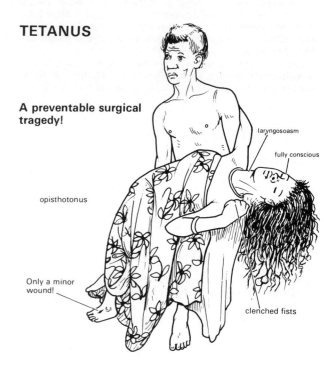

laryngosoasm

fully conscious

opisthotonus

Only a minor wound!

clenched fists

Fig. 54-12 SURGICAL TETANUS. A frightened farmer carries his wife, stricken with tetanus to the People's Health Centre in Savar, Bangladesh. Immunization with tetanus toxoid would have prevented this.

54.12 Treating tetanus

The warning signs that a patient is going to get tetanus are irritability, insomnia, increased muscle reflexes, a sore throat, dysphagia and difficulty starting urination. Tremors and spasm of the muscles near his wound follow. If he is fortunate, his disease remains localized, If it spreads, he has trismus, risus sardonicus, respiratory distress, and perhaps hyperpyrexia. Severe convulsions may follow even minor stimuli. Finally, he dies in opisthotonus with widespread muscle rigidity.

The method which follows is mainly that of Sanders and his colleagues from the Duncan Hospital in Bihar. They showed that the addition of low doses of intrathecal horse antitetanus serum (immune globulin was not available) to the standard regime could reduce the mortality from about 15% to about 5% in a crowded district hospital serving some of the world's poorest people. This regime is more likely to be practicable and may be as effective as attempting to paralyse a patient and ventilate him with intermittent positive pressure respiration (IPPR). If you can keep a patient alive for a month, he will probably recover, but you must sedate him and nurse him well.

Aim to: (1) Remove the source of the toxin by toileting his wound. (2) Sedate him heavily to control his spasms. (3) Nurse him devotedly for as long as is necessary, usually 3 to 4 weeks.

(4) Minimize the stimuli which may cause spasms by putting him in a quiet ward and disturbing him as little as possible. (5) Prevent aspiration pneumonia by trying to stop him aspirating his saliva and stomach contents, and by giving him penicillin. This will also prevent *Cl. tetani* from multiplying.

TREATING TETANUS

PROGNOSIS

Grade One The incubation period is over 14 days, trismus is the patient's only symptom, and comes on over 6 days. Sedation and oral feeding are the main means of treatment. His prognosis is good.

Grade Two The incubation period is 10 to 14 days. Symptoms come on over 3 to 6 days. Moderate trismus is combined with moderate dysphagia, rigidity and spasms. He may need nasogastric feeding, an intravenous drip, and a tracheostomy, or paralysis and IPPR.

Grade Three The incubation period is less than 10 days and symptoms develop over 3 days. Other features are similar to Grade Two but are more severe, or more urgent. If possible, transfer him to a hospital where IPPR and the analysis of blood gases are possible.

CAUTION ! Remember that a patient with tetanus is conscious and aware of all that is going on around him so talk to him and not about him.

CONFIRM THE DIAGNOSIS Examine the patient's nervous system thoroughly and do a lumbar puncture to exclude menigitis, encephalitis, and subarachnoid haemorrhage. Don't assume he has tetanus merely because he is in a surgical ward. Consider also epilepsy, rabies, and local disease of his temporomandibular joints. Disturb him as little as possible when you examine him.

SEDATION Sedate the patient heavily enough to control his spasms; each patient needs a different dose. Start with chlorpromazine 25 to 50 mg and diazepam 10 mg by intramuscular or intravenous injection, or orally, depending on his size and condition. An average dose is 100 mg 6 hourly. Continue with diazepam 10 mg, 8, 6, 4, or even 2 hourly, supplemented by chlorpromazine 25 mg 8 or 6 hourly. Or, use phenobarbitone.

If severe spasms cause him great distress, give him pethidine 50 to 100 mg as required.

CAUTION ! Continue sedation for 5 to 7 days, even if he appears to be improving, or he may relapse.

RESPIRATORY SYSTEM Raise the foot of his bed 30 cm to help postural drainage, until he can sit up and move about on his own. Turn him regularly. Suck out his mouth and nose as required. If necessary intubate him and suck out his trachea (A 13.2). You will probably find that managing a tracheostomy is impractical.

THE WOUND should already have been toileted (54.1). If the toilet has been inadequate, excise the patient's wound widely, remove all foreign bodies, pus, and clot. Handle it as little as possible. Leave it open and dress it with diluted hydrogen peroxide.

CAUTION ! Handling the wound may discharge the toxin in it into the circulation, so, give him antitoxin before you operate.

ANTISERA Ideally, give the patient human tetanus immune globulin (HTIG) 30-300 U/kg intramuscularly to fix the toxin.

Or, exclude hypersensitivity and give him antitetanus serum, 750 units intramuscularly or intravenously once daily for 3 days. Or, give him a single intramuscular dose of 20, 000 units. Intramuscular antitetanus serum is not of great value and regimes vary considerably.

Intrathecally as soon as he is adequately sedated, give him one dose of 200 units of antitetanus serum by lumbar puncture. Take this from the smallest ampoule obtainable (1500 units in 1 ml) and measure it with a tuberculin syringe.

ANTIBIOTICS Give him benzyl penicillin 1 megaunit intramuscularly every 6 hours. Culture the organisms from his respiratory tract and adjust his antibiotics accordingly.

STEROIDS The value of these are uncertain. Some surgeons give a patient betamethasone 8 mg initially, preferably intravenously, and repeat it 12 or 8 hourly.

NURSING Put the patient in the quietest part of the ward. Manage his bladder by continous catheter drainage with intermittent release (64.16). Prevent pressure sores, stop his mucosal surfaces drying, and prevent faecal impaction with suppositories or low enemata. Keep this up for several weeks.

FEEDING If possible, feed him by mouth. Even if he has trismus he can usually suck fluids through a straw. If necessary feed him through a nasogastric tube, or drip.

A suitable formula for the drip feed is: glucose 400 g, vegetable oil 100 g, dried skim milk 100 g, water 2.4 litres. This will make about 2.5 l of feed containing 12 MJ (2,900 kcals) or slightly more than an average adult's daily needs. Give him 200 ml 2 hourly.

54.13 Gas gangrene

This is an anaerobic infection of injured muscle caused by various species of clostridia. Suspect that it may occur if: (1) A patient has extensively lacerated muscles, or a missile wound, especially if this involves his buttocks, thighs, or axillae, or his retroperitoneal muscles following an injury to his colon. (2) The blood supply to these parts of his body has been interfered with. (3) His wound is grossly or deeply contaminated with soil.

Gas gangrene is probably developing *if he has been progressing satisfactorily, and then suddenly deteriorates.* Over a few hours he becomes anxious, frightened, or euphoric. His face (if he is Caucasian) becomes pale or livid, often with circumoral pallor. His injured limb feels uncomfortable and heavy. Although he has recovered from shock and is not bleeding, *his pulse rises.* It quickly becomes feeble as his blood pressure falls. He vomits.

Don't let these features mislead you: (1) He does not always smell of death, and even if he does, he may not have gas gangrene. (2) Gas in the tissues is a late sign, and even if it is present, it does not always mean gas gangrene.

One of the patient's muscles may be involved, or more often a group of them, or a whole limb, or part of it. Infection spreads up and down a muscle, and has less tendency to spread from one muscle to another. As infection progresses along a muscle, it changes from brick red to purplish black, as shown in Fig. 54-13. At first the wound is relatively dry; later, you can express from its edges a thin exudate with droplets of fat and gas bubbles, which becomes increasingly offensive. Stain this by Gram's method and look for Gram positive rods.

Prevent gas gangrene like this: (1) Do a thorough wound toilet, especially in all extensive muscle wounds of the buttock, thigh, calf, axilla or retroperitoneal tissues. (2) Give a patient with these wounds 1.5 megaunits of penicillin 4 hourly. If this is not possible, give him tetracycline. If you do a thorough wound toilet and give him penicillin, there is no need for prophylactic antiserum.

Once gas gangrene has developed, don't delay exploring a patient's wound because he is shocked. *Radical excision and massive doses of penicillin are his only hope.* You will be wise to excise too much muscle rather than too little.

ANY MUSCLE WOUND IS A POTENTIAL SITE FOR GAS GANGRENE

GAS GANGRENE

PREVENTION (1) Do a thorough wound toilet (54.1). (2) In high risk wounds (see above) give the patient penicillin 1.5 megaunits 4 hourly, or tetracycline. Start immediately after the injury.

GAS GANGRENE

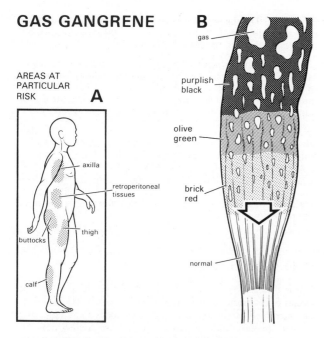

AREAS AT PARTICULAR RISK **A**

- axilla
- retroperitoneal tissues
- thigh
- buttocks
- calf

B
- gas
- purplish black
- olive green
- brick red
- normal

Fig. 54-13 MUSCLE CHANGES IN GAS GANGRENE. As the infection advances down a muscle, it changes from its normal purple, through brick red and olive green, to purplish black.

DIFFERENTIAL DIAGNOSIS Gas gangrene is not the only cause of gas in the tissues. Air sometimes escapes into them in surgical emphysema. In ischaemic gangrene, there is no toxaemia, unless the gangrenous tissue becomes secondarily infected. Neither of these should cause difficulty. There are however two other conditions where the diagnosis is not so obvious. Both require drainage and penicillin or tetracycline but neither needs radical muscle excision.

Suggesting anaerobic cellulitis Infection is limited to the patient's subcutaneous tissues. Spread may be rapid and there may be much subcutaneous gas. Sometimes his whole abdominal wall is involved. When you remove the affected tissue, the muscle underneath appears healthy, and bleeds and contracts normally. Remove the necrotic tissue, and drain the wound.

Suggesting anaerobic streptococcal myositis Spreading redness and swelling originating in a stinking discharging wound with Gram positive cocci and pus cells in its exudate. The patient's muscles are boggy and pale at first, then bright red and later pale and friable. The characteristic toxaemia of gas gangrene does not develop. Make radical incisions through his deep fascia to relieve tension and provide drainage.

TREATMENT FOR GAS GANGRENE

NURSING Isolate him from the other surgical patients. If possible, barrier nurse him.

ANTIBIOTICS Give the patient 10 megaunits of benzyl penicillin daily for 5 days as four 6 hourly doses.

Or, give him tetracycline 0.5 g intravenously or 1 g orally every 6 hours.

Culture his wound, do sensitivity tests, and if necessary change his antibiotics.

Although clostridia are not sensitive to metronidazole (2.7), some other anaerobic bacteria are, so give it.

ANTITOXIN There should be no need to use this in most wounds. If you give it, do a skin sensitivity test first. Then give him pentavalent gas gangrene antiserum intravenously and repeat it after 4 to 6 hours.

RESUSCITATION Transfuse him rapidly, and keep a drip running during the operation.

EXPLORATION Do this in a septic theatre, or even in the out–patient department, and not where clean cases go for operation.

Open the patient's wound, enlarge it if necessary, lengthwise in his limb, and cut his deep fascia throughout the whole length of the skin incision.

Excise all infected muscle widely. Remove: (1) Any black crumbling muscle. (2) Any muscle which is swollen and pale and looks as if it has been boiled. (3) Any muscle which does not contract when you pinch it. (4) Muscle which does not bleed. (5) Muscle which contains bubbles of gas. If necessary, remove whole muscles from their origin to insertion, part of a large muscle, or a whole group of muscles. Close his wound later by secondary suture.

AMPUTATION If a patient's limb is disorganized by injury or infection, amputate it, especially if he shows signs of severe toxaemia. X-ray it first to see how far the gas has reached. Amputate under a tourniquet. When you have amputated, his toxaemia should improve rapidly.

CAUTION ! Close the stump by delayed primary suture, even if you think you are amputating through healthy tissue.

POSTOPERATIVE CARE He may develop septic shock if he has not already done so (53.4). Expect, and treat as best you can, the dehydration, vomiting, delirium, jaundice, and anuria (53.3) that he may develop.

GAS GANGRENE

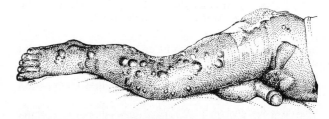

Fig. 54-14 SEVERE GAS GANGRENE. This followed an intramuscular injection by an unqualified person, but it could equally well have followed a severely contaminated wound. *Photograph by Dr. D. Fry, Cameroun. With the kind permission of the Editor of Tropical Doctor.*

55 Injuries to vessels, nerves and tendons

55.1 Immediate treatment for a severely bleeding wound

Preventing a patient's blood from leaving his circulation is one of the most urgent surgical tasks. He can lose a litre or more internally into his peritoneal (66.1) or pleural cavities (64.5), or around broken bones (76.1, 78.4). External bleeding is much easier to diagnose and stop. The most useful methods are to raise the wound and to press on it. The least useful method is a tourniquet. So when you teach first aid workers, stress the value of local pressure from a firm pack in the wound, combined with pressing firmly on the pressure points when necessary. Many surgeons feel that a tourniquet is so dangerous that no first aid worker should ever use one—you will however find a pneumatic tourniquet invaluable in the theatre (3.8).

IMMEDIATE TREATMENT FOR A BLEEDING
WOUND

ELEVATION If a patient's limb is bleeding, raise it. This will usually control venous bleeding. If his wound is in the upper part of his body, sitting him up may help, but be careful that he does not faint.

DIRECT PRESSURE Press a large dressing firmly over his wound and wait five minutes. This is usually much more effective than a haemostat. Don't do anything more until you have waited for at least five minutes, unless a torrent of blood pours from the dressing. If bleeding stops, be thankful and don't meddle with the dressing.

PRESSURE POINTS These are much less effective than direct pressure. Press: (1) the patient's carotid artery against the transverse process of his 6th cervical vertebra. (2) His temporal artery against his skull just in front of his ear. (3) His subclavian artery against his first rib. (4) His brachial artery against the middle of his humerus. (5) His femoral artery over his mid–inguinal point.

HAEMOSTATS If bleeding continues after after five minutes, a large vessel may have been injured, probably an artery, more likely from a tear rather than complete transection. When an artery is completely divided, bleeding usually stops. Secure the bleeding vessel with a haemostat. This is hardly ever necessary.
    CAUTION ! (1) Get proximal control by pressing on a pressure point first. (2) The vessel must be clearly visible. Don't jab the haemostat blindly into a pool of blood. Be sensible about where you apply a haemostat. Some vessels accompany important nerves. For example, don't crush a patient's ulnar nerve in trying to clamp his ulnar artery.
    When the haemostat is in place, incorporate it in the dressings. Don't remove it and try to tie the vessel until he is in the theatre.

PACKING Use this to control deep inaccessible bleeding when the above methods fail. Pack the wound with broad strips of folded gauze. If necessary, hold it in place with deep

sutures taking a bite of the uninjured tissue well wide of the edges of the wound.

TEMPORARY SUTURES In some situations, such as the face, temporary haemostatic sutures may be useful. Don't let them strangle the tissues.

FIRST AID TOURNIQUETS The few first aid indications for a tourniquet are: (1) When other methods of controlling bleeding have failed, bleeding threatens the patient's life, and the risk of losing his limb can be accepted. (2) A rapidly increasing arterial haematoma in a closed injury. (3) Some cases of snake bite.
    CAUTION ! (1) A tourniquet is too often applied by first aid workers in a way which impedes the venous return, and so *increases* bleeding instead of stopping it. (2) Record the time at which it was applied. (3) It must be supervised and released every 15 minutes.

If a patient arrives with an effective tourniquet that has been in place more than two hours (rare), he is in serious

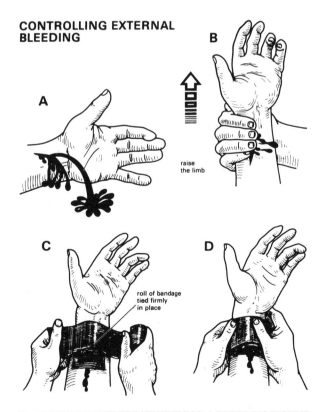

CONTROLLING EXTERNAL BLEEDING

A

B

raise the limb

C

roll of bandage tied firmly in place

D

Fig. 55-1 IMMEDIATE TREATMENT FOR A BLEEDING WOUND. A, the methods you see here will usually control arterial and venous bleeding from a wound like this one. B, raise the patient's bleeding limb and press on the wound. C, and D, apply a pressure dressing. A roll of bandage kept firmly in place is a convenient way of doing this.
Kindly contributed by Peter Safar

THE ARTERIES

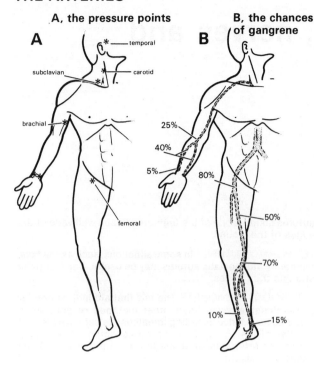

A, the pressure points

A

temporal

subclavian

carotid

brachial

femoral

**B, the chances
of gangrene**

B

25%

40%

5%

80%

50%

70%

10%

15%

**Fig. 55-2 THE SURGICAL ANATOMY OF THE ARTERIES. A, the
pressure points. If direct pressure on a wound fails to control bleeding,
press here to control it. B, the chances of gangrene if you tie an artery.**
Modified from 'Techniques Elementaires Pour Medecins Isoles' with kind permission.

danger of the crush syndrome. The sudden release into his
circulation of toxic metabolites, especially myoglobin from
his injured muscles, may cause renal failure and kill him. So,
if an effective tourniquet has been in place for many hours,
and his limb is ischaemic, amputate it at or above the level
of the tourniquet.

55.2 Definitive treatment for severe arterial bleeding

If you have temporarily controlled bleeding by the methods in
the previous section, you will now have to explore a patient's
wound and tie or try to repair his injured vessel, depending upon
its collateral circulation. You can usually safely tie: (1) The smaller
arteries below his elbow and his knee. (2) His profunda femoris
artery. (3) His internal iliac artery. (4) His subclavian artery. But
his limb may become gangrenous, especially if he is old, if you
tie: (1) his axillary artery, (2) his brachial artery, (3) his femoral
artery above the origin of its profunda branch, or (4) his popliteal
artery. Try to repair these if you can, by the methods in Section
55.6.

You may have great difficulty finding his injured artery, because
his wound may look just like so much meat, and his artery may
be contracted and very thin. To find it you may have to release
the tourniquet or the proximal clamp, and look for bleeding,
or feel for pulsation.

A LIMB ARTERY BLEEDS SEVERELY

IMMEDIATE TREATMENT Take the patient to the theatre, and
make sure you have good light. Place a pneumatic tourniquet
(3.8) loosely round his injured limb high above his wound so
that you can inflate it in a hurry later if you need to.
Anaesthetize and drape him. Drape any site you may need
to take a graft from. Gently remove the dressings, and explore
his wound.

If most bleeding has stopped, you will be able to explore
the wound without further trouble.

If his wound bleeds profusely, blow up the tourniquet while
you explore it. Try to find the torn artery. Try to apply an arterial
clamp above the tear.

If you cannot find the tear, enlarge the wound if necessary,
or release the proximal clamp, and feel for pulsation.

**If his wound is so high up his limb that you cannot apply
a tourniquet or a clamp,** be prepared to expose and temporarily
clamp his subclavian (3.4) or external iliac artery (3.5).

When you have controlled the bleeding and explored the
patient's wound, you will have to decide whether to tie his
injured artery or to try to repair it. Below his elbow and knee
tie it. Above them try to repair it (55.6).

ALTERNATIVELY, blow up the tourniquet from the start. If you
don't find the vessel (unusual), complete the wound toilet and
any other repairs, then deflate the tourniquet and look for
bleeding from the injured artery.

55.3 The cold blue injured limb

If a patient's limb is cold and blue (if he is Caucasian), its circulation is impaired and he is in danger of gangrene or the compartment syndrome followed by Volkmann's ischaemic
contracture (70.4). The commonest causes of these disasters are:
(1) An unsplit cast on a forearm fracture. (2) A supracondylar
fracture in a child. (3) A fractured tibia causing obstruction to
the anterior compartment of the leg (81.14). (4) Any badly treated
fracture, a crush injury, or a bullet wound.

The compartment syndrome is the easiest cause to treat. The
vessels of a patient's limb may be so tightly compressed by
exudate, blood, or swollen muscle that blood cannot pass through
them. Toileting his wound, incising the fascia, and exposing his
artery is often all that is necessary to restore his circulation. Or,
a local injury may be causing an artery to contract down so
tightly that no blood can pass through it. A tightly contracted
artery like this looks like a piece of solid cord. The distal part
of the brachial artery, the femoral, the popliteal, and the posterior
tibial arteries can all contract like this.

THE COLD BLUE INJURED LIMB See elsewhere for
ischaemia following a supracondylar fracture (72.8), or the
compartment syndrome in a patient's forearm (73.7) or lower
leg (81.14). If his injury is elsewhere, expose his injured vessel
through an adequate incision. This alone may be enough to
make it start pulsating again.

If it does not start pulsating, and part of it looks like a
piece of whipcord, expose the healthy artery above and below
the cord–like section. Expose it on all sides, so that there is
no tissue surrounding it.

If it fails to dilate, open an ampoule of 2% papaverine, or
less satisfactorily, pethidine, or 2% lignocaine (without
adrenaline), and flood this onto its contracted segment. Then
lay a warm moist pack on it, and wait 10 minutes. When you
return, you will probably find that the artery will have
increased in size and will have started to pulsate.

If it is still not pulsating, apply an arterial clamp above
the constriction, and inject 2% lignocaine with a little heparin,
between the clamp and the constriction. This may distend
it enough to make it start pulsating. Wait 10 minutes while
the heparin acts.

If it is torn, repair it (55.6). Only if these measures fail consider tying it, or if possible, resecting and anastomosing it.

CAUTION ! When you close the wound make sure that the
injured vessel is not exposed to the air; cover it with adjacent
tissue, or if necessary with split skin.

**WHEN IN DOUBT EXPOSE AND DECOMPRESS
WIDELY**

55.4 A stab wound close to a major artery

The common danger site for this emergency is the groin. Open and explore the wound early, so as to examine the artery and repair it if necessary. This will be easier than trying to deal with the arterial haematoma or aneurysm that may result from leaving it.

STAB WOUNDS NEAR MAJOR VESSELS Have blood for the patient cross matched. Take him to the theatre and explore his wound under general anaesthesia. Try to get proximal control of the vessel. If the artery and vein are injured, you may be able to close the hole by lateral suture as in Fig. 55-3. If necessary sew a patch of long saphenous vein over the hole, or do an end–to–end suture or graft.

ALWAYS EXPLORE STAB WOUNDS CLOSE TO ARTERIES

55.5 A pulsating (arterial) haematoma

Several things can happen if the blood from an injured artery cannot escape to the surface: (1) It may track widely in the patient's tissues. (2) It may form a tense local arterial haematoma, which may press on the collateral vessels, obstruct them, and cause gangrene. (3) The outer layers of the haematoma may later become organized and form a traumatic (false) arterial aneurysm. (4) If this aneurysm communicates with a vein, it will form an arteriovenous aneurysm. Initially, this may be difficult to diagnose. Suspect that such an an aneurysm is forming whenever a pulsating haematoma overlies a major artery and vein, particulary in the groin.

An arterial haematoma can form when an artery is injured by a penetrating wound or by a fracture. If it is rapidly expanding, it must be explored before it becomes an arterial aneurysm or an arteriovenous aneurysm, both of which are even more difficult to treat.

A PULSATING HAEMATOMA The patient has a pulsating swelling after an injury, perhaps only a minor one. If you cannot refer him, proceed as follows.

Where possible, apply a tourniquet proximally, to control bleeding. Then make an adequate incision to explore his wound. Expose the artery proximal to the injury, and control the flow of blood through it with an arterial clamp, or one of the other methods described below. Explore the haematoma, remove the clots, and tie his bleeding vessel. Finally, release the clamp or tourniquet cautiously to see if you have been successful.

If the haematoma is below his elbow or knee, tie the injured artery.

If the haematoma is above his elbow or knee, try to repair his injured artery (55.6). If you feel you cannot do this, or you don't have the necessary equipment, tie it as close to the injury as you can, and hope for the best. He may be lucky.

55.6 Repairing blood vessels

Vascular surgery is normally considered to be strictly the work of a specialist. But the patient must reach the specialist within 4 hours of his injury; if this is impossible, you will have to do as best you can yourself. If you operate carefully, and handle the patient's injured artery gently, you may succeed in repairing it. In doing so you may save his life, or his limb, so that you and he enjoy one of the most rewarding forms of fine surgical craftsmanship. *The penalty for failure will certainly not be worse than that of not trying.* You don't need any special equipment, but it will take you a long time. Use the finest instruments you have;

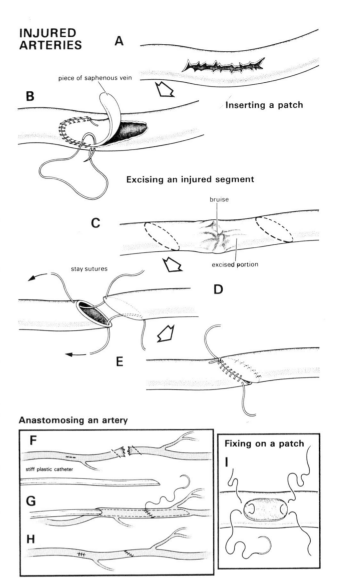

INJURED ARTERIES

Inserting a patch

Excising an injured segment

Anastomosing an artery

Fixing on a patch

Fig. 55-3 INJURIES TO ARTERIES. A, a lacerated artery. B, a piece of saphenous vein being sewn over the laceration. C, a bruised piece of artery being excised. D, and E, an oblique anastomosis. F, G, and H, you may be able to anastomose an artery by passing a stiff plastic catheter, such as that from an intravenous cannula, through an arteriotomy incision, and then using this as a stent over which to do the anastomosis. I, if you try to patch a vessel, start by fixing it with two sutures at either end like this. *From the Field Surgery Pocket Book, with the kind permission of Guy Blackburn. F, G, and H, kindly contributed by Naim Janmohammed.*

eye instruments are suitable if you treat them carefully, and so are eye sutures. But successful repairs have been done with quite coarse ones. You will also need good aseptic technique, a strong light, adequate anaesthesia, good eyesight, or magnifying spectacles, and a blood transfusion. Your repair may thrombose later, but it may stay open long enough to let an effective collateral circulation develop.

Arteries have to be clamped or tied proximally before you can repair them, either in the wound itself, or at one of the sites of election using either a tape, or an arterial clamp.

Never clamp an artery with a haemostat. Even rubber tubes over the jaws of a haemostat will not prevent them from injuring it. Instead: (1) use the special arterial clamps, or (2) the Rummel tourniquet shown in Fig. 55-4. This is merely a length of stout linen or cotton tape passed round the artery and then threaded through a rubber or plastic tube. If you pull the tape and push the tube down on the artery you will occlude it. (3)

Pass a fine rubber tube or catheter round the vessel, and hold it against your finger.

If the flow of blood in an artery stops, the blood in it is liable to clot, so stop it doing this by injecting dilute heparin into it proximal and distal to the clamp. Be careful never to inject more than one fifth of the anticoagulant dose of heparin for the whole patient (15,000 units in an adult).

Veins. In the limbs you can tie most veins without causing any disability. Veins bigger than the femoral should ideally be sutured. This is more difficult than suturing an artery. Torn veins are difficult to see because blood wells up into the wound, instead of spurting like an artery.

• *CLAMP, bulldog for arteries, Blalock cross action, assorted sizes, four only.* If you want to clamp an artery temporarily, apply one of these, not a haemostat.

END TO END ANASTOMOSIS

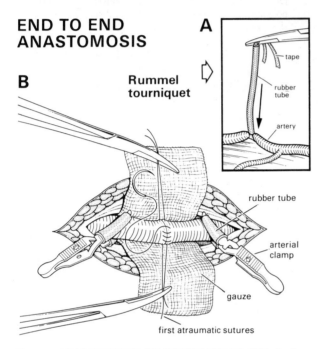

Fig. 55-4 ANASTOMOSING AN ARTERY END TO END. A, shows how an artery can be closed temporarily with a Rummel tourniquet. This is a piece of tape passed round the artery and then through a rubber tube. B, an artery being anastomosed. Note that the arterial clamps have rubber over their jaws. *Adapted from Hamilton Bailey by the kind permission of Hugh Dudley.*

REPAIRING BLOOD VESSELS

EQUIPMENT Arterial clamps. A very fine needle holder, and fine dissecting forceps such as Adson's or finer. Half circle round–bodied atraumatic needles (or better, a micropoint needle). 4/0 monofilament sutures or finer. Magnifying spectacles, such as the Bishop Harman loupe. Heparin (50 mg or 5000 units in 100 ml of saline), or use the citrate solution from a blood transfusion bottle or bag.

WOUND TOILET Do this carefully, and remove all dead or dying tissue from the patient's wound. If he has a fracture, allow its fragments to overlap while you repair his artery. Enlarge his wound as necessary, so that you can really get at his injured vessel easily, and inspect it.

TORN ARTERIES

If the patient's artery is only partly divided, or is cut longitudinally, you may be able to suture it directly.

If it has been nearly cut across, you may be able to anastomase its cut ends.

If a length of it is bruised or torn, you may have to cut out the ragged piece and bring clean cut ends together for anastomosis.

If its cut ends are ragged, excise them, so that you can bring two clean–cut ends together. You may be able to excise 2 cm or more and still bring the ends together. If they will not come together, you will have to insert a saphenous vein graft, as described in the next section.

If the adventitia (which looks like filmy cobwebs) projects beyond the other coats, trim it away. If you leave it, it will promote thrombosis in the suture line.

If there is a gap in one wall of the artery, you may be able to repair it with a saphenous vein patch graft, as in B, Fig. 55-3.

MOBILIZE THE ARTERY Arteries are elastic, so you will probably be able to free enough of the artery above and below the wound to let you work on it. Apply arterial clamps or Rummel tourniquets above and below the wound. In an emergency, ask your assistant to press the artery between his finger and thumb. Inject heparin into it on the far sides of each clamp or tourniquet.

Try to preserve any reasonably sized branches, because these will help to maintain the collateral circulation if the repair fails.

REPAIR Put something behind the injured vessel, such as a piece of gauze or half a glove, so that you can see what you are doing as in Fig. 55-4.

CAUTION ! Before you start the repair, allow the artery to bleed from both ends to remove any clot that may have formed. This will wash out the heparin, so inject more through fine catheters.

Squeeze any clot out of the cut ends of the artery and drip a few drops of heparin onto each of them.

Bring the cut ends of the artery together with two stay sutures at opposite sides. Two more at the top and bottom may help. Use these to steady the artery and rotate it, where necessary.

Either use horizontal mattress sutures to evert its cut edges, or use continuous sutures. Place them about 1 mm apart or less and 1 mm from the cut edges. Place the knots on the outside. Drop some heparin solution onto the artery while you suture it.

CAUTION ! Place the sutures carefully and avoid dog ears or the anastomosis will leak.

When the suture is complete, release the distal clamp first. This low pressure retrograde flow will show up any leaks. If necesary, stitch them.

Then press the anastomosis lightly with gauze and gradually release the proximal clamp. The repair will bleed, but the bleeding will usually stop spontaneously in a few minutes. If necessary, put in more sutures.

If the repair leaks, press it with a gauze pack for a few minutes. Blood may clot in the leaks and block them.

If you are successful there will be a pulse in the artery distal to the repair.

CAUTION ! Cover the repair with living muscle or subcutaneous tissue. Don't leave it exposed while waiting for delayed primary closure (54.4). Rotate a flap over it, or partly close the wound.

TORN VEINS Sponge holding forceps are useful in grasping a torn vein because they take large bites and flatten it. If possible use lateral occluding clamps which will let you see the edges of the tear and insert an everting layer of fine continous sutures.

Failing this, press firmly on the vein above and below the tear. This will empty it and show you the hole outlined against its posterior wall.

If all else fails, occlude the vein above and below the tear, and tie it.

POSTOPERATIVELY (all vascular injuries) Splint the patient's limb in the position of least tension on his injured vessel, and then gradually straighten it over several days. If there is a fracture, you have at least 10 days in which to align the bony fragments before they unite in the wrong position.

A SAPHENOUS VEIN GRAFT

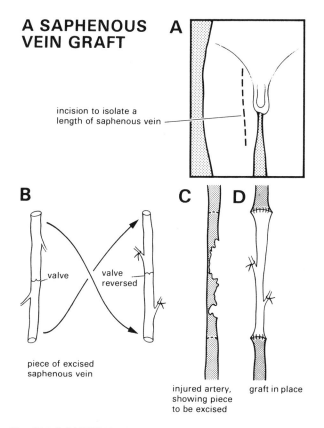

incision to isolate a length of saphenous vein

B

valve

valve reversed

piece of excised saphenous vein

C **D**

injured artery, showing piece to be excised

graft in place

Fig. 55-5 A SAPHENOUS VEIN GRAFT. A, the incision to expose the saphenous vien. B, the length of saphenous vien is being reversed, so that any valves it contains do not obstruct the blood flow. The grafted vein sewn in place and its side branches tied off. *Kindly contributed by Peter Bewes.*

55.7 Saphenous vein grafts

If such a large section of a patient's artery is injured that you cannot bring its ends together, you will have to join them with a piece of his saphenous vein, or refer him for this to be done. Although you are only using a vein, it will withstand his arterial blood pressure adequately, and will resist infection better than an artificial vessel. If repairing an artery is only possible under tension, insert a vein graft. This is a procedure for the caring operator who cannot refer a patient.

GRAFTING WITH THE SAPHENOUS VEIN

INDICATIONS An arterial injury, which cannot be repaired in any other way, and cannot be tied for fear of causing gangrene—see Section 55.2.

REVERSED SAPHENOUS VEIN GRAFT Expose the patient's saphenous vein through an adequate incision along its length.

Remove a suitable length of vein, and cut off all its side branches between 4/0 monofilament ligatures.

Remove the isolated segment of vein, clamp its distal end with a haemostat, and irrigate it with heparinized saline (55.6) under pressure. This will show up the leaks from any small side branches you may have have missed. It will also distend the vein most usefully, but take care not to distend it too much.

Leave it distended with heparin and lying in some heparin or blood while you prepare the artery to receive it.

Trim the ends of the veins and anastomose them to the artery, using the method described above for anastomosing an artery. The piece you take may have a valve in it, so make sure you reverse the direction of the flow of blood in it.

Remove the distal arterial clamp just before the last stitch or two, so that any air caught inside the repair can escape through the hole between your last two sutures.

Leave the repair under a warm saline pack while you wait 10 minutes. Inspect it, and if it looks satisfactory, cover it with adjacent tissue and close the wound, preferably by delayed primary closure.

SAPHENOUS VEIN PATCH GRAFT Take a piece of saphenous vein, open it out, make quite sure the intima faces inwards, and patch it in place with fine sutures. If you fail, you will have to tie the patient's injured vessel. If his limb becomes gangrenous, amputate it.

55.8 Examining the peripheral nerves

Whenever a patient has injured a limb, especially if he has a penetrating wound, test the function of its nerves and tendons *before you anaesthetize him* or refer him elsewhere. Test the most distal point supplied by each nerve. The following tests are so quick that you can do them all in a few seconds. Always record your results. It will then be certain that paralysis is not the result of treatment.

QUICK TESTS FOR PERIPHERAL NERVES
Record both power and sensation when you first see a patient, and after each subsequent examination. For the nerves of the hand goto Section 75.1.

AXILLARY (CIRCUMFLEX) NERVE This arises from the posterior cord of the bachial plexus, and winds round the neck of a patient's humerus to supply his deltoid and the skin over the lower part of this muscle. It is injured in dislocations of the shoulder.

Ask the patient to abduct his arm. Put the palm of your hand over his deltoid as he does so, as in A, Fig. 55-6. Even a flicker of contraction shows that his deltoid is working.

Test sensation with a pin on the outer part of his shoulder, over the insertion of his deltoid. If his axillary nerve has been injured, there will be a small patch of anaesthesia.

MUSCULOCUTANEOUS NERVE If this nerve has been injured there will be anaesthesia along the outer side of his forearm, and he will be almost unable to flex his arm.

SCIATIC NERVE This is sometimes injured by pelvic fractures. Test its peroneal and tibial branches as described below. Test the sensation of the dorsum of his foot.

COMMON PERONEAL BRANCH OF SCIATIC NERVE Paralysis causes foot drop. Can he walk on his heels with his forefoot raised? Test for anaesthesia in the distribution of his

TESTS FOR SOME PERIPHERAL NERVES

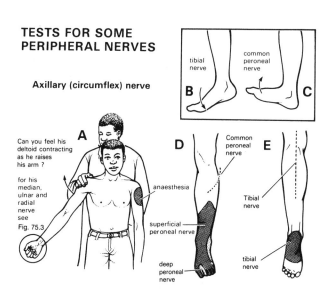

Axillary (circumflex) nerve

tibial nerve

common peroneal nerve

B **C**

Can you feel his deltoid contracting as he raises his arm ?

for his median, ulnar and radial nerve see Fig. 75.3

A **D**

anaesthesia

superficial peroneal nerve

deep peroneal nerve

E

Common peroneal nerve

Tibial nerve

tibial nerve

Fig. 55-6 SOME QUICK TESTS FOR PERIPHERAL NERVES. Test the function of an injured patient's nerves and tendons before you anaesthetize or refer him. Tests for the nerves of the hand are in Section 75.1.

deep peroneal nerve in the web between his big and second toe. His common peroneal nerve can be injured by Thomas splints, badly applied skin traction, or blows to the neck of his fibula.

TIBIAL BRANCH OF SCIATIC NERVE Ask him to plantar flex his ankle, or stand on tip toe.

EXAMINE HIS PERIPHERAL NERVES BEFORE YOU ANAESTHETIZE HIM

IS IT A NERVE OR A TENDON?

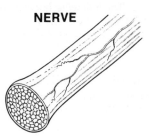

NERVE

yellowish, softer and more flexible, cut end bulges slightly, nerve fibres in bundles, vessel on the surface

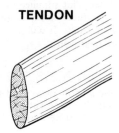

TENDON

bluish white, glistening, straighter, firmer, cut surface like wood

Fig. 55-7 IS IT A NERVE OR A TENDON? A nerve is yellowish and flexible, and you can make it lie in various positions. A tendon is bluish white and glistening, straighter and firmer and more difficult to deform by compression than a nerve. *Kindly contributed by Peter Bewes.*

55.9 Primary nerve repair

A patient's digital nerves, and his median and ulnar nerves commonly need repairing, but you may occasionally need to repair almost any nerve. Whenever you toilet a wound, inspect any nerves that might be injured, but don't try to repair them, unless they have been cut completely. Closed injuries usually only bruise nerves, so that they are able to recover in a few weeks.

One of your first problems will be to distinguish a nerve from a tendon deep in a wound. Even supposedly expert surgeons have sutured a nerve to a tendon, especially at the wrist.

A nerve is yellowish and flexible. You can make it lie in various positions, and if you press it, it will flatten fairly easily from side to side and from back to front. Its cut edge bulges slightly. Look at it carefully, if possible with a lens, and you will see its fibres lying in bundles, like fine macaroni. If it has been cut, you can easily see these bundles surrounded by connective tissue. A nerve often has a small tortuous vessel running along its surface. This is a rare on a tendon.

A tendon is bluish white and glistening, straighter and firmer and more difficult to deform by compression than a nerve. It has a flat smooth cut surface like wood cut across the grain, and its bundles are more difficult to see.

Nerve injuries are best referred immediately to an expert. But, if there is no expert, *make as good a primary repair as you possibly can yourself, and don't merely tack the cut ends of the patient's nerve together with black silk, which is now quite outmoded.* If a patient needs a secondary repair later, he will then be in a good position for it. In practice, an attempt at primary repair is likely to be more satisfactory than merely doing an approximate repair in the hope of being able to refer him later.

If, for any reason accurate primary repair has not been possible, the patient's wound should be re-explored and a secondary

repair done between 3 weeks and 3 months later. At 3 weeks fibrosis will no longer be proceeding proximally up his injured nerve and its sheath will be thicker, and better able to hold stitches. If secondary repair is necessary, *make this quite clear to the patient and to his relatives, and record it in his notes.* Mark the nerve ends with a non–absorbable suture.

DON'T SUTURE PALMARIS LONGUS TO THE MEDIAN NERVE!

PRIMARY NERVE REPAIR

INDICATIONS Any nerve which has been completely transected. If the wound is clean, attempt repair immediately. If it is grossly contaminated, control infection first.

EQUIPMENT Use your finest monofilament sutures, needles, and needle holder. Use 8/0 sutures on 3 mm atraumatic needles. Any suture larger than 6/0 is too big. Use ophthalmic forceps and needle holders, and operating spectacles such as the Bishop Harman loupe.

Don't use silk, catgut, human hair, or dexon because these are irritant. Coarse sutures may cause so much fibrosis that the nerve will never function again.

METHOD Explore the patient's wound as described in Section 54.1. Find the cut ends of the nerve. Put his limb in the position which will help to bring them together.

Trim back both the cut ends of the nerves with a new sterile razor blade as in A, Fig. 55-8. Usually about 2 mm is enough.

Match the cut ends in their correct anatomical positions, without rotation. There are usually very fine blood vessels on one side of a nerve which will enable you to distinguish its two sides. Study the cross section of its fasciculi carefully, and get the two cut ends to match.

Try to put all sutures into the outer sheath of the nerve. Sutures deep inside it will interfere with its function seriously. For clarity, the sutures in Fig. 55-8 are shown much larger than they really are.

Pass two stay sutures through the outer sheath of the nerve on either side. Tie them and leave the ends long (B). Carefully hold the two ends of the nerve together, and ask an assistant to hold the ends in artery forceps. Put one or two sutures into the front of the nerve (C).

Pass one of your stay sutures behind the anastomosis (D), and cross the other one in front of it, so that you rotate the nerve as you pull them and expose its back (E).

Put one or two sutures into the back of the nerve. It may be easier to repair the back of the nerve first.

CAUTION ! (1) Try not to put more than 8 sutures into the nerve, or there will be unnecessary fibrosis. (2) Don't let any nerve fibres stick out of the suture line.

Manage the wound as in Section 54.1. If you are leaving the wound open for delayed closure, try to cover the sutured nerve with muscle or skin, and don't leave it naked in the wound. If necessary, make relieving incisions, so that you can move skin over to cover the nerve, or cover it with a transposition flap, as in Fig. 55-9. Or, least satisfactorily, cover it with a split skin graft.

Splint the patient's limb in the position which best relieves tension on the nerve. If it is under tension, release the position of the splint slowly over several weeks. If you fail to do this, the sutures may pull out.

When you have removed the stiches from the patient's wound, and are waiting for his nerve to recover, splint his limb to prevent contractures, and tell him how to prevent trophic ulcers forming. If he intends to pick up something which might be hot, ask him to feel its temperature with his normal hand.

HAVE YOU SUCCEEDED? TINEL'S SIGN Tap the course of the nerve, if the patient feels pins and needles over its distribution, it is regenerating.

Examine and record the power of all the muscles that his injured nerve supplies. The most proximally innervated ones will recover first.

ANASTOMOSING A SEVERED NERVE

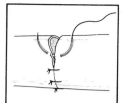
sutures pass through
epineurium only

for the sake of clarity, the sutures
have been drawn larger than in reality

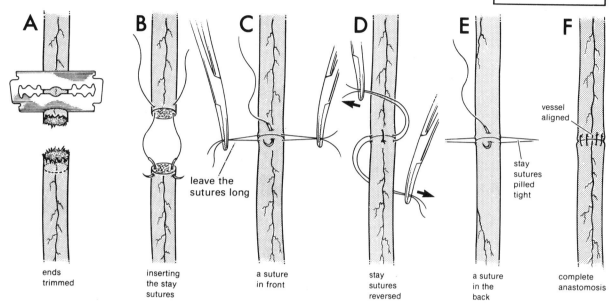

A	B	C	D	E	F
ends trimmed	inserting the stay sutures	a suture in front	stay sutures reversed	a suture in the back	complete anastomosis

leave the sutures long

vessel aligned

stay sutures pilled tight

Fig. 55-8 ANASTOMOSING A NERVE. A, the ends are trimmed with a razor blade. B, the stay sutures. C, an anterior suture. D, the stay sutures reversed. E, inserting a suture in the back of the nerve. F, the completed anastomosis, G, sutures pass through the epineurium only.
Kindly contributed by Peter Bewes

55.10 Secondary nerve repair by trial section

If you see a patient with an injured nerve late, or decide not to repair it at the time of the injury, the only way to repair it is by trial section and resuture. If you cannot refer him, you may have to do this yourself.

To begin with there is a blood clot between the fascicles of a recently cut nerve, as in A, Fig. 55-10. This soon becomes organized and invaded by fibrous tissue to form a rounded neuroma (B). You will have to cut this back in a succession of small slices until you reach healthy nerve (C). Sometimes a nerve is incompletely divided and although its ends are joined it is

deformed by bulbous neuromas (D). These too have to be cut back until you reach healthy nerve.

The best time for secondary repair is 3 weeks after the patient's initial injury. You may find that, when you have excised the retracted fibrosed cut ends of his nerve, it has to bridge quite a gap. Nerves are not very elastic, so this can be difficult. An expert may be able to bridge the gap with a graft. Your best hope is to explore the nerve through an enormous long incision, so that you can mobilize enough nerve to make it stretch the gap. For example, you may have to explore the ulnar nerve from the wrist to the elbow and down into the hand.

Another difficulty is finding the cut ends of the nerve deep in the scar of the wound. Look for them proximally and distally, and then follow both ends into the fibrous tissue of the wound. Be careful not to cut them as you look for them. Use blunt dissection, where you can. If you have to use a scalpel, cut in the length of the nerve, not across it.

TRANSPOSITION FLAP

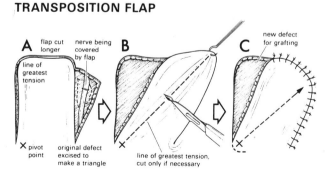

A flap cut longer nerve being covered by flap

line of greatest tension

B

new defect for grafting

C

X pivot point

original defect excised to make a triangle

line of greatest tension, cut only if necessary

Fig. 55-9 A TRANSPOSITION FLAP BEING USED TO COVER AN EXPOSED NERVE. You will have to graft the new defect, but you will have covered the nerve with full thickness skin. The incision in B, is dangerous, if you are not careful you may interfere with the blood supply of the flap *With the kind permission of James Smith.*

TRIAL SECTION AND RESUTURE

INDICATIONS (1) A nerve which was completely transsected at the time of the patient's original injury and was not repaired. (2) An injured nerve which is not recovering. If Tinel's sign (55.9) shows that *any recovery is taking place*, don't consider exploring a closed wound for several months. It is probably only contused, and will recover.

If possible refer the patient. If this is impossible, you may be justified in proceeding as follows.

Explore his healed wound and mobilize his injured nerve. Feel carefully for the parts of it that are hard and fibrosed.

Use a sharp scalpel, or a razor blade held in forceps, to cut thin slices across its thickest place.

SECONDARY NERVE REPAIR

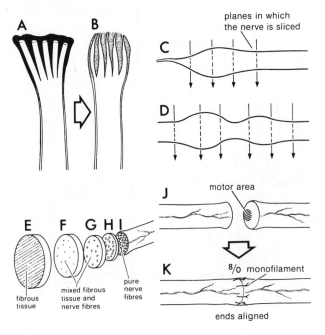

Fig. 55-10 SECONDARY NERVE REPAIR BY TRIAL SECTION. A, a ragged recently injured nerve surrounded by blood clot. B, later, when the clot has organized and become fibrous tissue. C, taking successive sections of the thickened end of a cut nerve. D, an incompletely divided nerve with two thickened swellings. E, to I, taking trial sections down a thickened nerve. J, the motor area in a cut nerve shown schematically. K, the cut ends of a nerve aligned, and sutured with fine monofilament. *Kindly contributed by Peter Bewes.*

The first slice you cut from the neuroma (E, in Fig. 55-10) may show a uniform slab of fibrous tissue. In the second slice (F) a few little dots of nervous tissue have started to appear. In the third slice (G) there are more little dots. The fourth slice is mostly nerve tissue (H). The final one (I) has the normal fibrillary structure of a nerve. This is the point to stop cutting back and do ananstomosis (J and K) as for primary nerve suture (55.9). Try to bring the ends together without rotation, so that the motor areas in each end correspond. One such area has been shown hatched in the diagram (J).

Section the distal end in the same way, then join the two ends as above.

PARTICULAR NERVES FOR SECONDARY REPAIR

Ulnar nerve Move the nerve anteriorly from behind the patient's medial epicondyle. This will give you the extra length you need to make the anastomosis. Keep his elbow and wrist flexed and try not to injure its branches to flexor carpi ulnaris, and the medial half of his flexor digitorium profundus.

Median nerve at the wrist Approach this by incising his carpal tunnel.

DIFFICULTIES WITH SECONDARY NERVE REPAIR

If the patient's **NERVE INJURY WAS NEVER DIAGNOSED** and his wound is now healing, explore it as soon as the danger of infection is over. The longer you delay after 2 months, the worse the result. If you feel a neuroma, the nerve has been seriously injured.

55.11 Tendon injuries

Rupture of the belly of a muscle usually causes little disability, but rupture of its tendon or the junction of tendon with muscle is usually serious. The result depends greatly on whether or not the tendon is surrounded by a sheath. For example, if one of the flexor tendons of a patient's wrist is cut, its ends retract, become rounded, fail to heal and lie loose inside their sheath. Repair will be easier and the result is better if a tendon has no sheath, as with the extensors of the wrist. Tendon injuries most commonly involve the hand, so they are further discussed in Sections 75.20 and 75.21. Here we only discuss the general principles. The main one is the method for inserting sutures.

REPAIRING TENDONS

See elsewhere for injuries of a patient's Achilles tendon (82.10), and his hand—his flexor tendons need special methods (75.21).

MATERIALS Non–irritating sutures, such as fine stainless steel wire, preferably braided, or monofilament nylon, preferably 5/0. Don't use catgut.

Thread both ends of a length of the suture material onto two straight needles, and pass this through the patient's cut tendon, as in A, Fig. 55-11.

Hold the cut end of the tendon in a pair of artery forceps and suture 1 or 2 cm down the tendon. Pass both needles through it diagonally two or three times.

Bring both ends of the suture out onto the cut ends of the tendon. Then thread them in a similar way into the cut surface of the other end of the tendon. Finally, pull the sutures tight and tie them.

CAUTION ! Take care to identify the cut ends correctly. Don't join a profundus to a sublimis tendon, or a nerve to a tendon!

POSTOPERATIVE CARE Immobilize the patient's limb for 3 weeks in the position which will cause least tension on his cut tendon. Encourage as much active movement as immobilization will allow.

The critical period for rupture of the repair is immediately you remove the splints. So start movements gradually, and try to devise some form of check strap to prevent sudden movements which may rupture his newly repaired tendon. His limb will be stiff and painful, but it should improve steadily over many weeks.

SUTURING A TENDON

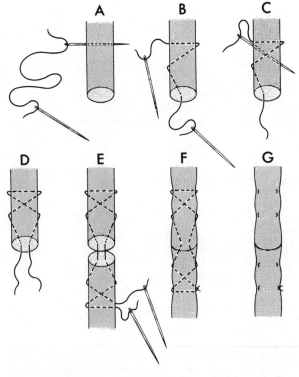

Fig. 55-11 SUTURING A TENDON. This method keeps the knots away from the cut ends of the tendon. *Kindly contributed by Peter Bewes.*

56 Amputations

56.1 The general method for amputations.

You will need to amputate a patient's leg about five times more often than his arm. Once you have cut off a limb there is no going back, so try to retain as much function as you can. The patient is unlikely to get an arm prosthesis, and it would be of little use even if he could get one. So aim instead for the longest possible stump of an arm. Every centimetre is useful, so is an elbow which he can use as a hook, and so is any kind of a wrist.

A patient's leg must have a prosthesis which will bear his weight. There are a limited number of these, and the stumps for them are standardized. *So always do one of the standard leg amputations.* There are three technological grades of prosthesis; of these the third is not necessarily the worst. A patient might have: (1) A sophisticated modern prosthesis costing $300 or more. (2) A simpler modern prosthesis costing $30, such as one of those developed by Huckstep for polio (26.2), which any bicycle mechanic can mend. Or, (3) the patient might have a traditional prosthesis, such as a pylon, a peg leg, or elephant boot. Don't despise these; when well made they last longer than any of the others, and are better than a modern prosthesis for working in the fields.

A leg prosthesis can: (1) Have a cup to bear weight on the sides of the stump, in which case the scar should be at the end. (2) Bear weight on the end of the stump, in which case the scar should be posterior. (3) Have a modern total contact socket in which the position of the scar is unimportant. Limb fitting centres vary in their scope and preferences, so visit your local one and find out what they like. A good prosthetist can fit any well constructed stump with a prosthesis.

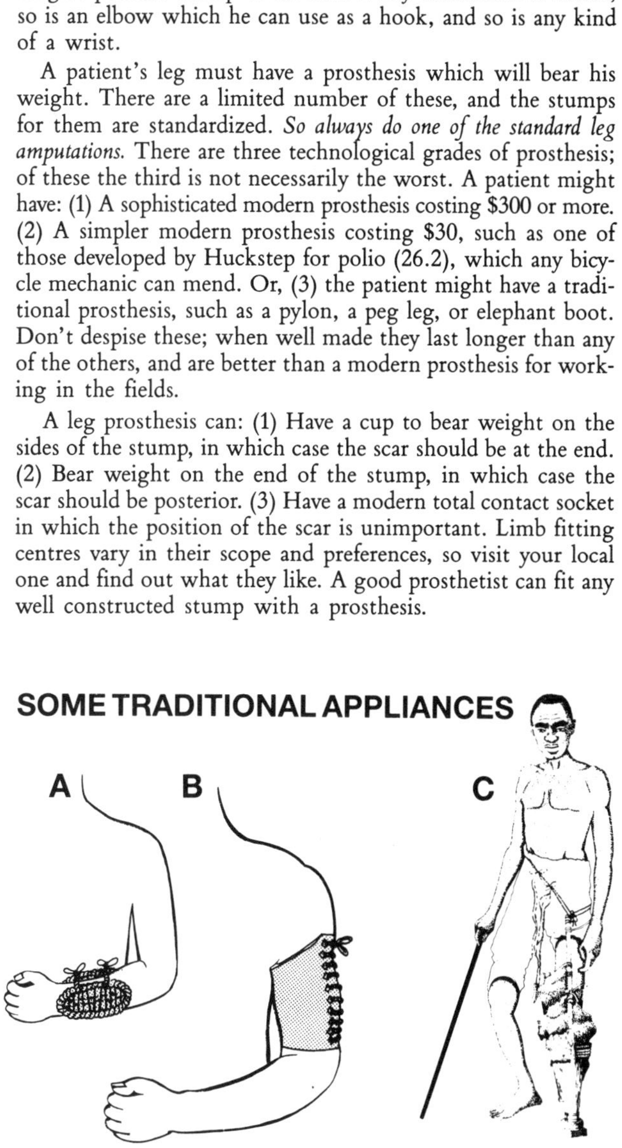

SOME TRADITIONAL APPLIANCES

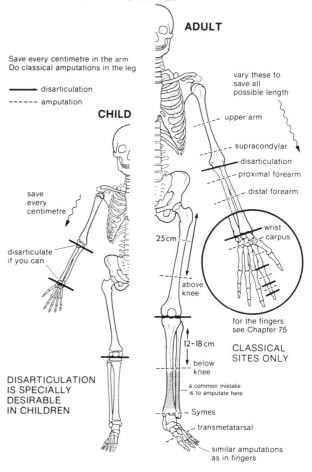

Fig. 56-1 SOME LOCALLY MADE APPLIANCES. A, a traditional splint for a child's forearm as used by the Pokot in Uganda. B, a Pokot splint for fractures of the shaft of the humerus—exactly what Section 71.17 would approve of! C, this Zimbabwian patient used his ingenuity in overcoming the disability of an amputation, and although the result is not beautiful and required constant attention, he was able to get around. *Kindly contributed by Kevin Rankin and Peter Cox.*

IN THE ARM CONSERVE EVERY CENTIMETRE
IN THE LEG DO A STANDARD AMPUTATION

In the abdomen poor surgical craftsmenship is hidden, but on an amputation stump it is there for everyone to see. In a perfect stump: (1) The scar is not exposed to pressure. (2) The skin slides easily over the bone. (3) The skin is not infolded. (4) There is no redundant soft tissue. (5) There is no protruding spur of bone. (6) The stump is painless. And, (7) the wound has healed by first intention. Most amputation stumps should be conical.

Fish mouth flaps As a general rule, cut the fish mouth flaps shown in Fig. 56-4. The alternative is a guillotine amputation, as described in Section 56.2. Fish mouth flaps must be long enough to cover the soft tissues of the stump, but not be so

WHERE TO AMPUTATE?

ADULT

Save every centimetre in the arm
Do classical amputations in the leg

—— disarticulation
----- amputation

CHILD

save every centimetre

disarticulate if you can

vary these to save all possible length

upper arm

supracondylar
disarticulation
proximal forearm
distal forearm

wrist
carpus

25cm

above knee

for the fingers see Chapter 75

CLASSICAL SITES ONLY

12-18 cm

below knee

a common mistake is to amputate here

Symes

transmetatarsal

similar amputations as in fingers

DISARTICULATION IS SPECIALLY DESIRABLE IN CHILDREN

Fig. 56-2 AMPUTATION SITES. In the arm save ever centimetre. In the leg amputate at the classical sites only.

long that their blood supply is inadequate and they necrose. If the flaps are equal, the scar will come at the end of a stump. If they are unequal the scar can come at the front or the back. Try to place the scar where it is not going to be pressed on. In the hand and the foot, place it dorsally. Higher up the arm the scar can be anywhere. In the leg, its site depends on the kind of prosthesis the patient is to have—end bearing, side bearing, or total contact. In the lower arm and leg transverse scars are better than anteroposterior ones because they do not get drawn up between the two bones.

Immediate suture or delayed primary closure? Delayed primary closure is always wise: (1) If the patient's limb is already infected, or might easily become so. (2) In all battle casualties. (3) If there is much soft tissue injury. (4) If the blood supply of the stump is uncertain. If you decide on delayed primary closure, cut the flaps long, to allow them to retract. Leave the patient's muscle and fascia unsutured, bandage the skin flaps over dry gauze swabs, don't put in any stitches, and bring him back to the theatre 3 to 5 days later. If his wound is not infected, close it. If it is infected, leave the flaps open for a week or longer, and close it later by secondary suture.

Postoperative care. Much depends on what happens to a patient after he leaves the theatre. His leg stump must be prepared for the prosthesis, and he needs to be taught how to use it. Firm bandaging will hasten to conversion of his stump from a bulky cylinder to a narrow cone, and exercises will strengthen its remaining muscles. So, give the stump something to do. After a lower leg amputation he can learn to kick a large rubber ball about.

How do amputations differ in children? Most of the same principles apply in a child. Disarticulate a joint if you can, especially at his knee, because this will preserve its epiphysis. Removing a limb by amputating through the shaft of a bone produces an effect which varies with the site. It can either cause excessive bony overgrowth with the need for a revision amputations later, or a short stump.

• *SAW, amputation, with hinged back, 230 mm, (a) saw, one only. (b) Spare blades for the above, three only.* The back of the saw stiffens it during the early part of the cut, but can be hinged back later to let the saw pass through.

• *SAW, Gigli, (a) pair of handles, one pair only. (b) Saw blades, 30 cm, 4 only.* A Gigli bone saw is a piece of wire with sharp teeth on it which you pull to and fro between two handles. Use it to cut bone in awkward places.

• *KNIFE, amputation, Liston 180 mm, one only.* If you don't have an amputation knife, sharpen a long kitchen knife and use that.

AMPUTATION EQUIPMENT

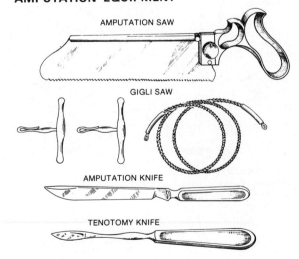

AMPUTATION SAW

GIGLI SAW

AMPUTATION KNIFE

TENOTOMY KNIFE

Fig. 56-3 EQUIPMENT FOR AMPUTATION. If necessary, you can use any saw or a domestic knife.

Here is the sequence of steps for all amputations. They are not repeated in the instructions for the specific sites described later. Follow the steps in the order in which we give them here.

GENERAL METHOD FOR AMPUTATIONS

INDICATIONS (1) An arm which is so severely injured that there is no chance of recovery of any part of the hand, fingers or thumb. (2) A leg which is so severely injured that you cannot restore the continuity of its vessels or nerves, especially when there is gross contamination or severe muscle or skin loss. Loss of bone alone without nerve or vascular injury does not usually justify amputation. (3) Gas gangrene. (4) Established gangrene due to vascular injury. (5) Continued infection with severe bone or nerve injury. (6) Secondary haemorrhage if all other measures fail. (7) Multiple injuries in a gravely ill shocked patient. Amputation may be the simplest and fastest way of removing large amounts of damaged muscle, and so saving his life. (8) Occasionally also for epitheliomas, bone tumours, or snake bites.

CAUTION ! If you amputate for a malignancy, biospy it first.

ANAESTHESIA Relaxation is unecessary. Ketamine is adequate (8.1). Subarachnoid (spinal) anaesthesia (A 7.4) is particularly useful for below knee amputations. Nobody likes hearing their bones being sawn through, so if a patient is conscious premedicate him heavily.

TOURNIQUET Use a tourniquet (3.8), except when you are amputating for ischaemia. Bleeding is a useful sign that a muscle is alive. If it is dead you may need to amputate higher up. A tourniquet may also make ischaemia worse. Release it *before* you suture the muscles, so that you can tie the bleeding vessels before you cover them.

When you use a tourniquet, exsanguinate the patient's limb with an Esmarch bandage first (3.8), except when you are amputating for sepsis or malignancy which it may spread.

CAUTION ! Don't rely on digital pressure over the main vessels to control bleeding.

CUTTING FISH MOUTH FLAPS FOR AN AMPUTATION

Decide where you are going to saw the bone (the point of section) and plan the flaps in relation to that point. Place the angle of the fish mouth at the site of bone section. Mark them out carefully with methylene blue or scratch marks.

If the flaps are equal, make the length of each of them equal to 3/4 of the diameter of the limb as in A, Fig. 56-4.

If the flaps are unequal, make the longer flap equal to the diameter of the limb, and the shorter one equal to half its diameter, as in B.

Cut through the skin down to the deep fascia, and reflect this up with the skin as part of the flap. The skin of the stump will need to slide over the deep fascia, so keep them together. If you are amputating for ischaemia *minimize trauma to the flaps.* Handle them with stay sutures rather than with forceps.

CAUTION ! (1) Start by making fish mouth flaps long. You can always trim them if they are too long later, but you cannot lengthen them if they are too short. (2) Cut them round not pointed. (3) Their combined length should be equal one and a half times the diameter of the limb at the site of bone section. (4) If you are amputating a severely lacerated limb, try to preserve all viable skin.

CONTROLLING BLEEDING DURING AN AMPUTATION

Early in the operation, find the major arteries and veins. Tie them separately with double transfixion ligatures (3.2) preferably linen. Then cut them between these ligatures. Later, after you have removed the limb, release the tourniquet slowly and tie the remaining smaller vessels. If the cut ends of the muscles bleed furiously, apply packs for five minutes.

If the amputation is very high, you may have to expose the main artery higher up at one of the classical sites described in Sections 3.4 to 3.7.

CAUTION ! (1) If you don't use a tourniquet, find and tie the major vessels *before* you cut them. (2) Don't clamp them, cut

THE GEOMETRY OF FISH MOUTH FLAPS

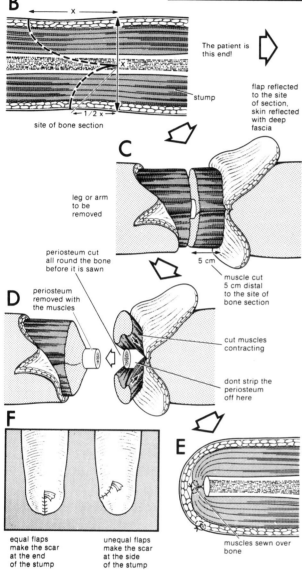

A EQUAL FLAPS

¾ x

UNEQUAL FLAPS

B

x

½ x

site of bone section

x

The patient is this end!

flap reflected to the site of section, skin reflected with deep fascia

stump

C

leg or arm to be removed

5 cm

muscle cut 5 cm distal to the site of bone section

periosteum cut all round the bone before it is sawn

D periosteum removed with the muscles

cut muscles contracting

dont strip the periosteum off here

F

E

equal flaps make the scar at the end of the stump

unequal flaps make the scar at the side of the stump

muscles sewn over bone

Fig. 56-4 FISH MOUTH FLAPS. Together, the flaps should be one and a half times the diameter of the limb. Either make them as two equal flaps, each ¾ of the diameter of the limb, or, make one flap equal to the whole diameter and the other flap equal to half of it. *Kindly contributed by Peter Bewes.*

them and then try to tie them. If a clamp slips there will be massive bleeding. (3) Careful haemostatsis of the stump is essential. If a clot forms, it is easily infected.

CUTTING MUSCLES DURING AN AMPUTATION

Muscles always contract, after you have cut them. So cut them transversely about 5 cm distal the site of bone section. Leave them a little longer if you are using delayed primary closure, because they will have more time to shrink.

Use a long sharp amputation knife or carving knife to cut the muscles straight down to the bone. Don't use a scalpel which makes many small cuts, and leaves shreds of injured muscle.

Sew the cut ends of the muscle securely together over the cut end of the bone, so that they cushion it, and are better able to move over the stump. Cut them long enough for this but don't leave so much muscle that the stump becomes bulbous.

CUTTING NERVES DURING AN AMPUTATION

Don't tie nerves. A painful neuroma will result, especially in the fingers. Instead, gently pull each nerve into the wound, cut it cleanly with a knife, then let it retract above the amputation site.

HOW TO COVER THE STUMP WHILE YOU SAW

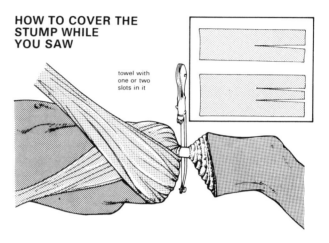

towel with one or two slots in it

Fig. 56-5 HOW TO COVER THE STUMP WHILE YOU SAW. The towel with two slots in it is for forearm and lower leg. The central flap goes between the bones. *From an unknown source.*

SAWING BONES DURING AN AMPUTATION

Clear the muscle from the site of section, and incise the periosteum all round it. Reflect this distally for one or two centimetres with the muscles, so as to leave bare bone for the saw.

Use a saw with well set teeth. Start by steadying it with your thumb. Draw it towards you across the bone a few times. When it has made a good slot in the bone, start sawing hard. Ask an assistant to hold the patient's limb to steady it, and pull gently to prevent the saw locking in the bone and splitting it. Finally, remove any spikes with bone forceps, and bevel any protruding edges with a coarse rasp.

CAUTION! (1) Don't reflect the periosteum proximally, because the bone under it will die, and a ring sequestrum will form. (2) Don't damage the surrounding muscle with the saw. Cut the muscle first, or retract it well out of the way with a towel wrapped round the limb, as in Fig. 56-5, then saw. (3) Bone dust from the saw acts as a foreign body, so wash it away with saline.

DEALING WITH FAT DURING AN AMPUTATION

If a patient's limb is very fat, cautiously remove as much subcutaneous fat as is necessary. Don't remove too much, especially near the edges of the flap, or it may necrose. Learn to design flaps so that they come together accurately without dog ears'. If they form, leave them, they will soon disappear.

CLOSING THE WOUND AFTER AN AMPUTATION

SUTURES As indicated above, delayed primary suture will be safer. Suture the skin and deep fascia separately.

Close the flaps without tension, without leaving gaping areas between the sutures, and without tying them too tight.

DRAINS If you use delayed primary suture, no drains are necessary. If you close a stump by immediate suture, insert a drain under the muscle flap (if there is one) over the end of the bone. If possible, use a suction drain. If you don't have one, insert a 2 cm corrugated rubber drain. Bring both its ends

CLOSING THE STUMP

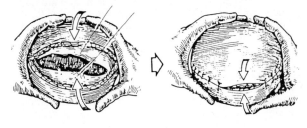

Fig. 56-6 CLOSING AN AMPUTATION STUMP. Close the deep fascia, then the skin.

out loosely through the two ends of the incision as shown in F, Fig. 56-4.

If no blood is oozing from the drains, remove them at 48 hours, if blood continues to flow, leave them for a further 24 hours.

DRESSINGS Dress the stump firmly, but not too tightly. A plaster covering will make it more comfortable. Change the dressings at 48 hours.

POSTOPERATIVE CARE FOR AN AMPUTATION

As soon as the skin has healed, bandage the stump. For the leg, sew two 15 cm crepe bandages end–to–end. For the arm, use one 10 cm bandage. Roll the bandage tightly, then wind it round the stump. Apply more tension to the end of the stump, than to its base, or it will become bulbous. Reapply the bandage several times a day until the prosthesis is fitted. Don't use adhesive strapping, or you may tear the skin of the stump.

THE FURTHER MANAGEMENT OF AN AMPUTATION

Read on for: guillotine amputations (56.2), amputating for gangrene (56.3), amputating through the upper arm and elbow (56.4), the lower arm and wrist (56.5), above the knee (56.6), through the knee (56.7), below the knee (56.8), Syme's amputation (56.9), and amputating through the foot and toes (56.10).

DIFFICULTIES WITH AMPUTATIONS

If a patient's LIMB IS TRAPPED in a falling building, you may have to amputate it on the spot. Give him ketamine or intravenous morphine (8.6), or infiltrate his tissues with a local anaesthetic. Control bleeding by pressing on the pressure point, or with a tourniquet and then tie the vessels. Cut through his trapped limb with an amputation knife and a saw, as far distally as you can, and apply a firm pressure dressing to the stump. Transfer him to hospital for a formal amputation at the next most suitable site higher up his limb, either immediately, or later.

If a patient is SEVERELY SHOCKED, you can do a quick provisional amputation distal to the site of election. Later, when his wound has healed, you can do a definitive amputation with immediate primary closure. He will no longer be shocked, his skin will be normal, and there will be less danger of infection.

If you amputate in an emergency for shock, or sepsis, or to remove a grossly crushed limb, don't do the final amputation until the stump is healing well.

If his STUMP BLEEDS SOME HOURS AFTER THE OPERA-TION (reactionary haemorrhage), take him back to the theatre, explore his wound, leave his wound open and sew it up secondarily. To prevent this happening: (1) tie the major vessels carefully, (2) release the tourniquet slowly, (3) control the vessels thoroughly, and (4), apply a pressure dressing.

If his STUMP BLEEDS SOME DAYS LATER (secondary haemorrhage), it is likely to be serious. Explore the wound. In desperation, open it, pack it with dry gauze, and remove the gauze 48 hours later.

If his STUMP BECOMES INFECTED, this may have been your fault. Did you: (1) Close the wound by immediate primary suture, when delayed primary suture would have been wiser? (2) Fail to control bleeding, before closing the flaps, so that the blood clot beneath them has become infected? (3) Strip up the periosteum from the stump so that a ring sequestrum has formed and become infected?

If a PERSISTENT SINUS develops in the stump, explore it; you may find a piece of necrotic tendon, or an area of osteomyelitis. Another possibility is a stitch sinus. If the offending stitch might be securing a vessel, don't remove it until you have tied the vessel higher up. Explore the stump, remove all dead and dying tissue, and pack it ready for secondary closure.

If the FLAPS BREAK DOWN, you probably cut them too short and closed them too tight. Wait until the granulation tissue is fit for grafting and then graft it. The final quality of the skin over the stump will be worse than it would have been if the flaps had survived, and it may break down later. Alternatively, you may have to amputate higher up.

If a PATCH OF GANGRENE forms in a flap, be careful, it may hide a larger area of necrosis underneath. You may be able to trim it away, or you may have to amputate again higher up, especially if a patient's limb is ischaemic. If it is not ischaemic, you may be able to excise the gangrenous area, allow granulations to develop, and apply a split skin graft.

If he has GAS GANGRENE, amputate high up, through his shoulder if need be, and leave the wound open.

If a PROSTHESIS CANNOT BE FITTED, you probably designed the stump wrong. The reasons include: (1) bone adherent to the scar, (2) a spicule of bone sticking out through the skin, (3) a flexion contracture in a below knee or above knee amputation, (4) too short a stump.

CUT FLAPS LONG
REFLECT THE DEEP FASCIA WITH THE SKIN
DELAYED PRIMARY CLOSURE IS SAFER

56.2 Guillotine amputations

If you amputate a severely infected limb, the infection may be spread to the stump, especially if you are amputating for gas gangrene. It will be less likely to do so if you: (1) Cut straight down to the bone all round the limb, and then saw the bone through at the same level, (2) leave the surface unsutured, and (3) revise the amputation later if necessary. A guillotine amputation is quick, and the flaps are less likely to necrose if the blood supply is poor. Some surgeons never use them.

GUILLOTINE AMPUTATIONS Apply a tourniquet. Cut the flaps as far distally as you can, so that you can refashion them later. Cut the patient's skin down to his deep fascia all round his limb 2 cm distal to the site of bone section. Let it retract. Then cut the muscle all round his limb down to the same site.

Tie and cut all the large vessels you meet. Cut all major nerves at least 2 cm proximal to the end of the stump. Dress the patient's stump with vaseline gauze and plenty of dry gauze. Bandage it, and let it granulate. When it has healed, or there is no further risk of infection, either: (1) revise the amputation higher up, or (2) graft it, or (3) refer him.

56.3 Amputating for ischaemic gangrene

Deciding where to amputate can be difficult. The lower you amputate, the greater the chance that the patient will walk again afterwards. But there is also more chance that the tissue through which you amputate will not be viable, so that his stump will become infected or gangrenous. Feel his pulses carefully, if you cannot feel his popliteal pulse, do an above knee amputation.

A GUILLOTINE AMPUTATION

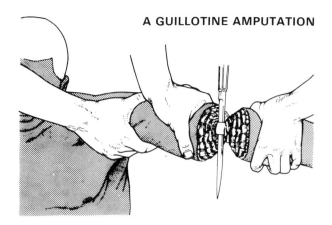

Fig. 56-7 A GUILLOTINE AMPUTATION. A guillotine amputation is quick, and the flaps are less likely to necrose if the blood supply is poor.

If his muscles do not look healthy when you cut them, abandon the operation at that site, and amputate higher up. Healthy muscle is a nice bright red, and has a good capillary ooze. Ischaemic muscle is a dusky bluish red, and bleeds little or not at all. The tissues of a diabetic are at particular risk, including those of his other limb. So handle the flaps with your fingers, not with forceps. Protect his other limb during the operation so as to make sure that pressure sores do not form. Control his diabetes as in A 17.7.

When you amputate for ischaemia, always close the wound by delayed primary closure (54.4).

56.4 Amputating through the upper arm and elbow

Save as much of the length of the patient's arm as you can, because he will probably have no prosthesis. If possible, disarticulate his elbow. If you amputate higher up, a convenient place is 18 to 20 cm below his acromion. If you can leave him with a reasonable length of humerus, he can use it to hold things by gripping them against his chest. If you have to amputate very high up, even a very short stump will preserve the outline of his shoulder. If he is to have a prosthesis, don't amputate through the lower 4 cm of his humerus, because it will be difficult to fit.

Remember that his brachial artery lies quite superficially, and is overlapped medially by his biceps.

AMPUTATING THROUGH THE UPPER ARM

For the general method see Section 56.1. Prepare the operation site, and abduct the patient's arm to about 80° on an arm board. Place a block under his arm just proximal to the amputation site. Apply a tourniquet as high as you can.

THE MID UPPER ARM AS AN AMPUTATION SITE

Start proximally at the site of bone section, and mark out equal anterior and posterior skin flaps. Make the length of each flap ¾ of the diameter of his arm at the site of section.

Find, doubly ligate, and cut his brachial artery and vein just above the site of section. Find, gently pull and cut the major nerves so that their ends retract well above the stump.

Cut the anterior muscles 1.5 cm distal to the site of section. Cut the triceps 4 cm distal to the site of section. Cut the periosteum all round the patient's humerus and saw it through. Rasp the end of his humerus smooth. Bevel his triceps to make a thin flap, reflect it anteriorly over the end

SUPRACONDYLAR AMPUTATION OF THE UPPER ARM

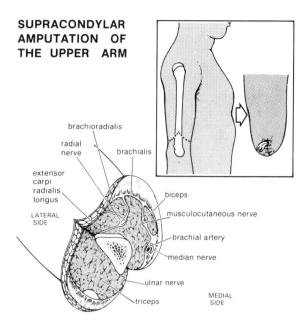

Fig. 56-8 AMPUTATING THROUGH THE UPPER ARM. If you can leave a patient with a reasonable length of humerus, he can use it to hold things by gripping them against his chest. *After Robb and Smith with the kind permission of Graham Stack.*

of his humerus, and sew it to the anterior muscle and fascia. Release the tourniquet, control bleeding, drain and close the stump as usual (56.1).

THE SUPRACONDYLAR REGION AS AN AMPUTATION SITE

Starting proximally at the site of bone section, mark out equal anterior and posterior skin flaps, each as long as 3/4 of the diameter of the patient's arm at the site of section, as in Fig. 56-8. Find, clamp, tie, and cut his brachial artery and vein just proximal to the site of section. Cut his median, ulnar, and radial nerves at a higher level so their ends retract well above the stump.

Cut the muscles in the anterior compartment of his arm 1.5 cm distal to the site of section. Free the insertion of his triceps tendon from his olecranon. Preserve his triceps fascia and muscle as a long flap.

If he has any hope of an elbow prosthesis, reflect this flap proximally and cut the periosteum all round his humerus at least 4 cm above his elbow joint to allow room for the elbow mechanisms of the prosthesis.

If he has no hope of an elbow prosthesis, leave as much bone as you can. Saw across his humerus at the level you choose, and rasp its end smooth. Trim his triceps tendon to make a long flap, carry it across the end of the bone, and sew it to the fascia over the anterior muscles.

Release the tourniquet, control bleeding, drain and close the stump as usual (56.1).

DISARTICULATING THE ELBOW

Make equal anterior and posterior skin flaps. Start at the level of the patient's epicondyles and curve the posterior flap 2.5 cm distal to the tip of his olecranon. Bring the anterior flap just distal to the insertion of his biceps tendon. If necessary make any suitable flap.

Reflect the flaps to the level of his epicondyles. Start on the medial side. Find and divide the lacertus fibrosus. Free the origin of his flexor muscles from his medial epicondyle and reflect it distally to expose the neurovascular bundle on the medial side of his biceps tendon. Tie and cut his brachial artery just above the joint. Gently pull his median nerve and cut it proximally. Find his ulnar nerve in its groove behind his medial epicondyle and cut it proximally in the same way.

Free his biceps tendon from his radius, and his brachialis tendon from the coronoid process of his ulna. Find his radial nerve in the groove between brachialis and brachioradialis, pull it, and cut it proximally.

On the lateral side of his elbow, cut his extensor muscles 6.5 cm distal to the joint, and reflect their origin proximally.

Cut the patient's triceps tendon near the tip of his olecranon. Cut the capsule on the front of the joint, complete the disarticulation, and remove his forearm.

Leave the articular surface of his humerus intact. Reflect his triceps tendon anteriorly and sew it to the tendons of his brachialis and biceps.

Make a thin flap from his extensor muscles, reflect it medially and sew it to the remains of his flexor muscles on his medial epicondyle. Suture the muscle mass to cover the bony prominences and exposed tendons at the end of his humerus. Put sutures through the periosteum when necessary. Close the flaps without tension.

Release the tourniquet, control bleeding, drain and close the stump as usual (56.1).

56.5 Amputating through the lower arm and wrist

Losing a hand is a tragedy. Minimize it by trying to preserve as much of the length of a patient's forearm as you can. An elbow with even a short length of forearm is better than none. If possible, amputate through his metacarpus or wrist, rather than higher up. Ischaemia is an exception. The circulation in the distal forearm, like that of the distal lower leg, is not good. So if his arm is ischaemic, an amputation higher up his forearm may be better than one lower down.

If you have to amputate through his wrist, a plastic surgeon may later be able to make an 'alligator mouth' out of his two forearm bones, so that he has something to grip with (Krukenberg's operation). Anteroposterior flaps are better than lateral ones, because the scar cannot retract between the bones.

AMPUTATING THROUGH THE FOREARM

For the general method see Section 56.1.

AMPUTATING THROUGH THE PROXIMAL FOREARM

Abduct the patient's arm on an arm board or side table, and place it supine. If you cut the flaps with his arm prone, they will later be twisted.

If there is enough good skin, make equal anterior and posterior flaps. If skin is scarce, make the best flaps you can.

Reflect the skin flaps with the deep fascia to the site of section. Tie, and cut his radial and ulnar arteries just above this site. Find his median, ulnar, and radial nerves, pull them gently, and cut them proximally. Cut his muscles transversely distal to the site of section, so that they retract above it. Trim away all excess muscle. Saw his radius and ulna and smooth their cut edges.

Release the tourniquet, control bleeding, drain and close the stump as usual.

Start elbow and shoulder movements as soon as possible.

AMPUTATING THROUGH THE DISTAL FOREARM

Start at the site of section and cut equal anterior and posterior flaps, as in Fig. 56-9. Make them as long as about one half the diameter of the forearm at the amputation site. Reflect the flaps proximally to the site of bone section.

Clamp, tie, and cut his radial and ulnar arteries just proximal to the site of section. Find his radial, ulnar, and median nerves, pull them gently and cut them high up so that they retract above the end of the stump. Saw both bones.

Release the tourniquet, control bleeding, drain and close his stump as usual (56.1).

DISARTICULATING THE WRIST

Make a long palmar and a short dorsal flap. Start the incision 1.5 cm distal to the patient's radial styloid, extend it distally

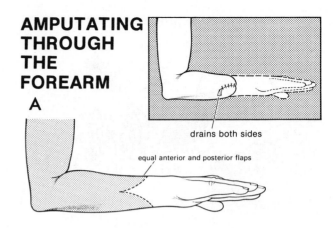

AMPUTATING THROUGH THE FOREARM

A

drains both sides

equal anterior and posterior flaps

B

retract the flaps

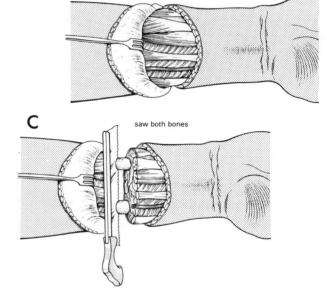

C

saw both bones

Fig. 56-9 AMPUTATING THROUGH THE FOREARM. Preserve as much length as you can. An elbow with even a short length of forearm is better than none. *After Robb and Smith, with the kind permission of Graham Stack.*

towards the base of his first metacarpal. Carry it distally across his palm, and then proximally to end 1.5 cm distal to his ulnar styloid. Make a short dorsal flap by joining the two ends of the palmar incision over the dorsum of his hand. Bring the dorsal flap distally level with the base of his middle metacarpal. If skin is scarce, vary the design of the flaps.

Reflect the flaps proximally with the underlying fascia to his wrist joint. Tie and cut his radial and ulnar arteries just proximal to the joint. Gently draw his median, ulnar, and radial nerves distally into the wound, and cut them short. Cut all tendons just above his wrist and let them to retract into his forearm. Cut round the capsule of his wrist joint and remove his hand.

Saw or nibble off his radial and ulnar styloids. Rasp the raw ends of the bones smooth and round.

CAUTION ! Don't injure his radioulnar joint or its triangular ligament. If you injure them, he will be unable to rotate his forearm, and the joint will be painful.

Release the tourniquet, control bleeding, drain and close the stump as usual (56.1).

AMPUTATING THROUGH THE CARPUS

Make a short dorsal flap and a palmar one twice as long. Reflect the flaps proximally to the site of bone section, and expose the soft tissues under them.

Pull the flexor and extensor tendons of his wrist distally, cut them, and allow them to retract into his forearm. Find the

DISARTICULATING THE WRIST

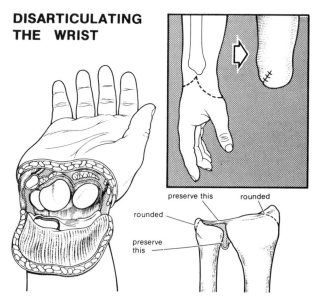

Fig. 56-10 DISARTICULATING THE WRIST. Try to preserve the patient's distal radio–ulnar joint and his triangular ligament. *After Campbell, with kind permission.*

four tendons which flex and extend his wrist (flexor and extensor carpi radialis and ulnaris), free their insertions, and reflect them proximally to the site of bone section.

Find his median and ulnar nerves and the fine filaments of his radial nerve. Pull them distally and cut them well proximal to the site of section. Tie and cut his radial and ulnar arteries proximal to the site of section.

Cut the remaining soft tissues down to bone. Saw across his carpal bones, and rasp all rough edges smooth. Anchor the tendons of his wrist flexors and extensors to his remaining carpal bones in line with their normal insertions.

Release the tourniquet, control bleeding, drain and close the stump as usual (56.1).

AMPUTATING THROUGH THE METACARPUS

Do this as for amputation through the carpus, but preserve what you can of the patient's metacarpals, and especially his thumb.

56.6 Amputating above the knee

Many above knee amputations for severe injuries could have been avoided, if only a below knee amputation had been done early enough, and not delayed. Provided the stump avoids the condyles of a patient's femur, the longer it is the better.

Be sure to exercise the stump immediately after the amputation, so as to strengthen: (1) the patient's remaining adductor muscles, and prevent the prosthesis moving outwards when he walks, and (2) his extensors, because they will have to extend both his hip and the prosthesis which is to form his knee. He will also have to learn to balance with his hip instead of his foot muscles.

Study the anatomy of his leg carefully, so that you can find his subsartorial canal fast, and tie his femoral artery. The canal and its vessels are described in Section 3.6.

AMPUTATING ABOVE THE KNEE

For the general method see Section 56.1. If the amputation is low enough, apply a tourniquet (3.8). Place a sandbag under the patient's buttock on the side to be operated on. Bandage his leg as far as his knee, so as to isolate it from the field of operation.

AMPUTATING ABOVE THE KNEE

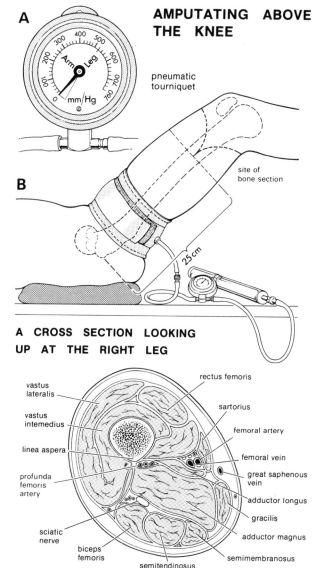

Fig. 56-11 AMPUTATING ABOVE THE KNEE. Provided the stump avoids the condyles of a patient's femur, the longer it is the better.

Prepare his thigh. Raise his leg so that you can prepare his upper thigh and groin. Put a drape behind it and another one in front.

Plan to leave 25 cm of his femur from the tip of his greater trochanter. If possible, make equal anterior and posterior flaps. If necessary, adapt them rather than amputating higher up. Start the anterior flap on the medial side of his thigh just proximal to the site of bone section. Curve it distally over the front of his thigh, to end on the lateral side opposite your starting point as in B, Fig. 56-11. Cut the posterior flap in a similar way. The combined length of the two flaps should be one and a half times the diameter of his thigh at the site of bone section.

Reflect the flaps to the site of section. Deepen the medial end of the anterior flap so as to expose his femoral artery underneath sartorius. Tie and divide his femoral artery and vein (3.6). Use two transfixion sutures for the artery. Begin the incision in his quadriceps along the line of the anterior flap, and bevel it proximally to the site of section, so as to make a muscle flap not more than 1.5 cm thick.

CAUTION ! If you are operating for arterial disease and the muscles do not seem viable (56.3), be prepared to amputate higher up.

Ask your assistant to raise the patient's leg while you cut across and bevel his posterior muscles distal to the site of section, in the same way as his anterior ones, so they retract to it. Trim away any excessively bulky muscle masses.

Find, clamp, and tie his profunda femoris artery on the posterior aspect of his femur adjacent to the linea aspera.

Find his sciatic nerve under his hamstring muscles, separate it from its bed without tension, pull it down, tie and cut it about 5 cm proximal to the end of his femur. Tie the artery that accompanies the sciatic nerve, but not the nerve itself.

CAUTION ! The collateral vessels which accompany his sciatic nerve can bleed profusely.

Cut the periosteum all round his femur and saw it across immediately distal to this cut. Rasp away the prominence of the linea aspera and smooth the end of the bone.

Slowly release the tourniquet, and tie bleeding vessels as they appear.

Sew the anterior muscle flap over the end of the bone. Sew its fascia to the posterior fascia of his thigh. Trim away any excess muscle or fascia. Insert drains deep to this flap.

Cover the stump with a crepe bandage and then apply a plaster cap. This will relieve pain, and its weight will help to prevent a flexion contracture developing.

CAUTION ! Don't let a flexion contracture develop.

PROSTHESES FOR AN ABOVE KNEE AMPUTATION

If the patient is a long time waiting for his prothesis, pad his stump well, make a cast round it and fit it into a sawn off thinned down crutch. Keep it in place with more plaster bandages. This will enable him to walk until his permanent prothesis is ready.

If you have to amputate both a patient's legs above his knees, consider the possibility of getting him short 'stumpy' protheses for both his legs. He may prefer them to a wheel chair, and they will be easier to balance with than prostheses of the standard length. He will however walk closer to the ground, and need two short sticks. 'Stumpy' prostheses are much easier to make, because they don't have jointed knees, and need only be sockets with simple boots on. Keep them in place with cords over his shoulder.

IF THERE IS A DANGER OF SEPSIS, USE DELAYED PRIMARY CLOSURE

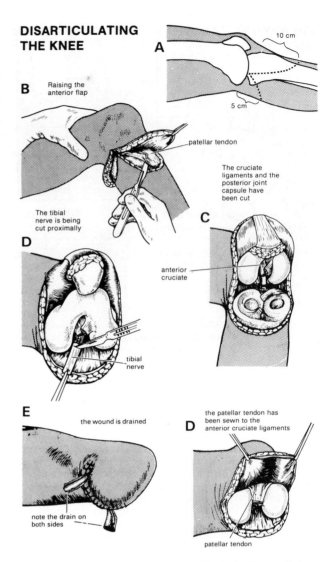

DISARTICULATING THE KNEE

A

10 cm

B Raising the anterior flap

5 cm

patellar tendon

The cruciate ligaments and the posterior joint capsule have been cut

The tibial nerve is being cut proximally

C

D

anterior cruciate

tibial nerve

E the wound is drained

D the patellar tendon has been sewn to the anterior cruciate ligaments

note the drain on both sides

patellar tendon

Fig. 56-12 DISARTICULATING THE KNEE. A, the flaps marked out. B, the flaps being raised. C, cutting the cruciate ligaments and the posterior joint capsule. D, cutting the tibial nerve. E, the patellar tendon sewn to the anterior cruciate ligaments. F, the stump with drains in place. *After Campbell, with kind permission.*

56.7 Disarticulating the knee

Disarticulating the knee: (1) Is one of the easier amputations. (2) Preserves the distal femoral epiphysis of a child, and so allows his stump to grow. (3) Cuts little muscle and no bone, so it is quick, there is little bleeding, and infection is unlikely. (4) Allows the normal weight bearing end of the bone to bear weight in the prosthesis. Although long flaps are necessary to bring the scar posteriorly, there are such excellent anastomoses round the knee that they seldom become gangrenous, so it is a good amputation for ischaemic patients. If you have a choice, disarticulating the knee is better than amputating above it. Good prostheses are now available for disarticulated knees.

DISARTICULATING THE KNEE

For the general method see Section 56.1.

ANAESTHESIA If possible, anaesthetize the patient, and then turn him onto his face, as in 'Primary Anaesthesia' Section 16.12.

METHOD Apply a tourniquet. Cut a long, broad anterior flap, and a shorter posterior one, as in A, Fig. 56-12. Mark these out with his knee flexed.

Start the anterior incision on the posteromedial side of his knee just proximal to the joint line. Extend it 10 cm below his tibial plateau, and then curve it proximally to end at a point just proximal to the joint line on the posterolateral side of his knee.

Start the posterior incision at the origin of the anterior one. Extend it 5 cm distal to the popliteal flexor crease. Then curve it proximally to meet the anterior incision.

CAUTION ! The anterior flap must have an adequate blood supply. If it might not, cut two equal medial and lateral flaps beginning just above the insertion of the patellar tendon.

Dissect the deep structures on the medial side of the patient's knee. Expose the tendons of his medial hamstrings and cut them as far distally as you can.

Find, tie and cut the main trunk of his popliteal artery just distal to its superior genicular branches. These arise high in the popliteal fossa. Tie his popliteal vein. Reflect the posterior flap, cut the fascia, and dissect downwards in the midline between his medial hamstrings on one side and his lateral ones on the other.

Cut the deep fascia along the border of the anterior skin flap. Cut his patellar tendon as close to its insertion into his tibia as you can. Reflect his skin, his fascia, his patellar tendon, and the synovial membranes as a single flap (B).

On the lateral aspect of his knee, expose and divide his biceps tendon and his iliotibial tract.

Find his common peroneal nerve below his biceps tendon, as it goes towards the head of his fibula. Cut it proximally so it retracts above the level of the amputation.

Reflect the short posterior flap and cut his collateral and cruciate ligaments near their attachments to his femur (C). Find his tibial nerve, draw it gently into the wound, and cut it proximally (D).

Dissect the posterior joint capsule from his tibia. Strip the heads of his gastrocnemius from his femur, and remove his leg.

CAUTION ! (1) The popliteal vessels lie very close to the posterior surface of the knee joint. If you have already tied them high up, they should not be in danger. (2) There is no need to disturb the articular cartilage of his femur, or to remove his patella.

Draw his patellar tendon posteriorly through the intercondylar notch of his femur, and sew it to the ends of his hamstring tendons with several interrupted sutures (E).

Stitch his sartorius and his iliotibial tract to the fascial part of his extensor mechanism. Remove the medial and lateral tubercles of the lower end of his femur. Remove the tourniquet, control bleeding, drain and close the stump as usual.

Prepare to fit a permanent prosthesis in 6 to 8 weeks.

56.8 Amputating below the knee

This is the most common amputation. If a patient has a good prothesis, he can do almost anything with it. The method described below, that of Perssen, as modified by Anderssen, uses two short equal medial and lateral flaps, and is especially suitable for leprosy and ischaemia. You can use it for all purposes, except when a guillotine incision would be wiser (56.2).

The best length of stump for a modern prosthesis is 12 to 18 cm below the patient's tibial tuberosity. If he is to have the traditional type of peg leg he needs a shorter 10 cm stump. A stump of only 5 cm too easily slips out of a prosthesis, so that he will be better with an amputation higher up. Don't amputate below the muscle area of his calf, because the tissue here has a poor blood supply.

AMPUTATING BELOW THE KNEE

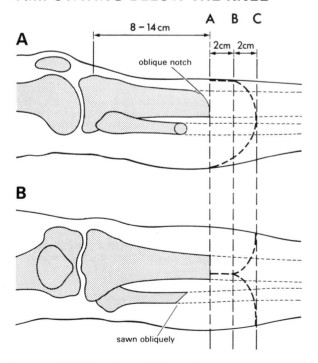

Fig. 56-13 AMPUTATING BELOW THE KNEE using two equal medial and lateral flaps. This is the most common amputation. If a patient has a good prothesis, he can do almost anything with it. *After Perssen and Anderssen.*

AMPUTATING BELOW THE KNEE
For the general method, see Section 56.1.

ANAESTHESIA It is a great help to be able to turn the patient onto his face, so a low subarachnoid anaesthetic (A 7.6) is suitable. If you cannot anaesthetize him lying on his face, bend his knee over the end of the table.

PREPARATION Wash, shave, and paint the operation site. Apply a tourniquet. As soon as he is anaesthetized, raise his leg steeply for a few minutes to drain the blood from it. Then bow up the tourniquet. Wrap his foot securely in a sterile towel.

Mark out the flaps.

Line 'A' is the site of bone section 8 to 14 cm distal to his tibial tubercle, 12 cm is optimal. This is about the length of your index finger, with the base of your second metacarpal on his tibial tubercle.

Line 'B' is 2 cm distal to 'A', and marks the point where the flaps divide anteriorly.

Line 'C' marks the distal extent of the flaps.

If you are not certain of the geometry of the flaps, cut them too long rather than too short.

Cut through the patient's skin, his subcutaneous tissue, and his deep fascia. Cut through the periosteum on the anterior surface of his tibia.

Raise two medial and lateral semicircular flaps to include the skin, subcutaneous tissue, deep fascia and the periosteum on the front of his tibia. Reflect them proximally for 2 cm only.

Divide the underlying muscle at this level, and tie the major vessels as you meet them.

Cut an oblique notch in the front of the tibia, then saw through it at line 'A'. The notch will be easier to make, if you saw it before you saw through the tibia.

Saw through the fibula obliquely 1 to 3 cm higher up.

Raise his leg, remove the tourniquet, find and tie the remaining vessels. Suture the fascia with interrupted monofilament sutures.

Don't try to suture the muscles. They are still attached to the deep fascia, and should fall neatly into place under the sutured layer of deep fascia.

CAUTION ! If there are any of the indications for delayed primary suture, as listed Section 56.1, this would probably be wiser. Otherwise, close his skin with interrupted monofilament sutures. Leave any dog ears.

If you have done a neat job, there should be no dead spaces in which a haematoma can collect. If you are not confident that you have eliminated any dead spaces, insert a drain.

Cover the stump, including the patient's knee, with generous gauze pads, and apply a firm pressure dressing. Mould a thin plaster shell round the stump, including the distal part of his thigh, with his knee fully extended, or apply a backslab. This is an effective way of preventing a flexion contracture.

Day 3. Keep the stump elevated. Start quadriceps exercises.

Day 14. Remove the plaster shell and the sutures. Bind the stump with a tight bandage. Start active knee exercises against resistance.

Day 28. Fit him with his first prosthesis.

CAUTION ! Watch for and prevent a flexion contracture, because it will prevent a prosthesis being fitted. If you are too late to prevent it, the best treatment may be to cut the stump even shorter, to allow the contacture to become even more severe, and then to fit a peg leg.

56.9 Syme's amputation

This is a disarticulation of a patient's ankle, adapted so that the stump can bear his weight. All the bones of his foot are removed, and his malleoli are sawn off, so that the end of his tibia is flat. A large full thickness heel flap is removed subperiosteally from his calcaneus, and brought forward to make a solid covering for the end of his tibia. He can walk about his house on it without a prosthesis or crutches, even though his leg is about 5 cm short. He can also wear a simple and durable elephant boot. His distal tibial epiphysis is preserved, so it is good amputation if he is a child.

This is an excellent amputation if it is well done, but it is also the most difficult of the amputations described here. If you are not skilled, amputating below his knee would be wiser. However, if a Syme's amputation fails, a below knee amputation is always possible.

A patient's posterior tibial vessels run into his foot just behind his medial malleolus. If you cut them too high, they cannot supply his heel flap. So: (1) Shell out his calcaneus from under the periosteum when you dissect the flap. If you can preserve the periosteum a useful piece of new bone will form in it. (2) Cut the vessels as far distally as you can. (3) Be sure to keep the heel flap correctly aligned postoperatively, so that the patient can walk on it.

SYMES AMPUTATION

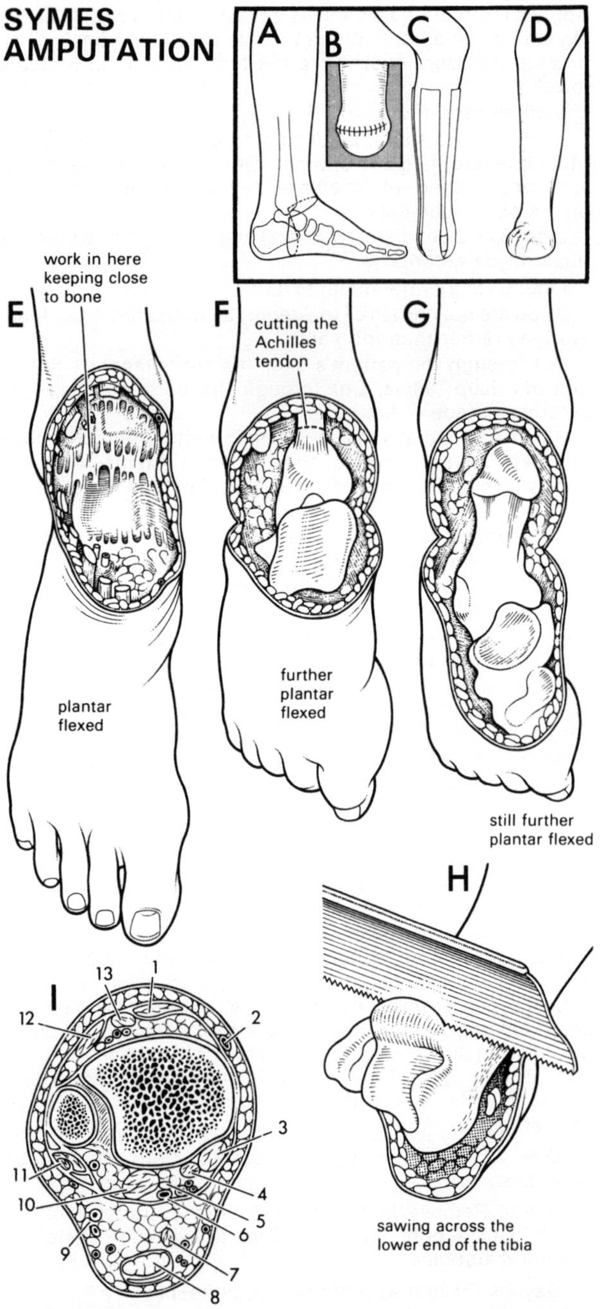

Fig. 56-14 SYME'S AMPUTATION. A shows the incision and B, the completed stump immediately after suture. C, shows how the stump can be held in place with strapping postoperatively. Ultimately, the stump should look like D. E, the patient's ankle joint has been exposed and its ligaments cut. F, his foot has been further plantar flexed and its Achilles tendon is about to be cut. G, extreme flexion allows his calcaneus to be dissected out of its surrounding tissues subperiosteally. H, the lower end of the tibia is being sawn through. I, shows a cross section of his ankle joint with the tibialis anterior tendon (1), the great saphenous vein (2), the tibialis posterior tendon (3), the flexor digitorum longus tendon (4), the tibial nerve (5), the posterior tibial artery and vein (6), the plantaris tendon (7), the Achilles tendon and its overlying bursa (8), the small saphenous vein (9), the flexor hallucis longus tendon (10), the peroneus longus and brevis tendons (11), the extensor digitorum tendon (12), and the tendon of extensor hallucis tongus (13).
After Campbell with kind permission.

SYME'S AMPUTATION

INDICATIONS Lesions confined to the forefoot only, when the operator is fairly skilled.

CONTRAINDICATIONS (1) Arterial disease, unless this is strictly confined to the distal part of the foot. One and preferably both ankle pulses should be present. (2) The need for an elegant prosthesis. A woman is likely to prefer a below knee amputation. (3) Infection. Syme's amputation has a special posterior flap and is not suitable for delayed primary closure. (4) A very inexperienced operator. (5) This is not a good amputation for leprosy.

METHOD For the general method, see Section 56.1. Apply a tourniquet to the patient's thigh (3.8), and let his ankle hang over the end of the table. Stand at the end of it facing his foot.

Mark out the flaps with methylene blue. Hold his ankle at 90°. Start the incision at the distal tip of his lateral malleolus. Bring it over the front of his ankle, level with the distal end of his tibia to a point one finger's breadth inferior to the tip of his medial malleolus. Then, bring the incision under the sole of his foot to the tip of his medial malleobus. Cut all structures down to the bone.

Forcibly plantar flex his foot and cut all anterior structures down to the bone. Put a knife into his ankle joint between his medial malleolus and his talus and cut his deltoid ligament. Do the same on the lateral side and cut his calcaneofibular ligaments.

Put a bone hook posteriorly in his talus to plantar flex his foot even more.

Using a new, sharp scalpel blade, dissect the tissues away from the medial and lateral sides of his talus and calcaneus, *keeping as close to the bone as you can, if possible within the periosteum.* Then cut his calcaneus out of his heel. Work at it from all sides keeping very close to the bones. When you get tired of one approach, start from another. *This is the most difficult and the most critical part of the operation.*

Pull his talus and calcaneus forward with a bone hook. Dissect posteriorly, and cut the posterior capsule of his ankle and his Achilles tendon. Then dissect subperiosteally round the ball of his heel, so as to free his calcaneus and reach the first incision on his sole. As you do so, steadily dislocate his foot downwards more and more, until you reach the distal end of the plantar skin flap and finally free it from his ankle.

CAUTION ! (1) Keep within the periosteum very close to the bone as you dissect his calcaneus out of his heel flap, or you will cut his posterior tibial and peroneal arteries which are very close to the back of the joint capsule. If necessary, remove his calcaneus piece by piece. (2) Don't trim away any muscle or fat in the heel pad, because he needs it to walk on. (3) Keep close to the bone, and don't button hole the heel flap.

Remove his whole foot except for the heel flap.

Dissect the heel flap from his malleoli, and reflect it posteriorly. Saw off his malleoli and the articular cartilage of his tibia in a single cut. Make sure that the ends of his tibia and fibula are accurately horizontal, so that he can bear weight squarely on the stump.

CAUTION ! (1) The cut surfaces of his bones must parallel to the ground when he stands. (2) If you are amputating in a child, don't destroy his distal tibial epiphysis.

Round and smooth all the sharp corners of his tibia and fibula. Cut his medial and lateral plantar nerves proximally.

Pull on any tendons you can see, cut them and let them retract proximally into his leg.

Tie and cut his posterior tibial artery and vein just proximal to the cut distal edge of the heel flap. Tie his anterior tibial artery in the anterior flap.

Using a step incision cut his Achilles tendon about 10 cm proximal to the heel flap. This will prevent the heel stump displacing. If you don't do this, his Achilles tendon is apt to pull up the back of the stump. Cut it high up, or you may injure his posterior tibial vessels.

Release the tourniquet, and control bleeding. Bring his heel flap forward to cover the ends of the bones.

CAUTION ! (1) Don't remove the dog ears, however big. They carry an important share of the flap's blood supply and will disappear later. (2) Prevent the heel pad from tilting out of alignment with the patient's tibia—this is a real disaster! Apply two long U–shaped strips of strapping as in C, Fig. 56-14. Put the first piece on starting below his knee posteriorly, bring it round the flap, and then anteriorly, so as to flex the flap over the stump. Apply the second strip from one side to the other. Keep these strips in place for at least three weeks, and replace them as necessary.

POSTOPERATIVE CARE FOR A SYME'S AMPUTATION

Check the strapping daily, to make sure that the patient's heel pad is centred over his tibia. Adjust it if necessary.

At **2 weeks** reapply the strapping, and put on a well moulded cast round the stump. He should not bear weight yet.

At **6 weeks** take the mould for the prosthesis. By now the stump has usually stuck firmly enough to the tibia to bear weight inside a cast, so apply a new one and let him bear weight on it.

At **10 to 12 weeks** he is ready for his definitive prosthesis, either an elephant boot, or a more sophisticated one.

56.10 Amputating through the foot and toes

This is one of the less useful amputations, its main use is in crush injuries of a patient's toes. Its advantage is that if he fills the front of his shoe with cotton wool, he can walk reasonably well without a prosthesis. Try to preserve as much of his metatarsals as you can. If you cannot preserve them, do a Syme's amputation, or amputate below his knee. If necessary, you can amputate as far back as their bases. Don't try to amputate through his tarsus, because the stump will tilt. If you can preserve his dorsiflexors, he will have a reasonable stump, if you lose them, his foot may go into plantar flexion.

Amputating through·the metatarsals is sometimes indicated in leprosy with very distal ulcers under the heads of the metatarsals. It is a poor amputation for arterial gangrene, which usually needs an amputation below the knee, or even above it.

Amputate toes in the same way as the fingers (75.24). Preserve a patient's big toe, if you can, because it has considerable functional value, particularly in the 'take off' of normal walking. Its most important part is the head of the first metatarsal, so preserve this if you can, even if it does mean cobbling up the remains of an injured foot. The distal phalanx of the big toe matters much less.

Amputating a patient's second toe soon causes severe hallux valgus, but amputating his third, fourth and fifth will cause him little disability.

AMPUTATING THROUGH THE FOOT AND TOES

METATARSAL AMPUTATION

INDICATIONS (1) Crush injuries of the patient's toes. (2) Occasionally, in leprosy when there are large and persistent ulcers due to osteitis. (3) Gross infections presenting late with osteitis.

CONTRAINDICATIONS The risk of failure is considerable if his toes are gangrenous, particularly if he is diabetic.

METHODS For the general method see Section 56.1. Make a long plantar and a short dorsal flap, as in Fig. 56-15. This will bring the suture line dorsally.

Start the dorsal incision at the site of bone section on the anteromedial aspect of the patient's foot. Curve it distally a little to reach the midpoint of the lateral side of his foot. Take the plantar incision distally beyond his metatarsal heads 1 cm proximal to the crease of his toes. The foot is thicker medially, so make the flap slightly longer on the medial than on the lateral side.

Cut the plantar flap to include his subcutaneous fat and a thin bevelled layer of his plantar muscles. Reflect the plantar flap proximally to the site of bone section and then use large bone cutters to divide his metatarsals. Find the nerves and cut them well proximally. Pull the tendons and cut them so that they retract into the stump of his foot.

Release the tourniquet, control bleeding, drain and close the stump as usual (56.1).

AMPUTATING AT THE BASE OF A PROXIMAL PHALANX

The big toe Make a long posteromedial flap. Start the incision at the base of the patient's big toe in the midline dorsally. Curve it distally over the medial side of his toe for a

METATARSAL AMPUTATION

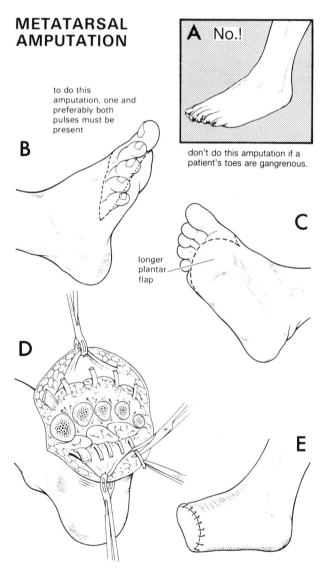

to do this amputation, one and preferably both pulses must be present

B

A No.!

don't do this amputation if a patient's toes are gangrenous.

C

longer plantar flap

D

E

Fig. 56-15 METATARSAL AMPUTATION. This is one of the less useful amputations, its main use is in crush injuries of a patient's toes. *After Rob and Smith with kind permission.*

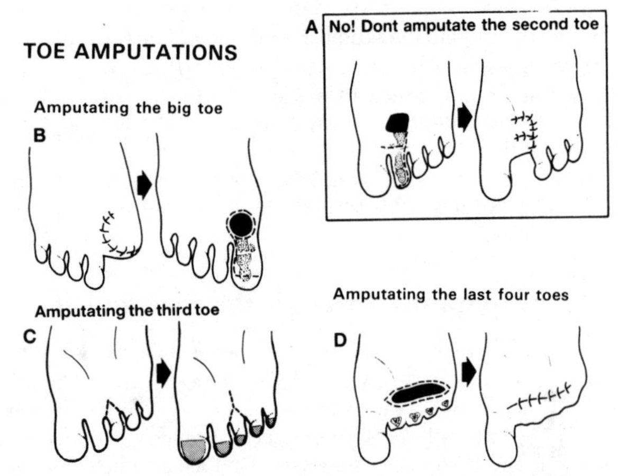

TOE AMPUTATIONS

Amputating the big toe

B

Amputating the third toe

C

A | No! Dont amputate the second toe

Amputating the last four toes

D

Fig. 56-16 TOE AMPUTATIONS. A, avoid amputating the second toe if you can. B, amputating the big toe. C, the incision for amputating the 3rd toe. D, amputating the stumps of the last four toes. *Partly from Techniques Elementaires pour Medecins Isolés, with kind permission.*

distance slightly greater than its dorsoplantar diameter. Then bring it proximally across the plantar surface. Section his flexor and extensor tendons and suture them together over the end of the bone to maintain the position of the sesamoids under the head of his first metatarsal.

Alternatively, some surgeons make a 'V' or a 'Y' on the medial side of the foot.

Second toe. Avoid amputating this.

The remaining toes Make a short dorsal racquet incision, proceed as in the corresponding amputation in the hand.

PLAN FLAPS LONG, YOU CAN ALWAYS SHORTEN THEM LATER

---

57 Skin grafts and flaps

57.1 Different kinds of graft

If a wound or a burn removes the whole thickness of a patient's skin, the natural way for his epidermis to cover it is by growing slowly inwards from the edges. If his wound is less than about 2 cm across, this is usually easy. But if it is larger than this, healing will take a long time. If you cannot bring the skin edges of a wound together by suturing them, you can close his wound in one of these three ways.

(1) You can slice the superficial part of some skin *(a split skin graft)* from another part of the patient's body (the donor area) and lay this on his wound (the recipient site). It will probably 'take' (live). The donor site will heal, because the whole of his epidermis can regenerate from the deeper parts of his sweat glands and hair follicles which you have left behind.

(2) You can take the whole thickness of some skin from another part of his body *(a full thickness graft)* and sew this into his wound. If the skin at the donor site is loose and the graft small, you can usually suture the edges of the donor site together to cover the gap. Or, you can cover it with a split skin graft.

Both split skin and full thickness grafts are completely deprived of their former blood supply. They are free grafts and have to be revascularised from the wound.

(3) You can move the whole thickness of his skin, complete with its blood supply, and sew it over his wound *(flaps and pedicle grafts)*. These are difficult and only the simpler kinds of flap (57.11) which move skin over a small distance are described here. Tubular pedicle flaps, in which the skin is moved widely about the body, are a job for an expert, with the possible exception of a groin flap for the back of the hand (75.27).

Split skin grafts are much the most useful kind of graft: (1) They can cover large areas of the body. (2) They take well. (3) They are easy to cut. (4) They resist infection moderately well, so you can put them on granulations which are not completely sterile. But they do have some disadvantages: (1) When they have healed, they don't look good or resist trauma well. (2) Because the dermis is missing, they shrink. (3) They also give a worse colour match than a full thickness graft. But in spite of all this, split skin grafting is one of the most useful methods in surgery, in the form of either immediate primary grafting (54.2), delayed primary grafting (54.4), or secondary grafting (54.6). *To leave graftable wounds ungrafted is a major surgical disgrace*, because it can do much to reduce suffering and disability.

Full thickness grafts: (1) Produce skin of much better colour and texture. (2) Resist pressure better. (3) Shrink less. But they have some great disadvantages: (1) They can only be small—usually only a few square centimetres. (2) They are a very sensitive to infection. (3) They are more difficult to apply. So they have a useful but much more limited role, mainly on the hands and face. Some surgeons consider that they have no place in a manual like this.

The equipment for cutting split skin grafts is simple—here it is:—

• *KNIFE, skin graft, Humby, modified by Blair and Watson, (a) knife only. (b) Set of 50 spare blades for the above, five sets only.* Sterilize only the knife, the blades are disposable and already sterile. Autoclaving will blunt them.

• *SKIN GRAFT KNIFE, miniature, as developed by H. L. Silver of Toronto, to use ordinary safety razor blades.* The advantage of this is that you can get the blades anywhere, its disadvantage is that it can only cut a narrow strip of skin.

• *RAZOR, for skin grafting, Gillette, modified as in Fig. 57-9, local adaptation, one only.* This modification is not yet made commercially so you will have to make it yourself.

• *HOOKS, skin, single point, Gilles, stainless steel, 200 mm, four only.* These are the least traumatic way of handling skin. They are not essential, and you can use fine dissecting forceps instead.

• *SKIN GRAFT BOARD, teak, with bevelled edge, 6×100×200 mm, two only.* These are rectangular hardwood boards with rounded edges. When you cut a graft, the skin must be held under tension in the line of the cut between two small boards, as in A Fig. 57-5. You can use any conveniently shaped board, or even a wooden spatula.

SKIN GRAFTING EQUIPMENT

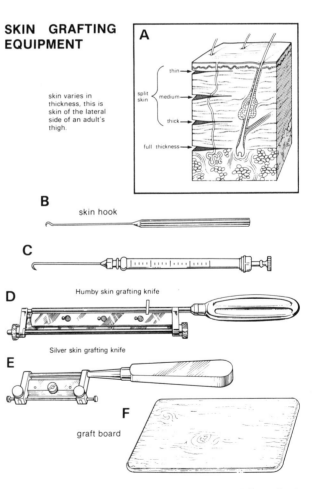

Fig. 57-1 EQUIPMENT FOR SKIN GRAFTING. A, **different kinds of graft. B, a skin hook. C, making a skin hook from a syringe. D, is the standard instrument. E, the advantage of this is that you can get the blades anywhere; its disadvantage is that it can only cut a narrow strip of skin. F, you can use almost any board, or even a spatula.** *With the kind permission of James Smith.*

57.2 Split skin grafting

You can cut split skin grafts thinner or thicker by varying the setting of the knife. A thinner split skin graft: (1) resists infection better, (2) takes more easily, (3) allows the donor area to recover quickly, which is useful if you want to cut a second crop of skin from the same place, and (4) is less likely to cause keloid formation in the donor area. But a thinner split skin graft also: (1) gives a worse colour match, (2) contracts more, (3) wears worse, and (4) is more difficult to sew in place. In practice, being able to vary the thickness of a graft is not important, and a graft of average or even varying thickness is enough for most purposes, except in large burns.

You can cut split skin grafts with many kinds of knife. Here we list the Humby knife as modified by Blair and Watson. This has disposable blades, but if you handle them carefully, you can use them several times. You can also cut skin grafts with an ordinary safety razor blade, a 'cut throat razor', or even with a carving knife (57-10), but they must all be sharp. You cannot cut a graft with a blunt blade.

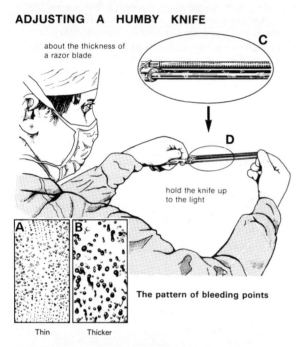

ADJUSTING A HUMBY KNIFE

about the thickness of a razor blade

C

D

hold the knife up to the light

The pattern of bleeding points

A — Thin   B — Thicker

Fig. 57-2 ADJUSTING A HUMBY KNIFE. A, and B, the pattern of bleeding points in the donor area. A, from a thinner graft. B, from a thicker one. C, and D, looking at the gap between the roller and the blade to adjust the thickness of the cut. *Kindly contributed by Ian McGregor and Peter Bewes*

You can apply split skin as: (1) Sheets which cover the wound completely. (2) Sheets which have been cut and expanded to make a mesh graft, as in Fig. 57-6. (3) Patches (stamp grafts). (4) Strips. The wound will only be completely covered if you use sheets of skin. In all other kinds of split skin graft, including mesh grafts, the epidermis has to grow across gaps. This it can easily do, but the cosmetic result will not be so good. So, use sheets if possible, because they give a better cosmetic result, and you can, if necessary, sew them in place.

Patch grafts are: (1) More resistant to infection because the exudate easily drains from under them. (2) Small enough to fit into the concavities of an irregular wound. (3) Easier to take.

But: (1) You cannot expand patch grafts into a mesh. (2) They do not require any less skin. (3) The wound takes longer to heal. (4) They are uglier than single sheet sheet grafts, so they are particularly contraindicated on the face. They are useful if, a wound is very irregular, or there is serious oozing, or infection is not completely controlled. They are very much better than

nothing, but avoid them if you can, and try to improve your technique, so that you can take sheet grafts. Once you can, you will seldom use patches again.

Strip grafts are intermediate in their properties between sheets and patches. One use of strip grafts is to be able to alternate strips of a severely burnt child's own skin, and his mother's skin. Another is in babies where a strip may be the only skin you can get.

IF POSSIBLE, USE SHEET GRAFTS

57.3 Preparing granulation tissue for grafting

Skin grafts may take on any surface that is sufficiently vascular, but they take best on granulation tissue which is in a favourable state for accepting them. This is why it is often best to wait 3 days for granulations to form on a wound, ulcer, or burn before you graft it. Here are the signs which tell you whether granulations will accept a graft or not. If there are several unfavourable signs, prepare the granulations first.

PREPARING GRANULATION TISSUE

FAVOURABLE GRANULATIONS **A graft is more likely to take if:** the granulations are young (48 to 72 hours), firm, flat, rough, bright red and bleed when you touch them; if there is the minimum of discharge which is not purulent; if there are no signs of infection in the skin round the wound; and if active epithelialization is taking place round the edges of the wound which are gently sloping.

UNFAVOURABLE GRANULATIONS **A graft is less likely to take if:** the granulations are old (more that 72 hours), pale and avascular, soft, heaped up above the surface of the wound; if they are thick, slimy, soggy, gelatinous, oedematous, or friable; if they do not bleed readily when you touch them; if there is a purulent discharge; if there is warm, red skin round the wound, or if there is lymphangitis or acute lymphadenitis.

PREPARING GRANULATIONS FOR GRAFTING Always scrape away most of the granulations from the base of a wound, unless they are very thin and are a good colour. This makes little difference to the chance of the graft taking, but much less fibrous tissue will form under it, the cosmetic result will be better and a contracture willl be less likely to form.

If granulations are in a very unfavorable state for grafting, you will have to prepare them first.

If the granulations are pale and avascular, excise and curette them, together with the fibrous base of the wound.

If the granulations are unfavourable in other ways, you can dress them. The important factor is not so much what dressing you put on, but how often you change it.

Apply dressings soaked in: (1) Saline, if possible changed 3 times daily. This is possibly the best. (2) Hypochlorite ('Eusol', or chlorinated lime and boric acid solution BPC). (3) 0.5% acetic acid. (4) Hydrogen peroxide.

LESS ORTHODOX APPLICATIONS FOR INFECTED WOUNDS often work, and may make granulation tissue fit for grafting. You may have nothing else. Scientific explanations can be postulated for some of them, particularly sugar. They include: (1) Mashed fresh papaya (paw paw) applied between layers of gauze. A slough will appear the following day and the skin round the wound will become red. (2) A 'swab and honey' applied honey side down. (3) Honey dripped into the wound (this is said to be useful in bed sores). (4) Sugar. (5) Salt. (6) Fresh placenta. (7) Amniotic membrane. (8) Yoghourt is particularly useful if a wound is very offensive. (9) Plaster of Paris over vaseline gauze or plain gauze.

If you use sugar, open the wound widely, dry it with gauze, completely fill it with granulated sugar, and add more sugar as this becomes diluted.

DON'T GRAFT GRANULATIONS WHICH HAVE RISEN ABOVE THE SKIN

57.4 Why grafts don't take—infection, bleeding, anaemia, and movement

All grafts should take on a wound you have yourself made, such as one for the relief of a contracture. On burns and other potentially infected wounds there are reasons why grafts don't take. The most important one is lack of preparation. So, prepare a wound carefully, so that you have a good chance of success. Besides preparing the granulations by the methods described just above, there are several other important factors. A graft will not take if:—

(1) The wound is more than minimally infected, particularly with *Strep. pyogenes*. This organism secretes an enzyme which destroys the fibrin that sticks the graft to the wound. Suspect that it is present if the growing epithelium at the side of the wound has a sharp edge, instead of a normal gently shelving one. Culture a wound, and if you find *Strep. pyogenes*, treat it first. If you cannot culture it, give the patient penicillin routinely before grafting. *Pseudomonas* infection can also prevent a graft taking. Gentamicin is likely to be the antibiotic of choice.

(2) The wound bleeds as you apply the graft. A little oozing is permissable, and a graft may help to stop it, but it must be thin, and it must be covered by a firm dressing.

(3) The patient is anaemic. If his haemoglobin is less than 6 g/dl transfuse him, or give him iron before grafting.

(4) The graft is separated from the wound. So keep it closely and firmly in contact. Within 20 minutes a layer of fibrin will form and stick it there. Later, capillaries will grow through this fibrin and vascularize it.

(5) The graft is pushed sideways over the wound. For, example it will not take on an actively moving leg.

(6) The graft is stretched too tight, or it lies loose in folds, or it is pressed on too firmly. On a smooth convex surface firm bandages are enough, but on an irregular one use plenty of well fluffed out gauze, cotton wool, or plastic foam, and cover these with a crepe bandage. Don't make the dressing too tight, especially over prominences such as the forehead, because too much pressure will stop it taking.

THE DRESSINGS ARE CRITICAL
DON'T ALLOW A GRAFT TO MOVE DURING BANDAGING OR AFTERWARDS

57.5 The general method for split skin grafting

You can take skin from any of the convex surfaces of a patient's body, but the most convenient places are the fronts of his thighs, each of which can provide a piece of skin 10×20 cm. The skin here is easy to prepare, and easy to dress. If you bend his hip and knee, you can also take skin from the back of his thigh, or from its medial and lateral surfaces, provided your assistant puts his hand behind it, and pushes it forwards so as to make it convex when you cut as in C, Fig. 57-5. You can also use

POSITIONS FOR CUTTING GRAFTS

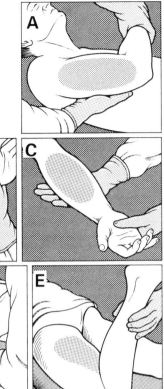

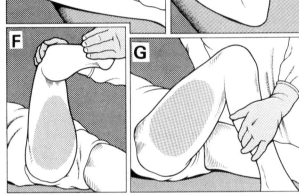

Fig. 57-3 POSITIONS FOR CUTTING GRAFTS. A, the outer side of the arm. B, the inner side of the arm. C, the forearm. D, the inner side of the thigh—usually the best place. E, the back of the thigh with the patient prone. F, the back of the thigh with the patient on his back. G, the outer side of the thigh. *With the kind permission of Ian McGregor.*

the antero—medial surface of his upper arm, which will match his face well. If he is extensively burnt, you may need to take grafts from his buttocks, his calves, his chest, or even his abdomen.

GENERAL METHOD FOR SPLIT SKIN GRAFTING

INDICATIONS (1) Immediate primary grafting, where skin has been lost, or where you can only bring the edges of a patient's wound together under excessive tension. (2) Delayed primary grafting. (3) Secondary grafting. Burns are the major indication.

Variations of these indications include: (1) The complete excision of a small recent deep burn (58.17). (2) All full thickness burns, bigger than 2 cm, usually between the 10th and 18th day. (3) To provide immediate skin cover where tissues lie exposed and nerves and tendons are near the surface. (4) Tropical ulcers (29.1).

Split skin grafts readily take on: (1) Favourable granulation tissue (57.3). (2) Healthy red tissue in a fresh wound. (3) Dermis. (4) Muscle. (5) Any vascular tissue or organ normally covered by aeolar tissue. This includes paratenon, nerves, fascia, and blood vessels. (6) The periosteum. (7) Cancellous bone. (8) The pleura. (9) The peritoneum. (10) The meninges. (11) The gut. (12) The shaft of the penis.

Grafts take less readily on: (1) Fat. (2) Joint capsules. (3) Ligaments.

Grafts fail to take on the following tissues, although they may be able to bridge a small gap: (1) Bare dry white tendon, except in young children. (2) Bare cortical bone. (3) Hyaline cartilage. (4) Open syovial joints.

CONTRAINDICATIONS Besides trying to graft a tissue which won't accept a graft, other contraindications include unfavourable granulations and untreated *Strep. pyogenes* or *Pseudomonas* in the wound.

Relative contraindications include the face. Split skin grafts look ugly here. They are less satisfactory than full thickness grafts, or pinch grafts, over areas which have to bear pressure, such as the heel.

CAUTION ! (1) Don't try to graft a patient while he is anaemic. Raise his haemoglobin above 6 g/dl first. (2) Don't try to graft too large an area at once, or he may bleed to death. 10% of his surface area is the absolute maximum at any one time.

ANTIBIOTICS If you are grafting a burn, especially a large one, give the patient penicillin for 2 days before grafting and 3 days afterwards to control possible streptococcal infection.

PREOPERATIVE PREPARATION Bathe the patient. Shaving the donor site is optional, but always scrub it well with soap and water.

EQUIPMENT A skin grafting knife, two graft boards, liquid paraffin, skin hooks, non–toothed forceps for handling the graft, vaseline gauze, a bowl of sterile saline to put the graft in, sterile cotton wool, and a sterile screw topped jar for storing excess graft.

Find two assistants.

ANAESTHESIA FOR SKIN GRAFTING If you have prepared the patient's wound adequately so that and it does not need scraping, and you are not going to sew the graft in place, you need not anaesthetize it. If possible, use local anaesthesia for the donor area because he is more likely to cooperate. (1) Use plenty of a very dilute local anaesthetic, such as 0.4% lignocaine with adrenaline, to puff out the skin all over the donor site. If you raise it like a plateau, it will be easier to cut. Raise blebs in suitable places and then infiltrate the whole area with a long needle just below the dermis, as in Fig. 57-4. This is the best method of local anaesthesia for the arm. (2) Take skin from his thigh by blocking both his femoral nerve and the lateral cutaneous nerve of his thigh (A 6.22). (3) If you are going to take an extensive graft from several sites, give him a general anaesthesic. (4) You can use ketamine; if you give him diazepam at the end of the operation (A 8.1), he is unlikely to thrash about as he recovers and so disturb the graft.

PREPARING A WOUND FOR GRAFTING

Start by preparing the wound, so it will have stopped bleeding when you come to apply the graft.

Clean the granulations with a saline swab and rub them firmly so that they bleed. Remove all slough, debris, grease, or pieces of vaseline gauze. Unless the granulations are very thin, scrape them with a piece of dry gauze or a wooden tongue depresser, or with a scalpel with the blade held at 90°. Scraping granulations like this will remove the tendency to subsequent fibrosis and contracture.

The wound should bleed well as you prepare it, but bleeding should stop before you apply the graft. So raise the patient's wound and apply warm packs, or dry gauze and a bandage. Don't use diathermy, or catgut. Instead, apply artery forceps to the small bleeders and twist them off.

If you cannot control bleeding by the above methods, apply the graft as a sheet, and see if this stops it. If it does not, mesh it to allow drainage. Or, put the graft back on the

LOCAL ANAESTHESIA FOR SKIN GRAFTING

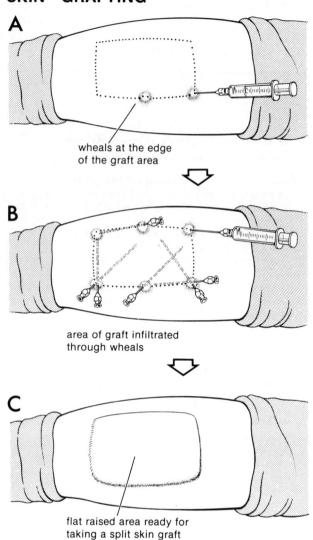

A

wheals at the edge of the graft area

B

area of graft infiltrated through wheals

C

flat raised area ready for taking a split skin graft

Fig. 57-4 LOCAL ANAESTHESIA FOR SPLIT SKIN GRAFTING. Use plenty of a very dilute local anaesthetic, such as 0.4% lignocaine with adrenaline, to puff out the skin all over the donor site. If you raise it like a plateau, it will be easier to cut. *With the kind permission of Peter London.*

donor site, and put dry gauze on the patient's wound. Two days later, under ketamine or light sedation, lift off the graft and reapply it to the wound.

PREPARING THE DONOR SITE FOR GRAFTING

Scrub the donor site with cetrimide and a scrubbing brush, and then swab it with a mild antiseptic, such as cetrimide or hexachlorophane soap. Don't use iodine or spirit, because they may kill the graft. Drape the donor site in towels.

PREPARING TO CUT Place yourself comfortably before starting.

The leg On the patient's right side, and assuming you are right handed, cut from below upwards, with a forehand stroke. On his left side cut from above downwards.

Ask your assistant to support the skin of the patient's thigh from underneath, as in C, Fig. 57-5, so as to make its upper surface flat, and under slight tension from side to side. This will allow you to make a smooth cut with neater edges.

The arm Abduct the patient's arm, and place it on a wide arm rest or table. Ask your assistant to put one of his gloved hands behind it, so as to stretch and flatten the skin on its antero–medial surface. Cut from his shoulder downwards.

SPLIT SKIN GRAFTING

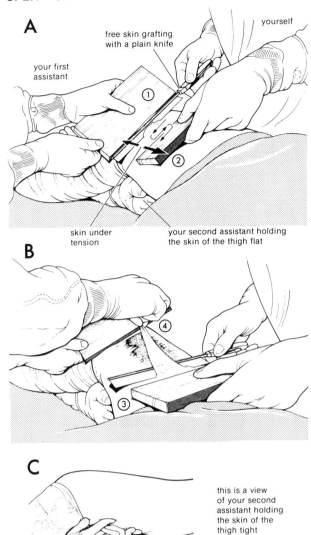

Fig. 57-5 TAKING A SPLIT SKIN GRAFT. This shows the use of two assistants. If you can only find one, ask him to hold the board in one hand and to stretch the skin of the patient's thigh with the other. *Kindly contributed by Peter Bewes.*

Stand inside his abducted right arm, or outside his abducted left arm.

CAUTION ! The skin of the upper arm is thin, so don't cut a full thickness graft by mistake.

The chest If necessary, fill out the skin from between the ribs of a thin patient by injecting his subcutaneous tissues with saline, so as to make a flat surface.

CUTTING THE GRAFT

ADJUSTING A HUMBY KNIFE In this knife the thickness of the skin to be cut is controlled by a rod. The position of this rod is controlled by a screw at one end, and a graduated lock nut at the other. You will have to learn by practice what thickness of graft these calibrations represent. Hold the knife up to the light and vary the distance between the blade and the rod. If you think you could just slip a razor blade between them (a little less than 0.5 mm), it is about right, perhaps a little narrow. Make it too narrow rather than too wide, because if the graft is too thin, you can always thicken it. If the rod touches the blade anywhere they are far too close. Make sure the screws and nuts are tight and the blade is locked.

The blade and the knife are flexible, so the thickness of the graft also depends on how hard you press.

Lubricate the back of the knife with liquid paraffin. Keep it clear of the roller, or it may cause the graft to wind round it.

Ask your assistant to hold one board behind the knife, to keep the board still, and to press on the skin so as to hold it flat and in tension as you move the knife, as in A, Fig. 57-5. Hold the second board in your left hand, cut towards it, and move it closely in front of the knife as you cut (B). Use the second board to keep the skin flattened in front of the advancing knife blade. Advance the board and the blade together along the limb (B). Apply the knife to the skin at a slight angle and use a regular sawing movement as if you were cutting a loaf of bread. Advance it slowly, and press gently. The graft usually collects in folds on the knife. If it does not, ask your assistant to pick its end up. When you get to the end of the graft, either cut it with scissors, or bring the knife to the surface.

CAUTION ! (1) Don't force the knife down the limb. (2) Don't stop or pull the knife backwards. (2) You will be wise to take more graft than you need and store it, so that you can apply it later to areas which do not take.

After you have cut about 1 cm of graft, inspect it for thickness. Assess this by: (1) Tranlucency. A very thin graft is translucent, like tissue paper. Thicker grafts are progressively more opaque. (2) The pattern of bleeding points. A thin graft produces many tiny points, a thicker graft fewer larger ones.

If the graft from a black skinned patient is a thin translucent grey, as it lies on the knife blade, it is the right thickness. If it is white and milky, and curls up vigorously, it is too thick.

If there are large bleeders every few millimetres, you have cut too deep. The donor area should bleed all over from fine bleeding points.

If you can see fat globules, you have cut much too deep, and have taken a full thickness graft. Stitch it back and start again somewhere else. Either to sew up the donor area, or better, to cover it with a very thin split skin graft from another site.

If a large area is to be covered, cut the sheet of skin as wide as possible, and up to 15 cm long. If necessary, cut several sheets. Cut the graft thin so that you can take another crop of skin from the same donor area 10 days later. You may be able to get three or four crops of skin from the back of a patient's thigh, or his buttocks, or the back of his trunk.

Keep the graft covered with saline soaked swabs until you are ready to store or apply it. If there is much delay, replace it temporarily on the donor area.

If you are worried that you may have cut too deep, start again a little way away at the same site. If you realy have cut too deeply, immediately apply a *thin* split skin graft from somewhere else.

CARING FOR THE DONOR SITE AFTER TAKING A GRAFT

The donor site always bleeds, and if it is large, the patient may lose much blood. Minimize this by immediately applying a hot moist pressure pack. Later, when you have applied the graft and dressed it, remove the pack and replace it by plain gauze or vaseline gauze, and a pressure bandage. You now have a choice of 3 methods.

The exposure method saves dressings. At 30 minutes to 48 hours remove the pressure dressing down to the inner layer of gauze. Leave the exposed area to dry and form a crust. The inner layer of gauze will separate with the crust at 10 days. Or, apply no gauze and dry the wound with a hair drier.

The occlusive method. Pad the wound *generously* to prevent blood soaking through, and bandage it, preferably with an elastic bandage. At 7 to 10 days remove the dressings.

The 'Op – site' method. 'Op – site' is an expensive self adhesive plastic sheet, permeable to water vapour but not to bacteria. It is the ideal way of caring for the donor area.

If the dressings have stuck to the donor site, leave them in place. If you tear them off, the wound will be very slow to heal.

If the donor site becomes infected, treat it like any other superficial wound with frequent cleaning and changes of dressings.

MESHING A SPLIT SKIN GRAFT

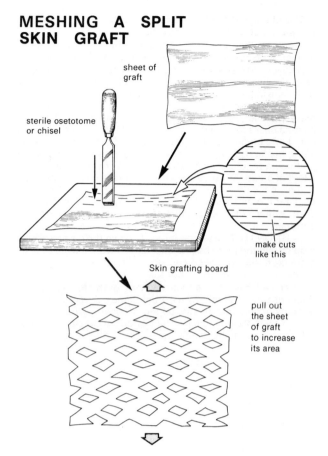

Fig. 57-6 MAKING A MESH GRAFT. Meshing a graft increases the area it can cover and helps it to take better. Use mesh grafts for extensive burns and difficult grafting problems. *Kindly contributed by Peter Bewes.*

APPLYING THE GRAFT

Drape the graft over the wound with forceps. If it curls up, lay a piece of vaseline gauze on one of the boards, and put the graft on it, *raw surface up.* The graft will stick to the vaseline gauze, which will stop it rolling up, and enable you to cut and handle it more easily.

CAUTION ! Be sure you apply the graft the right way up. The under side is shiny, the dull side must be on top as the graft lies on the wound.

SINGLE SHEET GRAFTS Always pierce some holes in the graft, so that the wound can drain through it. Trim it to shape. If you have to use several pieces of graft, lay them edge to edge, and let them overlap the edges of the wound a little. Make sure that they fit snugly to the bottom of any irregular areas, and do not bridge any concavities.

If the sheets of graft cross a joint, make sure that the joint between them (where a scar may form), goes *across a limb not along it*—this is CRITICALLY important.

Sewing a single sheet graft in place is optional. Some surgeons almost always sew grafts in place, and some almost never do. Sewing is particularly useful in the eyelids, the palmar surface of the fingers, the axilla, and the popliteal fossa. These are the places where a graft so easily slips. Use small curved needles and fine silk sutures. Insert the needle from within the graft outwards, as in B, Fig. 57-8.

If you see any blood clots under the graft, remove them. Wash them away from under it with saline, a syringe and a blunt needle. If some clots still remain, pull them out with non-toothed dissecting forceps. Immediately apply pressure to control further bleeding.

MESH GRAFTS are useful on rough surfaces. Don't use them on exposed areas, such as the face. Mesh a graft as in Fig. 57-6. Flatten it out on a piece of wood and use a No. 10 or

APPLYING AND REMOVING A DRESSING

One kind of dressing for a graft

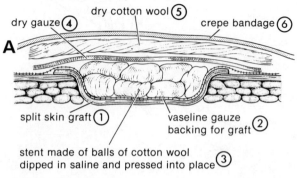

Removing a dressing

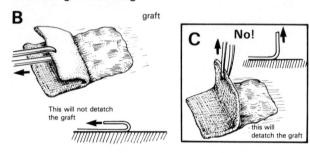

Fig. 57-7 APPLYING AND REMOVING A DRESSING. A, applying the dressing. The first layer is the graft itself (1), sticking to its backing of vaseline gauze (2). The vaseline gauze, but not the graft itself should come well beyond the edges of the wound. The next layer is the stent (3) which moulds the graft to the concavity of the wound. Make it by fluffing out some balls of cotton wool. Dip them into a bowl of saline, and while they are still dripping wet press them gently into place over the graft. They will mould themselves to any concavities in the graft. Make sure that the bandages applied subsequently can exert even pressure. Next apply a single layer of dry gauze (4), and let it overlap the edges of the wound. Then apply some dry cotton wool (5), and hold it in place with a crepe bandage (6). In children some turns of plaster bandage may be useful.

B, removing a dressing in the right way, so as not to pull newly adherent graft away from the surface. C, removing it in the wrong way, like this, may strip it from the surface. *A, with the kind permission of Peter London. B, from Yang Chich-chun with kind permission.*

15 blade, or an osteotome, to make the holes. If necessary, the bridges of skin making the mesh can be very narrow indeed.

STRIPS OR PATCH GRAFTS Take the whole of the graft, stick it on pieces of vaseline gauze, raw surface upwards, and cut this into strips, or patches the size of a small postage stamp. Apply these to the wound.

DRESSINGS FOR SPLIT SKIN GRAFTS

These are absolutely critical—it is the movement of a graft over its bed which stops it taking. There are several alternatives, and little agreement as to which is best.

THE FIRST METHOD is shown in Fig. 57-7 and uses a stent of cotton wool balls soaked in saline to keep the graft in place.

THE SECOND METHOD applies 5 mm of dry gauze between layers (2) and (3) of the first method in Fig. 57-7. It omits layer (4), and covers layer (5) with a single layer of gauze extending widely beyond the wound and stuck to the skin around it with tincture of benzoin.

THE THIRD METHOD applies vaseline gauze to the graft, followed by plenty of dry gauze and a bandage.

THE TIEOVER METHOD

(for split skin and full thickness grafts)

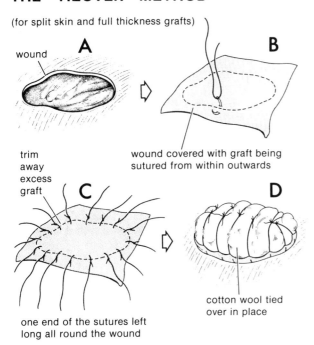

Fig. 57-8 THE TIEOVER METHOD is a useful way of dressing a graft that has been sewn in place. Use it for a patient's eyelids, his axilla, and for small intricate grafts, such as those over the tips of his fingers.
Kindly contributed by Peter Bewes.

THE FOURTH OR TIEOVER METHOD is very effective in difficult situations where a graft has been sewn in place. Use it as in A, Fig. 57-8, for a patient's eyelids, his axilla and for small intricate grafts, such as those over the tips of his fingers, and underneath his chin.

Stitch the graft in place all round the defect (B), but leave one end of each suture loose (C). Finally put a ball of moist cotton wool on the graft, and tie the loose ends of the sutures over it (D). The wool will keep the graft firmly applied to the wound.

POSTOPERATIVE CARE FOR SKIN GRAFTS

If a joint as to be grafted, a plaster cylinder over the dressings is very useful.

If a flexure has to be grafted, the position in which the patient's limb rests is critical, so see Figure 58-16, on the prevention of contractures in burns.

If a flexure does not have to be grafted, the position of the limb is not critical. Put a grafted arm in a sling, and put a grafted leg to bed and raise it.

CAUTION ! The graft must not move over its bed. This may be difficult to prevent. If necessary, you may have to strap a child to a frame, or apply a cast.

Leave the dressing on for 5 to 7 days unless there is some good reason for looking at it. Do the first dressing yourself, so that you can inspect your handiwork. At first remove only the superficial layers. Leave the layer of vaseline gauze which was used to spread the split skin. Remove this later when the graft is firmly adherent.

CAUTION ! Make sure your nurses remove any dressings with the greatest possible care, as in B, Fig. 57-7, or they may strip away the graft with the gauze. If necessary, soak the gauze away with saline. (2) Use vaseline gauze for the first dressing only. If you use it repeatedly, granulomas may form.

If there are any granulating areas, clean them with saline. If they are more than 1 cm in diameter, regraft them with stored skin (57.8).

If blisters appear, incise them, or aspirate them with a syringe.

If the donor or recipient areas are so painful and itchy that the patient scracthes them, sedate him, dress them, and consider applying a cast.

Start active joint movements a week after grafting. After 2 weeks you can usually remove all dressings.

57.6 The exposure method for dressing a graft

This method is well suited to warm countries, especially if dressings are scarce. There is no pressure on the capillaries under the graft. It is cooler, has a lower metabolic demand, and so is more likely to live. You can also observe a graft and express fluid from underneath it more easily. If possible, apply the graft while a patient is conscious, because success depends absolutely on his cooperation. He is much more likely to cooperate if you use local anaesthesia, and carefully explain everything to him. He is least likely to cooperate as he thrashes about while he is recovering from a general anaesthetic or ketamine. This is an excellent method for the caring surgeon applying a critical graft, *but it needs excellent nursing care:* (1) To make sure the patient does not absent—mindedly scratch away the graft when he is drowsy or confused, and (2) to swab away the exudate from under the graft 2 hourly.

THE EXPOSURE METHOD FOR SKIN GRAFTS

INDICATIONS (1) A very cooperative patient. (2) Small areas that can be grafted under local anaesthesia. (3) Large flat areas such as those on a patient's trunk. (4) Areas such as his perineum where applying a pressure dressing is difficult. (5) Chronic wounds such as varicose ulcers and leprosy ulcers where the underlying bed is poor. (6) Delayed primary grafting and secondary grafting.

CONDTRAINDICATIONS (1) An uncooperative patient. (2) Poor nursing.

METHOD Explain to the patient exactly what you are going to do. Take the graft as usual. If he is under general anaesthesia or ketamine, take the graft, store it and apply it in the ward later. If you are using local anaesthesia, apply the graft directly.

Try to control bleeding perfectly.

If bleeding is perfectly controlled, apply the graft immediately. The tissues underneath it will keep it moist. It may not need to be fixed. If it is thick, fix it with strips of adhesive paper.

If bleeding is not perfectly controlled, wait 24 to 48 hours before applying the graft to allow bleeding to stop completely. A nurse may be able to apply the stored graft.

Put a few sutures round its edges. Make sure there are no blood clots under it. You may be able to syringe out the underside of the graft until bleeding has stopped.

Keep the grafted part still and don't allow the patient to touch it. If flies are a problem, put him under a mosquito net or in a gauze cage.

Look at the graft after 4 hours, and lightly express any blood or serum from under it with a piece of sterile gauze or forceps. If necessary, repeat the syringing. Repeat this in the evening, and then daily until the graft has taken.

At 48 hours the graft should have stuck to its bed, so you can allow moderate movement. Leave it undisturbed for 7 days. If pus appears, dress it.

CAUTION ! (1) Regular gentle swabbing is absolutely essential. (2) Don't allow the graft to become dependent for at least 10 days.

57.7 Grafting with open knife or a razor

An expert can cut a skin graft with any very sharp knife and a block of wood to keep the skin tense, so can many auxiliaries. The best knife is an ordinary carbon steel carving knife, not a

GRAFTING WITH A MODIFIED SAFETY RAZOR

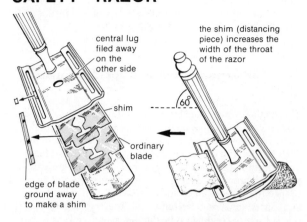

Fig. 57-9 CUTTING GRAFTS WITH A MODIFIED SAFETY RAZOR. File away the central lug. Make a shim (distancing piece) by grinding away the edges of an old blade. *Kindly contributed by Peter Bewes.*

stainless steel one, carefully sharpened. Take your knife to a barber, ask him to show you how to sharpen it. You will need two stones, a medium and a very fine one, and a strop. Sharpening the knife may take you an hour to begin with, but keeping it sharp subsequently only takes a moment. Keep the blade oiled.

GRAFTING WITH AN OPEN KNIFE Soak the knife in cetrimide for 30 minutes. Ask your assistant to kneel beside the patient, and to cradle the skin of the patient's thigh in his hands as in C, Fig. 57-5, to stretch it slightly, and to keep it flat.

Lay the knife on the patient's skin at about 5 to 15°. Steady the skin in front of it with a wooden block or tongue depressor. Then with short to and fro movements, move the knife forwards, and adjust the cutting angle as necessary.

57.8 Storing grafts

If necessary, you can store a graft in an ordinary refrigerator. Stick its upper surface to vaseline gauze. Roll it in gauze moistened with saline, with its raw moist surfaces together. Keep vaseline away from these surfaces, or it will prevent the graft taking. Put the roll in a sterile screw capped bottle labelled with the patient's name. No anaesthetic is needed to apply it, so you can do this in the ward. Unroll the bundle, cut the vaseline gauze to the required size, and lay the graft on his wound. The sooner

GRAFTING WITH A CARVING KNIFE

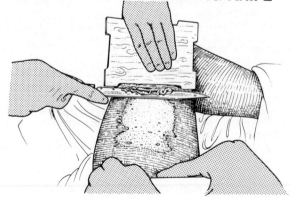

Fig. 57-10 CUTTING A SPLIT SKIN GRAFT WITH AN OPEN KNIFE. The best knife is an ordinary carbon steel carving knife, not a stainless steel one, carefully sharpened. *Kindly contributed by Peter Bewes.*

you apply it the better. You will be wise to discard grafts after eight days, although they may keep for 2 or 3 weeks.

If you take more graft than you need, you can also store it by putting it back on the donor site. If you use it within four days, you can usually lift it off again without cutting. Wise surgeons always take more graft than they need, so that, later, they can regraft any areas in which a graft has failed to take on the first occasion.

If you don't use a graft on the patient from which it came, you can use it to provide temporary cover as a homograft on other patients.

57.9 Pinch grafts

These are little pieces of skin nipped off the donor area and put on a wound. The centre of a pinch graft is full thickness skin, but its circumference is epidermis only, so a pinch graft is a combination of a full thickness and a split skin graft. Pinch grafts are easy to cut, they resist infection well, and because they contain some full thickness skin, they resist pressure better than a split skin graft; this makes them useful on the heel, or over the Achilles tendon. Pinch grafts have the disadvantage of making the donor site look ugly, unless you: (1) Make it look decorative and resemble tribial scarring. If so, explain that the graft will leave a scar and ask the patient what pattern he would like. (2) Excise the whole donor area in a strip of skin, as in H, Fig. 57-11.

GRAFTING WITH A RAZOR BLADE

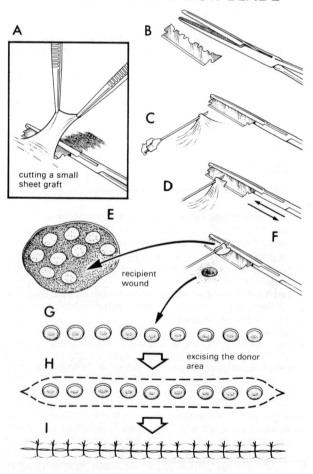

Fig. 57-11 GRAFTING WITH A RAZOR BLADE. A, shows how you can cut a narrow sheet graft with half the blade of a safety razor. B, to I, shows the stages in a pinch graft, including the excision of the donor area. *Kindly contributed by Peter Bewes.*

Because pinch grafts are so easy to take, and need so little equipment, they are particularly useful in health centres. Experienced surgeons rarely use them. Unless it is important for a graft to wear well, split skin is better.

PINCH GRAFTING

INDICATIONS (1) Pressure areas, such as a patient's heel or his Achilles tendon. (2) Health centre practice.

EQUIPMENT Local anaesthetic equipment (A 5.4). An intramuscular needle, a razor blade, and a pair of long straight artery forceps or a scalpel.

METHOD Pick up the skin in a needle and slice off a 4 to 5 mm piece of skin. Lay it on the granulating area. Go on until the area is mostly covered.

Alternatively, cut the pinch grafts in one long strip from the patient's thigh, then excise the whole perforated strip and suture its edges. This will greatly improve the appearance of donor area.

Cover the pinch grafts with a sheet of vaseline gauze, and then apply dressings and a bandage as above.

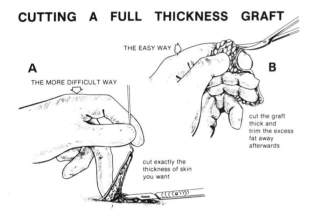

Fig. 57-12 CUTTING A FULL THICKNESS GRAFT. To begin with you may find it easier to cut the graft thickly, and then trim away any excess fat from underneath it afterwards like this. *With the kind permission of Peter London.*

57.10 Full thickness skin grafts

These are now only used for covering areas where the cosmetic appearance is important (a patient's face) or where trauma must be resisted (the palm of his hand). Even on the hand a thick split skin graft may be as good, besides being much easier. For wounds and burns, full thickness grafting is always a secondary procedure after the defect in his skin has already been closed, and when the risk of sepsis is minimal. *A full thickness graft will only take if it lies in the closest contact with the tissues underneath it, on a sterile vascular bed in which all bleeding has been controlled.* For all these reasons they are of very limited application under the circumstances for which this book is written (1.1).

Cut a full thickness graft through the fibrous layer of a patient's dermis, so that there is no fat on its under surface which will prevent it taking. This needs skill. To begin with you may find it is easier to cut the graft thickly, and then trim away any excess fat from underneath it afterwards as in B, Fig. 57-12. For an elegant result, sew it into place with the finest atraumatic sutures you have.

You can take skin from: (1) Behind a patient's ear. His skin here is hairless, and will match his face well. If you take skin from either side of his post auricular groove, it can provide a piece up to 4 cm in diameter. (2) His supraclavicular region. (3) His antecubital fossa. (4) His groin. Skin from his thigh will make a poor full thickness graft.

TAKING A FULL THICKNESS SKIN GRAFT FROM BEHIND THE EAR

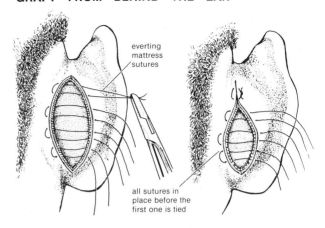

Fig. 57-13 TAKING SKIN FROM BEHIND THE EAR. You can also take a full thickness skin graft from a patient's supraclavicular region, his antecubital fossae, or his groins. *With the kind permission of Peter London.*

If a patient brings you the tip of his amputated finger or toe, you may be able to use this to make a full thickness graft. Carefully cut out the subcutaneous tissue from the interior of his finger tip, until you reach the right layer of the dermis for a full thickness graft, then sew it over the exposed stump. If you graft it complete with its pulp, it won't take.

FULL THICKNESS GRAFTS

INDICATIONS (1) A patient's face. (2) The palms of his hands; thick split skin grafts here are at least as good.

CONTRAINDICATIONS (1) Infection. (2) Granulating surfaces. (3) A bed of dense avascular scar tissue. (4) Any very irregular surface.

EQUIPMENT A fine sharp scalpel, small sharp curved scissors, aluminum foil, a sterile mapping pen and marking ink, if possible 4/0 or 5/0 atraumatic monofilament sutures.

ANAESTHESIA Use local anaesthesia if you can.

RECIPIENT SITE Excise all scar tissue. Control bleeding completely without using diathermy, or leaving any catgut or other suture material in the wound.

CUTTING THE GRAFT FROM THE DONOR SITE

Cut out the exact pattern of the defect in sterile aluminium foil, paper, or jaconet, place it on the donor site, and outline it in marking ink with a mapping pen or with scratch marks. Include orientation marks to make sure you get it the right way round. Include the graft in an ellipse, and remove the complete ellipse, so that you can close the wound more easily.

Incise the inked outline with a sharp knife. Cut only as deep as the thickness of his skin. You can remove it in either of the following two ways. The first is the easiest.

FIRST METHOD Cut the graft without trying to avoid the subcutaneous fat. Lie its raw surface upwards over the index finger of your left hand as in B, Fig. 57-12. Use small curved scissors to cut away any yellow fat until you get to clean white dermis.

Suture the donor area. If necessary, undermine its edges so that you can close it without tension.

SECOND METHOD Separate the graft through the fibrous layer of the dermis. Hold it with a skin hook to prevent it rolling up. Don't cut into the subcutaneous layer, and don't buttonhole it.

CAUTION ! Handle the graft with utmost care. Don't tear it with skin hooks, and use forceps as little as possible.

TAKING SKIN FROM ABOVE THE CLAVICLE

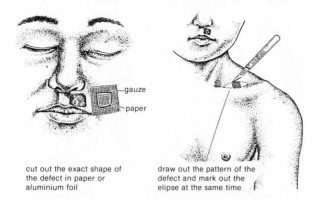

cut out the exact shape of the defect in paper or aluminium foil

draw out the pattern of the defect and mark out the ellipse at the same time

Fig. 57-14 TAKING SKIN FROM ABOVE THE CLAVICLE. Handle the graft with utmost care. Don't tear it with skin hooks, and use forceps as little as possible. *With the kind permission of Peter London.*

PARTICULAR DONOR SITES FOR FULL THICKNESS GRAFTS

Behind the ear Block the patient's greater auricular nerve (A 6.6). Sew up the skin with everting mattress sutures, as in Fig. 57-13. Put them all in place, then tie the first one under direct vision and the others blind, as his ear is pulled backwards. Alternatively, use a running subcuticular stitch. If sewing his ear back is difficult, cover the gap with a partial thickness graft from somewhere else, or bandage back his ear, and let the wound granulate.

SUTURING THE GRAFT IN PLACE

Lay the graft on the defect and sew it without tension to the margins of the wound using interrupted sutures of fine monofilament. If possible leave one end of each suture 10 cm long so that you can use the tieover method as in Fig. 57-8. An accurate edge to edge fit is essential. Sew from within outwards. Put your needle first into the graft and then into the dermis around the wound. This stretches the graft slightly and anchors it more firmly.

CAUTION ! (1) The graft must be firmly in contact with the wound over its whole area. (2) Don't insert a drain underneath it or it will slough.

Cover the graft with a layer of vaseline gauze, place a pad of saline soaked cotton wool, a dental roll, or a piece of plastic sponge on the wound. Tie the long ends of the sutures over it.

A SLIDING FLAP

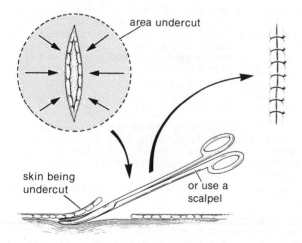

area undercut

skin being undercut

or use a scalpel

Fig. 57-15 A SLIDING FLAP. If you undercut the skin at the edges of a wound, you may be able to slide the skin edges across to cover it. *Kindly contributed by Peter Bewes.*

POSTOPERATIVE CARE Leave the graft for a week, then change the dressings, and remove alternate stitches. Remove the others a few days later.

If the graft fails to take: (1) The bed in which it lies may not have been sufficiently vascular. (2) You may have handled the graft roughly. (3) Blood clots may have formed underneath it. (4) It may have become infected. (5) You may have applied too much pressure.

57.11 Some of the simpler flaps

If you cannot bring the skin edges of a patient's wound together, an alternative to grafting it is to use a local skin flap which will wear better and look nicer than a graft. Flaps, even local flaps, are not as easy as split skin grafts, and are *for the careful, caring operator who: (1) is unable to refer patients who need them, and (2) has enough time to plan and do them well.*

Severe contractures (as from burns), or defects in important areas (such as the head and neck), or pressure sores in paraplegics, are often best managed by a myocutaneous flap. This is a single stage procedure in which a muscle and its overlying skin are moved to fill in the defect. For example, pectoralis major can be used on the face, or biceps femoris for a trochanteric ulcer. These methods are not described here so you will have to refer patients who need them. The most complex flap described here is the groin flap for the back of the hand (75.27).

Local flaps combine the principles of sliding, rotation, and transposition with a little ingenious geometry. The great danger in any flap is that its arterial and venous supply will not be adequate, so that it breaks down—venous obstruction easily kills a flap. *As a general rule, never make any flap longer than its base—the 1:1 ratio.*

(1) A sliding flap may be possible if a patient's skin is fairly elastic. If it is, you may be able to undercut the edges of his wound and slide the skin over it, as in Figures 57-15 and 54-6. This is easier on some parts of the body than on others, for example, it is be easier on the back of the hand than on its front.

(2) A rotation flap requires that you make the defect into a triangle, and then swing the skin around. It has to rotate on a pivot point, the radius of the arc of rotation being the line of the greatest tension, as in Fig. 57-16. You can only use rotation flaps on skin which has a good blood supply. They are particularly useful on the scalp, as in Figs. 63-13 and 63-15, but are unsuitable below the knee where the blood supply is poor. You can easily overestimate the elasticity of the skin, so make a rotation flap three times bigger than you think will be necessary.

MAKE A ROTATION FLAP THREE TIMES BIGGER THAN YOU THINK IS NECESSARY

A ROTATION FLAP

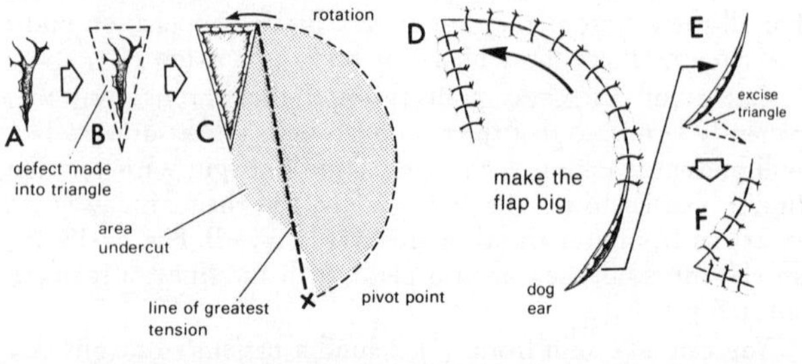

Fig 57-16 A ROTATION FLAP. The secret with this flap is to make it big. A, the wound. B, the wound excised. C, the position of the flap marked out, with the line of greatest tension and the area to be undercut. D, the flap rotated, unfortunately leaving a dog ear. E, and F, a triangle of skin excised to remove the dog ear.

TRANSPOSITON FLAPS

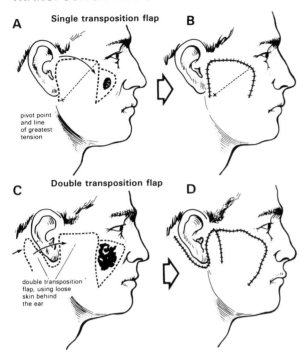

Single transposition flap

A   B

pivot point
and line
of greatest
tension

Double transposition flap

C   D

double transposition
flap, using loose
skin behind
the ear

Fig. 57-17 TRANSPOSITION FLAPS can have a single pedicle as in A, and B, or a double one as in C, and D. They are only for 'the careful, caring operator'. *With the kind permission of James Smith.*

(3) **A transposition flap** is made by moving a rectangle or square of skin and subcutaneous tissue on a pivot point to cover an immediately adjacent defect, as in Fig. 57-17. Make sure the end of the flap extends beyond the defect, as in this figure, and plan it carefully before you cut.

TWO MORE METHODS

A single pedicle advancement flap

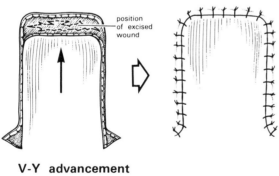

position
of excised
wound

V-Y advancement

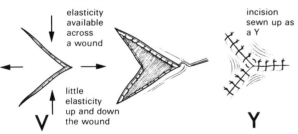

elasticity
available
across
a wound

incision
sewn up as
a Y

little
elasticity
up and down
the wound

V   Y

Fig. 57-18 TWO MORE METHODS. A V–Y procedure has many uses. Wherever you have a V–shaped incision, consider whether it might be better sewn up as a Y.

(4) **A single pedicle advancement flap** is done by moving skin as in Fig. 57-18. Excise the triangles as shown to equalize the length of the flaps and the adjacent wound edge.

(5) **A double pedicle advancement flap** requires an incision parallel to the long axis of the defect. Undermine the skin between the incision and defect, and advance the skin to cover it, as in Fig. 57-19.

(6) **A V–Y advancement** is useful if there is plenty of elasticity available across an incision, and you want elasticity up and down it. Do it by sewing up a V–shaped incision as a Y. Abundant elasticity across a wound is unusual, and even if it is present, it only provides a moderate amount of extra skin down the length of an incision. So don't overestimate what you can do.

SKIN FLAPS

GENERAL METHOD

PLANNING will be easier if you make a cloth pattern first, and use it to carry out the procedure of the actual operation in the reverse order, as in Fig. 57-20.

Sterilize an ordinary ink pen, and some ordinary ink or Bonney's blue. Draw on the patient's skin after you have prepared it for surgery. Transfer the pattern of the defect to a piece of cloth, preferably jaconet. Make sure you cut the pattern to include the base of the flap. Make it a little larger and wider than you think will be necessary. Try the pattern again, making sure that each time you move it you hold the base in a fixed position, without moving it with the flap. The final flap must be larger than is necessary, particularly in its length. You can easily trim a flap which is too large, but you cannot lengthen one which is too small.

DOUBLE PEDICLE ADVANCEMENT FLAPS

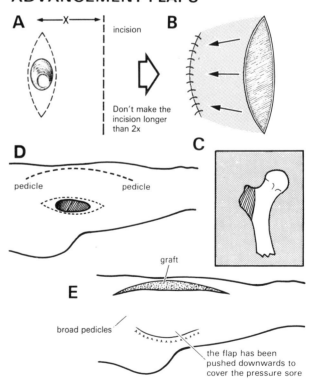

A   B

incision

Don't make the
incision longer
than 2x

D   C

pedicle   pedicle

graft

E

broad pedicles

the flap has been
pushed downwards to
cover the pressure sore

Fig. 57-19 A DOUBLE PEDICLE ADVANCEMENT FLAP. A, and B, show the principle of this flap. C, D, and E, show how it has been used to cover a pressure sore over the greater trochanter, part of which has been excised. Make the pedicles broad, and don't be tempted to use this flap on the skin of the face or the lower leg. *With the kind permission of James Smith.*

Undercut the flaps in the layers shown in Figure 54-6. You must leave some fat under the patient's skin, *if you undermine his skin alone, the flap will certainly break down.*

CAUTION ! (1) Make clean incisions with a sharp knife at right angles to the surface. (2) Handle *all* flaps with the greatest care, especially at the angles. Pick them up with skin hooks, or a silk stay suture. Don't use thumb forceps. (3) Cut the angles as bluntly as you can, preferably at less than 45°. (4) Use fine needles and sutures. (5) Make sure that a flap is not kinked, rotated, stressed or pressed on, and that there is no haematoma underneath it.

If bare areas remain when you have completed a flap, cover them with split skin grafts.

Leave the flap open in the early stages, so that you can inspect it and test its vascularity.

POSTOPERATIVE CARE Ask the nurses to roll a flap from its edge towards its base to evacuate static venous blood from it and free blood from underneath it.

PARTICULAR FLAPS

ROTATION FLAPS

INDICATIONS Large defects, especially triangular ones, if there is sufficient space to raise a large enough flap, especially on a patient's scalp, buttocks, thighs, or trunk.

CONTRAINDICATIONS (1) Parts of the body where a patient's skin is tight, or his circulation is poor, as in his hand and below his knee. (2) Don't make a rotation flap over bone (other than the skull) or over tendon.

PLANNING A TRANSPOSITION FLAP

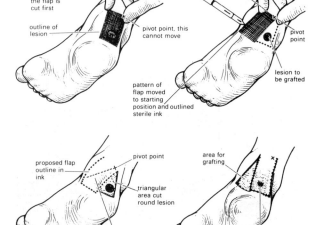

a cloth pattern of the flap is cut first

outline of lesion

pivot point, this cannot move

base of pattern held fixed

pivot point

lesion to be grafted

pattern of flap moved to starting position and outlined sterile ink

proposed flap outline in ink

pivot point

triangular area cut round lesion

line of greatest tension

area for grafting

flap sewn in place

Fig. 57-20 PLANNING A TRANSPOSITION FLAP. In the example here a lesion over the patient's heel has been excised and a flap moved across to cover it. The area where the flap has come from is larger and will have to be grafted, but it is no longer over a pressure area. Don't take skin from the ball of his heel—it is very specialized. The same method is applicable whenever you move skin from one place to another. *With the kind permission of James Smith.*

METHOD If possible, plan the flap so that its base is proximal. Give it as wide a base as possible so as to make sure it has an adequate blood supply and will not necrose.

CAUTION ! Don't let its base exceed its length.

Excise the defect cleanly to form a triangle as in Fig. 57-16. Extend the side of the triangle in a curved incision 4 to 5 times its length. Undermine the flap widely and twist it so as to distribute the tension in a wide area along the suture line.

If you cannot get the flap to rotate sufficiently, make a small right angled cut at the end of the curved line.

If a dog ear forms, don't excise it immediately, because this may compromise the blood supply to the flap. Leave it, and if necessary, excise it later. Or, cut a small triangle and sew it up as in E, and F. If there is a gap, close it with a split skin graft, or let it granulate.

DOUBLE PEDICLE ADVANCEMENT FLAPS

Make an incision parallel to the wound and some way away from it, so as to make a flap not more than twice the length of its base. Dissect the flap and the fat free and displace it as required. Close the secondary defect with a skin graft.

CAUTION ! (1) Don't make these on the lower leg, and particularly not on the shin, because the blood supply here is inadequate. (2) Don't exceed the 1:1 length to breadth ratio.

57.12 W−plasties

This is the only purely cosmetic procedure described here. You can camouflage a linear scar by cutting triangles of skin out of the edges of the incision and sewing it up as a series of Ws. This will not give you any added length in the direction of the scar, so it is of no use in releasing contractures, for which you may be able to use the Z−plasty described in Section 58.26.

W-PLASTY Remove the scar along with 1 cm equilateral triangles of skin on either side of it. If you make them bigger, they will be too conspicuous. Plan them with a pattern, and make sure they fit together.

CAUTION ! Plan the triangles carefully, and make the same number each side.

W-PLASTY

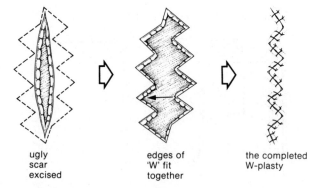

ugly scar excised

edges of 'W' fit together

the completed W-plasty

Fig. 57-21 A W-PLASTY is a cosmetic procedure which will make a scar less obvious. Use a pattern, and make sure that the triangles fit neatly together.

58 Burns

58.1 Caring for a severe burn

In many of the hospitals for which we write the problem of burns is a straightforward one—neglect, by both doctors and nurses! Burns may fill a third of your surgical beds. They are dirty, smelly cases, time consuming to treat properly and demoralizing for the patients, who are often full of complaints. It is so easy to pass a patient by with the thought, or the statement—'Just another burn!' So be sure to take a great interest in the detailed care of burns, and encourage the nurses to do so too. Although the emphasis of the early parts of this chapter is on the resuscitation of severe burns, they will only be a minority of your patients.

You should be able to: (1) Prevent infection turning a partial thickness burn into a full thickness one. This mostly means the correct early treatment. (2) Minimize the severity of all contractures, and prevent many of them completely. The important step is to graft full thickness burns early, usually between the 10th and 18th day. By doing this you will prevent a patient, especially a child, being unnecessarily disabled by what may be only a small burn. Tragedies, like those in Figure 58-1 are completely unnecessary. (3) Release and graft some of the contractures that you have not been able to prevent. If you have done your best to prevent contractures in the early stages, those that you will later need to release should not be too severe. Many

of the contractures that are still common in the developing world are the result of neglected early treatment, and would be the despair of plastic surgeons in the industrial world. (4) Prevent all deaths from shock in the first 48 hours, except in the most extensive burns. (5) Save the lives of most adults with 30 to 40% burns, and of most children with burns of 20 to 25%.

THE GENERAL METHOD FOR A SEVERE BURN

Only an occasional patient will require the full regime described here. Most patients have lesser burns.

IMMEDIATE FIRST AID Pouring cold water on a burn immediately after the accident, or putting a burnt limb in water during the first few seconds, cools the patient's burnt tissue. It relieves his pain and can prevent superficial burns becoming deep, especially when the agent is hot fluid like porridge or syrup.

Cover the burn with the cleanest thing available, such as a recently washed sheet. Don't apply any ointments or local remedies.

PRIORITIES IN CARING FOR BURNS If a patient's eyelids or hands are burnt, make saving his sight and the use of his hands your priorities.

THE FIRST 24 HOURS AFTER A BURN

ADMISSION The indications for admission include: (1) All patients liable to shock (that is all burns over 10%). (2) Any patient who has burnt his face, eyes, hands, feet or perineum, whatever the size of his burn. ALWAYS admit a child with a burnt hand. (3) All patients who have inhaled smoke. If possible, refer all these patients.

SECURE THE PATIENT'S AIRWAY This is the first priority if a patient has burnt his face or inhaled smoke—see Section 58.27. Only do a tracheostomy if it is absolutely necessary and intubation fails (52.1). But, if it is necessary, do one. Asphyxia will kill a patient quicker than hypovolaemia or infection.

If his breathing is noisy, his airway is obstructed. Hoarseness and stridor occur late in the shock stage and are important signs of impending airway obstruction.

If there is a contracting eschar round his neck, you may have to do a tracheostomy to remove the obstruction and an escharotomy to relieve the constriction.

If his face is swollen, suspect oedema and obstruction of his nasopharynx.

If his respiratory tract might be burnt, look for burnt nasal vibrissae, soot in his nostrils, and burns on his tongue, oral mucosa, palate, and pharynx. Is there any soot in his sputum?

WHEN WAS THE PATIENT BURNT? Record the exact time of the burn—*time your fluid replacement plan from that moment and not from the time of admission.*

HOW WAS HE BURNT? Question his relatives, or the ambulance men carefully. They will have been to the scene of the accident.

A NEGLECTED BURN

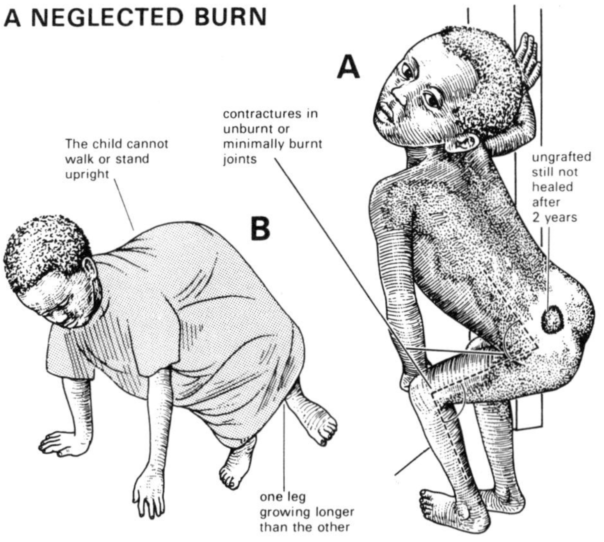

Fig. 58-1 THE FOCUS OF THIS CHAPTER is on the treatment of less severe burns like this one. Pepita was thrown into a fire by another child two years previously and received an 8% burn of her lower back, which was at first thought to be superficial, but is still open and has never been grafted. She cannot stand upright (A) because she has flexion contractures of both hips and one knee. Instead, she has to crawl (B). Her groins were not burnt, and the burn on her knee was only a minor one. Her contractures are the result of failing to make sure that she used her unburnt and minimally burnt limbs during the acute stage of her injury. She has now been abandoned by her family. Early grafting and elementary physiotherapy would have prevented this tragedy.

SET UP A GOOD DRIP Do this for all burns over 15% in adults and 10% in children under 3 years, taking careful aseptic precautions. Start with Ringer's lactate, or 0.9% saline—NOT 5% dextrose! Look for a good arm vein, and if necessary cut through burnt skin. If possible use the veins in a patient's forearm and avoid his long saphenous vein at his ankle. This vein usually goes into spasm, and is a bad one to use in shocked patients. If you can leave it intact, it may be very useful later.

Put in as big a cannula as you can, and fix it firmly. The best way to keep a drip running is to make sure it never stops. If the blood enters the cannula and clots there, his lifeline has gone. So make sure that nobody turns off the drip while waiting for a fresh bottle.

As you put the cannula in, take blood for a haematocrit (or haemoglobin), and for grouping and cross matching.

MORPHINE AFTER A SEVERE BURN If a patient has been severely burnt, pain may not be very marked after 2 hours, especially if the surface of his burn has been cooled. He will often present later than this.

If he is restless, but not in great pain, he needs fluids, not morphine.

If he is in severe pain, and has not inhaled smoke, give him *intravenous* morphine in the doses advised in section A 8.7.

If there is any danger that he has burnt his lungs, avoid morphine and other opioids.

When you give morphine, give a small dilute dose intravenously slowly over several minutes. Observe his respiration and his relief from pain. Give him as much morphine as he needs and no more. You may be able to give it through a small vein on the back of his hand. It is most urgently needed in shallow burns and fatal ones.

WEIGH HIM If this is impractical, guess his weight. Weigh him at least once a week subsequently.

IF NECESSARY (58.4), CATHETERIZE THE PATIENT'S BLADDER. Pass an indwelling catheter. Use a small self–retaining catheter, empty his bladder, and start to measure his urine, every hour on the hour. Keep early urine specimens to compare with later ones. If he develops haemoglobinuria, you will know if this is getting worse or not. Start a fluid balance chart (A 15.5).

Try to measure the volume of urine actually produced by his kidneys during the previous hour. The urine bag should be small and it must have a short tube (not more than 10 cm), or urine will accumulate and make measurements inaccurate. If this is impractical, particularly in a child, collect it in a bed-pan or urine bottle and measure it 4 hourly.

HOW BIG AND HOW DEEP IS HIS BURN? Use the chart in Fig. 58-4, or the rule of nines or sevens (58.3). For small or scattered burns, estimate how many times the area of his hand (1%) would fit on his burn. Draw the burn on a photocopy of Fig. 58-4, and sketch in the areas of each depth (58.9).

HOW MUCH FLUID AFTER A SEVERE BURN?
Calculate this from the formula in Fig. 58-5 as discussed in Section 58.4. Decide how much intravenous fluid to give him during the next hour and write down the appropriate infusion rate. If he has a burn of over 30%, he needs some of his fluid requirement as colloids, such as dextran or plasma, so prescribe them (58.7).

If he is thirsty and wants to drink, let him do so.

TETANUS PROPHYLAYIS Give all burns patients tetanus tox-oid (54.11).

OTHER MEASURES If a patient's burn is large, give him penicillin for five days to prevent streptococcal infection (57.3) and assist in the prevention of tetanus. Prescribe the necessary sedatives.

If he has lost blood from other injuries, make as good an estimate as you can of this, based on Fig. 53-3. If possible measure his central venous pressure (A 19.2). Transfuse him as necessary and keep it between 4 and 8 cm of water. It must not exceed 15 cm.

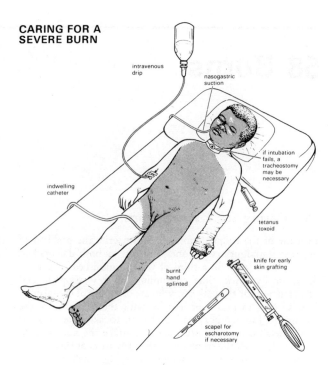

CARING FOR A SEVERE BURN

intravenous drip

nasogastric suction

indwelling catheter

if intubation fails, a tracheostomy may be necessary

tetanus toxoid

knife for early skin grafting

burnt hand splinted

scapel for escharotomy if necessary

Fig. 58-2 THE SECRETS OF SUCCESS in treating a severely burnt patient include :(1) A drip for early rapid transfusion. (2) A catheter for monitoring his urine output. (3) A knife for grafting his skin. The fourth secret, unbounded enthusiasm and commitment, is not shown. Many hospitals have everything else, but because nobody really cares, their patients die. If a fifth were to be added, it would be blood for transfusing him. A patient may also need nasogastric suction, tracheostomy, and escharotomy. If he is admitted late, he needs tetanus toxoid. *With the kind permission of James Smith.*

LOOK FOR OTHER INJURIES Look especially for fractures of his pelvis (76.1), ribs (65.1), and spine (64.1). These are often missed.

LOOK FOR OTHER DISEASES Especially in children who are often burnt partly because they are ill and fretful with some other disease, such as diarrhoea or an upper respiratory infection.

CAUTION ! Don't apply splints, dressings, or casts too tightly over burnt tissue, because it is going to swell. Wait until the swelling has gone down.

Burns over a fracture may be an indication for traction rather than for an external splint.

ESCHAROTOMY If this is necessary (58.18), it will be necessary immediately.

X-RAYS If a patient might have inhaled smoke, X-ray his lungs.

NURSING A SEVERE BURN
Place the patient on a clean sheet under which is a layer of plastic to prevent the mattress being soiled. If possible don't let him lie on the burn. Keep the bed clothes off him with a cradle.

If he is conscious, lie him supine or prone (depending on the site of the burn) and raise his legs or the foot of his bed. Don't give him a pillow or let him sit up until shock is over.

If he is unconscious, lie him on his side, head down in the recovery position (51-2).

CAUTION ! Wash your hands before and after touching him. If possible use sterile disposable gloves. Try to make sure the nurses do so too.

Keep him mobilized as much as you can. If his burns are extensive, move him to different positions every two hours to prevent chest complications, bed sores, thrombosis, and embolism.

NASOGASTRIC TUBE If a patient's burn is very severe, or he is nauseated or vomits, or his abdomen is distended and his bowel sounds are scanty, pass a nasogastric tube. He may inhale his vomit at any time, particularly if he is weak or semiconscious. Intravenous chlorpromazine, 0.5 mg/kg 6 hourly, may ease his nausea.

MAKE A PLAN FOR HIM Where appropriate, tell the patient and his relatives what you expect to happen and when. Record it in his notes.

AFTER THE FIRST 8-HOUR PERIOD AND AFTER EACH SUBSEQUENT 8 HOUR PERIOD

Reassess the patient after the first hour and at the end of each of the 8 hour periods in Fig. 58-5. Is his urine volume adequate? Did he get the fluid he should have had during the previous eight hours? Give clear instructions to the nurses for the next 8 hours. For example, "If he will not drink, give. . ., If his urine volume is less than X ml for two hours or more, do. . ." etc.

NEXT DAY AFTER A SEVERE BURN

Reassess the extent of the patient's burn. Areas which showed only erythema yesterday may have blisters today and need to be included in the area of partial thickness skin loss.

LATER, WATCH FOR THE COMPLICATIONS OF BURNS

Anuria and oliguria are serious complications. Check the urine collected from the patient's catheter (58.10).

Haemoglobinuria is common in burns and contributes to renal failure.

Pulmonary oedema is due to too much fluid, perhaps combined with lung damage, so reduce the infusion rate; give him frusemide and perhaps steroids.

Anaemia Watch for this and treat it as necessaary (58.10).

Contractures and joint stiffness Anticipate the places where contractures will form and nurse him in the positions which will prevent them, as in Fig. 58-16. Splint his joints appropriately, and mobilize them as soon as the skin over them has healed (58.24). Keep burnt hands in a plastic bag (58.29) and encourage full movements from the start.

THE FURTHER MANAGMENT OF A SEVERE BURN

Read on—to learn about prevention and physiology (58.2), to measure the extent of a patient's burn (58.3), to assess his fluid needs during shock (58.4), the kind of fluid he needs (58.5), whether you should allow him to drink or not (58.6), his need for colloids or blood (58.7), resuscitating him if he was admitted late (58.8), his fluid needs when shock is over (58.9), problems with fluid and blood replacment (58.10), feeding him (58.11), assessing the depth of his burn (58.12), choosing a method to treat his burn (58.13), the exposure method (58.14), the occlusive dressing method (58.15), the saline method (58.16), early excision of a burn (58.17), sloughs and eschars (58.18), grafting (58.19), preventing infection (58.20), antibiotics (58.21), topical agents (58.22), treating an infected burn (58.23), preventing contractures (58.24), relieving broad contractures (58.25), relieving narrow contractures with a Z–plasty (58.26), burnt lungs (58.27), burnt eyes (58.28), burnt hands and feet (58.29), burnt face and ears (58.30), burns of the trunk (58.31), burnt bones and joints (58.32).

**THE FIRST DAY AFTER A SEVERE BURN IS CRITICAL
EXAMINE THE PATIENT OFTEN**

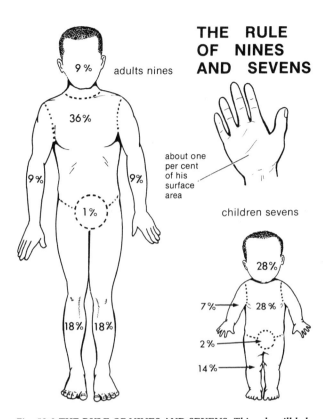

Fig. 58-3 THE RULE OF NINES AND SEVENS. This rule will help you to remember how to calculate the surface area of a burn. An adult's head and each of his arms makes up 9% of his surface area. His legs each make up 18% (2×9). In a child the unit is 7%, but his proportionally larger head makes up 28%.

tion would prevent many burns, so would the improved control of epilepsy.

The skin is the largest structure in the body. It isolates a patient's inside from his outside, chemically, thermally, mechanically, and biologically. A burn destroys these functions, so that treatment is mainly an attempt to restore them. A severe burn is a three dimensional rather than a two dimensional lesion. It opens up a huge surface through which the body loses water, electrolytes, proteins, and heat, and across which bacteria and drugs can enter. The immediate result of a burn is severe shock which lasts about 48 hours. This is followed by a period of 2 or 3 weeks during which the slough over a deep burn separates, allowing you to graft it. During this period sepsis is the major problem.

The *area* of a burn determines the volume of fluid lost and the volume you must give a patient in the first few hours to replace it and prevent shock. The *depth* of his burn determines how you should treat it, and especially if you need to graft it. Its *position* determines how you should nurse him and especially how you should prevent contractures. Between them the area, depth, and position of a patient's burn determine what will happen to him.

AREA, DEPTH AND POSITION DETERMINE THE OUTCOME OF A BURN

58.2 Prevention and physiology

Many burnt patients are children who have pulled cooking pots over themselves, or fallen into the fire. Most are poor, and many are malnourished. Some are epileptics who have fallen into the fire during a fit. An increasing number come from factories where safety precautions are not observed. Enforcing such precau-

58.3 What percentage of a patient's body surface has been burnt?

The proportions of parts of the body differ in adults and children. Estimate them with the chart in Fig. 58-4, which is also included as a 'tear out page' at the end of the book. This table is difficult to remember, so memorize the rule of nines in adults and the rule of sevens in children, in Fig. 58-3. Remember that the area of a patient's hand (not yours!) is about 1% of the total area of his body. When you calculate the area of a burn, don't include the area of erythema in a white skin (it is not visible in a black one). Blisters may not appear for 24 hours, so revise your estimate if more appear after you have first examined a patient. Burns are easily underestimated in a black skin, and over–estimated in a white one.

There is an upper limit to the severity of a burn above which a patient is almost sure to die, and if he does live his life will only be a burden to him. In anything but the most sophisticated burns units a patient with a burn of 60% or more is so unlikely to live that compassionate palliation may be the only logical treatment for him. Morphine and a drip to prevent him suffering thirst will make his last days more comfortable. Scarce facilities are probably better kept for patients with a greater chance of life.

58.4 How much fluid does a shocked patient need?

A patient loses much fluid into tissues which have been burnt, but not actually killed—*most of it is lost during the first 8 hours.* He loses more fluid this way than by evaporation from the surface of his burns, or into blisters. The loss of this fluid sends him into shock and raises his haematocrit. At the same time he also loses water and electrolytes in his urine, and water through his lungs and his normal skin. *Treat him by replacing all this fluid.*

Severe injuries, as from a road accident, for example, cause shock immediately, but the shock following a burn develops more slowly. Half an hour after a severe burn a patient may look suprisingly well, but four hours later he will be deeply shocked. Try to prevent this and resuscitate him *before he becomes shocked.* If you delay, he may die.

A BURN CHART

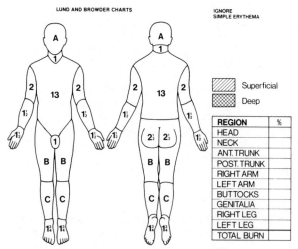

Fig. 58-4 A BURNS CHART is a more accurate way of estimating the area of a burn. It is reproduced again on one of the end papers, so that you can photocopy it and sketch in a patient's burns. *After Lund and Browder.*

A FORMULA FOR FLUIDS

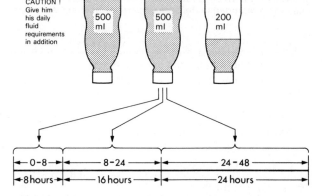

Weight in kg × area of burn = ml of fluid
Give this volume of fluid in each of these time periods

Example

A 60 kg man with a 20 per cent burn needs 60 × 20 = 1200 ml of fluid in each time period

Fig. 58-5 A FORMULA FOR TREATING SHOCK IN BURNS. Give a patient his daily fluid requirements in addition to this. Calculate these from Scale E in the next figure.

A burn of over 15% in an adult, or 10% in a child, causes shock. Burns of this severity always need a drip, lesser ones may do, especially in children. Besides childhood, old age, malnutrition, and anaemia can also reduce a patient's ability to withstand a burn and increase his liability to shock.

Many formulae are used. Although some centres use plasma and colloids, there is no evidence that a patient does better. They are expensive, so only crystalloids are described here. *Give an adult 1 ml of fluid for each 1% of his body burnt, for each kilo of his weight.* Thus a 60-kg man with a 20% burn needs 60 × 1 × 20 = 1,200 ml of fluid. *Give a child under six years twice as much. Give him 2 ml of fluid for each 1% of his body surface burnt for each kilo of his weight.* Thus a 6-kg child with a 20% burn needs 6 × 2 × 20 = 240 ml of fluid. Both adults and children need these volumes of fluid once in the first eight hours following the burn, once in the next 16 hours, and once again in the following 24 hours.

This formula is designed for use with Ringer's lactate or 0.9% saline, or if necessary Darrow's solution, and is more generous than those designed for use with colloids.

After 48 hours you can usually take a patient's drip down, but only provided that his urine output is satisfactory and he is drinking well. There is a danger of overhydration if fluids are continued unnecessarily after 48 hours.

Calculate a patient's fluid needs from the time of the burn, *not* from the time of admission. If admission is delayed, you will need to give the fluid correspondingly faster (58.8).

CALCULATE A PATIENT'S FLUID NEEDS FROM THE MOMENT OF THE BURN

The formula above accounts only for the fluid loss from the burn itself, *and not for a patient's ordinary daily fluid requirements (metabolic water needs),* which vary with his size and the ambient temperature and are given in Scale E Fig. 58-6. So give him this volume of fluid in addition to the fluid you give him to treat the shock his burns have caused. Give him his daily fluid requirements (metabolic water needs) as 5% dextrose intravenously, or as water by mouth, as in the next section.

IMMEDIATE FLUID REPLACEMENT IN BURNS

DOES THE PATIENT NEED A CATHETER? All patients with burns of over 30% need a catheter to measure their urine output. Patients with burns of less than 10% never do. Patients with burns of between 10% and 30% only need one if their urinary output is poor. A patient also needs a catheter if his perineum has been burnt. Catheters have their risks, so observe this intermediate group of patients carefuly. It is tragic for a patient with a minor burn to die later from a urinary infection.

IS HE GETTING ENOUGH FLUID? A patient's urine flow is the most reliable indication as to whether you have treated his shock adequately or not. But: (1) His bladder must be empty before collection starts. (2) The formula is a rough guide only, so adjust it according to how he responds. Watch his jugular venous pressure, and listen to the bases of his lungs. Adjust the rate of infusion and the volume of fluid you give him like this:—

If he is already shocked, give the initial transfusion fast over 10 or 15 minutes. A severely shocked patient may have lost a third of his blood volume, so be prepared to give him up to a third of his blood volume fast. You will need to know what his blood volume is, so consult Scale C, in Fig. 58-6. Thus a child with a blood volume of a litre may need up to 330 ml of fluid. As soon as he starts to recover, slow the drip.

If treatment starts late, give more fluid than the formula indicates.

A PHYSIOLOGICAL NOMOGRAM

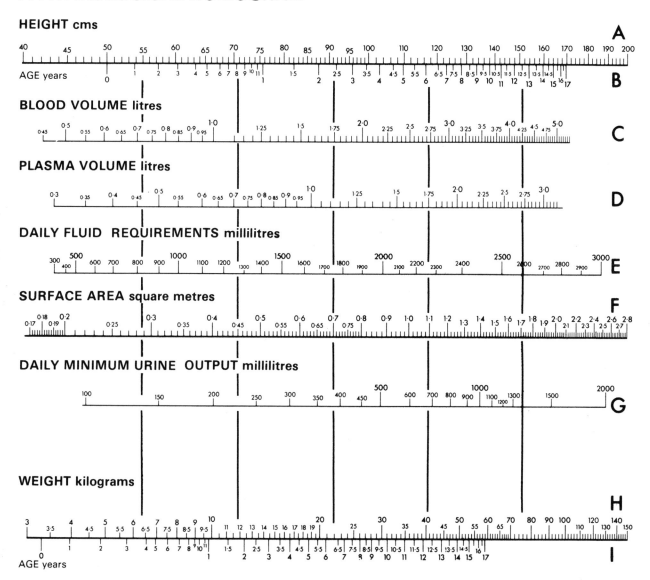

Fig. 58-6 A PHYSIOLOGICAL NOMOGRAM. Don't be defeated by this—it is really quite easy! A patient's blood volume, his plasma volume, his fluid requirements, and his minimum urine output are all proportional to his surface area. This in turn is proportional to his weight and height.

First, align his height and weight with a ruler, this will cross Scale F, at a point which indicates his surface area. Then hold the ruler vertically at this point (hold it parallel to the thick vertical lines) and read off his blood volume etc. For further instructions, see the next figure.
Drawn at the suggestion of Peter Bewes using data from the Ciba–Geigy Scientific Tables.

USING THE PREVIOUS FIGURE

Step two, using his surface area to find other variables

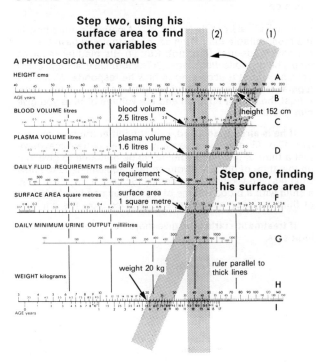

Fig. 58-7 HOW TO USE THE PREVIOUS FIGURE. Measure the patient's height and weigh him. (1) Align your ruler with his height (scale A) and weight (scale H). Read off his surface area from scale F. Next, (2) hold your ruler vertical at the figure for his surface area and read off his blood volume (scale C), his plasma volume (scale D), his daily fluid requirements (scale E), and his minimum urine output (scale G).

For example, say he was 152 cm tall and weighed 20 kg. He would have a surface area of 1 square metre, a blood volume of 2.5 litres (scale C), and a plasma volume of about 1.6 litres (scale D). His fluid requirement would be about 2150 ml (scale E), and his minimum daily urine output about 600 ml (scale G). If you cannot weigh and measure him, estimate his approximate height and weight from his age. This will be much less accurate.

If shock is not controlled, give more fluid than the formula indicates. Here are the signs that shock is not controlled and that he needs more fluid: restlessness, cold hands or feet, a rising pulse rate, thirst, sweating, collapsed veins, or a falling blood pressure. A common error is to give morphine instead of fluid to relieve restlessness.

A patient should secrete between 0.5 to 1.0 ml/kg of urine an hour. For a 70 kg adult this is between 35 and 70 ml per hour. Scale G, in Fig. 58-6 is drawn at 0.5 ml per hour, so this is his *minimum* output. If he is secreting less urine than this, he usually needs more fluid, but he may need less if he has renal failure (58.10). The minimum volume of urine required to excrete the solutes produced by metabolism is about 300 ml in a normal person and 600 to 800 ml in a burns patient.

If you are not giving colloids, **his urine flow is the best indication of adequate fluid replacement.**

If you are giving him colloids, **combine estimation of his urine output with: (1) inspection of his jugular venous pressure, (2) the filling of his peripheral veins, (3) the colour and temperature of his skin, and (4) the capillary filling of his nail beds.**

If his jugular venous pressure rises and there are basal crepitations, you are over-infusing him (which is a less common error than under-infusion), so reduce his fluid intake drastically. As he loses fluid from the surface of his burn he should improve.

If you can measure his microhaematocrit, measure it 2 hourly for the first 8 hours, then 8 hourly thereafter. Fill two capillary tubes from a pin prick in his ear (in case one breaks), and plot the readings immediately on his fluid balance chart.

Provided he was not anaemic or polycythaemic before treatment began, changes in his haematocrit will be a useful guide to fluid replacement. A high haematocrit shows that he needs more fluid and vice versa. Don't be a slave to it, and consider it with other signs.

A PATIENT SHOULD EXCRETE 0.5 TO 1 ml/kg OF URINE PER HOUR
(35 to 70 ml per hour for adults)

58.5 What kinds of fluid does a severely burnt patient need?

A severely burnt patient needs fluid for two purposes, and for each of them the fluid must be different.

(1) A patient needs fluid to replace his fluid loss and treat shock. Besides losing water, he loses sodium from his extracellular fluid into the cells of the unburnt part of his body, so that his plasma sodium falls and must be replaced. If you replace this fluid with plain water, or 5% dextrose intravenously, he may become confused and die from water intoxication (58.10), especially if he is a child, due to excess water and not enough sodium. So, give him Ringer's lactate or 0.9% saline intravenously. If necessary, you can give him Darrow's solution

When you replace a patient's fluid losses by mouth, give him saline or oral rehydration fluid, or milk *not plain water or tea.* This is especially important with young children. To make a suitable solution, add a teaspoonful of salt, and another one of sodium bicarbonate, to a litre of water. If you add fruit juice, and serve the mixture cold from the fridge, no child will refuse it.

(2) A patient needs fluids to fulfil his basal (metabolic) water loss. For this he needs water without sodium, so estimate this need from scale E, (his daily fluid requirements) in Figure 58-6. Give him the water he needs as 5% dextrose intravenously, or as water by mouth.

58.6 Should you let a burns patient drink?

Intravenous fluids are expensive and may be scarce, so it is convenient to let a patient take his fluids by mouth, if he can. This may be possible if his burns are not too extensive, but it can cause problems. He may drink too little or too much. Nausea, gastric dilatation, and ileus may occur in severe burns. Shock, on the other hand, makes him thirsty, and he may be tempted to drink too much. If he does, he may vomit severely, so manage him like this:

SHOULD A BURNS PATIENT DRINK? If he is thirsty and wants to drink, let him do so, even if he is being given intravenous fluids.

If his burn is under 10% let him take all his fluids by mouth as bicarbonate saline (58.5), or milk.

If his burn is between 10% and 15%, he is on the borderline. Treat him with supervised oral fluids, if you can.

If his burn is more than 15%, give him his calculated fluid needs intravenously. If intravenous fluids are very scarce and you want to try treating him orally, pass a nasogastric tube and empty his stomach hourly before giving test quantities of oral fluids.

If his stomach empties normally, **give him up to 75% of his fluid requirements by mouth.**

If his stomach does not empty normally, **stop oral fluids and give him all his fluid requirements intravenously.**

58.7 Does a burns patient need blood?

If a deep burn is more than 10% in a child, or 20% in an adult, give the patient some blood, especially if his burn is full thickness. Give it on the second day at the end of the shock phase, and repeat it as necessary. Give him one per cent of his blood volume for each one per cent of a deep burn. Thus a 60 kg patient with a 30% burn needs 30% of 4.4 litres (this is his blood volume as read off from Scale C, in Fig. 58-6) or about 1300 ml of blood. A simpler way of estimating the blood that a severely burnt patient needs is to give him 25 ml/kg. Signs which suggest that blood is indicated are: (1) Evidence of blood loss such as haematemesis, melaena, or delayed haemoglobinuria (18 to 36 hours after burning). (2) A falling haematocrit, when plasma or crystalloid infusions have not been excessive.

58.8 If resuscitation starts late

Don't be deceived if a patient who arrives early looks quite well. His severe pain may have gone and the ill effects of hypovolaemia may not be manifest yet. If transport in your district is difficult, most of your patients will arrive late. If a patient with a severe burn takes more than three hours to reach you, he will arrive severely shocked. The longer the delay the worse his shock, and the more important it is for you to correct his fluid deficit *quickly*, and the more difficult this will be without overloading his circulation. Suppose that a 70 kg adult has a 40% burn, and is admitted four hours later. During the eight hour period following the burn he should have $40 \times 70 = 2800$ ml. Four hours of this period has already elapsed, so he needs this volume of fluid during the remaining 4 hours, or 700 ml an hour. Because his burn is over 40%, he will need some of this fluid as colloids. Here is some guidance for managing these difficult cases.

RESUSCITATION STARTS LATE Calculate a patient's fluid deficit as in Fig. 58-5. Start by giving him saline, until he becomes conscious, or his peripheral pulses return.

After an hour give him chlorpromazine 0.5 mg/kg and look for a fall in his jugular venous pressure. Chlorpromazine will reduce vasconstriction and enable you to proceed with giving him the rest of his calculated fluid requirements.

Monitor his his urine volume carefully, and if possible, his central venous pressure also (A 19.2).

58.9 How much fluid does a burns patient need when shock is over?

If a patient has a comparatively minor burn, he will probably start to eat and drink normally when shock is over. He will then be able to adjust his fluid and electrolytes himself without difficulty, so that you can take his drip down at about 48 hours, and start giving him a high protein diet about the third or fourth day. But, if his burn is extensive and he is not drinking for any reason, you will have to control his fluid and electrolyte intake for him. Two things are particularly important at this stage—water and sodium.

Water Although little plasma will leak from a patient's burn after 48 hours when shock is over, he will continue to lose fluid by evaporation from its wet surface. In a 30% burn he may lose 2 litres of fluid a day in addition to his loss by other routes. The result is that he can easily become dehydrated, hyper-

natraemic, wasted, and oliguric. His serum osmolarity will rise and he may die from circulatory failure. So, keep a careful watch on his fluid balance chart, even if he is taking fluids by mouth. Calculate the water loss from his burn from Fig. 58-8. It is based on his surface area. Read this off from Fig. 58-6.

Fig. 58-8 is only a rough guide to the fluid a patient needs. Add it to his daily fluid requirements (scale E in Fig. 58-6), and adjust the fluid you give him in the light of the following factors.

(1) The ambient temperature. He will need more fluid if the weather is hot.

(2) The stage of healing of his burn. His fluid requirements will become less as it heals.

(3) Oedema is not a good guide to his electrolyte and fluid needs, because he can be both oedematous and salt depleted.

(4) His urinary output. Unfortunately, this too is an imperfect guide because a diuretic phase commonly follows the shock phase.

Sodium A patient can also lose much sodium from a severe burn. Calculate his sodium loss from Fig. 58-8. To find out how many mmols of sodium there are in the commonly used fluids, consult Fig. A 15-6 in *Primary Anaesthesia*.

If your laboratory tests are limited, the safest fluid to give him will be 0.18% saline in 5% dextrose for *maintenance* (for 'shock' he needs Ringer's lactate or 0.9% saline). *Take care not to overload young children and cause water intoxication as described in the next section.*

58.10 Difficulties with fluid and blood replacement

There are many of these. Here are some of the more common ones. One of your more serious problems is likely to be lack of fluids. If so, Section 58.6 should be some help.

DIFFICULTIES WITH FLUIDS IN A SEVERELY BURNT PATIENT

If a burns patient PASSES NO URINE, suspect that there is probably a drainage problem with the catheter. Even in acute renal failure the kidneys can usually manage to produce some urine

FLUID AND SODIUM NEEDS WHEN SHOCK IS OVER

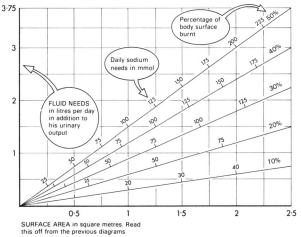

Fig. 58-8 FLUID AND SODIUM NEEDS WHEN SHOCK IS OVER. **Calculate a patient's surface area from Fig. 58-6. Read off his daily fluid needs. This covers the evaporation from his burn and his respiratory losses, BUT NOT HIS URINE. Read off the sodium he requires in mmol. For example, if his surface area is 2 square metres, and he has a 50% burn and is passing 1500 ml of urine, he will need 3000 ml + 1500 = 4500 ml of fluid a day. He will also need 200 mmol of sodium.** *Data from Cason.*

If his URINE FLOW FALLS below 0.5 ml/kg per hour after the first 12 hours, this is likely to be serious. During the first 12 hours a low urine flow is not of great significance. But after 12 hours a urine volume of less than 35 ml an hour in an adult (10 ml/hr in an infant) is a clear sign that a patient's kidneys are not being adequately perfused, or are failing. If it is less than this for two consecutive hours, give an adult a test dose of a litre of saline over half an hour. Before you do so, make sure that the bases of his lungs are not wet.

If a test dose of a litre of saline increases his urine output, previous transfusion was inadequate.

If a test dose of a litre of saline fails to increase his urine output, give him 15% mannitol (1 g/kg) or frusemide. If this does not increase his urine output, his kidneys are failing, so consider referring him for renal dialysis. Even if this is possible, his prognosis is so bad that it may not be justified.

Acute renal failure occurs in about 5% of patients with extensive burns, and usually kills them. Half of them are oliguric. The other half pass a normal volume of urine, but cannot concentrate it. A burns patient normally passes a concentrated urine, so a fixed specific gravity of 1.010 indicates renal failure, even if his urine volume is normal. Remember that protein or dextran in it will raise its specific gravity, and make it appear normal when it is not.

If RENAL FAILURE is established, and you cannot refer a patient, don't stop transfusion treatment for shock, or he will be grossly hypovolaemic at the end of the 48 hour shock period. After 48 hours he will only need oral or intravenous fluid to replace water loss from his burns, plus his insensible loss (Scale E in Fig. 58-6).

If a burnt child becomes irritable, vomits, twitches, has fits, becomes apathetic or comatose, has hyperpyrexia, goes blue, and breathes slowly and shallowly, suspect that he is HYPONATRAEMIC. Although all these signs are unlikely to occur in the same child, when several of them occur together, they suggest that he may have cerebral oedema caused by water intoxication which may kill him. It is the result of not giving him enough sodium in the fluid used to correct shock. Because it is due to inadequate treatment, it should never happen. Watch for 'twitches', if he has them, give him diazepam. He may have a generalized convulsion at any moment. If he does have convulsions, control them with diazepam or barbiturates, and give him chlorpromazine, or some more powerful vasodilator. Correct his hyperpyrexia gently. Don't try to correct it with fans, because by increasing vasocontraction they may reduce heat loss, and raise his temperature. Correct his hyponatraemia by giving sodium in the following quantity:—:

mmol of sodium needed = (140 minus his serum sodium in mmol/l)×(60% of his body weight in kg).

If you cannot estimate his serum sodium, assume it is 125 mmol/1. Be cautious, give half the calculated dose to begin with, and observe his response.

If a severely burnt patient: (1) vomits, or feels nauseated, (2) has absent bowel sounds and abdominal distension (indicating PARALYTIC ILEUS) or (3) has GASTRIC DISTENSION, pass a nasogastric tube, and leave it down. Paralytic ileus and gastric distention are common after severe burns. Aspirate the tube and give him his hourly oral fluid requirement. If this is returned when you aspirate at the next hour, then he is not absorbing fluid from his gut, and needs intravenous fluid. Continue to aspirate his stomach hourly. This will not prevent acute dilatation of his stomach, but it will control it and prevent vomiting.

Make sure that his potassium intake is adequate and, as far as is possible, exclude hyponatraemia, hypovolaemia, septicaemia, and constipation.

If a patient becomes OEDEMATOUS, this is unlikely to be serious, and will soon go if his kidneys are functioning normally and a high protein diet starts on the 3rd or 4th day.

If a burns patient becomes becomes ANAEMIC, the reasons include: (1) Destruction of his red cells at the time of burn. (2) Depression of his bone marrow as the result of sepsis. (3) Loss of blood from the burnt area each time it is cleaned or desloughed. If his haemoglobin falls below 10 g/dl, healing slows, and grafts do not take, so transfuse him when necessary, but remember that one unit of blood will only raise an adult's haemoglobin by 1 g/dl. When his haemoglobin has

fallen to 75%, he will need transfusions equal to 25% of his blood volume. A severely burnt adult may need 10 units of blood and perhaps more.

A burn of a given percentage will reduce a patient's haemoglobin by an approximately equal one. Damaged red cells are inefficient, so, if he needs blood, give it early. His haemoglobin may fall to 5 g/dl or less a week or more after severe burn, so measure it often.

MEASURE A PATIENT'S HAEMOGLOBIN REGULARLY

58.11 Feeding a burn patient (or any severely injured patient who can eat)

Fluid infusions during the first 48 hours may increase the weight of a severely burnt patient by 20%. Thereafter he may steadily lose up to 40% of it and die. Losses of 10% and 20% are common, and often overlooked. They are the result of the intense tissue catabolism that follows a burn, combined with sepsis and malnutrition. So weigh him, if you can, on admission, and each week thereafter. You can prevent most of this loss and improve his chances of recovery *if you can feed him enough.* His needs are huge, and are given below. You may not be able to achieve all of them, but the less weight he loses, the more likely he is to live, so persist in your efforts to get food into him. He should not be losing weight when you graft him.

Intravenous feeding is expensive, impractical, and seldom necessary. So you have two choices: (1) You can try to make a patient eat larger quantities of ordinary foods. (2) You can have diets for tube feeding made with a blender in your hospital kitchen. The lists below give the composition of some of the foods you may be able to blend. Eggs are likely to be the most practical high protein food. Anorexia, vomiting, and diarrhoea are the main difficulties. If a patient has diarrhoea, try reducing the carbohydrate content of his feed to reduce its osmolarity.

DON'T LET ANYONE CONNECT A PATIENT'S FOOD DRIP TO HIS INTRAVENOUS LINE

FEEDING

INDICATIONS (1) A severely burnt patient. (2) Any severely injured patient.

If what follows is too difficult, at least make sure that every day a severely burnt adult has at least 2 eggs, 500 ml of reconstituted milk, and the vitamins listed below. It also applies to any severely injured patient who is able to eat, whatever the nature of his injuries.

If he cannot take food by mouth, try to give him at least some of his energy needs as 10%, 25%, or 50% dextrose through a central venous line (A 19.2).

Here are the needs of adults and children:

ADULTS

Energy 80 kJ/kg (20 kcal/kg) of body weight + 300 kJ (70 kcal) for each 1% of the burn.

Protein 1 g/kg + 3 g for each 1% of the burn.

CHILDREN

Energy 250 kJ/kg (60 kcal/kg) + 150 kJ (35 kcal) for each 1% of the burn.

Protein 3 g/kg + 1 g for each 1% of the burn.

A FOOD TABLE

In the following list the first figure is the weight of food containing 40 g of reference protein, while the second is the weight containing 10 MJ (about 2,500 kcal), these being a normal adult's daily requirements.

Dried skim milk powder 150 g, 660 g; full cream powder 210 g, 480 g; cow's milk 1500 g, 3,700 g; soya beans 210 g, 590 g; beans (dry) 430 g, 700 g; peas (dry) 410 g, 690 g; shelled groundnuts 360 g, 440 g; meat (beef) 320, 1,100 g; liver 390, 1,700 g; eggs 330 g, 1,700 g; maize meal 910 g, 660 g; margarine nil, 330 g; cooking oil or fat nil, 270 g.

NASOGASTRIC FEEDS FOR BURNS

These are mostly needed in children.

If a patient has no bowel sounds, you cannot feed him by mouth. Intravenous feeding is his only hope.

If he has got bowel sounds, but is unable to eat normally (because he is too weak, too old or too sick to feed himself by mouth, or is unconscious), pass a small nasogastric tube (2.5 mm 8 Ch in a child or about 4.5 mm 14 Ch in an adult).

CAUTION ! Make sure that the tube is in the patient's stomach, and not in his trachea, by the methods in Section 4.9. (2) Always aspirate the stomach before giving a feed, to make sure that it is emptying properly. In an unconscious patient, overdistension may cause regurgitation and aspiration of feed.

If the patient has previously not been eating, start with half or quarter strength feeds initially, until you are sure that he has adapted adequately to his new method of feeding.

Give him some water by mouth to lubricate his oesophagus. Give him small blenderized feeds to start with, well spaced throughout the day and night. Filter them through gauze to prevent them clogging the tube and give them as a continous drip from a drip set. If the feed clogs the drip set, give it intermittently with a syringe. Remember that the fluid part of the feed is part of his daily intake. Before giving them aspirate his stomach to detect retention. If you aspirate 100 ml, reduce the next tube feed by this amount.

Work up to his required intake over several days. 15 MJ (3,500 calories) and 180 g of protein are about as much as an adult can take by mouth. If he can eat, encourage him to do so, with the incentive that his tube will be removed as soon as he eats normally. Reduce his intake as his burn heals.

Give him enough water (about 30 ml/kg) in addition to his non–renal losses to excrete the breakdown products of his diet.

Give him at least 10% of his energy needs as fat. You will probably be unable to estimate his urinary potassium losses which may be large. As a rough guide, give him 100 mmol a day by mouth. This is 100 ml of the commonly used potassium solution containing 1 mmol/ml (A15.1).

CAUTION ! (1) A blenderized feed is readily infected, so boil it and keep it cold. (2) Don't add salt or you will overload him with sodium.

Alternatively, give him 250 ml of feed with a 50 ml syringe every 3 hours, followed by 25 to 50 ml of water to flush out the tube and make up the daily fluid requirements.

VITAMINS Each day give the patient capsules of vitamins B, A, and D, 600 mg of ascorbic acid, and 600 mg of ferrous sulphate.

DIFFICULTIES WITH TUBE FEEDING

If you DON'T HAVE A BLENDER, you will have to give a patient milk, eggs, and sugar, vegetable oil, and gruel of various kinds.

If he gets DIARRHOEA, the feed may be hypertonic. Try diluting it.

If he REGURGITATES AND ASPIRATES the feed (which may be fatal), you probably failed to check that his stomach was being emptied, before giving him more feed. So, check on his gastric residue, and raise the head of his bed.

FEED HIM UP
GIVE HIM SMALL REGULAR FEEDS
DON'T FORGET THE VITAMINS

THE DEPTH OF A BURN

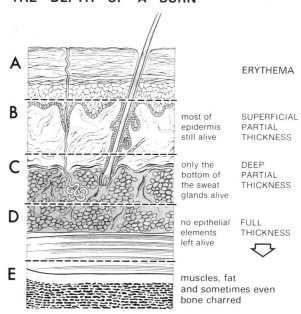

Fig. 58-9 THE DEPTH OF A BURN. Burns are usually classified into superficial, superficial partial thickness, deep partial thickness, and full thickness. Here we have given them the letters A, B, C, D, and E.

58.12 How deep are the patient's burns?

The depth of a patient's burns will determine whether or not you need to graft them. His sweat glands and hair follicles are epidermal structures and penetrate deep into his dermis. If his epidermis is destroyed it can regenerate from these deep epidermal structures—provided that his burn is not so deep that it has destroyed them also. There is still no universally accepted way of classifying burns, so we will call them types A, B, C D, and E.

Type A In the mildest burns (first degree) there is erythema only and no blistering. Protect them from infection.

Type B In slightly more severe burns, blisters form within 24 hours and break to leave a wet pink surface. These are burns with superficial partial thickness skin loss (psl). Most of the deep epidermal structures are still alive, so burns of this type heal in less than three weeks. The pain fibres in the skin are also still alive, so they are sensitive to the of prick of a sterile needle. Most flash burns and scalds are of this type.

Type C Burns of the next grade of severity kill all a patient's epidermis except for the bottoms of his sweat glands. Although they may look like a burn of Type B above, they take 6 weeks to heal because the epithelial cells at the bottom of his sweat glands take this long to grow out and cover his dermis. When they eventually do so, the quality of the skin they produce is poor, so burns of type C are sometimes better grafted, especially if the the patient has a black skin. The skin that regenerates is pink, of poor quality, and prone to epitheliomas later. The nerves in the dermis are destroyed, so burns of this type are insensitive to pin prick. They are an important type of burn, because some of them may be suitable for excision and grafting at 3 to 5 days. They show deep partial thickness loss (dpsl). Burns of types B and C are sometimes classified as second degree burns.

Type D In these burns the whole thickness of a patient's epidermis, including the bottom of his sweat glands, has been killed. Unless his burn is very small, you will have to graft it. His dead skin looks white, or greyish brown, and is completely insensitive to pin prick.

Type E The deepest burns char a patient's fat and muscles, and sometimes even his bones and joints. Types D and E are third degree burns, full thickness burns, or burns showing whole thickness skin loss (wsl).

In practice, it is often convenient to use this classification loosely, and to disregard burns of type A entirely. The critical distinction (which is often difficult) is between: (1) Superficial burns (B and C above) in which enough of the epidermis remains to regrow without grafting, even if it grows slowly and (2) deep burns (D and E) in which the epidermis is totally destroyed, and which need grafting.

Unfortunately, you often cannot diagnose the depth of a burn. The most certain way is to wait and see what happens. If the crust separates to leave clean new skin underneath, the burn was superficial. If no epidermis appears to cover a wet granulating surface, or if a slough or eschar remains firmly stuck, it is deep. *A burn which is sensitive to pin prick (B) never needs grafting*, but one which is insensitive (C, D, or E), may or may not do so. *The ability to feel a pin is thus more significant when it is present than when it is absent.*

Burns are dynamic injuries, so that the distinction between superficial burns and deep ones is not permanent. The deep epidermal structures which survived after a partial thickness burn *can easily be destroyed by infection later.* One of your main aims must be to prevent this. The signs which follow are very approximate. You will be most interested in knowing the depth of small deep burns which you might be able to excise and graft early (58.17). You can assess the depth of a burn most reliably at about the 7th day.

HOW DEEP ARE A PATIENT'S BURNS?

Burns of types A and E are easily diagnosed. You are most interested in the differences between B and C. Be guided by these signs.

What was the temperature of the agent and the time of exposure? The depth of a patient's burn is a function of both.

The thickness of the burnt skin The thin skin on the back of his hand is more likely to be deeply burnt than the thick skin on the front.

How alert was he at the time of the burn? His burns are more likely to be deep if he is or was drunk, drugged, paralysed, feeble, or very old, or if he was burnt in an epileptic fit.

Blisters usually indicate a superficial burn.

Red fat If haemoglobin from destroyed red cells has stained his subcutaneous fat, his burn is deep.

Thrombosed veins visible through translucent subcutaneous fat, or hairs which can easily be pulled out, are both signs of a full thickness burn.

Speckling If at 2 weeks you see fine dots (skin regenerating from the bottom of sweat glands), a patient's burn is partial thickness (D). These dots are grey in a black skin and red in a white one.

If his burn has shrunk below the level of the surrounding skin, it is probably full thickness.

THE PIN PRICK TEST This is a test of pin prick, not pin pressure. The patient must be conscious and cooperative, and understand the difference between pain and pressure.

Take a sterile hypodermic needle and practise first on normal skin by asking him if he can feel its sharp or blunt ends. Then test the burn.

If he mostly says "sharp", the burn is almost certainly Type B (superficial partial thickness) and it will heal in less than three weeks without grafting.

If he mostly says "blunt", the test is of less significance it might be Type C (deep partial thickness) or type D (full thickness).

If the pin pricks bleed, this is a useful sign that his burn is superficial (B).

58.13 How should the burn itself be treated?

You will probably find yourself treating burns in overcrowded wards with more than one patient in the same bed, with few imperfectly trained nurses, and with the minimum of dressings drugs and equipment. Which methods are best suited to these extreme limitations? Here are the possibilities: (1) The open (exposure) method which leaves a burn open to the air and encourages it to form a dry crust. (2) The closed (occlusive) method in which the burn is isolated from the environment by thick dressings. (3) A method in which the burn is kept continously wet with saline. (4) The plastic bag method for burnt hands or feet. (5) Early excision and grafting. Each method has its own advantages and disadvantages, and there is no 'best method'. Instead, combine the best of all methods to suit the needs of a particular patient. *The combination that you are likely to find best is the exposure method for a patient's superficial burns, saline soaks for his deep ones, and the plastic bag method for his hands and feet.*

HOW SHOULD A BURN BE TREATED?

These indications apply to conditions where nursing care and dressings are minimal. Where they are not, the closed method has wider indications.

THE EXPOSURE METHOD FOR BURNS

INDICATIONS (1) Scalds. (2) Burns of a patient's face. (3) Large partial thickness burns anywhere except his hands. (4) Full thickness burns anywhere except his hands, when dressings are scarce or nursing care minimal. (5) The exposure method or the saline method are mandatory if a severely burnt patient is hyperpyrexic.

CONTRAINDICATIONS An extensive burn in a cold environment with lack of adequate heating.

THE CLOSED (OCCLUSIVE DRESSING) METHOD FOR BURNS

INDICATIONS (1) Smaller burns if a patient is to be treated as an outpatient, especially if the burns are on his limbs. (2) Smaller burns of his hands. (3) A larger burn for which he has to be transported elsewhere.

CONTRAINDICATIONS All other burns.

THE SALINE METHOD FOR BURNS

INDICATIONS This is probably the best method for all burns which are severe enough to be admitted, but if nursing skills are scarce, reserve it for deep ones.

THE PLASTIC BAG METHOD FOR BURNT HANDS AND FEET
All but the most minor burns of the hands.

EARLY EXCISION AND GRAFTING FOR BURNS

INDICATIONS Small (less than 2%) full thickness burns during the first 3 days, if you have plenty of blood and are good at skin grafting.

58.14 The exposure method

In this method nothing touches a patient's burn except air, and preferably an antibacterial agent, such as povidone iodine. Air keeps it cool and encourages the dry eschar to form, both of which minimize the growth of bacteria. The exposure method is excellent if his burn is superficial and the climate warm. It is economical in nursing time, you can examine it easily; it avoids expensive dressings, it is useful for parts of his body which cannot easily be dressed, such as his face, buttocks, and perineum, and it is less dependent on local antibacterial agents than is the

TWO METHODS FOR BURNS

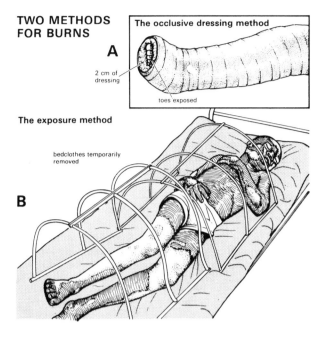

Fig. 58-10 TWO METHODS COMPARED. In the closed method note: (1) the thickness of the dressing, and (2) that the patient's toes are exposed so that their circulation can be monitored. In the open method the bed clothes are being kept away from the burn with a cradle. *A, from Yang Chih-chun withkind permission.*

THE EXPOSURE METHOD

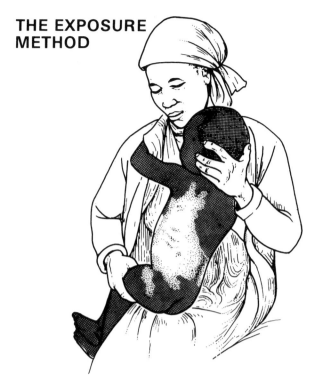

Fig. 58-11 THE EXPOSURE METHOD is the most practical one for most burns in the hospitals for which we write.

occlusive method. If you manage the exposure method properly, flies are seldom a problem, but if they are, you can put the patient under a mosquito net.

In a superficial burn, the crust separates like the skin of a snake to leave new, pink, well healed skin underneath.

In a deep burn the dead tissues form a tough eschar (sometimes with pools of pus underneath it), or less often they remain as a moist slough. You can leave these sloughs and eschars open to the air, but the best way to treat them is to cover them with saline soaks. Dry or moist, the dead tissue will have to be removed and the burn grafted.

A common modification of the exposure method is to put vaseline gauze over the whole burn, and then expose this to the air. The exudate flows through the holes in the gauze and dries. This is no longer strictly the exposure method, and there is no evidence that it is any better than the unmodified exposure method, except perhaps on the flexures. Nor is it certain that impregnating vaseline gauze with expensive antibiotics, such as soframycin, improves it in any way. Some experienced surgeons say that to modify the exposure method, by applying vaseline gauze, is a compromise which combines the disadvantages of both the open and the closed methods.

Patients treated by the exposure method should ideally be barrier nursed. Unfortunately, this is quite impossible in the hospitals for which we write. Even if they cannot be barrier nursed, *the exposure or saline method is likely to be better than the occlusive method done badly*—which is the common alternative.

The following description describes the care of a child by the exposure method, because children so often need this treatment.

THE EXPOSURE METHOD FOR BURNS

INDICATIONS See Section 58.12.

EQUIPMENT The equipment for cleaning a burn is simple, but it must be sterile. It includes aqueous chlorhexidine solution or saline (conveniently from a bottle of intravenous saline), a gallipot, and a sterile glove.

METHOD Sedate the child with chloral hydrate or ketamine. Put him on a sterile mackintosh in a clean bed. Put a sterile theatre drape or a clean sheet on top of this. Leave the burn alone, the heat will have sterilized the burnt surface. Don't prick the blisters unless they are tense and painful.

Local antibacterial agents are desirable, but not absolutely necessary. Some workers apply povidine iodine or cetrimide.

Put a cradle over the child and cover this with another sterile drape.

TEMPERATURE The room should be warm and moist (40°C and 40% relative humidity is ideal). Monitor his temperature carefully. Feel his extremities. If necessary, close the windows and put a heater beside him. Electric fans heaters are the best, but with suitable precautions you can use a charcoal brazier. Don't put him in the sun, except for short periods, because pink depigmented skin burns easily.

THE THIRD OR FOURTH DAY ONWARDS

Don't do anything to the *dry* surface of a superficial burn after the first day. Continually dressing and scraping its surface interferes with healing. Tell the nurses that it is being dressed, but that it is being dressed with air! Let any dry part of the burn remain dry. If more blisters form, prick them. Try to preserve the dry crust until it falls off naturally. *Clean only parts which remain wet.* Use gauze swabs and chlorhexidine, or sterile saline, as for the initial toilet.

CAUTION ! If there is any danger that a tight crust or eschar might be obstructing the child's circulation, split it immediately (58.18).

You may not know if a burn is superficial or full thickness until about the 7th day.

SUPERFICIAL AND DEEP PARTIAL THICKNESS BURNS (B and C in Fig. 58-9) dry to form an eschar which falls off in 7 to 12 days in type B, or 10 to 21 days in type C, with little bleeding. They heal in 3 to 4 weeks.

FULL THICKNESS BURNS (D, and E) form thick sloughs and eschars. Choose between the following methods.

(1) Leave the eschar open to the air. Remove it in the theatre at 10 to 18 days, and then graft.

(2) Much the best, start the saline method at 48 hours. Either put the burnt part in a bowl of half strength saline 4 hourly or pour saline on the dressings 4 hourly (58.16). Some slough will come away in the dressings, remove large pieces by 'sloughectomy' in the theatre, then graft.

DIFFICULTIES WITH THE EXPOSURE METHOD FOR BURNS

If a DEEP BURN CROSSES A FLEXURE, splint the patient's limb in extension. You can safely do this for 3 weeks in an adult or 6 weeks in a child while the skin over it heals. Then mobilize it—see Section 58.24. Skeletal traction as in Fig. 58-15 may be the best way to maintain extension.

CAUTION ! Appropriate splinting is essential to prevent contractures: (1) To prevent movement of the joint while the graft takes. (2) To maintain the positions in Fig. 58-16 until the burn has healed.

If DRY ESCHARS CRACK over a patient's flexures, such as those of his elbows or axillae, splinting is required, so change methods.

If his burn is deep use the saline or the closed method for the deep part of it, and if necessary, excise the slough.

If it is superficial, apply vaseline gauze or silver sulphadiazine cream. In deep burns the skin under these cracks always needs grafting and you will have to take great care to prevent contractures. You may also have to graft cracks in burns which are superficial elsewhere.

If he has EXTENSIVE BURNS ON HIS TRUNK, arrange his position so that he lies on normal skin, not on his burn. If his back and buttocks are burnt, turn him hourly, if he has burns all round his body, the only way to nurse him by this method is in a string hammock. His burns will probably be at least 50%, so his chances of surviving are not good.

If his BUTTOCKS AND PERINEUM HAVE BEEN BURNT, put him in gallows traction (78.2), if he is under 5, and expose his burn. If necessary, (and it seldom is) catheterize him, and don't let overflow incontinence develop. Urine does not harm a burn, but moisture promotes infection. His perineum will be difficult to graft, and perineal grafts usually fail, so you may need to repeat them several times.

If his AXILLA has been burnt, try holding his arm above his head with skin traction—this is not easy.

If he SCRATCHES HIS EXPOSED BURNS, try to prevent him doing so, because scratching can easily convert a superficial burn into a deep one. Immobilize both his elbows in padded plaster cylinders to keep them extended. Sedate him. Don't try tying his hands to the sides of his cot, because this is cruel and dangerous.

If PUS APPPEARS, send a swab for culture daily. Dip a swab in sterile broth (or saline) and rub it widely over the burn.

DON'T DISTURB THE CRUST, LET IT SEPARATE SPONTANEOUSLY
DON'T LET HIM GET COLD

58.15 The closed (occlusive dressing) method

At the moment of burning a burn is sterile. The aim of the closed method is to keep it so, as far as possible, by sealing it off from the environment with an effective dressing, *before* it has become seriously contaminated. The bigger the burn, the more difficult this is. To be effective the dressing which covers a burn must be about 2 cm thick as in A, Fig. 58-10, so that it absorbs the exudate and prevents it reaching the surface where it can become infected. Gauze is more absorbent than cotton wool, but is more expensive. In practice, asepsis is difficult to achieve, especially with larger burns, so you should put some local antiseptic agent on the burn (58.22). Some surgeons would say you must do this. The best local agents are silver

sulphadiazine cream or 0.5% silver nitrate with 0.2% chlorhexidine.

The closed method: (1) Demands more and better nursing care than the exposure method. (2) Needs abundant dressings. (3) Is more dependant on a local antiseptic agent than the exposure method. (5) Can cause hyperpyrexia in large burns in hot environments.

Done *well*, the closed method can be wonderfully successful. When you remove a dressing from a partial thickness burn which you have left undisturbed for 10 days, you may find perfect new skin underneath. But this method can be very dangerous if you forget that: (1) Dressing a burn is a surgical procedure, which must be done aseptically. (2) The aim of the dressings is to contain exudates, and prevent organisms reaching the burn. This means that you must change them on the indications given below.

Done badly, this method is a disaster, and too easily converts a partial thickness burn into a full thickness one. Doing it badly includes: (1) Not applying enough dressings (sometimes only a thin layer of gauze). (2) Letting exudates soak through without changing them. (3) Not bringing the dressing well beyond the edges of the wound.

Unfortunately, the closed method, badly done, is in widespread use. As such, it is painful, messy, expensive, and hinders healing. There should be no compromise—either a burn should be left open with nothing on it at all, or it requires 2 cm of dressings. *There is a strong body of opinion which considers that the closed method has no place whatever for inpatients in the hospitals for which we write.* Under our circumstances it is only suitable for parts of the body where the necessary dressings will stay in place. In effect, this means the limbs. In practice, because of the cost of the dressings and the labour involved, you will only find the closed method suitable for *superfical* small burns on the extremities of outpatients. It becomes increasingly difficult with larger burns, and on the trunk.

THE MERE APPLICATION OF A FEW 'DRESSINGS' IS NOT THE CLOSED METHOD

THE CLOSED (OCCLUSIVE) METHOD
FOR BURNS

LOCAL ANTISEPTIC AGENTS are highly desirable for larger burns. Use: (1) Silver sulphadiazine cream. (2) 0.5% silver nitrate with 0.2% chlorhexidine changed every 4 days. (3) Povidone iodine. Or, less satisfactorily, use (4) cetrimide, or (5) chlorhexidine. In practice, you will probably have to use no antiseptic, or one of these last two.

APPLYING THE DRESSINGS FOR THE OCCLUSIVE METHOD

Use a 'no touch technique'. Use sterile forceps or sterile disposable gloves so that no human hand touches the burn or the dressings, and no sterile glove touches anything else in the room. If necessary, sedate the patient, or give him ketamine. Clean his burn and the skin around it with chlorhexidine solution. There is no need to puncture the blisters.

If a deep burn encircles a limb, you may need to do an escharotomy before applying a dressing.

Using a sterile spatula, spread one of the local antiseptic agents listed above on sterile gauze and apply this to the burn. Alternatively, and less satisfactorily, apply vaseline gauze.

Cover this with 2.5 cm of cotton wool and a crepe bandage. The dressing must extend 10 cm beyond the wound margins. If there is a wound over a flexure, apply the dressing with the joint in extension to prevent contractures (58.24). A thin plaster cast may prevent a child from removing his dressings.

CHANGING THE DRESSINGS WITH THE OCCLUSIVE METHOD

Partial thickness burns If you are sure that a burn really is only partial thickness, you can leave the dressing on for 10 days, unless the indications given below require that you should remove it. When you remove the dressing the burn should be healed.

Full thickness burns The limit for leaving a dressing on is about 4 days which is about the limit of the effectiveness of the local antibacterial agent. This is the usual interval for changing the dressings of minor burns in outpatients. Remove the dressing earlier than this on the following indications: (1) If the exudate soaks through the dressings. (2) Smell. (3) Swelling. (4) Pain. (5) Fever. (6) Regional lymphadenitis. (7) Restriction of the distal circulation. (8) Hyperpyrexia (this is only a danger in large burns). If changing the dressing is painful, give the patient ketamine (A 8.1).

If you are using 0.5% silver nitrate, change the dressing daily.

If the inner layer of a dressing sticks to the wound and is not stinking, leave it, or it will tear off valuable epithelium as you try to remove it. Allow it to come off by itself later. If it stinks, soak it with saline and remove it. Dab the wound dry, don't rub it.

Deep burns may shed their sloughs in the dressings. If sloughs have not separated in 2 weeks, remove them surgically under anaesthesia.

BACTERIOLOGY If possible, send a swab for culture each time you change a dressing.

IF THE DRESSINGS HAVE STUCK AND DO NOT STINK, LEAVE THEM

58.16 The saline method for burns

The aim of this method is to keep a burn constantly wet with half strength saline until it heals—full strength physiological saline is painful. As usually described this method requires that the burnt part be dipped into a bath of saline. If it is large, this is inconvenient. A simpler alternative is to pour saline over the burn from a jug, and catch the excess in a mackintosh. This makes the saline method practical in a ward, rather than always in a sluice room.

The saline method: (1) Reduces the time in hospital compared with the exposure method. (2) Uses the minimum of equipment and materials. (3) Is painless, and so enables a patient to start moving his joints early, thus minimizing stiffness and contractures. (4) Allows partial thickness burns to heal promptly and eschars to separate early, leaving healthy granulation tissue nearly ready for grafting. (5) Uses the minimum of dressings and no topical antiseptics. (6) Is popular with mothers and nurses.

This is probably the best method for deep burns in district hospitals, especially if they are extensive—provided: (1) your nursing care is not too bad, (2) your sluice arrangements are reasonable, (3) the climate or the ward is warm (about 28°C). *In practice, you will find the saline method very useful for full thickness burns, while using the exposure method for superficial ones.*

Early on, a wide variety of organisms are likely to be present including *Pseudomonas*. Later on, the predominant organisms will probably be Staphylococci. These are unlikely to need treating unless a patient has symptoms of generalized infection. If he does, he will be easier to treat than he would be if he were infected by *Pseudomonas*.

THE SALINE METHOD FOR BURNS

EQUIPMENT A mackintosh sheet and a variety of buckets, jugs, and basins.

SALINE Make half strength (0.5%) saline. You can make small quantities by dissolving a teaspoon of salt in a litre of ordinary tap water. Make larger ones by dissolving some suitable measure of salt in a much larger quantity of water. Learn what half strength saline should taste like, and test its concentration by tasting it first.

TEMPERATURE Keep the room comfortably warm. A patient should not go out into a cold bathroom.

METHOD Start at 48 hours with minor burns, and as soon as shock is over with major ones. Meanwhile, keep the burn moist with saline.

If you are using a jug, put a thick gauze dressing on the burn, and put a plastic sheet under it. If convenient, arrange this so that saline poured over the burn flows into a bucket. Keep the saline in a jug beside the patient's bed. If he is a child, ask his mother to pour a little saline over the burn every hour or so to keep it wet. Renew the dressing and clean the wound 4 hourly. Some sloughs will come off in the dressing.
CAUTION ! Keep the sloughs wet.

If you are going to immerse a burn, find some suitably sized container, such as a baby's bath, fill this with saline. Encourage the patient to keep dipping his burnt limb into it. Renew the saline at least daily. If you cannot let him have his own bath all the time, let him dip his burn into a bath of saline for 20 minutes twice a day. Let him exercise his burnt joints passively and actively while his burn is in the bath. If he has a deep burn, apply soaks between the baths.

The sloughs on a deep burn will usually separate about the the 12th day, and be ready for grafting on about the 15th to 17th day. As soon as the granulations are favourable, graft them (58.19). If possible, do regular culture and sensitivity tests.

DIFFICULTIES WITH THE SALINE METHOD

If SLOUGHS DO NOT COME OFF COMPLETELY in the dressings, take the patient to the theatre for 'sloughectomy' (58.18).

If BATHING A BURN IS PAINFUL, sedate him first. Make sure the saline is not too strong.

If he has EXTENSIVE BURNS, he should ideally be lowered into a stainless steel bath.

If his FACE IS BURNT, wash it in saline gently and continually.

If he is in danger of DEVELOPING CONTRACTURES, splint his limb appropriately (58.24).

58.17 Early excision and grafting for a full thickness burn

A logical method of treating a deep burn is to excise the dead tissue in the first few days before it becomes infected and then to graft it immediately, instead of waiting to deslough at about 14 days. Skilled surgeons in well equipped hospitals can do this in stages for burns of up to 30%. If you try it, you would be wise to use it in special sites only, such as the back of the hand, and in burns of less than 2% in which there is no shock.

There are difficulties: (1) Knowing which burns it is suitable for. You must be sure the burn is full thickness by the criteria in Section 58.12. If you excise and graft a partial thickness burn which is going to recover without grafting, you worsen the patient's chances of recovery. You can easily sacrifice living tissues, and injure important structures, such as tendons and cutaneous nerves. (2) Severe bleeding is the main danger and can be fatal, so the burn must be small, and even so, you must have plenty of blood for transfusion. (3) Early excision and grafting is only practical early, before the slough separates, usually at 3 to 5 days, sometimes up to 7 days.

There are various methods of early excision and grafting. The one described below is the only one which deserves to be used more widely in district hospitals. It is often a very effective method for deep burns on the palm of the hand. If left to themselves these may take many weeks to heal.

THE EARLY EXCISION OF A FULL THICKNESS BURN

INDICATIONS This method is only indicated if *all* these indications apply. (1) You are sure the burn is full thickness. (2) You can do the excision within the first 3 days. (3) The burn is small, certainly less than 10% and preferably only 2%. (4) You have plenty of blood for transfusion. (5) You are a good skin grafter.

METHOD Use a scalpel or, better, bend the blade of a Humby knife and use it to shave away thin layers of burnt tissue until you reach a layer which you know is alive because it bleeds.

If the bed is suitable, graft the burn immediately, or by delayed primary grafting at 3 days.

If the bed is unsuitable, for example, if it is formed by dead bone, you may have to refer the patient for the wound to be covered with a flap. Alternatively, gouge down to healthy cancellous bone, wait 3 days to allow granulations to start forming, and then graft.

58.18 Sloughs and eschars

The dead tissues over the surface of a burn have to separate. If the burn is superficial, they peel off as pieces of dry membrane. If it is deep, they either form: (1) a slough, which is moist, soft, grey, and stinking. Or, (2) they form an eschar which is dry,

hard, and dark and which may be so brittle that it cracks. There is no sharp distinction between sloughs and eschars, the main difference being how dry or how wet they are. The exposure method tends to form eschars, while the occlusive and saline methods form sloughs. Pieces of slough and eschar can: (1) Fall off spontaneously, if you wait long enough for infection to rot them. Even burnt bone will sequestrate eventually. (2) Come off in small pieces in the dressings of the occlusive method. (3) Be removed by escharotomy or 'sloughectomy' in the theatre. However sloughs and eschars separate, they leave wet granulations underneath them, which you must graft. Maggots also deslough most effectively, although few people have the courage to use them deliberately.

Sloughs and eschars have three dangers: (1) Eschars (but not sloughs), may restrict the circulation. Both eschars and sloughs may, (2) become infected, or (3) cause severe bleeding when you remove them, especially if you remove them from a large area.

A thick, tough, dry eschar can act like a tourniquet, and may constrict a patient's neck, or his chest, or the circulation in his limbs or his fingers. His oedematous tissue swells, but the eschar round it is rigid and cannot expand. Escharotomy can thus be an emergency procedure.

If only a patient's skin is dry and dead, the underlying tissues can remain uninfected for several weeks, during which the patient's fat liquefies. But if muscle is dead, infection occurs much more easily, and a rise in temperature about the 10th day usually shows that it has started. Infection under an eschar is difficult to localize, but pain is a useful sign. When infection is further advanced, you may be able to feel a dry eschar floating in a pool of pus. If there is much dead muscle, beware of anaerobic infection, particularly gas gangrene and tetanus, and deslough early.

**ESCHAROTOMY CAN BE AN ACUTE EMERGENCY
BEWARE OF PUS BENEATH THE ESCHAR
IF MUSCLE IS DEAD, DESLOUGH EARLY**

Manipulating any infected tissue may cause bacteraemia, and removing an extensive slough or eschar may shower so many bacteria into a patient's circulation that it causes septic shock (53.4). So, if a burn is severely infected, deslough it under antibiotic cover. Usually, this is not necessary.

Sloughs and particularly eschars don't usually bleed until you try to remove them. Then they may bleed massively, especially if the area is large. So remove them a little at a time, in stages separated by a day or two. Remove them gently, and stop when

EMERGENCY ESCHAROTOMY

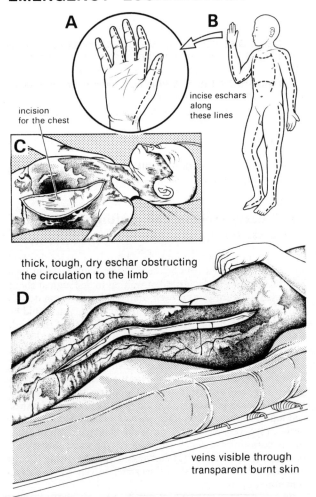

Fig. 58-12 EMERGENCY ESCHAROTOMY. A, incisions for the hand. B, those for the rest of the body. C, an emergency escharotomy for a burn of the chest. D, an emergency escharotomy for the thigh. *D, was kindly contributed by Peter Bewes.*

DESLOUGHING

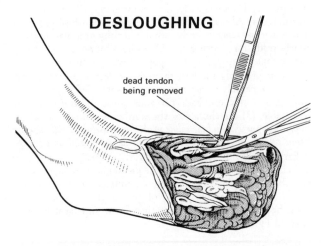

Fig. 58-13 DESLOUGHING A BURNT FOOT. This is the foot of a charming old grandmother who fell into a fire dead drunk. Her tendons and part of her metatarsals have sloughed. Pieces of her dead tendons are being removed prior to grafting. She went home walking. *Dr. Naim Janmohammed's patient.*

the patient has had enough. Be guided in how much to remove by his pulse and blood pressure, and by the amount of blood he loses.

After you have removed a slough, you can either graft the raw area immediately, if the surface is suitable, or you can wait until there are favourable granulations. Control infection first.

Desloughing can vary from a minor procedure, if a burn is small, to an extensive 'sloughectomy' in the theatre, if it is large and deep. Most desloughing is done piecemeal by the nurses as they dress a wound, especially when they apply saline soaks. *One of the commonest mistakes is not to deslough a burn—as long as any slough remains, you cannot graft it.*

REMOVE SLOUGH WHICH SEPARATES EASILY
DON'T REMOVE TOO MUCH SLOUGH AT ONCE

'SLOUGHECTOMY' AND ESCHAROTOMY FOR A DEEP BURN

ANTIBIOTIC COVER is essential if the patient's slough or eschar is severely infected. If Streptococci are present, use penicillin, if Pseudomonas are present they may be sensitive to gentamicin. If possible do sensitivity tests.

INDICATIONS Full thickness burns only. (1) A constricting eschar needs immediate splitting as an emergency procedure. (2) Most other eschars are best removed at about 2 weeks. There is usually a clear line of demarcation for surgical desloughing at this time. (3) Fever (which is not malarial) and toxaemia.

ANAESTHESIA Full thickness burns have no sensation, so anaesthesia is theoretically unnecessary. But be kind and give the patient ketamine, or morphine. If he feels pain, either an escharotomy is not necessary because the burn is only superficial, or you are cutting in the wrong place.

SLOUGHECTOMY Clean the burnt areas with chlorhexidine. Use any convenient instrument, such as scissors, a scalpel, or an elevator. Or, open the gap between the blade and roller of a Humby knife and shave away the slough.

EMERGENCY ESCHAROTOMY Incise the eschar down the length of the patient's limb; if necessary in two or more sites, and avoiding tendons and vessels. You may have to incise any burnt area, and cut across joints, so don't be limited by Figure 58-12.

ROUTINE ESCHAROTOMY Cut very lightly partly through the tough thickened dermis. Thrust the points of artery forceps through into the subcutaneous fat, then separate them to open the incision. Like this, you will avoid cutting vessels. Pull off the tough stinking pieces of eschar. The patient's wound will gape open, and bleed, perhaps for some hours, so watch him carefully.

CAUTION ! (1) Don't make deep cuts. (2) Never deslough more than 10% of the surface of his body at one time.

Bleeding may be troublesome. Control it with pressure and warm packs, or hydrogen peroxide (10 vols %), and tie or undersew larger vessels. If necessary, apply haemostatic gauze. Raise his limb.

If the raw area is suitable (57.3), graft immediately. This is the best choice if it is practical.

If his burns are not clean or if there is excessive bleeding, either: (1) Apply an antibacterial dressing or vaseling gauze and send him back to the ward. Clean his wounds with saline baths three times daily for a week. Then bring him back to the theatre later for grafting. Or, (2) take skin grafts now, store them (57.8), and apply them a few days later in the ward when his wound is clean.

Alternatively, use soaks, as in the saline method (58.16).

58.19 Grafting burns

Grafting is described in Chapter 57. All full thickness burns more than 2 cm in diameter need it. Before you can graft a burn, the dead tissue over it has to be removed. You can do this in two ways: (1) In some small deep burns you can, *very occasionally,* excise the wound and graft it, either immediately or in the first 3 days, as in Section 58.17. Or, (2) you can allow the dead tissue to demarcate itself, and graft the wound after desloughing, *usually between the 10th and 18th day.* There is thus an early and a late period for grafting, and seldom any indication to graft between the 3rd and 10th day. As a general rule, *don't delay beyond the 18th day.* One of the commonest errors is not to graft early enough, or not to graft at all!

Is the patient's skin regenerating naturally? Don't graft his burn if you can see that the skin is starting to regenerate. This is easy to see in a black skin—look for little greyish patches of regenerating skin at regular intervals in the depths of the burn. In a white skin, look for dull white or pink patches the size of a pin's head or larger ('leopard spots'.)

Graft any burn where grafting might possibly help, and don't delay merely because skin is slowly growing inwards from the edges. If you wait to allow a large burn to heal from the edges, you may have to wait a long time and when skin does finally cover the burnt area, it will be thin, pale, and more likely to become cancerous, or to break down later. Grafts take best on favourable granulation tissue (57.3), especially if this forms on the remains of the dermis. They take badly on yellow fat, and are likely to take better on the deep fascia. If granulations are favourable, a graft will probably take. If they are unfavourable, apply saline dressings (if possible three times daily), or 1% acetic acid, or hypochlorite ('Eusol'). If you are not sure the graft is going to take, be sure to mesh it.

Timing is critical. If you graft too early, you may occasionally graft unnecessarily. If you wait too long, you may find that in a few burns grafting was not necessary after all, but in most cases the granulations will be older, the graft will take less well, and the fibrosis and contractures will be worse. *Make the mistake of grafting too often rather than not often enough.*

When you have grafted a full thickness burn, it may look rather nice to begin with, but during the following months the scar is likely to become larger, ugly, bumpy, vascular, red, and itchy. If a patient is fortunate during the following years, it will

PRIORITY AREAS FOR GRAFTING

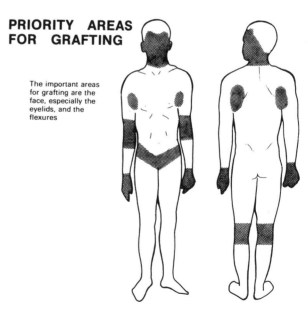

The important areas for grafting are the face, especially the eyelids, and the flexures

Fig. 58-14. THE PRIORITY AREAS FOR GRAFTING are a patient's eyelids, the front of his neck, his axillae, the front of his elbows, his hands, his groin, his popliteal fossae, and his ankles. His scalp, beard area, the back of his elbows, or the front of his knees have a low priority.
Kindly contributed by Jack Cason

becomes flatter and paler, and stop itching. If he is unfortunate, a keloid will form and grow.

**THE TIMING OF A GRAFT IS CRITICAL
DON'T GRAFT MORE THAN 10% OF THE BODY AT
ONE OPERATION**

GRAFTING BURNS

If skin for grafting is scarce, use it as patches or mesh (56-7), *except over joints where sheet grafts will be better at preventing contractures.* Place these sheets so that the joins between them go across a joint rather than along it, and thus minimize the risk of a serious contracture forming. You will use the grafts most efficiently if you leave a little space between them, because the epithelium will grow across the spaces.

If there is not enough skin to graft all a patient's burns, give priority to the areas in Fig. 58-14, because these are the places where contractures are most likely to develop.

Skin readily regenerates from the scalp and the beard area, so these have a low priority for grafting. In practice, you will usually find yourself grafting whatever area is fit for it.

CAUTION ! Never graft more than 10% of a patient's surface area at one operation (unless you are expert and have good facilities), or he may die from hypovolaemic shock. An adult may lose a litre of blood, or more, when you graft a 10% burn, so have blood ready. Before you graft, make sure his haemoglobin is more than 10 g/dl, and that he is not losing weight.

58.20 Preventing infection in burns

It is here that crowded district hospitals differ most significantly from the sophisticated burns units of the industrial world, although these too have problems with infection. You may have no facilities for barrier nursing, or even for boiling the linen.

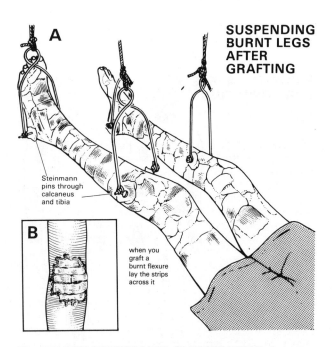

SUSPENDING BURNT LEGS AFTER GRAFTING

A

Steinmann pins through calcaneus and tibia

B

when you graft a burnt flexure lay the strips across it

Fig. 58-15 TWO METHODS FOR GRAFTING BURNS. A, suspending a patient's legs. The entire circumference of his legs has been burnt, so Steinmann pins have been passed through his tibia and calcaneus on both sides, with the aim of keeping pressure off them and avoiding touching them. B, if a flexure needs grafting, lay strips of graft across it. The scars that form between them will then go across the flexure rather than along it. *Kindly contributed by Jack Cason.*

Sterile supplies, gloves, dressing, and sometimes even soap and water may be scarce. You will probably have few nurses, who change rapidly, and have only hazy ideas about bacteria and how they spread. The care of burns is an enormous burden to them. The patient's relatives may be at the bedside 24 hours a day, bringing with them bacteria from the outside world. How can you improve your present practice? What is the bare minimum of preventive measures that you should insist on? Here are some ideas.

PREVENTING INFECTION

Cover raw burnt surfaces as soon as possible with: (1) a dry crust (the exposure method), or (2) a clean dressing (the occlusive method), or (3) a biological dressing (skin grafting).

Make sure the staff know how bacteria spread (1) by staff–to–patient and patient–to–patient contact, and (2) by flies. So exclude flies with mosquito nets, or gauze on the windows, and make the staff wash their hands before and after touching any patient or his bed. Set the example by doing it yourself.

Keep a separate plastic apron for each patient. Make the staff wear this when they handle him. If possible, they should wear disposable plastic gloves when they do so.

Use antiseptic rather than antibacterial topical agents, because resistance is less likely to develop to them. Don't rely on antibiotics. Have an antibiotic policy (2.7), and change the antibiotics, and particularly the topical agents you use every few months.

WASH YOUR HANDS !

58.21 Systemic antibiotics for burns

Organisms are found on all burns, so their mere presence in a burn is not an indication for chemotherapy (the only exception is *Strep. pyogenes*). The signs of clinical infection are fever, cellulitis, lymphangitis, lymphadenitis, and septicaemia. Of the patients who die from infection, about half die from septicaemia, and the rest from bronchopneumonia.

There is no evidence that prophylactic antibiotics are effective, so only give them when there are signs of systemic infection, such as fever or toxicity. Penicillin is perhaps the only exception, so give all severe burns a five day course immediately on admission, and then stop it. This will help to control Streptococci, and Clostridia, including *Cl tetani*. If you isolate or suspect *Pseudomonas* infection, and have only been using gentamicin sparingly, it is likely to be the antibiotic of choice.

Above all, don't forget to let out pus! If it is under an eschar, drain it. If it is under a failed occlusive dressing, remove the dressing. If pus is present and is not removed, antibiotics will not help!

58.22 Local (topical) antibacterial agents

Local antibacterial agents (chlorhexidine, povidone iodine, and silver sulphadiazine, etc.) are not essential, and *local antibiotics (soframycin, etc.) are useless.* Local antibacterial agents must be safe, because they can readily be absorbed through the surface of a burn. The cheapest local application for a burn is open air, which the exposure method makes good use of. Another is saline (58.16). Soap and water are useful, preferably as a shower, rather than a bath, because of the risk of cross infection.

Vaseline gauze is sometimes useful for its physical rather than its antibacterial properties, and if you don't have any, make it. For use on burns it should if possible be impregnated with with an antibacterial agent, such as 0.5% chlorhexidine. In any wound you can use vaseline gauze once only, *but not again.* If you use it repeatedly, enough small pieces may be left behind to form a granuloma. Instead, use plain gauze and soak it off.

The occlusive method of treating a burn should have an antibacterial agent to control the growth of bacteria under it. The few useful ones are expensive and include: (1) 1% silver sulphadiazine cream. This has most of the advantages of silver nitrate, without its disadvantages. Unfortunately, few hospitals can afford it. It is cheaper if your pharmacy can make it as described below. Don't rely on it because it is laborious to make and big burns need a lot of it. (2) 0.5% silver nitrate alone or with 0.2% chlorhexidine. The difficulty with silver nitrate is that it is very messy and stains everything brown. You may have to discard all stained linen and blankets. If it were not for this it would be much more widely used.

Outpatients need a dressing on their burns. If you don't put something on a child's burn, his mother will treat it herself, and she may even use dung. Make sure that his burn has a satisfactory dressing, and that she knows how to care for it.

TOPICAL ANTIBIOTICS HAVE NO PLACE IN BURNS

MAKING DRESSINGS FOR BURNS

VASELINE GAUZE

Spread vaseline onto layers of ordinary gauze. Place them in a tin and autoclave them.

SILVER SULPHADIAZINE FOR BURNS

REAGENTS Sulphadiazine (or sulphadimidine) 146 500 mg tabs. Silver nitrate crystals 48.5 g. Sodium hydroxide pellets 11.5 g. Glycerine 1440 ml. Liquid paraffin 560 ml. Non–ionic emulsifying wax 1100 g. Hibitane solution (ICI), 5% 320 ml. Sterile distilled water as required.

METHOD Find a 10 litre bucket, a mixer, a mixing rod, a beaker, and a heater.

Dissolve the sodium hydroxide in about 100 ml of water. Dissolve the silver nitrate in 4000 ml of water.

Suspend the sulphadiazine tabs in 1000 ml water and stir. Heat to boiling point and add to the suspension the solution of sodium hydroxide while stirring.

Slowly add the solution of silver nitrate to the suspension of sulphadimidine and sodium hydroxide. A white precipitate of silver sulphadiazine will form.

Stop adding more silver nitrate when a brown precipitate of silver oxide shows that the formation of silver sulphadiazine is complete. Boil for some minutes to make the precipitate finer and more easily filterable.

Separate the precipitate: (1) by centrifugation, or (2) with an old glass filter, or (3) by letting it stand overnight, and pouring off the supernatant. Wash the precipitate many times with water until you can detect no more silver ions in the supernatant (add a few drops to some saline and watch for a white precipitate of silver chlride).

Mix together the glycerine, the liquid paraffin, and the, emulsfying wax, and sterilize them at 150°C for an hour. Let them cool and add the Hibitane solution warmed to 80°C.

Mix the two preparations and stir vigorously to obtain a fine pink cream. Put the bucket into cold water and mix until cold. Meanwhile, add enough distilled water to bring the volume up to 8 litres before the preparation becomes cold.

58.23 Difficulties with infected burns

If a patient's temperature rises, watch his temperature chart. Fever is the first sign of infection. In adults, it often indicates septicaemia, but a child may have an intercurrent viral infection.

Sometimes, a patient's temperature does not rise when he becomes septicaemic, so the diagnosis can be difficult.

Other causes of fever include: (1) Infection of the burn itself. (2) Infection of an infusion site (change the drip). (3) Urinary infection (examine his urine). (4) Respiratory infection (X-ray his chest). Septicaemia may follow infection by any of these routes, and causes many deaths in severe burns. Even a small burn can be a source of infection. Fever continuously over 39.5°C with mental confusion makes a diagnosis of septicaemia likely. Petechial haemorrhages in unburnt areas and an enlarged spleen are rare in the septicaemia caused by burns, so don't expect to find them.

If possible, take a blood culture, and culture the burn before giving the patient any antibiotic. At least stain a film and find out if he has predominantly Gram positive cocci, or Gram negative bacilli. This will be some help in deciding which antibiotic to give (2.7). *Pseudomonas* is a common and deadly invader. Give the most appropriate antibiotic intravenously in high doses.

DIFFICULTIES WITH INFECTED BURNS

If a CHILD IS APATHETIC and is obviously NOT WELL, look for petechial haemorrhages in his burn. If you find them suspect streptococcal infection, and give him penicillin—urgently!

If you DON'T KNOW THE ORGANISMS, give him intravenous gentamicin, unless you know you have gentamicin resistant organisms in the ward. If so amikacin is an alternative. If possible, isolate him.

If a patient's TEMPERATURE RISES to 39.5°C, and you have no other way of reducing his fever, expose his burn and turn a fan on it. He may develop hyperpyrexia. Chlorpromazine may help if his blood pressure is adequate.

If RIGORS AND FEVER are followed by a sudden fall in blood pressure, mental confusion, and apathy, with occasionally diarrhoea hypothermia, oliguria, and hypotension, he is probably in septic shock (53.4).

If he shows SIGNS OF SEPTICAEMIA OR SEPTIC SHOCK and there is a GREEN STAIN on the dressings, suspect *Pseudomonas* septicaemia. give him gentamicin, and apply hypochlorite ('Eusol') to the burn.

If SEPSIS IS EXTENDING and is going deeper, the possible agents which might control it are silver sulphadiazine, or silver nitrate.

58.24 Preventing contractures

You can minimize all contractures and prevent many of them completely by using quite simple methods. *Failure to apply these methods is one of the commonest mistakes in treating burns.* Some of them have already been discussed: (1) Prevent full thickness skin loss where possible, by preventing infection from making superficial burns into deep ones (58.20). (2) If skin for grafting is scarce, make sure you always graft burnt joints (58.19). (3) When you graft them use sheets, rather than patch grafts or mesh. (4) Arrange the sheets of grafted skin so that the joins between them go across the flexor surface of a joint rather than along it (58-15). This will avoid lines of healing along a joint that will later form contractures. (5) Before you graft, scrape away most of the granulation tissue, so that only a thin layer remains. This will reduce the subsequent fibrosis under the graft.

The scar tissue that forms a contracture was once granulation tissue. The deeper a patient's burn, and the longer you leave it ungrafted, the more granulation tissue there will be, the worse his scar, and the greater the risk of contracture—*so graft early!*

UNGRAFTED
GRANULATIONS→FIBROSIS→CONTRACTURES

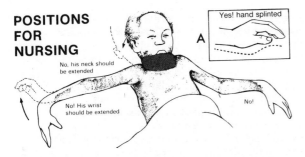

POSITIONS FOR NURSING

No, his neck should be extended

Yes! hand splinted

A

No! His wrist should be extended

No!

Failure to follow these simple procedures is one of the commonest errors in treating burns

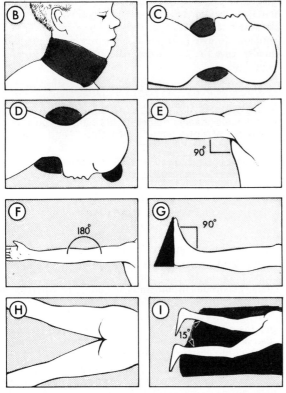

Fig. 58-16 THE POSITIONS FOR NURSING to prevent contractures are critically important. This is one of the most important figures in this chapter. Nurse a burnt neck in extension, either on a pillow or with a collar as in B, C, and D. The neck of patient A, is not extended enough, nor are his wrists extended enough. If a patient's axilla is burnt, abduct his burnt arm to 90° (A, and E), or extend it above his head. If his cubital fossa is burnt, extend his elbows (F) using splints or sandbags. Keep his burnt ankle at 90° (G). Extend his burnt hips and knees (H, and I). If his popliteal fossa is burnt, persuade him to keep his knee straight, as much as possible, for several months after discharge, even when he is sitting in a chair. *Modified from a contribution by Jack Cason.*

The great danger of a scar is that as it contracts it will pull part of the patient's body into an abnormal position, particularly if he is a child, because he will grow but his scar will not. The abnormal position is usually the position of rest, and a bad one for function. Most contractures are the result of burns on the flexor surfaces—they flex a patient's elbows, his hips, his knees, and his neck, and they adduct his arms, as in A, Fig. 58-18. The exceptions are the extensor contractures of his wrist and fingers, which commonly follow deep burns on the back of his hand.

Preventing contractures is usually a compromise between: (1) Splinting a patient's burnt joint in extension for several months, which will prevent the contracture, but may stiffen the joint permanently, often in a bad position for function. And, (2) trying to mobilize a burnt joint early, which will increase its mobility, but will not prevent the contracture. The best compromise between splinting and mobility depends on the joint

and how cooperative its owner is. For example, a hand has priority for early grafting, and should be mobilized as soon as it is healed. An intelligent and cooperative patient, who can be trusted to exercise and mobilize his burnt joint, and will apply a night splint, can be told to do so. A less intelligent and cooperative one will be best with his joint in a cast in the extended position. For example, go for mobility with a burnt finger of a teacher, but, if an epileptic of subnormal intelligence has burnt his popliteal fossa, put him in a plaster cylinder for several months. These represent the extremes, with other cases you will have to achieve a compromise.

Stiffness is seldom serious until a joint has been immobilized for 3 weeks in an adult or 6 weeks in a child, so *the usual compromise is to splint a joint in extension continously for not more than 3 weeks in an adult (6 weeks if necessary in a child), while the skin over it heals, and then to mobilize it.* After this it can be splinted only at night for a few more weeks, if the patient is fortunate, or for many months if he is not. Three weeks immobility allows partial thickness burns to heal, so contractures should not form. It is deep burns which take longer to heal that are at risk.

Use splints and traction to keep a patient's limb in the opposite position from that of the expected contracture. Use any simple splint that will do this. The dynamic splints in Fig. 58-19, are ideal in the later stages, but in the earlier ones *any simple splint is much better than nothing.* No two burns are exactly the same, so you will need considerable ingenuity. There are two important kinds of splint: (1)Those applied initially which a patient wears all the time, and (2) those applied later which he only wears at night. Splints need care—don't let them cause ulcers in newly grafted skin!

A patient's contractures may continue to form for a year or more after discharge, so continue the appropriate night splinting while he is an outpatient, and see him regularly. Even splinting for a year may be followed by contractures during the next six months. *Earlier on, they can form in a few days.* If he is the child of a village mother, try hard to make her understand what a night splint is for, and why she must apply it. Only too often you will see a contracture, which you have carefully released, recur, because she did not understand or use the night splint you gave her.

You will need the continued help of a physiotherapist, and if you don't have one, you will have to train somebody to fill this role. Make sure he understands what he has to do.

Hypertrophic scars can be prevented by applying a pressure garment for several years if necessary, but you will probably find this impractical.

Finally, remember that if a patient lies continually in the same position because of a burn elsewhere, contractures can form in his *unburnt* limbs, as happened to Pepita in Fig. 58-1!

PREVENTING CONTRACTURES

NURSING BURNT JOINTS

Nurse a burns patient in the positions shown in Fig. 58-16. Protect all his bony points from pressure sores—his elbows, trochanters, ischial tuberosities, and his heels. Use a combination of padding, pillows, frequent turning, and splinting. Putting him in the right position to begin with may be painful, so, if necessary, sedate him, or give him ketamine while you do it.

CAUTION ! Pressure sores can form in a burnt patient almost as easily as in a paraplegic.

SPECIAL SITES FOR CONTRACTURES IN BURNS PATIENTS

NECK Try to keep a patient's burnt neck away from his chest. Put a pad under his shoulders to extend his neck, as in C, Fig. 58-16. If he is lying on his front, put a pad under his forehead to extend his neck and free his airway (D). Examine his back and the front of his head repeatedly for pressure sores.

SKIN TRACTION FOR A BURNS CONTRACTURE

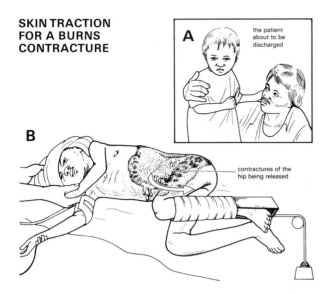

Fig. 58-17 SKIN TRACTION FOR A BURNS CONTRACTURE. When you treat a knee make sure that pressure over the head of the patient's fibula does not cause foot drop. Some loss of flexion in a knee is not important, and is probably inevitable anyway. But you must preserve full extension. If necessary, apply a plaster cylinder for 12 weeks or longer. *Kindly contributed by Gerald Hankins.*

Or, place a mattress under him only as far as his shoulders, so that his head falls backwards. If you raise the head of his bed, he will probably tolerate this well.

Continue with a bulky neck bandage for 6 to 12 months, or use a plastic foam collar, or a neck cast, watching carefully for pressure sores.

AXILLA Abduct his arm to 90°. In a child try forearm traction as in Fig. 72-11, or use traction to raise his arm above his head.

ELBOW Extend the patient's elbow, and apply a splint, or maintain this position with pillows and sandbags.

CAUTION ! (1) Don't let his arm fall backwards, because the head of his humerus may be forced forwards and injure his brachial plexus. (2) Don't let pressure cause sores on his elbow, or an ulnar paralysis.

HANDS See Section 58.29.

HIPS AND KNEES Extend a patient's hips and knees and abduct his legs about 15°. Use roller towels held in place by sandbags, or a plaster splint between his lower legs.

Ask him to keep his hips and knees as straight as he can for several weeks, and don't let him flex his knees when sitting on a chair. If necessary, fit him with a posterior plaster slab for a few weeks.

CAUTION ! (1) Make sure that pressure over the head of his fibula does not cause foot drop. (2) Some loss of flexion in a knee is not important, and is probably inevitable anyway. But you *must* preserve full extension. If necessary, apply a plaster cylinder for 12 weeks or longer.

FEET AND ANKLES Prevent foot drop or contractures behind a patient's heels. Keep his feet at 90° with right angle splints or foot blocks or sand bags. Support his thighs and legs on pillows to prevent pressure sores forming on his heels. In infants use blocks of plastic foam as pillows.

If contractures are starting to form, serial casting (26.1) may correct them.

KEEP THE LIMB IN THE OPPOSITE POSITION TO THE CONTRACTURE
PREVENT STIFFNESS BY MOBILIZING BURNT JOINTS EARLY
PREVENT CONTRACTURES BY EARLY SPLINTING IN EXTENSION

SOME SEVERE CONTRACTURES

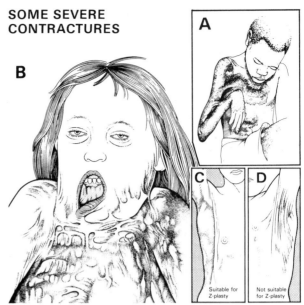

Fig. 58-18 A CONTRACTURE OF THE NECK AND AXILLA. The girl has contractures of her neck and axilla; the boy has contractures of his axilla, elbow, and wrist. If their joints had been splinted in the positions shown in Fig. 58-16, their contractures would probably have been prevented. They would certainly be much less severe. Note the web contractures adducting patient A's shoulder and flexing his elbow. C, a narrow contracture which is suitable for Z—plasty and D, a broad one which is not. *Kindly contributed by Jack Cason, Ian McGregor, and Peter Bewes.*

58.25 Treating broad burns contractures

You might be surprised that as a 'generalist' you should ever have to release a burns contracture! Unfortunately, if you don't, it is likely that nobody else will, because your nearest plastic surgeon will probably have a waiting list which is years long. *While a child is waiting for a bed in a referral hospital, his contracture is likely to become an incurable deformity.* In the district hospital studied in Section 1.4, releasing contractures formed 2% of all the operations done under general anaesthesia, so this is not an uncommon task. If you are persistent and careful, you will not find them as difficult as you might expect. You have skin loss to cope with, so they are more difficult than polio contractures (26.2). Postoperative care is half the battle.

Contractures of a patient's larger joints are not too difficult, but those of his hand are tasks for an expert, yet you may have to try. They are certainly not the contractures to start with. If you do have to attempt them, gain experience with larger joints first. Contractures on the palm are slightly less difficult than those on the back of the hand, where a patient's MP joints readily become hyperextended, as part of a claw hand. They are close to the surface and are easily burnt. Fortunately, a child's joints don't become stiff nearly so easily as those of an adult. After you have grafted the flexor surfaces of a child's fingers, you can safely immobilize them in extension.

Contractures may be linear or, more commonly, broad. Aim to: (1) Excise linear ones with a Z—plasty (58.26). (2) Release broad ones widely without excising them, then graft the bare area with a medium or thick split skin graft. Splint the patient's limb in a position opposite from the contracture, and start exercises as soon as the graft has taken.

We advise you to graft with sheets of thick split skin. If the graft is large and you are inexpert, you may be wise to mesh them. Experts seldom do this and often use full thickness grafts, especially for hands.

Make children your first priority, you will be much less successful with adults. *Don't try to relieve burns contractures by using serial casts (26.1)!*

THE GENERAL METHOD FOR A BROAD
CONTRACTURE

Wait until the patient's burn has healed completely.

ANAESTHESIA Ketamine or general anaesthesia. This is not a task for the minor theatre. Check that the patient's haemoglobin is over 10 g/dl. Have blood cross matched.

Start by taking skin from the donor site. When his contracture is straightened out, you will need more skin than you expect.

Infiltrate into and under the contracture a mixture of saline 80 ml, 2% lignocaine 20 ml, adrenaline 1:1000 0.5 ml, and preferably hyaluronidase 1 ampoule ('jungle juice' see A 5.4). This solution will: (1) Demonstrate the tissue planes more clearly. (2) Allow you to separate the scar more easily. (3) Control bleeding. (4) Reduce the amount of general anaesthetic he needs.

Cut through the scar down to the patient's subcutaneous tissue, in the middle of the contracture. Keep it under tension as you do so. If necessary, cut right down to his tendons. *If possible, separate the scar from his deeper tissues by blunt dissection. Push your scissors into the tissues, then open them.* This will help you to avoid any superficial veins. You will probably be wise not to try to excise the scar, either in the main part of the contracture, or at its upper or lower ends.

CAUTION! (1) Release the contracture first, and then decide if you need to excise any scar tissue. (2) Don't cut his deep fascia, unless the scar tissue extends right through it. (3) Contractures will take longer to release than you expect. (4) Beware of congested veins, especially in his axilla and neck.

Carry the incision beyond the limits of the scar tissue, and beyond the axes of the joint on each side. If you don't do this, the contracture will recur. Or, make a double–Y, as in Fig. 58-21; this will reduce the length of the incision you need to make.

Cover the bare area with a sheet split skin graft, and sew it in place. If you are worried about it taking, mesh it.

CAUTION ! Graft the exposed raw areas immediately, especially over joints. This will reduce the risk of the contracture recurring, and the risk of infecting the joint.

Splint the patient's limb in the opposite position to the contracture, until the graft has taken. When the time comes to remove the dressing, do this yourself. Keep him in a night splint *for at least 3 months.* Review him regularly and add more skin as necessary.

NECK CONTRACTURES FOR RELEASE

If a patient's chin is contracted down on his sternum as in Fig. 58-18, refer him if you possibly can. His anaesthetic problems are considerable.

ANAESTHESIA You cannot intubate a patient while he has a contracture of his neck. So, give him ketamine, infiltrate the scar with anaesthetic solution, release it, and then, if necessary, intubate him.

METHOD Incise the scar transversely, if necessary almost from ear to ear. Carefully release the scar tissue by blunt dissection to reveal a huge gap in the front and sides of the patient's neck.

Apply a sheet of split skin graft and a wet cotton wool dressing, as for the axilla. Immobilize his neck with his head well extended. To prevent recurrence, keep his neck in extension. Apply a soft collar as soon as his skin is soundly healed, and leave it there for at least 6 months. He must wear a night splint for several more months.

If necessary, repeat the procedure, several times if required, to obtain a little more movement each time.

AXILLARY CONTRACTURES FOR RELEASE

Try to restore full abduction and elevation in a single operation. A Z–plasty will probably be best if the contracture is narrow (58.26).

If the patient has a broad contracture, incise the scar as above, and abduct his arm. Apply a large medium thickness split skin graft to the bare areas, and dress it with wet wool (57-7), so as to fill the dome of his axilla. Cover this with plenty of dry wool, and bandage this (preferably with crepe bandages) to include his whole arm as well as his axilla and chest.

If he is a small child, a large ball of cotton wool bandaged into his axilla may hold his arm in the right position.

If he is an older child or an adult, raise his head and back on a suitable support (as for a hip spica Fig. 77-4), and apply a plaster shoulder spica to include his arm and hand, with his arm at 90° from his chest, his elbow flexed, and his wrist dorsiflexed. This is the most comfortable position.

CAUTION ! (1) Don't injure a patient's axillary vessels or nerves. (2) Don't hyperabduct his shoulder, or you may paralyse his brachial plexus.

ELBOW CONTRACTURES FOR RELEASE

A large scar may involve the whole flexor surface of a patient's elbow. Make a cautious transverse incision across the fold of his elbow, starting laterally, and trying to avoid any congested veins. If the whole width of his elbow is involved, extend the incision into healthy tissue beyond the axis of the joint on each side.

Find a fatty layer and then work gently medially. If you have found the right fatty plane, you should be able to slide the scar tissue up and down his arm. When the incision is complete, divide any deeper strands of fibrous tissue.

Fill the large diamond shaped gap with a medium thickness split skin graft. Cover it with a wet cotton wool stent, as in Fig. 57-7. Immobilize his extended and supinated elbow in a cast which should also immobilize his hand. Dress the graft at 7 to 10 days. When it has taken, apply a cast in extension, for at least 6 to 12 weeks. You are operating for a flexion contracture, so lack of flexion will not be a problem.

HAND CONTRACTURES FOR RELEASE

Try one of the dynamic splints in Fig. 58-19. If the patient's contracture is mild, this may cure it. If it is severe, a dynamic

DYNAMIC SPLINTS

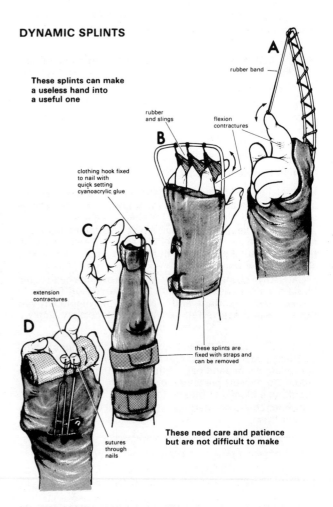

These splints can make a useful hand into a useful one

rubber band

rubber and slings

flexion contractures

clothing hook fixed to nail with quick setting cyanoacrylic glue

extension contractures

these splints are fixed with straps and can be removed

sutures through nails

These need care and patience but are not difficult to make

Fig. 58-19 SOME DYNAMIC SPLINTS. These are a great help in preventing the disastrously contracted hands in Fig. 58-26. *Kindly contributed by Jack Cason.*

splint may partially correct the deformity, so that operation will be easier.

If a patient's metacarpophalangeal joints are hyperextended as part of a claw hand, try to refer him, particularly if he presents late with a gross deformity. This is a particularly difficult contracture, because the capsules of his joints may need opening up and freeing. If you cannot refer him, make transverse incisions over their dorsal surfaces, flex them, graft the gap, and splint his hand in the position of function.

If his wrist is hyperextended, and he presents reasonably early, divide the scar transversely, and apply a medium thickness split skin graft—beware of his median nerve and ulnar artery!

If he has contractures on the flexor surfaces of his fingers, incise them transversely well beyond the axis of the joint, and fill the gap with a full thickness graft, or a thick split skin graft sewn into place.

If he is a child, splint his fingers in extension for 3 months, or the contracture will recur. To help the cast stay in place, apply it with his wrist extended. Examine the cast daily at first, and later weekly, to make sure it has not slipped.

If he is an adult, don't immobilize his extended fingers for more than 10 days. If necessary, use dynamic splints as in Fig. 58-19, and night splints.

If a patient has a very severe finger deformity, you may need to amputate a finger, or arthrodese it in the position of function.

GROIN, KNEE, ANKLE, AND FOOT CONTRACTURES FOR RELEASE

Follow the general method, as described above, taking care to extend the incision well beyond the axis of the joint.

DIFFICULTIES WITH BURNS CONTRACTURES

If you CANNOT GET SUFFICIENT RELEASE of a contracture in a single stage, release it as much as you can; consider splinting it, leaving it open, trying to release it further in a few day's time, and then grafting it.

If there is an ULCER within a scar, excise it.

MANY SEVERE CONTRACTURES ARE LARGELY THE RESULT OF POOR CARE

58.26 Z–plasties for narrow contractures

A Z–plasty is a useful way of releasing a patient's contracture—if it is narrow enough. It is not an easy method, but if your result is not perfect, you can always graft any bare areas that remain. Good results are easier to achieve than with a wide contracture which needs inset grafts. Make a Z–plasty by excising the scar and then cutting two flaps in the form of equilateral triangles which share one common limb, and so form a Z. When you extend the patient's limb, the triangular flaps will change their positions spontaneously.

Initially, the two triangles together form a parallelogram, with its shorter diagonal in the line of the contracture, and its longer diagonal transversely across it, as in C, Fig. 58-20. Releasing the contracture and transposing the two triangles changes the shape of the parallelogram, so that the new contracture diagonal is the same length as the transverse diagonal was before, as in D, in this figure. The difference in length between the two diagonals determines the amount of lengthening in one direction and shortening in the other.

Transposing the triangular flaps: (1) Gains length in the line where the contracture was and so relieves it. (2) Makes any extra elasticity that there may be across a scar available up and down it. It may extend the length of the contracture diagonal by a least a third, at the expense of the skin on either side. (3) Changes the direction of a scar, from one which runs along a flexure to

one which runs across it. Expert plastic surgeons find this useful for changing the direction of a facial scar, so that it lies in a line of election (61-3).

If you make one large 'Z', all the transverse shortening, and all the tension is concentrated in one transverse diagonal (E, and F, in Fig. 58-20). But, if you make multiple 'Zs', the lengthening is additive, because all the contracture diagonals are in the same line, but the transverse shortening is spread out over several smaller 'Zs' (G, and H). In practice, you will not achieve quite as much lengthening with multiple 'Zs' as you would expect, but it is still a very useful method.

Unfortunately, most burns usually cause scarring in all directions, so that there is no lax tissue at either side, and a Z–plasty is unsuitable. But in those burns where it is suitable, it is very effective.

Z–PLASTIES

INDICATIONS The occasional patient with a narrow contracture of his axilla, elbows, fingers, knee, or neck, especially

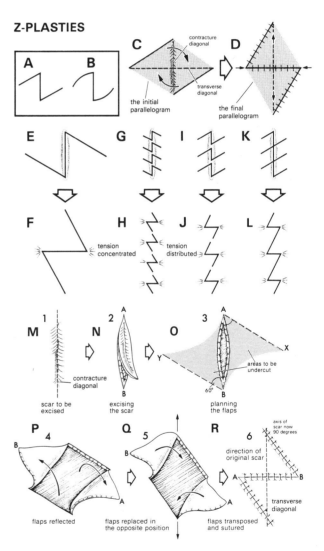

Fig. 58-20 Z-PLASTIES. A, how flaps are usually cut. B, how to cut them if you are doubtful about their blood supply. C, the initial parallelogram before transposition of the flaps. D, the final parallelogram after transposition. Note that the contracture and transverse diagonals have exchanged lengths. E, and F, a single 'Z' showing how the lateral tension is concentrated in a single line. G, and H, multiple 'Zs' distributing the lateral tension. I, and J, the same but with fewer larger 'Zs'. K, and L, the 'Zs' joined up. M, the scar. N, the scar excised. O, the flaps planned. P, the flaps raised. Q, the flaps transposed. R, the flaps in place. *With the kind permission of Ian McGregor*

one of the bowstring type, provided the surrounding tissues are reasonably lax and undamaged. Only a few burns contractures are of this kind. If there is no transverse slack tissue to start with, a Z–plasty will not work.

A single 'Z' extending the whole length of the patient's contracture. There is a large quantity of lax tissue to be brought in from the sides, and the the bowstring is sufficiently deep for the base of the flaps not to extend much onto the surrounding flat skin—if they do, multiple 'Zs' would be wiser.

Multiple 'Zs' The available lax tissue is not available at one point, but is spread out along the length of the scar.

CONTRAINDICATIONS (1) Narrow contractures, when the surrounding tissues are not reasonably lax, or the flaps would be scarred. (2) Broad contractures.

If you cannot refer the patient, proceed as follows.

SINGLE 'Z' Use a pen to draw the position of the central limb on the patient's skin, the longer it is the more length you will gain. Its length will however be limited by the amount of loose tissue available at the sides.

You have two alternative ways of choosing the flaps. Select the best one like this. Draw equilateral triangles on either side of the central limb, in both of the possible ways. Choose the flaps which: (1) have the better blood supply, (2) avoid scarring across the base, (3) will give the best cosmetic result, and (4) are likely to rotate most easily. If you complete the quadrilateral, with its contractural and transverse diagonals, you will see how much increase in length you can expect, after you have transposed the flaps.

CAUTION ! (1) Angle the flaps as near to 60° as you can. Use a precut 60° pattern. Remember that the angles of an equilateral triangle are 60°. (2) Make the sides the same length as the central limb, except that if one flap is scarred, cut it a little longer than the other. (3) If you are worried about the possible viability of a flap, curve it a little, as in B, Fig. 58-20. (4) The tip of a 'Z' is most likely to necrose, so make sure you cut it deep enough. If necessary include some of the underlying scar tissue.

Check the geometry of your flaps by joining their free ends. The transverse diagonal should pass through the middle of the contracture diagonal.

Extend the patient's limb to show the full extent of the scar, and then excise it in a narrow elliptical incision. Don't make the flaps out of the scarred band itself, or they will slough.

Undermine the triangles so formed, so as to raise two flaps as thickly as the tissue will allow, while obeying the rules in Fig. 58-20. Extend the patient's limb so as to allow the flaps to fall into the opposite positions, and stitch them up with fine monofilament. At the tips use a half buried horizontal mattress suture (54-8).

If you have designed the flaps properly, you will not need to transpose them actively; they will fall naturally into position.

CAUTION ! (1) Handle flaps with skin hooks. (2) Control bleeding meticulously. (3) If bare areas remain (as they often do), don't close the plasty under tension, instead graft them. (4) Bandage the limb in the mid position, not at the extreme of extension, or you will impair the circulation in the flaps.

MULTIPLE 'Zs' Cut these in the same way. Either keep the Zs' separate, as in G, and I, or join them together, as in K, and L.

SPECIAL SITES FOR Z–PLASTIES

AXILLA The contracture must be linear, on one or other of the axillary folds, usually the anterior one, as in A, Fig. 58-18. If possible, avoid transferring axilliary skin, which contains hair and apocrine glands, outside the patient's axilla. Incise the scar longitudinally. If it is thick and rigid, excise it, with a 'Z' release at either end. Bring one limb of the 'Z' anteriorly, and the other one posteriorly.

If you cannot get sufficient abduction with a Z–plasty, make it in the central part of the web, and make V–shaped incisions at either end. When the patient's elbow is fully abducted, these will leave bare areas which you will have to graft.

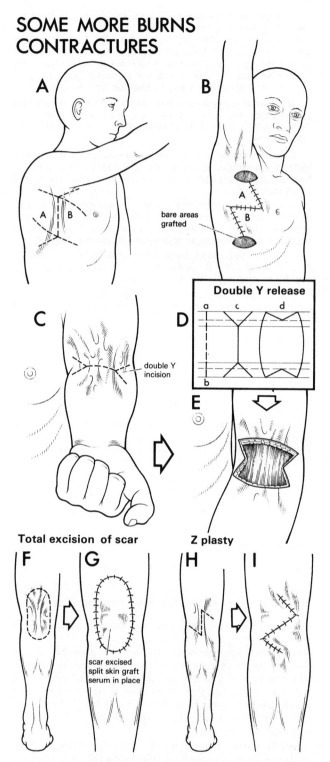

SOME MORE BURNS CONTRACTURES

bare areas grafted

Double Y release

double Y incision

Total excision of scar

Z plasty

scar excised split skin graft serum in place

Fig. 58-21 MORE METHODS FOR BURNS CONTRACTURES. A, and B, combining Z–plasties and skin grafting; a Z–plasty has been made with transverse incisions at each end of it. These have been opened to leave raw surfaces ready for grafting. C, a contracture of the elbow showing a 'double Y' release incision. D, 'a double Y' release. This will release the ends of the contracture maximally, without increasing its length: (a) to (b) the width of the scar, (c) the 'double Y' drawn to cover its full width, (d) the full release of the incision. E, a 'double Y' incision ready for grafting. F, and G, total excision of a scar with a split skin graft sewn in place. H, and I, a Z–plasty used to treat a narrow popliteal contracture. *By the kind permission of Irving Feller and William C. Grabb of the US National Institute of Burns Medicine.*

If you HAVE TO GRAFT BARE AREAS, sew the grafts in place with fine monofilament, and apply a firm dressing.

58.27 Burnt respiratory tract

Most people who are removed from a smoke filled building cough, retch, and then recover in 48 hours or less. But a burnt patient can injure his respiratory tract by inhaling smoke, and die from asphyxia due to laryngeal oedema. He can also die from pulmonary oedema, or from respiratory infection. Bronchopneumonia after burns is common, even if a patient's respiratory tract was not burnt, and unfortunately antibiotics don't prevent it. The danger signs to watch for are *severe dyspnoea and wheezing 12 to 36 hours after a burn.* If this does not respond to simple measures, there is usually little to be done.

RESPIRATORY BURNS

Admit the patient to a small room with steam from a steam kettle, or humidification from a cold humidifier. Record his pulse, temperature, and respiration 4 hourly. Take a baseline X-ray on admission and another 24 hours later. Watch for multiple fluffy shadows (the snow storm effect), interlobar shadows, hilar flare, fine linear crescentic shadows, and pneumothoraces (following explosions). Examine his sputum for soot.

If he has no abnormal signs, discharge him at 48 hours.

THE COMPLICATIONS OF RESPIRATORY BURNS.

If a patient's temperature rises, give him a broad spectrum antibiotic. If he is producing sputum, examine this and prescribe the appropriate antibiotic. Often, the same organism causes both chest and skin infections.

If he has mild signs of respiratory discomfort, encourage him to cough effectively and do breathing exercises; try postural drainage and suck out secretions.

If physiotherapy fails to clear the secretions from his respiratory tract, intubate him and apply suction using careful sterile precautions. If this fails, his only hope is tracheostomy.

SEVERE FACIAL BURNS

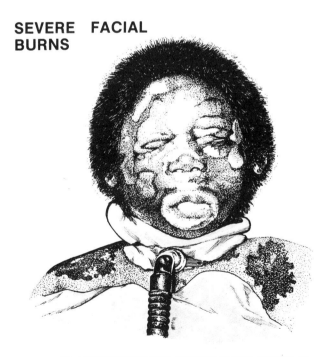

Fig. 58-22 TRACHEOSTOMY FOR SEVERE FACIAL BURNS. If a patient with facial burns has stridor, or shows inspiratory intercostal, supraclavicular or abdominal recession, try to intubate him. If this fails, do a tracheostomy.

If intubation is going to be necessary, try to do it in the first few hours, before his face has a chance to swell. Early prophylactic intubation is better than intubation later. It may save a tracheostomy, or make it easier.

If he has inspiratory stridor or wheezing, or shows inspiratory intercostal, supraclavicular, or abdominal recession, intubate him. If this fails, do a tracheostomy.

If he wheezes, or shows prolonged expiration and rales or crepitations, his bronchi are in spasm. If these signs are mild, give him bronchodilators, such as salbutamol or aminophylline. If they are severe, give one dose only of hydrocortisone or methyl predisolone under antibiotic cover. But avoid steroids if you can.

If he shows signs of pulmonary oedema, restrict his fluid intake, give him frusemide, and repeat it after some hours if necessary.

If he shows increasing respiratory distress, with dyspnoea, tachypnoea, cyanosis, tachycardia, inability to cough, exhaustion, restlessness, and altered consciousness, he will probably die. He needs mechanical ventilation and oxygen. If he also has pulmonary oedema, try PEEP (A 19.4).

CAUTION ! Don't give him too much oxygen because this may precipitate the adult respiratory distress syndrome and make him worse. 2 to 4 l/min is enough.

58.28 Burnt eyes

Burnt eyelids are much more common than burnt eyes. A patient is usually able to shut his eyes before the fire burns his corneae, so his sight is more often in danger from the burns to his lids, or from the late effects of scarring. His burnt swollen lids make his eyes shut for a few days, after which they open again.

At any time from 3 weeks onwards, his eyelids, particularly the lower ones, may start to contract and expose his cornea (ectropion). This causes conjunctivitis, exposure keratitis, corneal ulceration, perforation, and finally infection of his globe. *Try to prevent this deadly sequence by making sure that his corneae are always covered and moist.* The easiest way to do this is to keep them covered with an antibiotic eye ointment. The most radical way is to sew his eyelids together (tarsorrhaphy).

If the full thickness of the skin of his eyelids is burnt, graft them. Grafts take well on eyelids, so that grafting them is not as difficult as you might think.

If contractures start to occur, you may have to release them, do a tarsorrhaphy and then graft them. Unfortunately, this is usually only partially successful.

Treat chemical burns in the same way. The most important measure is to apply quantities of water to burnt eyes at the earliest possible moment.

BURNT EYES

EXAMINATION Examine the patient's eyes early, before they start to swell. While his eyes are closed, he will be very anxious, so see that the ward staff talk to him often.

If they have already closed, you may be able to open them using gauze and sterile gloves, or eyelid retractors. A bright shiny cornea is a good sign. Stain the patient's conjunctivae with fluorescein and look for ulcers. There are 4 grades of corneal injury. In the first two his prognosis is good.

Grade One. There is epithelial injury only.

Grade Two. The patient's cornea is hazy but you can see the details of his iris clearly.

Grade Three. There is total epithelial loss, and stromal haze. You cannot see the details of his iris. His sight will probably be impaired, but perforation is rare.

Grade Four. His opaque cornea completely obscures his iris and his pupil. His globe will probably perforate.

THE TREATMENT OF BURNT EYES

If a patient's cornea is hazy, apply chloramphenicol ointment, and atropine or homatropine eye drops.

If there are particles in his eyes, irrigate them away with saline.

If his punctae or canaliculae are damaged, pass a style or indwelling suture through them to keep them open while they scar.

If his palpebral and ocular conjunctivae start sticking to one another, separate them with a smooth glass rod, or the movements of his globe will later be limited.

If his eyelids are not completely destroyed, they will protect his eyes for about 3 weeks, before they disintegrate. Refer him early for reconstruction of his eyelids.

If all or most of his eyelids have been destroyed, dissect the conjunctiva of both lids free of his orbicularis muscle and his tarsal plates, and cover his globes by suturing the remains of his lids together. Graft their exposed surfaces. Refer him to an expert later. If necessary, use his conjunctivae only, as in Fig. 60-2.

If an eye is hopelessly damaged, it will have to be removed at some stage.

KEEPING AN EXPOSED CORNEA MOIST AFTER AN INJURY

If a patient's cornea is exposed, try the following methods of keeping it moist, in the order you see below. If one is not successful, try the next down the list.

EARLY TARSORRHAPHY

pass the sutures through the edges of his lids and keep them away from his cornea

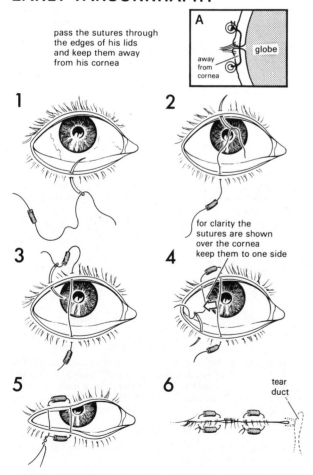

for clarity the sutures are shown over the cornea keep them to one side

tear duct

Fig. 58-23 TEMPORARY TARSORRHAPHY. A, shows how sutures pass through the opposed edged of a patient's lids, and so avoid his cornea. For ease of illustration the sutures are shown crossing the centre of his cornea. Try to keep them away from it at each side of his eye. *Kindly contributed by Peter Bewes.*

(1) Fill the patient's cornea with chloramphenicol ointment, and renew it four times daily. This is all that most patients need.

(2) Seal goggles over his orbit with adhesive strapping and cream. These will keep his cornea moist for 12 to 24 hours, but don't use them for longer, because they will macerate his whole orbit.

(3) If his eyelids are charred and tight, make relaxation incisions, if necessary combined with traction sutures from his cheeks. Try to prevent retraction of his upper eyelids, because these are the ones that protect his cornea in sleep.

(4) If these methods fail, consider an early inlay split skin graft, it may avoid tarsorraphy.

CAUTION ! (1) Don't use steroids. (2) Never apply an eye pad directly to a patient's cornea, because it may rub and ulcerate through. Even vaseline gauze can cause ulceration. If his cornea cannot be covered with its own lids, an open eye covered with antibiotic cream is safer.

TEMPORARY TARSORRHAPHY FOR AN INJURED EYE

INDICATIONS If you have kept a patient's cornea moist by the above methods, tarsorrhaphy should very rarely be necessary. It is unnecessary in the early days when his oedematous lids cover his cornea, and is unsatisfactory if his lids have been severely damaged.

ANAESTHESIA Ketamine.

METHOD Use fine monofilament and a curved needle. Make two horizontal mattress sutures through the patient's eyelids as in Fig. 58-23. Site them away from his cornea. Pass them through the skin, and out through the flat free margin of one lid, across to the flat free margin of the other lid, and then through small pieces of plastic tube.

If the burn prevents you getting his lids together, make relaxing incisions in each lid, as in A, Fig. 58-24. Cover the bare areas with split skin grafts and hold them in place by the tieover method (57-8).

CAUTION ! (1) Make sure that the sutures do not rub against his cornea, or cross it at the grey line. If possible, place them to one side of his cornea. (2) Make sure that the sutures avoid

CONTRACTURES OF THE LIDS

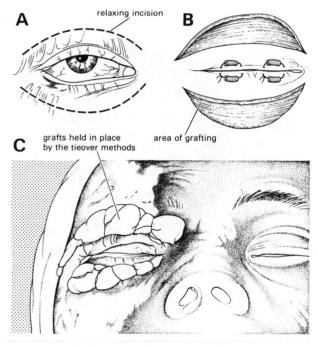

Fig. 58-24 CONTRACTURES OF THE EYELIDS. A, retraction of scar tissue has everted this patient's eyelid and exposed his cornea. **B,** relaxing incisions have been made and are ready for grafting. **C,** shows the grafts held in place by the tieover method. *Kindly contributed by Randolph Whitfield II.*

his punctuae and his canaliculae. (3) Make sure that no eyelashes press against his cornea. If he feels any scratching sensation, re-examine his eyelids immediately.

All the time that his lids are closed, irrigate his eyes with saline every 12 hours. Don't open his lids for 12 weeks.

If a patient's eyelids are burnt, graft them. If convenient, put a thick split skin graft over both lids, and cut the lids apart later. You can do this under local anaesthesia.

CONTRACTURES OF THE LIDS

INDICATIONS If contractures are already starting to expose a patient's eyelids and expose his corneae, you may have to release his lids and graft them.

Put stay sutures through his lids (23-2), so that you can move them up or down as necessary. Make the relaxation incisions shown in Fig. 58-24.

When you have prepared a satisfactory bed for the graft, and controlled bleeding, stretch it, apply a piece of split skin graft, and hold it in place with tieover sutures, or 4/0 monofilament.

If the graft contracts a few weeks later, apply another one. Don't worry too much about what the patient's eye looks like at this stage. What matters is that his cornea should not be exposed.

CAUTION ! Stretch the lid first so that there will be some slack tissue when it contracts later. The thinner the graft, the more the shrinkage. If you are skilled, apply a full thickness graft.

Primary skin grafting will not prevent ectropion, and you may need 2 or 3 operations to insert enough skin.

DON'T DELAY GRAFTING THE LIDS

RELEASING CONTRACTURES OF THE FACE

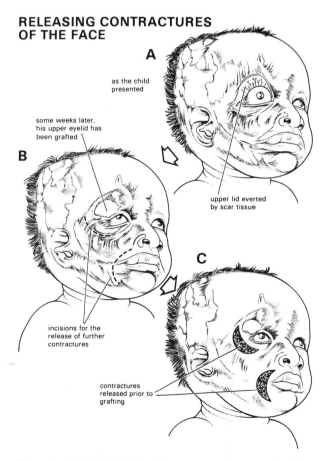

Fig. 58-25 RELEASING CONTRACTURES ON THE FACE. If you are going to graft patients like this, make sure your grafts are big enough. These grafts are on the small side, particularly the first one. *Kindly contributed by Randolph Whitfield II.*

58.29 Burnt hands and feet

The thick skin on the palms of a patient's hands usually protects them, so most burns are on the back. This swells, and as the oedema organizes his hand stiffens. Minimize this oedema by raising his burnt hand. Hang it from a drip pole, as in A, in Fig. 75-1, or put it in a St. John's sling as in C, in that Figure.

Severely burnt hands are not suited to the exposure treatment because the crust cracks when a patient's uses his fingers; nor are they well suited to the occlusive method because he cannot exercise his hand inside a big bulky dressing. The plastic bag method is usually best. This keeps his fingers moist and mobile, and makes even a severe burn almost completely painless. Even if both his hands are burnt he can still do many things for himself. An antiseptic in the bag is desirable but not essential. *If you use one, you can leave his hand in the bag for more than a day. If you don't use one you will have to remove his hand and wash it daily.*

Recognizing the depth of a burn is difficult in the hand, but is important, because small deep burns may be best treated by immediate excision and grafting (58.17).

RAISE ALL BURNT HANDS AT ALL TIMES

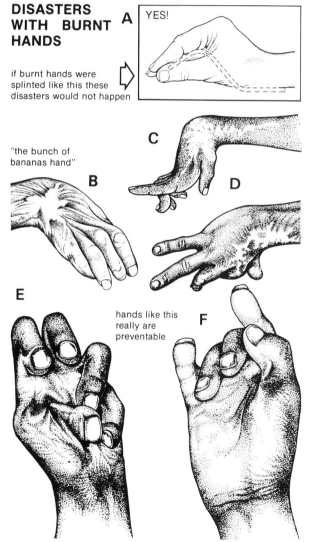

Fig. 58-26 DISASTERS WITH BURNT HANDS. If the methods described here had been applied almost none of these disabilities and deformities would have occurred.

When grafting a burnt hand is needed, graft early, or the patient will lose the function in his hand unnecessarily. His next most urgent need is a splint to prevent contractures, especially if he is a child. The common deformities that can follow are the 'bunch of bananas hand' B, Fig 58-26, or in its more extreme form the 'claw hand' shown as E, and F, in this figure. The patient's wrist extends, his MP joints extend and adduct, and his IP joints flex. Sometimes, his proximal interphalangeal joint is flexed and the distal one extended, producing the boutonniere deformity shown in Fig. 75-22.

If you are aware of the deformities that can happen, you can usually prevent them, by: (1) Splinting a patient's burnt hand in the position of safety as in A, in Fig. 58-26, and Fig. 75-8. (2) Starting physiotherapy as early as is practical. There is no universal splint for a burnt hand, so consider each patient's needs separately.

SPLINT A PATIENT'S HAND WITH HIS WRIST IN DORSIFLEXION

Dynamic (lively) splints are ideal when a patient's hand starts to recover, so change his fixed splint for one which allows him to move his fingers, but still holds his hand in the best position when it is resting. The easiest way to make a dynamic splint is to make a plaster cock–up splint, and to fix a piece of thick wire to it as shown in B, Fig. 58-19. Attach rubber bands to the wire and pass these round his proximal phalanges to allow him to exercise his fingers.

BURNT HANDS

WHICH METHOD IS BEST FOR A BURNT HAND?

Superficial burns. the exposure method or the occlusive dressing method is best.

THE PLASTIC BAG METHOD

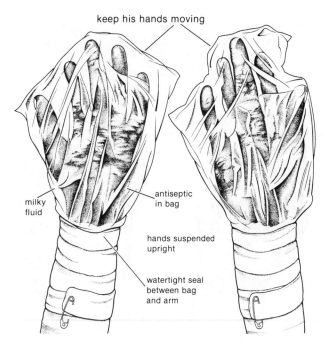

keep his hands moving

milky fluid

antiseptic in bag

hands suspended upright

watertight seal between bag and arm

Fig. 58-27 THE PLASTIC BAG METHOD for treating burnt hands keeps a patient's fingers moist and mobile and is almost completely painless. It is also very simple.

Deep partial thickness burns on the dorsal surfaces. Use the handbag method, or if you are skilled, treat the patient's burn by tangential excision and grafting in 3 to 5 days (58.17).

Small (less than 20 mm) full thickness burns. Excise the patient's burn, especially if it is on the palmar surface, and apply a split skin graft. If you are not very skilled, the hand bag method might be wiser.

Burns with bare tendon, bone, cartilage, or joints. The patient is usually in so much pain that you cannot find out if his nerves and tendons have been injured or not. His hand requires skin flaps which is a highly skilled task, so refer him. Before doing so, remove any obviously burnt tissue from the remains of his hand.

If referral is impossible, you will have to: (1) treat him by the hand bag method. Meanwhile, (2) wait for the exposed tissues to slough, and for his wound to granulate, and then, (3) graft what is left of it.

If a burn is very severe, you may have to amputate, but don't do this unless it is absolutely necessary. You may be able to graft the stumps of his fingers, and preserve some useful function. The same indications for amputation apply in burns as in other hand injuries (75.24).

If you are in doubt to what to do, use the hand bag method until granulations appear, and then graft.

THE HAND (OR FOOT) BAG FOR SEVERE BURNS

MATERIALS Any big clean plastic bag of a suitable size. There must be plenty of room for the patient's hand to move about inside it. Don't use a plastic glove. If possible, use one of the following antiseptics: (1) Silver sulphadiazine 0.5% changed every 1 or 2 days. Or, (2) povidone iodine.

METHOD Smear the patient's hands with silver sulphadiazine, or povidone iodine.

Wrap a piece of gauze round his wrist and hold it in place with a piece of strapping. Place his hand in the bag with some more antiseptic, and secure the bag round his wrist with a bandage. The gauze already round his wrist will help to form a watertight joint, or sweat band, and prevent the exudate in the bag from dripping down his raised forearm.

CAUTION ! A burnt hand swells alarmingly, so suspend it beside his head, by the method in Fig. 75-1.

Encourage the patient to move and use his hand inside the bag right from the start. Let him feed himself, and shave, etc. Large volumes of a murky fluid will collect in the bag. If this alarms him, explain that it is normal. Change the bag each day. Take his hand out of the bag, wash it with soap and running water. Apply more antiseptic, and put it back in a new bag, or in the old bag washed clean.

CAUTION ! (1) Early movement is important. If he is reluctant to use his hand, encourage him. (2) If silver sulphadiazine or some other antiseptic is not available, daily washing is absolutely essential. (3) Full thickness burns of the digits inside a plastic bag may still need an escharotomy (58.18), so observe the circulation in his fingers carefully.

DESLOUGHING A BURNT HAND Sloughs will usually fall off in pieces into the bag by themselves, so that desloughing with scissors is usually unnecessary.

GRAFTING A BURNT HAND Small islands of new skin will appear in a superficial burn. If these are not enough to cover the raw areas, graft them. Graft early, before three weeks. A hand which stays uncovered with skin longer than this is more likely to become stiff.

If you put a patient's grafted hand back in the bag, the grafts may float off, or be rubbed off. So take his hand out of the bag, graft it, splint it (a wire frame is convenient), and treat it by the exposure method (58.14) or with an occlusive dressing (58.15).

If you are in doubt as to whether to graft or not, (this is common with the bag method), keep his hand in the bag, wait for granulations to appear, and then graft his wound with split skin.

SPLINTS FOR A BURNT HAND A plaster cock-up splint is generally the most useful one. Place it outside the dressing or the plastic bag and then bandage it in place. Keep a pad or splint in the space between the patient's thumb and index to prevent an adduction deformity.

If the dorsum of a patient's hand is burnt, so that it is likely to assume the deformity in C, Fig. 58-26, splint his hand with his MP joints flexed and widely abducted, his IP joints in 15° of flexion, and his thumb widely abducted and forward of his palm (the position of safety in Fig. 75-8).

If his palm is burnt, splint his MP joints in 30° of flexion, and his IP joints in 15° of flexion.

To begin with he should wear his splint day and night. Later, he will only need it at night. Splinting may need to last three months.

THE OCCLUSIVE METHOD FOR A BURNT HAND

Apply this as in Section 58.15. Put gauze between the patient's fingers to prevent webs forming between them. Cover each finger separately to prevent them sticking together, and change the dressings daily. Dress his hand in the position of safety.

DIFFICULTIES WITH A BURNT HAND

If the JOINTS OF A PATIENT'S HAND ARE EXPOSED, aim for an arthrodesis in the position of function (usually 30° of flexion of his IP and MP joints). Remove any dead cartilage and fix the position with crossed Kirschner wires, left in place for 3 weeks.

If ONE FINGER REMAINS STIFF, consider amputating it.

If ALL A PATIENT'S FINGER JOINTS HAVE BEEN DAMAGED, fix his ring and little fingers well flexed to act as hooks for carrying, and his index and middle finger only mildly flexed, so that his thumb can grasp things against them.

58.30 Burnt face and ears

Burnt face Warn the patient's family that massive oedema may greatly distort his face, but that this will disappear. Raise his head to 30° and have intubation and tracheostomy equipment ready. If you have to do a tracheostomy, do it in the theatre after intubating him first. Oedema will be at its maximum 12 to 24 hours after the burn, so watch him carefully, because respiratory obstruction may be sudden.

Full thickness burns of the beard area are rare, because the hair follicles extend so deep. Use thin split skin sheet grafts, not mesh grafts, and apply them to complete anatomic areas of his face. Sew the grafts in place, and hold them by the tieover method (57-8). The most common cause of failure to take is not keeping the graft still. So try to stop him talking and give him liquid food.

Burnt ears Inflammation of the cartilages of the ears can occur 2 to 5 weeks after a severe facial burn, when the skin over a patient's ear may have healed. His burnt ear becomes acutely, painful, red, and tender, because its cartilage has become necrotic. If you don't excise the dead cartilage, it becomes infected and sloughs. Once this has happened he will need his ear reconstructed.

CHONDRITIS OF THE EAR

PREVENTION Treat a burnt ear carefully. When you dress it, put a pad of gauze behind it to prevent it bending.

If a collection of fluid gathers on a patient's ear, incise it urgently, if necessary, more than once. If you leave it, the cartilage under it may necrose.

If his ear cartilage becomes necrotic, block his greater auricular and auriculotemporal nerves with lignocaine (A 6.6). Incise the outer border of his ear, so as to separate its anterior and posterior surfaces. Remove any soft yellow cartilage which lacks the normal resilience of healthy hyaline cartilage. Pack his ear with fine gauze, being careful not to bend it. Keep it moist with saline. Examine it 24 hours later, under local anaesthesia. If necessary, remove more necrotic cartilage.

If there is sepsis and abscess formation, drain the septic area with a wide incision, and remove all necrotic cartilage. If you fail to do this, the whole cartilage will become infected.

REMOVING NECROTIC CARTILAGE

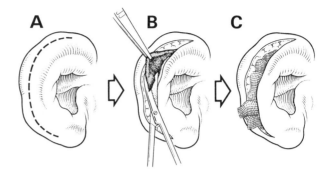

Fig. 58-28 BURNS OF THE EARS. If the cartilage of a patient's ear becomes necrotic, you may have to remove it.

58.31 Burns of the trunk

Follow up a child with severe burns of the trunk carefully. As growth occurs, they may prevent the normal development of his (or her) breasts, abdominal wall, or buttocks.

Follow up a little girl with burns of the front of her chest until her breasts develop at puberty. Severe scarring may distort them and require further grafting. A scar on the abdominal wall of a pregnant mother may need to be released as her abdomen expands.

GRAFTING A DEVELOPING BREAST If you cannot refer the girl, make a semilunar incision just below her contracted breast. Continue it into her intermammary cleft. Cut down to the deep fascia, lift her breast upwards, and correct its position by gauze and scalpel dissection. Apply split skin grafts, and hold them in place with tieover sutures over wet wool. Cover them with dry wool and crepe bandages. Lie her flat until the grafts have taken.

If her nipples have been destroyed and she becomes pregnant, you may need to suppress lactation.

58.32 Burnt bones and joints

The tibia, the ulna, and the skull are often burnt when an epileptic falls into the fire. If the tissues over his periosteum are burnt, it dies, and so does the bone under it, even if it escaped being burnt directly. As the slough falls away you may see greyish yellow bone protruding from among pink granulations round the edge of the burn. Granulations don't form on dead bone, although they sometimes form under it as it separates, so speed up this process by chiseling it away.

BURNT BONES AND JOINTS

As soon as you see that a patient's bone is dead, chisel it away, until you see some bleeding which shows that you have reached living bone. Wait for granulations to form, usually in 5 to 10 days. Then apply split skin grafts.

If a patient's skull has been burnt, its outer table is usually dead. Chisel this away, and graft the granulations that form on the inner table. If the whole thickness of his skull has been burnt, graft his dura.

If a burnt joint becomes infected and pus pours from it, nibble away its articular cartilage and let an arthrodesis form in the position of function (7-16). If it does not fuse spontaneously, refer the patient for a formal arthrodesis; this may require the use of a compression clamp.

If an amputation is necessary, graft the stump.

IF HE IS EPILEPTIC, HAVE YOU CONTROLLED HIS FITS ADEQUATELY?

---

59 Atomic trauma

'The living will envy the dead'.

Nikita Khrushchev

59.1 The final challenge to preventive surgery

Thermonuclear annihilation is the ultimate in trauma, both in the severity of a single injury, and in the number of casualties. There are three dangers which are commonly confused: (1) Those associated with atomic power. (2) The release of a single atomic bomb by accident or design. (3) A multimegaton exchange of intercontinental ballistic missiles. The consequences of the first are comparatively minor, those of the second are survivable by mankind as a whole, as indeed were the bombs at Nagasaki and Hiroshima. The last is truely terrifying. If we in the Third World do not actually perish, we will see our sources of drugs, equipment, and spares, and much of our tenuous hope of development, vanish instantly.

Firstly, some facts, many of them in the words of *The Lancet*.

The arsenals of the world now contain the equivalent of a million bombs of the kind that fell on Hiroshima, and are equal to about 4 tons of TNT for everyone of us here on earth. More energy can now be released by one weapon in one microsecond than in all the conventional wars of history. In the nations directly attacked tens to hundreds of millions of people would be killed instantly. Hundreds of millions more might starve to death. Millions might die from cancer caused by nuclear radiation.

Radioactive contamination would spread to vast areas and pollute the biosphere. *The natural protective ozone layer round the earth might be damaged, with unpredictable consequences to all forms of life, and possibly even the extinction of the human species. Mankind might indeed destroy itself.* At the very least, the social, cultural, environmental, and medical damage in the aftermath of a nuclear war would persist for generations.

---

4 TONS OF TNT FOR EVERY ONE OF US ON EARTH

Among those who might survive the initial effects of blast, fire, and radiation, many would endure prolonged agony and a slow death. Untold numbers would die from injuries for which no adequate medical care could be provided. Widespread starvation, epidemics, and civil disorder would be inevitable. The people who would not be immediately vaporized would suffer from radiation, and from many of the injuries discussed elsewhere in this manual. A 'nuclear winter' might end all life on earth. Medically, the terms 'limited' and 'winning' have no meaning in the context of nuclear war.

Mounting military expenditures and the intensification of the arms race heighten the tension, and each new crisis worsens the threat. World military spending in real terms, corrected for inflation, has increased four fold since World War Two. In the 1970's it approached $5 trillion, or about $500 thousand million a year—a sum larger than that of the total goods and services

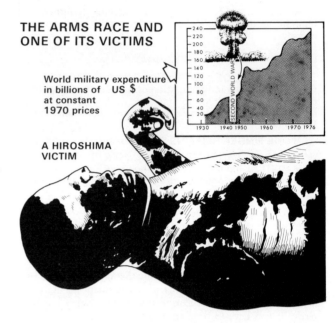

THE ARMS RACE AND ONE OF ITS VICTIMS

World military expenditure in billions of US $ at constant 1970 prices

A HIROSHIMA VICTIM

Fig. 59-1 ATOMIC CATASTROPHY. The second world war ended with the atomic explosions at Hiroshima and Nagasaki. Here is one of the victims. The graph shows the world's military expenditure in $US billion at 1970 constant prices. Most of this expenditure is designed to produce death from the very injuries we describe here.

created by mankind in one year. *Most of this expenditure is carefully designed to cause the very injuries we describe here, if not death itself.* It is also killing people now by diverting scarce resources from urgent health needs. Twenty times as much is spent on arms as on development aid. To provide everyone on earth with clean water and sanitation would cost less than the equivalent of seven months of the arms race. Smallpox was eradicated from the world for a cost equal to only five hours of it. One year of it would more than abolish all the international debts of the Third World. One nuclear aircraft carrier, the Ohio, launched in 1979, cost $6 billion—more than the total government budgets of Kenya, Tanzania and Uganda combined.

'Overkill' is now such that 1000 times more bombs are available then are required to kill everyone on the other side. The balance of terror becomes daily more frightening. It is sometimes argued that it has kept Europe free of war for nearly 40 years. This is not correct since there has never been a sufficient cause for war during this period. If war does break out it will only be by accident; if it does it will annihilate most of the industrial world and perhaps all mankind.

Not only is there a very real chance that all this will happen, but *such is the unreliability of military computer systems that it is quite possible that it might even happen by mistake.* The growth in sheer numbers of nuclear weapons and the increasing complexity and sophistication of their delivery systems increase the possibility that a nuclear conflict may be triggered by some tragic accident. Any technological system is liable to malfunction, and

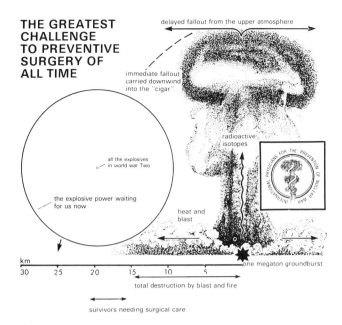

THE GREATEST CHALLENGE TO PREVENTIVE SURGERY OF ALL TIME

delayed fallout from the upper atmosphere

immediate fallout carried downwind into the "cigar"

radioactive isotopes

all the explosives in world war Two

the explosive power waiting for us now

heat and blast

one megaton groundburst

km
30   25   20   15   10   5

total destruction by blast and fire

survivors needing surgical care

Fig. 59-2 NUCLEAR ARSENALS. The area of the small circle represents the power of all the explosives used in World War Two. The area of the larger circle represents the nuclear arsenals of the world now which are about 5,000 times greater. The scales at the bottom of the figure show zones of total destruction and of the survivors needing surgical care; they are those following a 1 megaton groundburst. The Hippocratic serpent symbolically surmounting the mushroom cloud is the the emblem of International Physicians for the Prevention of Nuclear War (IPPNW).

the people who direct them can easily make mistakes, or be sick, or mentally deranged, or tired, stressed, drunk, drugged, or senile. Until now their errors could kill only a few people. Now they can endanger the very existence of humanity.

The strategy of mutually assured destruction ('MAD') was bad enough. Even more terrifying are the attractions of a 'premptive first strike' to overwhelm the command, control and intelligence systems of the other side. The risk now is that, at a time of international tension, a defensive response by one side mignt be taken as an offensive one by the other side in a series of escalating responses that would culminate in catastrophe. The system itself may indeed have been mistakenly designed so that it cannot operate safely. For example, the carrying out of necessary additional defensive procedures during a high level alert may give the opposing side the mistaken impression that it is about to be attacked. Instead of escalation taking weeks as it did in the first world war, following the assination of an obscure archduke in Sarajevo, it might only take minutes—a "nuclear Sarajevo".

Hitherto it has been asumed that the ultimate authority for pressing the button to release the holocaust would lie, in the West, with the President of the United States. There are however good grounds for believing that he has already given 'preauthorisation' to end life on this earth to his generals in their bunker. If the Strategic Defence Initiative ('Star wars') is implemented, they will have to be given this authority, and may in turn have to hand it on to a computer. In matters of military technology the East usually follows the West . . .

In the face of this unimaginable calamity, our response, as mere humans, is to deny reality and to try to forget it, and to hope that it won't happen. Most of us can just cope with the little tragedies of our daily lives, but a cataclysm of this kind is too much for us. We become apathetic, and our response is in no way appropriate to the magnitude of the threat that faces us.

Perhaps this is not surprising. We have slowly evolved over millennia, yet in the space of only one lifetime, we have found ourselves able to fly, to unravel the chemistry of our own genes, to reach for the moon, to probe the very limits of the universe— and to destroy ourselves. Unfortunately, with it we retain an attitude to war which is at best mediaeval. Many of us even enjoy some aspects of it. We need time, much time, in which to adapt to our new powers. *Above all, we need to look into the future with a much longer time perspective.* Instead of seeing it in terms of years, or tens of years, we must look at it, not in the span of our own lifetime, but of that of our children's children, far into the centuries ahead.

A HUMAN PERSPECTIVE OF MILLENNIA

Both East and West see themselves, almost certainly falsely, ss being about to be overrun, but even if they were, they should take comfort from the fact that all previous dominations have ultimately come to an end, often suprisingly quickly. Against such a longer time perspective, what happens in the next decade or two will not matter very much. Both sides—and mankind— will ultimately survive. So will our beautiful green earth.

Henceforward, the greatest threat to man's life and health may not be the diseases with which medicine presently concerns itself, but his propensity to make war and destroy himself. If so, the greatest challenge to preventive medicine (and preventive surgery) in the closing years of this millennium and the next one (if we reach it), must be the prevention of war, both between East and West, and between the countries of the Third World. In some countries one person in 20 is a health worker, so if every health worker could become a 'peace worker', the massive challenge of 'global health education for a nuclear age' is not an impossible one. In the Third world it would allow money spent on arms to be spent on development.

Paradoxically, this is less a challenge to our intellects than to our courage, to our imagination, and to our willingness to face reality. We have yet to realize that the real courage required of us now is not courage in battles as it used to be, but courage to stand against the opinions of our fellows, who have yet to see things as clearly as we think we do, and conceivably, when the time comes, to resist domination—not violently but with an even greater kind of courage. The weapons of today are not tritium and plutonium but vision, hope, courage, perseverance, and indomitableness, together with the solidarity and good humour which several nations are already showing to magnificent effect against just such domination. If an atomic holocaust is the ultimate challenge to preventive traumatology, then these are our vaccines against global trauma and insane suicide, the "new community medicine (and surgery). . .".

IT *MIGHT* ALL HAPPEN BY MISTAKE!
COURAGE,   PERSEVERANCE,   HOPE

NEAR DISASTERS There have indeed been many mistakes: (1) In 1961 near Goldsboro, North Carolina a B-52 bomber broke up in flight, releasing two 24 megaton bombs. Airforce experts found that on one of the bombs five of the six interconnecting safety devices had been set off by the fall, leaving only one to prevent an explosion. (2) In September 1980 a technician working on a Titan II intercontinental ballistic missile droppped a socket wrench onto a fuel tank below. The tank lost fuel and some hours later exploded, blasting open the silo's 740 ton door and shooting the 9–megaton warhead 600 feet into the air. Frantic radio messages were overheard as the survivors tried to find the missing warhead. (3) In November 1979, a war game training tape was accidentally fed into a NORAD computer, and was accepted as real, initiating a low level nuclear war alert as personnel prepared launch procedures. (4) On another occasion the military systems of the USA were alerted, B-52s took to the air and readied to counter attack. Within six minutes of the time that this was to happen, the hostile missiles identified on the radar screens were seen to be only a flock of Canadian geese. . . East and West had come to within 6 minutes of destroying one another, and perhaps the Third World too. This happened when the superpowers faced one another over the poles, where missiles have a journey of half an hour. Now that they confront one another in Europe, where there are only three minutes in which to react, the possiblities of a mistake are ever more frightening. LESSONS ''You may reasonably expect a man to walk along a tightrope safely for ten minutes, it would be unreasonable to expect him to do so without accident for two hundred years''. The risks have grown greatly since Bertrand Russell wrote this.

Not only are all thinking people in the West frightened, but from many accounts those in the East are even more so. If it does happen by mistake, or intention, and you do have the fortune or misfortune to survive, here is an atomic ABC.

THE GREATEST CHALLENGE TO MEDICINE IN THE NEXT MILLENIUM
(and the rest of this one)
''EVERY HEALTH WORKER A PEACE WORKER''

59.2 Trauma from heat, blast, and radiation

Atomic bombs release energy in four forms. Like any chemical explosion, they cause: (1) heat and (2) blast, which produce the burns, fractures, and crush injuries described on other pages. (3) Radiation in the form of neutrons, X-rays, gamma rays, and alpha and beta particles. This radiation takes two forms: (a) the initial radiation, mostly neutrons and gamma rays, which ends within a minute of the explosion, and falls off with distance according to the inverse square law, and (b) the fall out radiation emitted by a mixture of radioactive isotopes, some with a half life of centuries. This fallout occurs in two forms, immediate and delayed, and is described below. (4) There is also an intense pulse of electromagnetic energy at the moment of the explosion capable of destroying communications and all electromagnetically stored data over a huge area.

The heat and blast from bombs of one megaton and larger kill almost everyone who might possibly have survived the initial radiation. As bombs get smaller, their radiation becomes more important than their blast. This is the principle of the small, neutron bomb, which kills by radiation without causing much heat or blast.

A 10 megaton bomb exploded at a height of 2000 metres (an airburst) produces an intensely hot luminous fireball, and a blast wave which travels at supersonic speed. It produces no crater, and therefore little fallout.

The same bomb exploded on the surface (a groundburst) makes a crater nearly a kilometre wide. In doing so it makes thousands of tons of earth radioactive by irradiating them with neutrons, and draws them up into the air as the 'mushroom cloud' in Fig. 59-2. This huge quantity of radioactive material then descends to the earth as fallout in two forms; (1) Immediate fall out which occurs in the first few days, and is comparatively localized, the larger particles falling nearby, and the finer ones progressively further downwind. The pattern of this fallout is determined by the speed and direction of the prevailing wind. The large particles are deposited close to the site of the explosion as a fine visible radioactive sand. (2) Delayed fallout in the form of much smaller particles. These reach the upper atmosphere and descend only slowly to be added to the natural background radiation of the biosphere.

Assuming that the ozone layer and the biosphere itself survive a major nuclear exchange (and there is good reason to think that they might not), it is the delayed fallout which matters to countries which are not directly attacked, and particularly to us in the Third World. This fallout is ultimately distributed round the earth, although fortunately for us, most of it falls in the hemisphere in which it is released.

The heat and blast from a one megaton bomb destroys everything within about 14 km. Within this area heat causes severe burns and ignites anything combustible. Innumerable fires are started, and if the weather conditions are right, these produce a firestorm, like that at Hiroshima which destroyed 12 sq km of the city. A powerful vertical upstream of hot air draws cool air in from the periphery until everything which can burn has burnt. In doing so it creates temperatures of 1,000°C, that melt glass and metal. The Dresden firestorm, caused by conventional incendiary bombs during the second world war, killed 100,000 helpless people, many of them women and children, in one night.

59.3 Radiation injury

Radiation imparts energy to the electrons of living tissues. This allows harmful chemical reactions to take place, particularly in DNA. Extreme radiation damage kills cells, particularly those in rapidly multiplying tissues, like the mucosa of the gut and the marrow. Lesser damage causes: (1) mutations, which can only express themselves when cells divide, and are responsible for cancer in the survivors, and (2) genetic deformities in their children.

The absorbed energy is measured in rads. In tissue at or near the surface of the body, an exposure of one roentgen of radiation energy results in the absorption of one rad (100 ergs/gram). Clinically, this absorbed energy expresses itself in the short term as the 'radiation sickness' described below. If irradiation is spread over weeks or months the body can tolerate more.

'RADIATION SICKNESS'

This is the response to whole–body radiation delivered over 48 hours or less.

0 to 100 rads. Men lose fertility at 20 to 50 rads

100 to 200 rads. After 3 to 6 hours there is nausea and vomiting which lasts for less than a day. After a latent period of up to 2 weeks, symptoms recur for 4 weeks. Leucopenia develops.
There are few deaths below 200 rads.

200 to 600 rads. Nausea and vomiting lasting 1 to 2 days are followed by the recurrence of symptoms for up to 8 weeks.

THE FALLOUT PATTERN

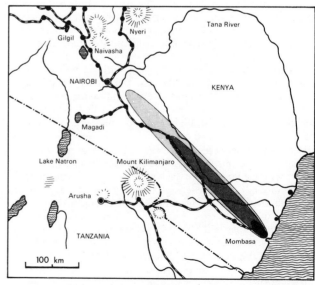

Fig. 59-3 THE EXPECTED FALL OUT PATTERN after a one–megaton surface burst on Mombasa, assuming a uniform southeasterly wind of 30 km/hr. The contours indicate seven day accumulated doses of 900, 300, and 90 rads to unprotected people. A dose of 500 rads will kill about half of those exposed to it.

There is severe leucopenia, purpura, and haemorrhage, often with infection. Above 300 rads the hair is lost.

The death rate is 0 to 90% in 2 to 12 weeks from haemorrhage or infection.

600 to 1000 rads. Nausea and vomiting start within half an hour and last 2 days. There is a latent phase of 5 to 10 days, followed by the same symptoms as with 200 to 600 rads which last 1 to 4 weeks.

The death rate is 90 to 100% in 6 weeks from haemorrhage and infection.

1000 to 5000 rads. Nausea and vomiting start within half an hour and last one day. A latent phase of under 7 days is followed by fever and diarrhoea lasting 2 to 14 days.

Everyone dies within 14 days from circulatory collapse.

More than 5000 rads. Almost immediate nausea and vomiting are followed by convulsions, tremor, ataxia, and lethargy.

Everyone dies within 48 hours from respiratory failure or cerebral oedema.

Anyone within 1.5 km of a 1 megaton bomb could expect to receive a dose of the initial radiation with a 50% chance of killing him (about 500 rads)—should he survive the initial heat and blast.

The dose from fallout decays exponentially by a factor of 10 for every sevenfold increase in time. If it is 3000 roentgens per hour at one hour, it will be 300 at 7 hours; at 49 hours (7×7) it will be only 30 roentgens an hour. In practice, radiation from fallout is difficult to calculate, and has to be measured. Here is an example. After a one megaton ground burst with a uniform wind of 24 km an hour, the fallout plume that would expose an unprotected person to a fatal cumulative dose (about 500 rads) in the first week after the explosion would be 240 km long and 32 km wide.

The longer the fission products remain in the mushroom cloud, the less radioactive they will be when they fall to the ground. They are likely to arrive in dangerous concentrations for at least 24 hours. If you are in the path of the plume, there will be an interval before the fallout arrives, which will depend on your distance from ground zero and on the wind speed. When it first arrives, the dose rate is small. It then builds up over a day or two and decays.

Whereas there is little effective protection from the heat and blast, except perhaps in a deep bunker, some protection is possible from the fine radioactive dust of the fallout.

SOME POSSIBLE MEASURES

These are the preventive measures you can take to protect yourself from the fallout.

PREVENTION Build a fallout shelter for yourself and your family, preferably in a basement. The further this is from any dust that might fall outside, the better. The more material of any kind you can put between yourself and the falling dust the better. Pile 50 cm of earth against the windows and any unexposed walls. Fit your shelter with a simple ventilation system that will keep dust out. Carefully seal it against dust, and provide it with a toilet. Furnish it with enough food and water for at least two weeks.

CAUTION ! Get into your shelter before any fallout descends, and don't come out!

IF YOU ARE CAUGHT IN THE FALLOUT change your clothes and wash any dust from your skin and hair. Dust particles in contact with your skin will cause beta burns. Don't eat or drink anything contaminated with fallout.

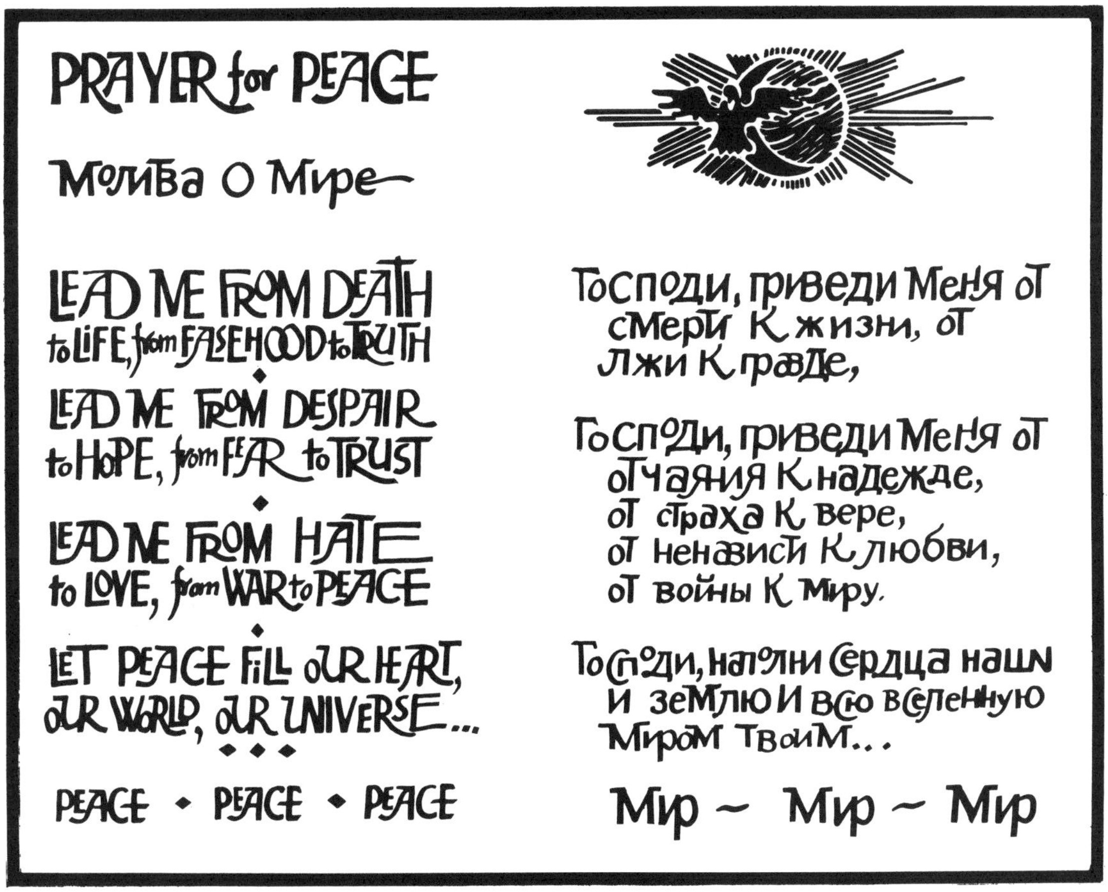

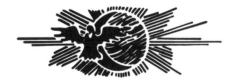

PRAYER for PEACE

Молива О Мире—

LEAD ME FROM DEATH
to LIFE, from FALSEHOOD to TRUTH

LEAD ME FROM DESPAIR
to HOPE, from FEAR to TRUST

LEAD ME FROM HATE
to LOVE, from WAR to PEACE

LET PEACE FILL OUR HEART,
OUR WORLD, OUR UNIVERSE...

PEACE • PEACE • PEACE

Господи, приведи меня от
смерти к жизни, от
лжи к правде,

Господи, приведи меня от
отчаяния к надежде,
от страха к вере,
от ненависти к любви,
от войны к миру.

Господи, наполни сердца наши
и землю и всю вселенную
миром твоим...

Мир ~ Мир ~ Мир

Fig.51 59-4 PREVENTIVE MEDICINE FOR MANKIND'S FINAL EPIDEMIC. *Kindly contributed by Donald Swan.*

HOW LONG TO STAY INSIDE? If you don't have a radiation monitor, there is no means of knowing. Stay for at least two weeks.

WHEN YOU COME OUT expect millions of your countrymen to be dead; power, communication, water, and sewage to be disrupted, pestilence and famine to be widespread, the economy to be in ruins, and civil disorder rife.

Perhaps, when (and if) you do come out you will agree with Nikita Kruschev that it might have been better not to have done so. Perhaps you will realize that you might have done more to prevent it? If so, read on.

59.4 A nuclear Hippocratic oath

As physicians (and surgeons), our calling is to prevent sickness where we can, to cure it when we cannot prevent it, and to comfort the sick whom we cannot cure. Our challenge now is to make the ultimate supreme effort in the history of our profession—to do our bit to prevent mankind, all 4.3 billion of us, from destroying ourselves in the ultimate catastrophic act of global suicide—with the obscene possibility that it might all happen by mistake. 'International Physicians for the Prevention of Nuclear War' (225 Longwood Avenue, Boston, MA 02115, USA) have suggested that we should adapt our Hippocratic Oath to the atomic age like this:—

As a physician of the 20th century, I recognize that nuclear weapons have presented my profession with a challenge of unprecedented proportions, and that a nuclear war would be the final epidemic for mankind. I will do all in my power to work for the prevention of nuclear war.

Thompson James, 'Psychological aspects of nuclear war' (1985) Published by the British Psychological Society, and John Wiley and Sons, Ltd.

60 Eye injuries

60.1 The general method for eye injuries

There is no branch of surgery which the non−specialist is more afraid to enter than ophthalmology. All operations inside a patient's eye are work for an expert, but you should be able to repair most injuries to his lids. If you cannot refer him, you may have to suture his cornea, or his sclera. Even if his eye seems to be hopelessly injured, there is much that you can do to preserve some useful sight in it.

As with the skull, the chest, and the abdomen, there are two main kinds of injury—blunt ones which leave his cornea and his sclera intact, and penetrating ones which go through them.

A blunt injury, such as that from a fist, resembles a head injury. It can cause serious internal lesions, including bleeding, with few external signs.

Penetrating eye injuries are always serious and differ geographically. In rural areas many of them are caused by thorns striking the eyes of people walking in the bush, or by young children pushing things into one another's eyes. Injuries of this kind are difficult to prevent, but you should try to make sure that: (1) goggles are worn by everyone whose work might injure their eyes, and (2) seat belts are always worn in cars.

The purpose of an eye is to see with, so always start by testing (and recording) a patient's visual acuity. An eye injury can be terrifying. If he cannot see, make sure he knows what has happened, understands any treatment you give him, and is told the prognosis for his sight.

An injured eye is always an emergency, but it is not quite so urgent as a ruptured spleen, or an extradural haematoma. After the necessary emergency treatment, you usually have 2 or 3 days in which to refer him. If you do have to operate, make sure you go to the theatre having made the diagnosis and knowing exactly what you are going to do. You will need fine instruments and sutures and a magnifying loupe. These are listed in Section 23.1.

JAMES (8 years) was referred with a swollen eye and a diagnosis of rupture of the globe. His visual acuity was tested and found to be normal. Examination of his upper conjunctival fornix showed a piece of wood. LESSON Always test the visual acuity. In this patient it made the original diagnosis of rupture of the globe impossible.

GENERAL METHOD FOR AN INJURED EYE

For burns of the eye, see Section 58.28. For the basic methods, see Section 23.1.

REFERRAL If you decide to refer a patient with an eye injury, instil antibiotic drops into his eye, fit his eye with a protective shield (23-1), and refer him lying down. If the journey is long, or is likely to be delayed, give him oral chloramphenicol 500 mg initially, followed by 250 mg 6 hourly for 5 days.

HISTORY Take as careful a history as you can.

LOCAL ANAESTHESIA FOR EXAMINATION Pain will make a patient keep his injured eye shut. Local anaesthesia will make it easier to examine. Retract his lower lid and instil 2 drops of local anaesthetic. This can be 2% or 4% lignocaine, or decicaine 1%, or tetracaine hydrochloride 1%, or propara-

caine hydrochloride 0.5%, or cocaine 4% to 10%. You may have to make many instillations before anaesthesia is effective—see A 5.8.

CAUTION ! (1) Don't put ointments ito a patient's eye, they will make it difficult to examine later. (2) Topical anaesthetics, dyes, and drugs *must be sterile*. They can readily become infected, especially with *Ps. pyocyaneus*. Tetracaine and fluorescein can be autoclaved repeatedly. (3) Don't give a patient a local anaesthetic to take home—he may injure his anaesthetic cornea, and the drug may delay healing.

THE EXAMINATION OF AN INJURED EYE

Start by examining the visual acuity of both the patient's eyes, his normal one first. Lie him down, examine him in a good light and use whatever means of magnification you have.

If he cannot open his eye himself, gently open his lower lid by pulling down the skin over his zygomatic arch. Instil local anaesthetic. This will probably relieve his pain enough to let him open it himself.

If he is still unable to open his eye, put a Desmarre's retractor gently under his upper lid, and lift it upwards away from the globe. Or, use a retractor made from two bent and sterilized paper clips.

If even this fails, you may have to wait until you anaesthetize him before operating.

CAUTION ! Avoid pressure, either by squeezing his eye, or by letting him squeeze his eye with his lid. If his globe is perforated, pressure may squeeze the contents out of it.

SIGNS OF INJURY IN THE EYE

Examine the patient's lids carefully. A tiny laceration may be the opening of a track which penetrates his globe, as in Fig. 60-9. Examine his conjunctiva for haemorrhage, foreign bodies, or tears. Note the depth and clarity of his anterior chamber. Compare the size, shape, and light reaction of his pupils.

If his globe is intact, examine the fornices of his conjunctiva and evert his upper lid, as in Fig. 23-2. Dilate his pupils and examine his fundus with an ophthalmoscope.

Examine his lens, his vitreous, and his retina for signs of haemorrhage, or retinal detatchment.

Examine his cornea and his sclera for wounds and abrasions. Put drops of fluorescein into his conjunctiva. Don't try to feel the tension in his globe, because if you do, you may squeeze out its contents. You will however get some idea of its tension as you examine it.

If there is blood under a patient's conjunctiva, be careful: (1) Even a very small bruise may mark the site where a small foreign body has entered his sclera, as in Fig. 60-9. (2) Haemorrhage at the limbus is itself unimportant. It is only likely to be serious if it extends far posteriorly, when it may indicate a fracture of the base of his skull (62.1).

If his anterior chamber is shallow, he has a penetrating injury of his cornea, which has allowed his aqueous to leak.

If his iris trembles when his eye moves, his lens may have dislocated.

If there is a greyish area in his cornea with swollen margins, his cornea has perforated. In severe cases he may have no anterior chamber, so that his iris touches his cornea.

If a black mass of tissue bulges through the lips of a wound, as in B, Fig. 60-7, his iris or his choroid has prolapsed.

If the wound is in his cornea, his pupil will be irregular and drawn towards it as in J, Fig. 60-6.

If his eye feels soft, his globe has probably ruptured. The rupture is nearly always curved, parallel to the limbus, and about 5 mm behind it. Feel the bony borders of his orbit. X-ray his skull and his orbit.

If you can see the edge of his lens with an ophthalmoscope, and he has some visual impairment, the suspensory ligament of his lens is partly ruptured. If it is also tipped the pressure in his eye may rise. If this happens, give him acetazolamide and refer him.

If his lens is completely dislocated, you may see it lying in his anterior chamber, or at the bottom of his vitreous. He will also have a severe visual impairment. There may be no immediate reaction. But an inflammatory response and a secondary rise in pressure are common. Give him acetazolamide and refer him. His lens may need removing.

If he has severe proptosis, goto Section 62.1. He has a retrobulbar haematoma.

If his eye is hopelessly injured, don't consider enucleating it, unless he is unaware of any sensation of light whatever, when you shine a *strong* light into it. This light must be strong, because it may have to shine through the clot in his eye. If he has any perception of even a strong light, a suprising amount of vision may have returned 6 months later.

ANAESTHESIA Remember that the patient's stomach may be full. Any rise in the pressure in his globe may make the injury worse. You can use ketamine. If his eyes move about, give him a little more. Be sure to premedicate him.

Don't use a retrobulbar block, because if it happens to bleed and his globe is ruptured, the clot may force the contents of his eye out of the wound.

THE FURTHER MANAGEMENT OF AN INJURED EYE

Read on for 'black eye' (60.2), injuries of a patient's eyelids canaliculae and conjunctiva (60.3), injuries of his cornea and sclera (60.4), injuries of his iris (60.5), penetrating injuries (60.6), blunt injuries of his globe (60.7), bleeding into an injured eye (60.8), foreign bodies (60.9), and endophthalmitis (60.10).

YOU MUST HAVE A BRIGHT LIGHT AND GOOD MAGNIFICATION

SUTURING THE EYELIDS

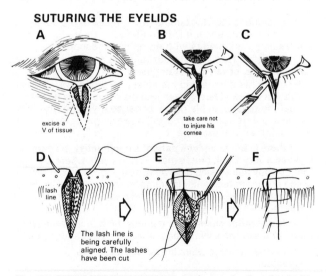

Fig. 60-1 SUTURING THE EYELIDS. Little tissue has been lost in this injury, so that bringing the edges of the patient's lids together is not too difficult. A, B, and C, show the steps in making a clean edge to the wound. Take care not to injure his cornea with the tip of your scalpel.
Partly after Hill with kind permission.

60.2 Haematoma of the eyelid ('black eye')

A black eye is the result of a blow by a blunt object. By itself it is not serious. But: (1) it may be part of a head injury (63.1), or a maxillofacial injury (62.1). (2) The patient's globe may have ruptured. This may be difficult to diagnose if there is much swelling, so anaesthetize him and use eyelid retractors. If his globe has not been injured, no treatment is necessary. If it has been injured, goto Section 60.7. Mild ptosis (drooping of the lid) is common after a black eye. If it lasts more than a month, refer him.

60.3 Injuries of the eyelids, canaliculi, and conjunctiva

Injuries to a patient's eyelids are common, and can be serious because of the danger to his eyes under them, either immediately, or later if scar tissue distorts his lids and exposes his cornea. The injury can involve part of the thickness of a lid, or its whole thickness, including its tarsal plate, sometimes with tissue loss.

When you repair a torn eyelid, start by putting a suture in the lash line immediately behind the patient's eyelashes. If you align his lash line correctly, it will align the other structures. *The secret of success is multiple small sutures and accurate repair.* The common mistake is to use large instruments and coarse sutures.

INJURIES OF THE EYELIDS

This extends the general method for an injured eye in Section 60.1. Examine the patient's eye to see exactly what structures are involved. Make sure his globe has not been injured. If he has a severe injury to his lids, refer him if you can.

Toilet his injured lids. Don't remove any skin, unless it is obviously dead or detached. Infection is unusual, so you can always close his wound by immediate primary suture. Use fine instruments, and 6/0 silk or monofilament on his skin. If the edges of the wound are irregular, try to fit them together with great care.

CAUTION ! Take great care to keep his lid against his globe, and don't allow it to become inverted or everted.

If the edge of the patient's eyelid is intact, you can treat his injury in the same way as any other skin laceration.

If the injury has involved the whole thickness of his lid, approximate the tarsal plate, the muscle layer and then the skin. Disregard his conjunctiva. It is stuck to his tarsal plate, and if you align this, it will align itself.

If the wound gapes, it will do so because the fibres of his orbicularis muscle have been cut. Use 5/0 buried catgut to bring the edges of the muscle together, before you suture the skin.

If he has lost some of the skin on his eyelid, graft it. Use split skin, and hold the graft in place by the tieover method (57-8).

If less than a quarter of the margin of a lid is involved, as in Fig. 60-1 and B, and C, Fig. 60-2, freshen the lacerated edges by making incisions perpendicular to the skin margins through the full height of the tarsus to excise an 'I' of tissue. Close the patient's tarsus with interrupted catgut sutures. Align the lid margin with 7/0 silk sutures, one in the posterior margin through the orifices of his meibomian glands, and another in the anterior margin through the lash line. Allow the sutures to remain 5 mm long and tie them over his skin to prevent them abrading his cornea.

CAUTION ! Bring the edge of his lids together accurately by aligning the lash line. If you repair them with their edges notched, part of his cornea may not be covered, so that it will dry out and ulcerate.

If between a quarter and a third of either lid margin has been lost, make a small incision just lateral to the patient's eye, as in D, and E, Fig. 60-2. Divide the upper or lower bifurcation (depending on which lid is being repaired) of the Y–shaped outer canthal ligament in Fig. 60-3 which anchors

WHEN TISSUE HAS BEEN LOST FROM AN EYELID

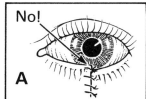

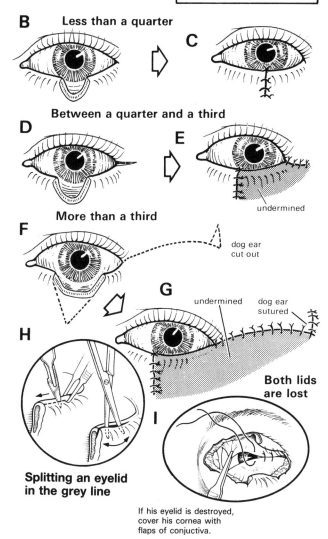

B Less than a quarter

C

Between a quarter and a third

D

E

undermined

More than a third

F

dog ear cut out

G

undermined

dog ear sutured

H

Both lids are lost

Splitting an eyelid in the grey line

I

If his eyelid is destroyed, cover his cornea with flaps of conjuctiva.

Fig. 60-2 WHEN TISSUE HAS BEEN LOST FROM AN EYELID. A, don't notch the edge of the patient's lid. B, and C, if less than a third has been lost, close the wound directly. D, and E, if between a quarter and a third has been lost, make a lateral relaxation incision, and divide his lateral canthal ligament, as in the next figure. F, and G, if more than a third has been lost, you will have to make a long relaxing incision, and undermine the tissues of his cheek. H, incising the lower eyelid in the lash line, and in front of the tarsus. I, if there is not enough eyelid left to cover a patient's cornea, cover it with flaps of his conjunctiva. *Partly after Mustardé, with kind permission.*

his eyelids to his orbit. If you don't divide this Y–shaped ligament when you need to, there will be too much pull medially on the lachrymal apparatus. Don't divide the main stem of this ligament, or a severe deformity will result.

Before you can move an eyelid across, you will have to split it and undermine the shaded areas in Figs. 60-2 and 60-3. Hold the patient's injured eyelid with forceps, and incise it in the lash line for 3 mm with a scalpel. Then split it by inserting scissors and spreading them. This will give you the right plane of dissection without injuring his tarsus or his orbicularis muscle. Moving his lower eyelid across will leave a fold of

skin in his upper eyelid which you will have to excise and suture.

CAUTION ! Don't try to move the medial part of his lid, or you will interfere with the drainage of tears through his lachrymal apparatus.

If more than a third of a patient's eyelid is lost, refer him. If you cannot refer him make a longer relaxation incision, as in F, and G, Fig. 60-2.

If a deep horizontal laceration of the patient's upper lid divides his levator palpabrae muscle, or its attachment to his tarsal plate, try to suture it. This filmy muscle is hard to find in the bloody mess of an acute injury. If you fail to suture it, ptosis will follow.

If you cannot cover his cornea by any of these methods, do a tarsorrhaphy. The simplest way of doing this is to 'raw' the edges of his lids, and suture them with fine silk, as in Fig. 58-23.

DIVIDING THE OUTER CANTHAL LIGAMENT

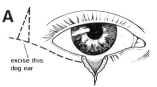
excise this dog ear

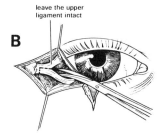
leave the upper ligament intact

B

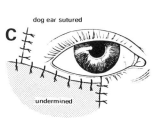
dog ear sutured

C

undermined

Fig. 60-3 DIVIDING THE OUTER CANTHAL LIGAMENT. A, Make the incision several millimetres below the lash margin. B, find the lateral canthal tendon and divide it. C, undermine the skin flap and repair the defect. *After Peyman, Sanders, and Goldberg.*

If there is not enough of his eyelids left to do a tarsor-rhaphy, grasp his conjunctiva at the upper fornix, with forceps, pass a suture through it, bring it down, and pass it through a similar fold from his lower fornix, in the same vertical line. Use several interrupted sutures to bring a double thickness of conjunctiva across his globe, as in I, Fig. 60-2.

If he presents late when his lid is greatly swollen, toilet his wound, excise the minimum amount of tissue, give him antibiotics, and repair his lid when the swelling has subsided.

INJURIES OF THE CANALICULI

If his upper canaliculus is injured, ignore it. It only drains 10% of his tears.

If his lower lid has been lacerated medial to the punctum, search for the divided cut ends of his inferior canaliculus. It needs microsurgical repair by an expert, so refer him.

If you cannot refer him, take a fine polyethylene or silastic catheter or a monofilament suture, pass this through the punctum, out through the wound and across his divided canaliculus and into his lachrymal sac just below the attachment of his medial canthal ligament to his nasal bones. Suture the wound and leave the monofilament suture in place for a week.

CAUTION ! If you don't repair his lower canaliculus, his tears will flow continually.

INJURIES OF THE CONJUNCTIVA

Most conjunctival lacerations will heal without suturing.

If a laceration is extensive, expose the patient's eye with lid sutures (23-2). Dissect his conjunctiva away from his globe and search it for a perforating wound. If you find one, go to the next Section. Gently probe the wound and extend it if

SUTURING THE CONJUNCTIVA

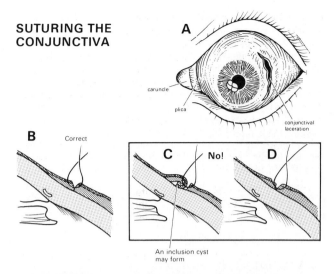

Fig. 60-4 SUTURING THE CONJUNCTIVA. Don't suture small lacerations. A, preserve the caruncle and the plica if you can. B, a correctly placed suture. C, if the conjunctiva is folded over like this, an inclusion cyst may develop. D, this suture will allow Tenon's capsule to herniate into the wound. *After Peyman, with kind permission.*

necessary. Suture his conjunctiva with continuous sutures of 5/0 silk or plain catgut. Silk sutures are more comfortable, but you will have to remove them later. Catgut will be absorbed.

CAUTION ! (1) Sometimes a major injury is hidden under a small conjunctival wound, so probe it carefully. (2) Don't probe around inside a patient's eye. Only probe to see if his sclera has been perforated.

60.4 Injuries of the cornea and sclera

The common corneal injuries are abrasions and lacerations. The danger of an abrasion is that it may become infected, so that a corneal ulcer forms, followed perhaps by endophthalmitis. A corneal laceration is the most difficult eye injury that you may have to treat.

If a laceration goes right through a patient's cornea so that his aqueous escapes, his iris may move up against its posterior surface, or prolapse outside it (J, 60-6). If a laceration is small, and its edges are not separated, you may not need to suture it. A clean wound of the cornea heals rapidly, especially if only the epithelium is injured. If a wound goes deeper than this, a scar always forms.

INJURIES OF THE CORNEA AND SCLERA

CORNEAL ABRASIONS

This extends the general method for an eye injury in Section 60.1.

The patient's eye is red and watery and his lids tightly closed. He may have ciliary injection, but his visual acuity is normal. After looking at his eye carefully, you can find no foreign bodies on the surface of his cornea, or underneath his upper lid. Instead, you see an abrasion, which you may only find after you have stained it with fluorescein.

If an abrasion is clean, and is only visible after staining with fluorescein, and there are no signs of infection, instil chloramphenicol eye drops and shield the patient's eye (23.1). Check it daily, and instil chloramphenicol, until it no longer stains with fluorescein.

If his cornea becomes cloudy, it is infected. He now has a corneal ulcer so see below.

TWO CORNEAL INJURIES

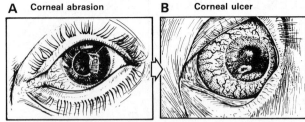

Fig. 60-5 TWO CORNEAL LESIONS. A, a corneal abrasion. B, a corneal ulcer. If you are not careful, an ulcer can follow an abrasion.

CAUTION ! To prevent infection, always instil chloramphenicol eye drops after any corneal abrasion and shield the eye.

CORNEAL ULCERS

There is a hazy white spot on the patient's cornea; it may be hollowed out, and there may be a yellowish area, or pus in his anterior chamber. His eye is painful, photobic and red with ciliary injection.

If possible, send a pus swab from the ulcer for bacteriological and fungal examination.

Instil atropine drops, topical broad spectrum antibiotic drops (neomycin, bacitracin, or chloramphenicol) and inject subconjunctival chloramphenicol or gentamycin 500 mg once or twice daily for several days (23.1).

CORNEAL LACERATIONS

If a corneal laceration is less than 1 mm, the patient's anterior chamber is normally deep, and there is no iris in the wound, don't suture it.

If the normal curve of the patient's cornea is maintained and the edges of the wound are close together, you can probably leave his laceration unsutured.

If the normal curve of his cornea is not maintained, so that his cornea is angled or tented, suture it. If you don't, and the laceration is central, he will have a severe refractive error.

If his anterior chamber is shallow or his iris has prolapsed into his corneal wound, remove the prolapsed iris and suture his cornea, as described below.

If a small amount of corneal stroma has been lost from the edge of the wound, repair it by inserting a tight horizontal mattress suture.

SUTURE If you can refer a patient to an expert within 2 days of his injury, do so.

If you have to suture his cornea yourself, use sutures of 7/0 or 8/0 atraumatic silk, or monofilament. You will find this difficult task easier if you use interrupted sutures. Experts always use continuous ones. One length of atraumatic suture material will be enough for the whole injury.

CAUTION ! Don't suture the cornea with catgut because the wound will take 6 weeks to heal, and by that time the catgut will have dissolved.

Use a small curved cutting needle. Grasp it at its mid point, so that the convexity of the jaws of the needle holder is towards the tip of the needle. This will give you more control over it.

CAUTION ! Aim to bring the cut edges of the endothelium on the posterior surface of the cornea together, without actually going through it. The way to do this is to pass the needle across the wound in its posterior third. The whole thickness of the cornea is only about 1 mm, so that this will not be easy. If your sutures are too superficial they will pull out; if they are too deep, they will enter the anterior chamber and damage the endothelium on the back of the cornea. You will need a steady hand, so support your wrist on the patient's forehead, or on a sandbag underneath the drapes beside his head. Or, support your wrist on your assistant's fist.

SUTURING THE CORNEA AND SCLERA

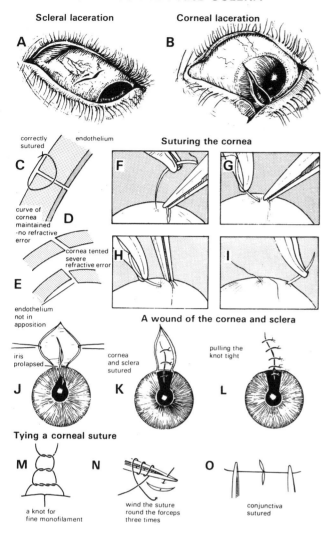

Fig. 60-6 SUTURING THE CORNEA AND SCLERA. A, a laceration of the patient's sclera. B, a laceration of his cornea and his eyelid. C, try to make the suture cross his cornea in its posterior third. It is only about 1 mm thick, so this will not be easy. If the normal curve of his cornea is maintained (D), there is less need to suture it than when it is deformed or tented (E). The cut edges of the endothelium on the posterior surface of his cornea should be in contact. F, the needle entering at 90° to his cornea. G, the needle about to cross the wound. H, entering the other side of the wound. I, pulling out the needle.

J, this patient's conjunctiva retracted to show a wound of his cornea and sclera with prolapse of his iris. K, his prolapsed iris has been excised, and his cornea and sclera have been sutured. L, his cornea has been closed over the wound.

M, a knot for tying 9/0 mofilament. N, wind the suture three times round the forceps. O, pulling the suture tight. *Partly after Galbraith, with kind permission.*

Hold the edge of the wound (not the whole thickness of the cornea) obliquely with fine toothed forceps, so that one blade enters the wound as in G, Fig. 60-6.

While you are holding the edge of the wound undistorted with forceps, insert the needle at almost 90° into the cornea 1.5 mm from the edge of the wound. As the needle goes through it, let the needle holder follow its curve. Aim the needle to enter the wound in the posterior one third of the cornea. It should then pass across the wound to the matching opposite edge, and come out at 90° to the cornea.

If the wound is vertical, bring the stitch out 0.5 mm from its edge. If it is oblique, bring it out 1 mm from the wound edge.

Pull the suture material through the wound, until only about 1 cm remains. Tie the suture in three throws by winding the

monofilament round the needle holder or the suture tying forceps. Use three turns for the first throw, then one, and then another one, (M, and N, 60-6).

CAUTION ! Don't pass sutures through a patient's iris. If you find that a suture has gone through his iris, remove it.

Use the first throw to bring the tissues together without any tension. Leave a tiny loop between the first and second throws to make sure that no undesirable tension is transmitted to the first throw. Pull the third throw down and hold it down so that it can mould into a knot.

Pull one side of the suture, as it emerges from the cornea so that the knot just enters the needle track. This will make the patient more comfortable while his eye heals. Instil atropine drops.

CAUTION ! Don't try to reconstitute his anterior chamber by injecting air or saline. This is a highly skilled task, and you are likely to do more harm than good.

SCLERAL LACERATIONS

Suture a patient's sclera in the same way as his cornea, but use 4/0 or 5/0 sutures of atraumatic silk or monofilament. Cover the sutures in his sclera by repairing the conjunctiva over them with fine silk (6 to 8/0), as in L, Fig. 60-6. Leave the scleral sutures in place, but remove those in his conjunctiva.

If vitreous prolapses through a wound in the sclera, excise it. Dip a swab into the wound and lift the vitreous away. If a strand of vitreous is pulled from the wound, cut it off with scissors. The proximal end of the strand will retract into the patient's eye. Repeat this until you have removed all the vitreous that has escaped from his globe. If some still oozes out or sits on the wound, aspirate it using a wide bore needle. Then suture the sclera as described above.

CAUTION ! Don't allow vitreous to remain trapped at the edges of the wound, because the complication rate increases, and wound healing will be poor.

POSTOPERATIVE CARE FOR CORNEAL AND SCLERAL LACERATIONS

Instil atropine, pad and bandage the patient's eye.

If the wound is near the edge of the patient's cornea, remove the sutures at 2 weeks.

If the wound is more central in his cornea, leave the sutures in for 2 months if his eye is comfortable and quiet. To remove them, lie him flat, instil local anaesthetic and insert a speculum. Using good magnification, pull the superficial arm of the suture to the surface with a fine hook, and cut it with the tip of a No.11 scalpel blade. If necessary, make a fine hook by tapping a 6 mm needle on a metal surface so that its tip becomes burred.

60.5 Injuries of the iris

A patient's iris can be torn, or detached from his ciliary body, or it can herniate through a wound in his cornea or sclera. He usually has a hyphaema and other eye injuries also. Sometimes, his lens is dislocated at the same time and you may be able to see his vitreous herniating into his anterior chamber. If his iris or ciliary body remain prolapsed in his wound, it will greatly increase the risk of infection and sympathetic ophthalmitis (60.10).

INJURIES OF THE IRIS

This extends the general method for an eye injury in Section 60.1.

If a patient's iris has prolapsed through a corneal wound, as in J, Fig. 60-6, less than 24 hours ago, and it is clean, put it back in his eye with an iris spatula. Try to separate his iris from the rest of the wound, to prevent the formation of anterior synechiae (adhesions). This is difficult. Excision as described below is simple, and may be wiser.

If his iris is obviously damaged or contaminated, excise it. Grasp it with fine toothed forceps, draw it a little further out of the wound, and cut it with spring scissors flush with his cornea. Stroke the wound, so that the cut edges of his iris retract back. Or, gently push them back with an iris spatula. Provided there is no blood in his anterior chamber, instil atropine 1% twice daily—the atropine must be sterile.

If the cut edge of his iris bleeds, put a drop of 1/1000 adrenaline into his conjunctiva. It will control bleeding and dilate his pupil.

POSTOPERATIVELY shield the patient's eye for three days, or until pain stops. If light disturbs him, pad both his eyes.

60.6 Penetrating injuries of the globe

The anterior part of a patient's globe is most at risk. His lens may be injured, and there may be a foreign body in his globe (60.9). Try to diagnose and treat him within 24 hours; delay worsens the prognosis for his sight. You may see the injury, and if it is in his cornea, it may be plugged by iris. It may be small, so look carefully. All you may see is a tiny hole in his iris and an opacity in his lens. Provided you are sure that there is no foreign body, suture any lacerations by the methods in Section 60.4

60.7 Blunt injuries of the globe

A blow to a patient's eye can:—

(1) Burst his globe parallel to and just behind his limbus. When this happens, you will see black uveal tissue prolapsing through it, as in B, Fig. 60-7. The conjunctiva over it may or may not be torn.

(2) Burst his globe near his optic nerve. You may see this injury with an ophthalmoscope, but there is nothing you can do, and useful vision is unlikely to return.

(3) Tear his choroid and his retina without bursting his sclera. Again, the common sites are near the optic disc, and peripherally near the limbus, where the retina is inserted into the ciliary body. You can only see the central third of a patient's fundus with an ophthalmoscope, so you will see tears near his optic disc, but not peripheral ones. To begin with, blood in his vitreous may obscure a central tear, but when this has cleared you will see it as a semicircular slit in his retina exposing the white of his sclera, as in A, Fig. 60-7. Keep him in bed until the blood has cleared. A retinal tear never heals and is almost always followed by detachment of his retina from his choroid, perhaps years later. No repair is possible.

(4) Detach his retina without tearing his choroid. The detached part of the retina is grey, instead of its normal red colour, and the vessels over it are dark, almost black.

BLUNT INJURIES OF THE GLOBE
This extends the general method for an eye injury in Section 60.1

If a patient's eye is so hopelessly injured that any useful sight is impossible, you may need to enucleate it (60.1).

If his globe is less severely injured, expose his scleral wound by making an opening through his conjunctiva parallel to it. Divide Tenon's capsule, and clean its lips.

Gently replace any undamaged prolapsed uveal tissue with a blunt spatula. Excise any damaged tissue and remove any prolapsed vitreous. Close his sclera with interrupted sutures as in Section 60.4, then suture his conjunctiva.

CAUTION ! Don't try injecting air into his eye to restore its intraocular pressure.

Give him a course of subconjunctival antibiotics (23.1).

If you suspect that a patient has a retinal injury, observe him for 3 months, and tell him to report back immediately if he notices shadows, black spots, or flashes of light in his field of vision. They indicate actual or impending detachment of his retina. A detached retina is grey, instead of its normal red colour, and the vessels over it are dark, almost black. Provided his macula is not involved, his retina can be repaired.

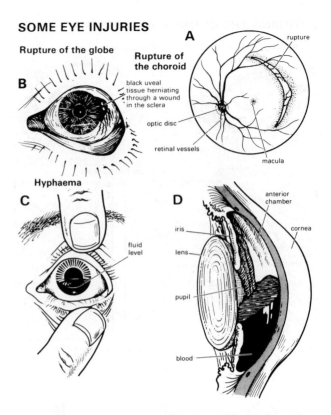

SOME EYE INJURIES

Fig. 60-7 SOME BLUNT EYE INJURIES. A, a blow to the patient's eye has ruptured his choroid and exposed the white of his sclera. B, his globe has burst just behind his limbus. His iris and ciliary body have prolapsed through the tear and lie under his conjunctiva. C, and D, show a hyphaema; an obvious fluid level like this is unusual.

Refer him with his eye properly padded as soon as you can—the sooner his retinal detactment is repaired, the better his prognosis.

If he develops a traumatic cataract after a blunt injury, his lens may need to be removed. An eye with no lens may however be a greater problem than an eye with a cataract.

60.8 Bleeding into an injured eye

Bleeding from a patient's iris into his anterior chamber (hyphaema) is common, and can occur immediately after the injury, or not for some hours or days. It can be mild, or it can fill his anterior chamber with blood. The blood may clot and obscure his anterior chamber completely, or it may occasionally form a fluid level as in C, and D, Fig. 60-7. The tear in his iris (which may be obscured by blood) can be partial or complete.

The patient complains of poor vision after a blunt injury. When you examine him, you may see: (1) Only a diffuse reddish haze in his anterior chamber. (2) A settled layer of blood. (3) His anterior chamber so full of blood that you can see nothing behind it. His eye may feel abnormally hard or soft.

Fortunately, bleeding into the anterior chamber usually stops spontaneously, but in 20% of cases it starts again during the following week. If it does start again, it is likely to be more severe than after the original injury. A hyphaema is not an acute emergency, so that you usually have a week in which to see if it is going to absorb, and in which to refer the patient. Meanwhile, give him acetazolamide to keep the pressure in his globe low, and reduce the chance of secondary glaucoma, which is the major complication. Operating on a hyphaema is an expert task and results are often not good.

There is little you or anyone else can do for bleeding into the vitreous of the posterior chamber, so pad both the patient's eyes and put him to bed.

BLEEDING INTO THE EYE

This extends the general method for an eye injury in Section 60.1.

If the patient is a reliable adult with minimal hyphaema, ask him to rest quietly at home.

If his hyphaema is more than minimal, admit him, and put him to bed with his trunk raised at 30°. This will lower the venous pressure in his head and thus his intraocular pressure. If you can see through his pupil, examine his fundus for vitreous haemorrhage and other damage.

Sedate him. Pad both his eyes. Give him acetazolamide 250 mg 6 hourly. Don't give him any eye drops. Ask him to avoid moving his head, and especially to avoid bending down. Monitor the tension in his globe carefully. The blood usually absorbs in a few days; if it does, you can discharge him.

If bleeding starts again, keep him in bed for a further week from the time of the bleed. If he has a massive further bleed causing an almost black hyphaema, and making his eye hard and his cornea oedematous, the blood in his eye needs evacuating urgently.

If the blood does not absorb in a week, refer him.

If the tension in his globe rises, he may be developing secondary glaucoma. Control it with acetazolamide 500 mg initially, and 250 mg 6 hourly. If he does not improve after two days, refer him because he may need paracentesis of his anterior chamber.

60.9 Foreign bodies in the eye

Foreign bodies are often missed, because nobody looks for them. They can be embedded in a patient's cornea, or lodged in his upper conjunctival fornix, so that they can only be seen when his eye is everted. Always instil some anaesthetic drops into his eye before you try to remove them. The risk with any foreign body is that the eye will become infected.

Fortunately, most foreign bodies don't go deeper than the conjunctiva or sclera. The commonest one to go right inside the eye is a piece of steel that breaks off a cold chisel when the patient hammers it. When this happens, he may have a stained area in his cornea, a tiny hole in his iris, and signs of an early cataract. He may also have been misdiagnosed as conjunctivitis. His history, and the fact that his eye remains red and watery should however make you suspicious. *If a patient has a painful eye and he has been doing anything which might have caused a foreign body to enter it, assume that he has a foreign body in his eye until you have proved that he has not.*

MIGHT HE HAVE A FOREIGN BODY INSIDE HIS EYE?

FOREIGN BODIES IN THE EYE

This extends the general method for an eye injury in Section 60.1. Look for an entry wound in: (1) the patient's lids, (2) his sclera, or (3) his cornea. Stain his cornea. Feel the tension in his globe. Examine his anterior chamber for a hyphema, and his iris for a tear. Look for the foreign body with an ophthalmoscope.

CAUTION ! The entry wound in his cornea may be a very small one indeed. Look for a tiny haemorrhage.

CONJUNCTIVAL FOREIGN BODIES

If a patient complains that something has got into his eye, you will probably find it in his upper or lower conjunctival fornix, usually the upper one. Search both, and evert his upper lid, as in B, Fig. 60-8. You will probably find the foreign body about 3 mm from the margin of his lid, about half way along, where it is most concave. Brush the foreign body away with a cotton wool swab on a match stick. Don't be content with only finding one; expect to find several more.

If he complains of a foreign body but you cannot see it, be sure to instil fluorescein. You may see an abrasion, a laceration, or a foreign body.

If the foreign body is embedded in his conjunctiva, instil a few drops of local anaesthetic, pick it up with forceps and snip it out with the overlying conjunctiva.

If fragments of spectacle glass have gone into his eye, remove them with forceps, and sweep them out of his fornices with a cotton wool swab on a match stick.

CAUTION ! Always examine a patient's cornea carefully, and stain it with fluorescein, even if you find a foreign body in his conjunctiva.

CORNEAL FOREIGN BODIES

The patient's eye is painful, red, tearful, and photophobic. You will need great care, a steady hand, 5% cocaine, or 4% or 2% lignocaine, good magnification, and a strong light. The sun is ideal. Stain his cornea with fluorescein, hold his eye open, and examine his cornea.

If you can see a corneal foreign body, wipe it away with a swab or moist cotton tipped applicator.

If the foreign body is firmly attached to his cornea, put the tip of a sterile disposable hypodermic needle under it, and lift it out of its small pit in his cornea.

CAUTION ! (1) Don't damage the surrounding normal cornea. (2) The cornea is thin (1 mm) and tough, so don't push the foreign body through it into his anterior chamber. (3) Use a fine sharp needle, not a corneal spud.

If fluorescein shows vertical corneal stains, a foreign body has stuck to the deep surface of the patient's upper lid, and is scratching his cornea. Evert his upper lid, and remove the foreign body by rubbing it with a swab.

If an iron containing foreign body has remained in the cornea for any length of time, a ring of rust forms. You must remove the foreign body, but if you cannot easily lift out the rust ring, leave it.

CAUTION ! Whenever there is or has been a foreign body in a patient's eye, instil antibiotic drops, and pad it.

POSTOPERATIVELY On the following day, stain the patient's cornea with fluorescein.

If there is any area of staining and his eye looks irritated, dilate his pupil with 1% atropine and bandage his eye.

INTRAOCULAR FOREIGN BODIES Take lateral double exposure X-rays of the patient's orbit with his eye in two posi-

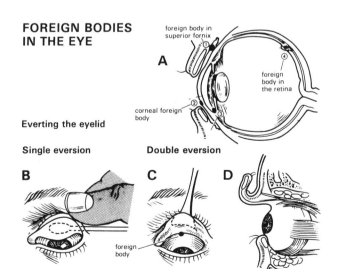

FOREIGN BODIES IN THE EYE

Everting the eyelid

Single eversion   Double eversion

Fig. 60-8. FOREIGN BODIES. A, common sites for foreign bodies. (1) The conjunctival fornix. (2) The cornea. Foreign bodies here usually lie within the fissure formed by the lids. (3) The anterior chamber. (4) The retina. B, single eversion of the lid. C, and D, double eversion. *After Peyman, with kind permission.*

103

tions, looking up and down. If the foreign body changes its position in these two views, it is probably inside his eye. If it is a metallic foreign body, refer him for its removal. This highly specialized procedure is beyond the competence even of most ophthalmic surgeons. If it is a small splinter of sand or glass, leave it.

ORBITAL FOREIGN BODIES If possible, leave them.

A PENETRATING EYE INJURY

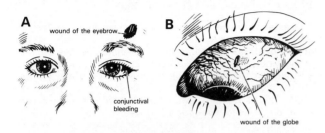

Fig. 60-9 A PENETRATING INJURY OF THE GLOBE. This patient has a penetrating injury well above his eye. The bleeding into his conjunctiva should however make you suspicious. Only when he looks downwards and inwards (B) do you see the injury of his globe. *After Goldberg and Tessler.*

60.10 Endophthalmitis after an injury

This takes two forms, the first is very common and the second very rare.

(1) Bacteria can invade a patient's eye through even a minor injury, which is one of the reasons why these injuries should be treated so carefully.

(2) An immune reaction (sympathetic opthalmia) can involve his normal eye 4 to 8 weeks after the original injury. When this happens, it becomes sensitive to light, red (with ciliary injection), and painful; its near vision is transiently blurred. Don't remove his injured eye; it may in the end have better vision than his other one. Give him steroids.

BACTERIAL ENDOPTHALMITIS This extends the general method for an eye injury in Section 60.1. If: (1) a patient's cornea is cloudy, or (2) there is an abscess in it, or (3) there is pus in his anterior chamber, start a course of subconjunctival chloramphenicol or gentamicin (23.1). If possible, culture his conjunctiva. Instil drops of atropine 1% into his conjunctiva. If you treat him energetically, you may save his sight.

61 Lesser face injuries

61.1 The general method for lesser face injuries

The appearance of a wound is nowhere more important than on a patient's face. He is unlikely to be able to consult a plastic surgeon later, so your main task is to minimize his disfigurement. This mostly means a careful toilet and accurate repair with numerous fine sutures. Plastic surgeons have few skills which you don't have for the immediate care of a face wound—their remarkable achievements are mostly the result of careful attention to detail. So, handle a patient's tissues gently, and be prepared to take enough time. Don't operate on his face with equipment designed for abdominal or orthopaedic surgery, or apply artery forceps to the skin edges; use skin hooks. Your scissors should be sharp. The face has an excellent blood supply, and heals well, so: (1) Save all injured tissue that might survive. (2) Make immediate primary suture the rule in all except late or severely contaminated wounds.

The common errors are: (1) Not removing all dirt, and so leaving an area of tatooed scarring. (2) A scar with unnecessarily gross suture marks. (3) Failure to replace the wound edges in the correct position, especially those which involve the edges of the eyelids, eyebrows, lips, or nose, like that in A, Fig. 61-2.

GENERAL METHOD FOR LESSER FACE WOUNDS

If a patient's eyelids and eyebrows are injured, turn to the previous chapter (60.3). If he has a severe maxillofacial injury, turn to the next one. Read on for injuries of his lips, gums, and tongue (61.2), injuries to his facial nerve and parotid gland (61.3), and for injuries to his ears and nose (61.4).

You will probably be able to treat him as an out-patient, but if repair is likely to take 2 hours or more, or you have to graft him, admit him.

EQUIPMENT A No. 5 scalpel handle, No.15 scalpel blades, Metzenbaum scissors, Glasgow pattern scissors, Adson's dissecting forceps, Derf needle holder, 2 skin hooks, mosquito haemostats, skin graft knife and board, fine needles, and 4/0 chromic and monofilament sutures.

BLEEDING Try to control this by direct pressure, and avoid buried ligatures if you can.

EXAMINATION If a patient's facial nerve might have been injured, test its function before you anaesthetize him. Ask him to smile, and see if his smile is symmetrical. Don't forget to examine his eyes (23.1).

ANAESTHESIA (1) Ketamine. (2) General anaesthesia with intubation. (3) Local nerve blocks, which are better than local infiltration because they will not distort the tissues. Where possible, use a mental nerve block (A 6.3), or an infraorbital or supraorbital nerve block (A 6.5). If you do use local infiltration, add hyaluronidase (1500 units in 10 ml) to help the solution spread through the tissues and minimize swelling.

If you sedate a patient with diazepam or chlorpromazine, he may fall asleep during the operation. A child will usually cooperate if you reassure him authoritatively and sedate him adequately. If you can, do the repair quickly. You may be able to do it while you restrain him. If necessary, wrap his arms and legs in a sheet as in Figure A 18-1.

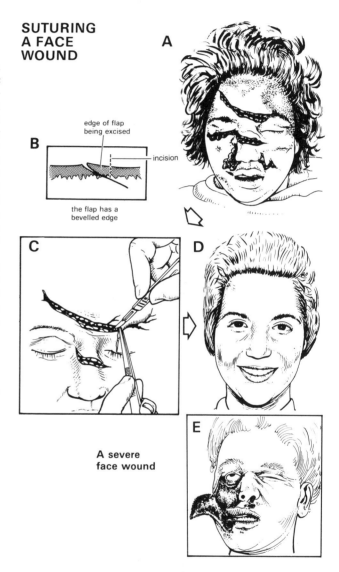

SUTURING A FACE WOUND

B edge of flap being excised / incision

the flap has a bevelled edge

C

D

E

A severe face wound

Fig. 61-1 SUTURING A SEVERE FACE WOUND. This patient was thrown against the windscreen of her car. The flap on her forehead has a bevelled edge, so B, and C, show the thin edge of this flap being excised before suture. D, the final result. E, if a patient's face looks like this, make sure you suture his tissues back in their proper places.
With the kind permission of James Smith.

TOILET If necessary, shave the patient's scalp, moustache, and beard, but leave his eyebrows. A wound can be difficult to align without them. Do a social and, when necessary, a surgical toilet (54.1). Clean his wound adequately, irrigate it copiously, and explore it. You may find a fracture, or foreign bodies, such as glass from a broken windscreeen, or grit from the road.

Where possible, plan the suture lines in or parallel to the

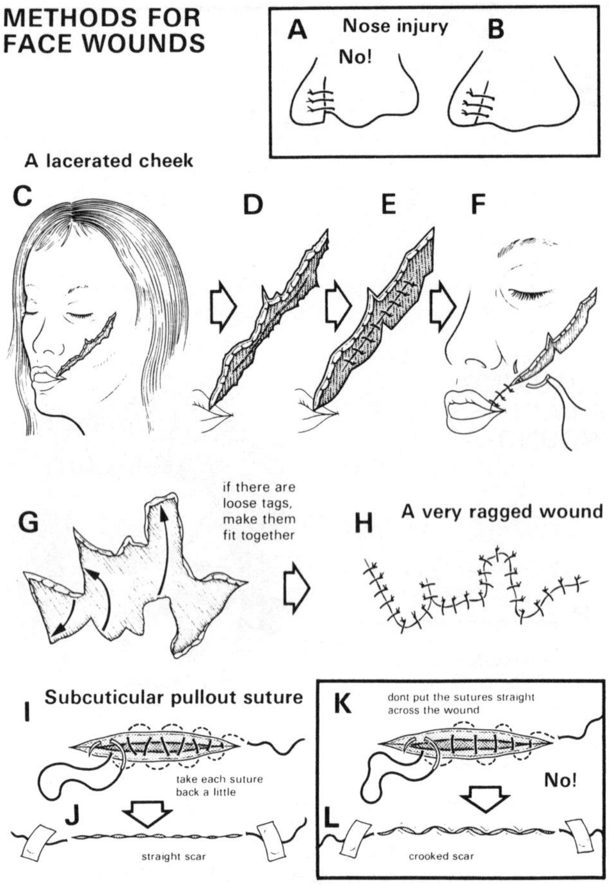

METHODS FOR FACE WOUNDS

A Nose injury No! B

A lacerated cheek

C D E F

G if there are loose tags, make them fit together H A very ragged wound

I Subcuticular pullout suture K dont put the sutures straight across the wound

take each suture back a little

J straight scar No!

L crooked scar

Fig. 61-2 METHODS FOR FACE WOUNDS. When you suture a patient's nose, don't leave a notch as in A; make sure there is no kink in the edge, as in B. If his wound is jagged, excise its edges and make them fit together, as in C, to F, and G, and H. Don't make sutures too tight, or they will leave an ugly scar. If a suture has to be tight, a subcuticular suture (I and J) will leave a better scar. The scar will be neater if you take each subcuticular suture back a little (I), and don't put sutures straight across a wound, as in K, and L. *Partly after 'Techniques Elementaires pour Medecins Isolés', with kind permission.*

skin lines as in Fig. 61-3. This will greatly improve the look of the scar.

If the wound edges are ragged or bruised, excise the minimum amount of skin, to give them a clean edge. Small tags of the skin which you would remove in other parts of the body will usually survive on the face, so replace them carefully.

CAUTION ! If you remove too much tissue, you will make a plastic repair later more difficult.

If the patient's wound is very extensive, be conservative and only remove dirt and obviously dead tissue. The scar will inevitably be ugly, but he may be able to have it revised later.

If his skin is grossly contaminated with dirt, only excise it if there is no other way of removing the dirt.

If the edge of the laceration is steeply bevelled, as in B, Fig. 61-1, and you leave it like this, the scar will be ugly. So cut off the thin edge of the flap to make it perpendicular. The best wound edges for suture are vertical.

If two lacerations are closely parallel, the final scar may be neater if you excise the bridge of tissue between them.

If a piece of the patient's cheek is missing, as in B, Fig. 61-4, suture his skin to his mucous membrane, and refer him for a plastic repair later.

If his wound is ugly and you can excise it along the skin lines, do so.

If an extensive wound has distorted his anatomy, so that you do not know how to suture it, as in F, Fig. 61-1, look for a landmark at either side of his wound. Match these and the rest of the jig saw will fit together.

CAUTION ! Time spent fitting the jig saw together is never wasted.

If his face has been extensively destroyed, fit the pieces that remain into their correct places. This will help you to see what has been lost.

IMMEDIATE PRIMARY SUTURE Don't close the skin until you have done all that is necessary to the structures underneath it. If you have done an adequate toilet, you can close most wounds by immediate primary suture.

Close the wound accurately at all points and in all planes. There must be no dead spaces. So, if necessary, insert tissue sutures of fine catgut to prevent cavities. If the patient's muscles of facial expression have been injured, try to bring them together to avoid dimples. Control bleeding, preferably by pressure, before you start to suture the wound.

Repair muscle, mucosa, and subcutaneous tissue with 4/0 chromic catgut, and skin with fine interrupted sutures of 4/0 monofilament. Place them 2 to 4 mm from the edge of the wound, but let them take an adequate bite of deeper tissue. Tie them only just tight enough to bring the skin edges together because the wound will probably swell and make them tighter. Tight sutures will leave the stitch marks.

If you cannot bring the skin edges together, cautiously undercut them and insert fat stitches.

CAUTION ! The level at which you undercut the face is important. Cut just deep to the dermis, superficial to the branches of the facial nerve, as in A, Fig. 54-6.

If you have to suture a wound under moderate tension, you will have to leave sutures in for 2 or 3 weeks, or the wound will burst open. Leaving ordinary stitches in as long as this will cause ugly stitch marks. Instead, insert subcuticular sutures. If you are not suturing a wound under tension, ordinary sutures give a better result.

If you cannot bring the skin edges together, even by undermining them or by suturing under moderate tension, graft the bare area with split skin. This will provide the best conditions for plastic surgery later.

CAUTION ! (1) Don't allow the wound to close by spontaneous scarring. (2) Don't try to rotate any flap as a primary procedure, or try to graft with full thickness skin. These are both secondary procedures after a wound has healed and its scar has been excised. (3) Don't make 'relaxing incisions'.

If a small haematoma develops, evacuate it after removing a suture.

ANTIBIOTICS If a wound is more than 6 hours old give the patient a systemic antibiotic.

PARTICULAR FACE INJURIES

HAEMATOMAS If necessary, aspirate these with a wide bore needle.

SKIN LINES ON THE FACE

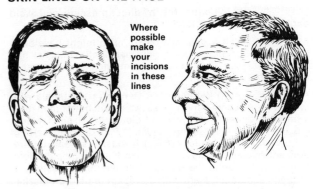

Where possible make your incisions in these lines

Fig. 61-3 THE SKIN LINES OF THE FACE. The scar on a patient's face will be less obvious if you can make it in or parallel to one of his natural wrinkle lines. These are the lines of election for a scar. *With the kind permission of James Smith.*

106

ACCIDENTAL TATTOOS If grit or foreign bodies have been rubbed into the patient's skin, remove them with a stiff sterile nail brush. Use small circular movements, and press hard. If oil or grease has been rubbed into his wound, remove it with a little ether. If you leave foreign material in place in his skin, it will leave a permanent ugly scar.

AVULSION FLAPS After repairing the wound, apply a pressure dressing for several weeks, if necessary. This will minimise haematoma formation under the flap and will improve the scar.

BITES of any kind, especially human bites, are very likely to become infected. Excise the wound margins, and give the patient an antibiotic (2.7).

POSTOPERATIVE CARE OF FACE INJURIES

To minimize stitch marks, remove alternate stitiches after 3 days and the remaining ones 4 to 8 days later (except on the ears).

Reassure the patient that the scars on his face will soften and improve with time. He will not know what he is finally going to look like until at least a year after the accident. Don't refer him for revision of the scars for a year or more.

INJURIES OF THE LIPS

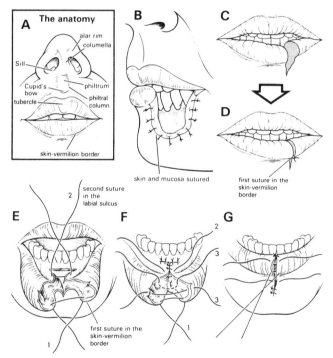

Fig. 61-4 WOUNDS OF THE LIPS. A, shows the anatomy you should try to preserve in a wound of a patient's nose and lips. Try especially to preserve his skin–vermilion border and his philtral columns. B, if a large piece of his lip is missing, suture his skin to his mucosa. C, and D, show the first suture placed in his skin–vermilion border. E, F, and G, show the sequence of steps in repairing a severe laceration of his lip. Note that the first stitch brings his skin–vermilion border together, and the second one is in his labial sulcus. *With the kind permission of Peter London.*

61.2 Injuries of the lips, the gums, and the tongue

When you suture a patient's lip: (1) Try to align the border between the skin and the vermilion part of his lip exactly. If you fail, he will look very ugly. (2) Try to prevent a scar forming, because this may notch the margin of his lip, shorten it, and evert it. Try also to restore his Cupid's bow and his philtral columns. Mark them before you infiltrate or manipulate his

wound, and align them with guide sutures before you infiltrate the rest of it.

His tongue can be injured if he is hit on the jaw when his tongue is out, or if he bites his tongue during a convulsion.

INJURIES OF THE LIPS, GUMS, AND TONGUE

LIP INJURIES

Tears of a patient's lips are often caused by his teeth. If a piece of tooth is missing, feel for it inside his lip. Small tears on the inner surfaces of his lips don't need suturing. Suture larger lacerations in layers. Close his mucosa as a separate layer.

If a laceration crosses his skin–vermilion border, mark it with a felt pen *before* you inject the local anaesthetic because the anaesthetic will blanch it and make accurate alignment difficult. Use the first fine monofilament stitch to draw his skin–vermilion border together, as in D, and E, Fig. 61-4. Traction on this will cause the other structures to fall into line.

If a laceration involves his labial sulcus, put your second suture into this, so as to align it. If you don't, it may be obliterated later.

If his orbicularis oris muscle is divided, suture it first with 3/0 catgut. Then bring his skin–vermilion border together. Finally, suture his mucosa with fine catgut.

CAUTION ! Preserve the line of his skin–vermilion border.

If up to one quarter of his lip is missing, you can repair it by primary suture without great deformity.

If so much of his lip is missing that you cannot close it by primary repair, suture skin to mucous membrane, as in B Fig. 61-4, and apply a vaseline gauze pack held by adhesive strapping. Refer him.

GUM INJURIES

If a laceration of a patient's gum retracts and exposes the margin of his alveolus, suture it. Dressings are not required. Remove skin sutures on day 4, and sutures in the mucous membrane on day 8.

TONGUE INJURIES

If a laceration does not involve the edge of a patient's tongue, or leave a free flap, you may not need to do anything to it. Otherwise, suture it with catgut. If it is on the tip, suture it using ketamine and suction, or use local anaesthesia. If it is on the dorsum, he may need a general anaesthetic with nasotracheal intubation (A 13.4). Children may need a general anaesthetic.

If the anterior two thirds of an injured tongue bleeds, hold it in a piece of gauze and pinch it between your finger and thumb behind the tear. Put in a mouth gag and repair it with fine silk. If deeper sutures are needed, use catgut.

If the tip of a patient's tongue is almost completely avulsed, try to repair it. It will probably live.

If the posterior third of his tongue is bleeding, put your index finger over it, and press it down against his mandible.

If you cannot reach a severe tongue wound, do a tracheostomy under local anaesthesia. Pack the patient's pharynx and repair his wound with deep stitches.

INJURIES INSIDE THE CHEEK
Repair these with catgut.

61.3 Injuries of the cheek, the facial nerve, and the parotid gland.

Deep lacerations of a patient's cheek may cut his facial nerve or his parotid duct, or both. Asymmetry in his smile will tell you that his facial nerve has been cut. Its temporal branch is the most important one because this supplies his eyelids, and division of it may expose his cornea. Division of its marginal mandibular branch will make his lip droop.

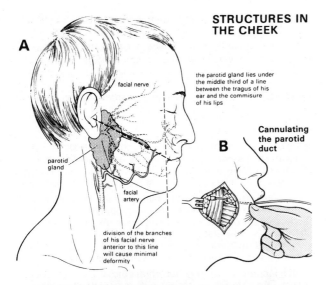

STRUCTURES IN THE CHEEK

the parotid gland lies under the middle third of a line between the tragus of his ear and the commisure of his lips

Cannulating the parotid duct

parotid gland

facial nerve

facial artery

division of the branches of his facial nerve anterior to this line will cause minimal deformity

Fig. 61-5 STRUCTURES IN THE CHEEK. If you fail to repair an injury to a patient's parotid duct, a salivary fistula will form. A, the anatomy of his parotid gland, parotid duct, and facial nerve. B, cannulating an injured parotid duct. *Partly after Hill, with kind permission.*

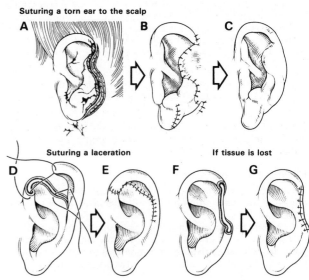

EAR INJURIES

Suturing a torn ear to the scalp

Suturing a laceration

If tissue is lost

Fig. 61-6 WOUNDS OF THE EARS. A, B, and C, if part of a patient's ear is missing and there is any hope of referring him for plastic surgery later, you can make an incision in his scalp (A), suture his ear to the edges of this incision (B), and refer him for plastic surgery (C). D, and E, when you suture this kind of laceration, put the first suture in the edge of his ear. *With the kind permission of Peter London.*

The parotid gland and its duct lie more superficially than the facial nerve, and are more easily injured.

STRUCTURES IN THE CHEEK

Repair the patient's muscles of mastication and facial expression with buried chromic catgut.

FACIAL NERVE INJURIES

If the laceration is anterior to a line dropped vertically from the lateral canthus of the patient's eye, only the peripheral branches of his facial nerve can have been injured. Deformity will be minimal and repair impractical.

If major branches of his facial nerve have been cut posterior to the vertical line, explore his wound and try to repair them by the methods in Section 55.9.

PAROTID GLAND INJURIES

If fluid leaks from a posterior wound of a patient's cheek, his parotid gland has been injured. Suture the wound as usual. If a fistulous leak of saliva does develop, it will probably heal spontaneously within a few days, and almost always does so within a month.

PAROTID DUCT INJURIES

If you fail to repair an injury to a patient's parotid duct, he will have a persistent flow of saliva from his cheek. The duct runs under the middle third of a line from the tragus of his ear to the commisure of his lips.

If his parotid duct is injured, repair it with fine silk or catgut over a polythene catheter leading into his mouth and fixed to his buccal mucosa. Pass the catheter, as in B, Fig. 61-5, from his wound, or from the opening of the duct inside his mouth. This is opposite the crown of his second upper molar tooth. Passing the catheter will be easier if you retract his cheek outwards to straighten the duct.

Keep the catheter in place by looping it out of his mouth and taping it to his chin to encourage the flow of saliva. Leave it in for a week.

Alternatively: (1) reimplant the proximal end of the duct through a new opening into his mouth, or (2) tie the duct. This will cause the gland to atrophy.

61.4 Injuries of the ears and the nose

An injured ear has some special problems: (1) It curves in three dimensions and is difficult to repair. (2) Its lacerations are usually jagged and skin or cartilage may be missing. (3) It has an unfortunate tendency to form haematomas which may become organized as a 'cauliflower ear'. (5) Exposed cartilage readily becomes infected causing major deformity. (6) Secondary reconstruction is unsatisfactory and is likely to be impossible, so do what you can when you first see an injured ear. Fortunately, the ear has a good blood supply, so flaps with even a short pedicle will live.

EAR AND NOSE INJURIES

EAR INJURIES

If there is any devitalized skin on the patient's ear, remove it. Don't leave cartilage uncovered! The skin over the ear is not very mobile, so you may have to graft it or excise the injury. Depending on the site, you may be able to remove up to 5 mm without this being noticeable.

If a patient's ear has been incised, insert the first stitch at the edge of the helix. This will avoid a ridge forming which can be very conspicuous when his wound has healed. Then align his antihelix. Try to repair his ear by suturing its perichondrium. If you have to suture the cartilage, use fine monofilament.

If a minor part of a patient's pinna is missing, suture the skin edges together, over the edge of the cartilage. Refer him for a plastic repair later.

If a major part of his pinna is missing, toilet the wound, spread the injured pinna slightly, and suture it in two layers to an incision immediately beneath it in his postauricular scalp, as in A, B, and C, Fig. 61-6. Refer him for a plastic repair later. Alternatively, suture the skin of his ear together over its cartilage, as in F, and G, in that figure.

If you are worried about the formation of a haematoma, pack his ear with moist cotton wool to maintain its shape, and bandage it firmly.

Leave most wounds exposed, don't dress them. Remove his stitches at 14 days.

If a haematoma forms, with or without a laceration, aspirate it and apply a pressure dressing. If it recurs following aspiration, incise it and insert a short length of rubber band for a drain.

NOSE INJURIES

See also Section 62.4. Try to align the edge of the patient's nose accurately, as in B, Fig. 61-2. Insert the first suture at the edge.

If an injury penetrates all layers of a patient's nose, repair the mucous membrane first using 4/0 catgut. Bring his nasal cartilages together, and try to hold them in place by suturing the skin with fine monofilament.

Only pack his nose if a pack is necessary to hold it in place. Avoid leaving packs in place, if you can.

CAUTION ! If he has a septal haematoma, evacuate it immediately through a small mucosal incision. If you fail to do this it will be absorbed, but in doing so, it will destroy his septal cartilage and cause a saddle nose.

62 Maxillofacial injuries

62.1 The general method for maxillofacial injuries

A patient with a severe facial injury is a very distressing sight—so distressing that you may feel that you can do nothing for him. In fact, you can do much, and maxillofacial injuries are no more difficult (or easy) than any others. They are usually the result of road accidents, and seat belts prevent most of them.

Not suprisingly, the parts of the face which stick out are those which are most often injured—a patient's nose, his zygoma, or his mandible. Fortunately, their injuries are usually not too difficult to treat. Much greater force has to be applied to fracture his maxilla, with the result that maxillary injuries are less common, but much more difficult. Although we describe each injury separately here, a patient is likely to have several of them, and other injuries also, especially injuries to his head and eyes.

Fractures of the middle third of the face are so complex that we shall not attempt to classify them except to say that the usual classification is that of Le Fort, who divided them into Types One, Two, and Three, as shown in Fig. 62-1. In a Type One fracture the alveolus, or tooth bearing part of the patient's upper jaw, breaks off, and may drop onto his lower teeth. In Types Two and Three the fracture lines are higher up in his maxilla. These fracture types may be combined, and may occur on one or both sides. The radiology, reduction, and fixation of the more difficult Le Fort fractures is beyond a district hospital. But prompt treatment, particularly in securing a patient's airway, may save his life, after which you have several days in which to refer him for expert reduction and fixation. Failure to reduce one of these fractures can cause severe deformities, which include a jaw which does not close, 'dish face', and diplopia. If you cannot refer a patient, we describe some of the easier methods you can use.

WHAT OTHER INJURIES DOES THE PATIENT HAVE?

The critical displacement in Le Fort fractures of Types Two and Three is the downward movement of the bones of the middle of the patient's face, as shown in Fig. 62-2. The strong front of his cranium forms an inclined plane, down which his facial skeleton slides. (1) This lengthens his face. (2) It pushes his upper molars down onto his lower ones so that they gag (prevent his jaw closing properly). (3) It pushes his soft palate down onto his tongue and prevents him breathing through this mouth. At the same time, his fracture bleeds severely, and his nose is obstructed by blood clot. The result is that he may suffocate, so *the immediate life saving procedure is to hook two of your fingers round the back of his hard palate, and pull his maxilla back up the inclined plane of his skull.* This will allow him to breathe. His breathing can also be obstructed by bilateral fractures of his lower jaw which allow his tongue to fall back against his pharynx.

Fractures of the middle third of a patient's face have several other unfortunate features: (1) They are always multiple, sometimes with 50 or more fragments. (2) Several of his cranial nerves may be injured, especially his infraorbital and superior dental nerves. (3) His ethmoid may be fractured and his dura

FRACTURES OF THE MIDDLE THIRD OF THE FACE

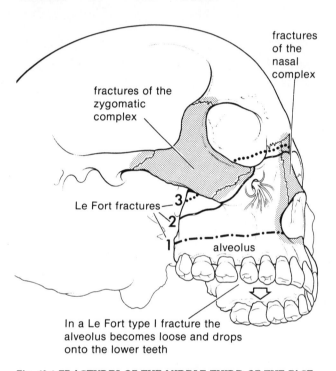

fractures of the nasal complex

fractures of the zygomatic complex

Le Fort fractures

alveolus

In a Le Fort type I fracture the alveolus becomes loose and drops onto the lower teeth

Fig. 62-1 FRACTURES OF THE MIDDLE THIRD OF THE FACE. In a Type One fracture the alveolus, or tooth bearing part of the patient's upper jaw, breaks off, and may drop onto his lower teeth. In Types Two and Three the bones of the middle of the patient's face slide downwards, as shown in the next figure. These fracture types may be combined and may occur on one or both sides.

torn, so that CSF leaks from his nose. (4) His orbit may be fractured (Fig. 62-3), sometimes with the displacement of its contents into his maxillary sinuses (the orbital blow—out syndrome). (5) The circulation to his eye may be obstructed and make him blind if the obstruction is not relieved within minutes of the accident (the ophthalmic canal syndrome). (6) His maxillary sinuses may fill with blood. (7) His nasolachrymal ducts may be injured and cause a flow of tears.

When you treat such a patient aim to: (1) Restore his airway. (2) Control bleeding. (3) Make his teeth bite normally. You should be able to do this with most fractures of his mandible, and some fractures of his maxilla. If either his maxilla or his mandible is intact, you can use one of them to splint the other. *If you can make his bite normal, reduction will be perfect.* (4) Prevent some deformities by reducing fractures of his nose and zygoma.

If you can refer a patient, do so early because the longer you wait, the more difficult reduction will become. If you cannot refer him, you can certainly save his life, but he may have to live with his deformities. Soon after the injury his face will look distressingly swollen, so do your best to reassure him and his

DOWNWARD DISPLACEMENT OF THE MAXILLA

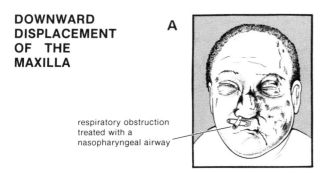

A

respiratory obstruction treated with a nasopharyngeal airway

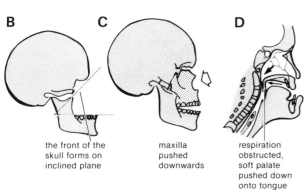

B

C

D

the front of the skull forms on inclined plane

maxilla pushed downwards

respiration obstructed, soft palate pushed down onto tongue

Fig. 62-2 DOWNWARD DISPLACEMENT OF THE MAXILLA. A, if the patient's respiration is obstructed, push a nasopharyngeal airway down one or both sides of his nose. B, C, and D, show how the front of his skull forms an inclined plane down which his maxilla can be pushed. *After Killey, with kind permission.*

family. The face has a good blood supply and will heal well, so that they can expect him to improve remarkably. But it can also swell quickly and hide underlying deformities, so examine him with care when you first see him.

The methods we describe assume you don't have a dental laboratory, and so cannot make cap splints, etc. You will however need a drill and some soft stainless steel wire (70.9). Occasionally an arch bar is useful. If you can get the help of a dentist, always do so.

• *ARCH BAR, stainless steel, five only.* Sometimes, the most convenient way to fix the fragments of a patient's upper or lower jaw is

THE ORBITAL BLOW-OUT SYNDROME

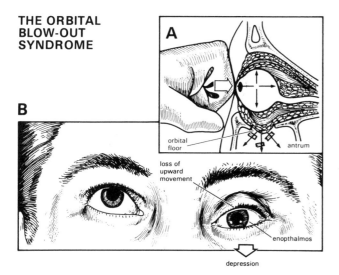

A

B

orbital floor

antrum

loss of upward movement

enopthalmos

depression

Fig. 62-3 THE ORBITAL BLOW–OUT SYNDROME. A, a blow to the patient's orbit has broken its floor, so that its contents have prolapsed into his antrum. B, unless you refer him to have it repaired, he may have permanent enophthalmos, diplopia and loss of upward eye movement. *From Rutherford, Nelson, Weston and Wilson with kind permission.*

to bend a metal bar, to shape it, and to wire it to his teeth. If you don't have a proper arch bar, you can use any tough piece of stainless steel wire, or even some paper clips twisted together.

A SWOLLEN FACE CAN CONCEAL A MAJOR INJURY

THE GENERAL METHOD FOR A MAXILLOFACIAL INJURY

This extends Section 51.3 on the care of a severely injured patient. Injuries to his lower jaw are described in Section 62.7.

IMMEDIATE TREATMENT

CAN THE PATIENT BREATHE? If his breathing is difficult, look into his mouth to see if: (1) his airway has been obstructed by blood and vomit, (2) his soft palate has been driven down onto his tongue by displaced Le Fort fractures, or if, (3) his tongue has fallen backwards after a mandibular fracture?

If his soft palate has been driven onto his tongue, hook your fingers round the back of his hard palate, and pull the bones of the middle of his face gently upwards and forwards, so as to restore his airway and perhaps the circulation to his eyes. Reduction may not be easy, and you may need considerable force. If the fracture is impacted and you fail to reduce it, he may need a tracheostomy, as described below.

If necessary, grip his maxillary alveolus with the special forceps (Rowe's) for this purpose, or with suitable strong sharp toothed forceps, and rock it to disimpact the fragments.

If his tongue or lower jaw has fallen backwards, put some sutures or a towel clip through it, and gently pull it forwards. Lying him on his side will also help. When you transport him, lie him on his side.

If he has a severe jaw injury with much tissue loss, transport him lying on his front with his head over the end of the stretcher and his forehead supported by bandages between its handles, as in Fig. 62-4.

If he feels more comfortable sitting up, let him do so. His airway may improve remarkably when he does this.

Suck out his mouth, remove blood clots, debris, loose teeth, vomit, and foreign bodies.

A Guedel airway does not help, so don't waste time trying to insert one. Tracheal intubation is usually impractical.

If his nose is severely injured and bleeding, suck it clear and insert a nasopharyngeal tube, or any similar thick rubber tube, down one side. Put a safety pin through it to stop it slipping, as in A, Fig. 62-2.

CAUTION ! A nasopharyngeal tube does not always ensure a clear airway because it may kink or block against the posterior pharyngeal wall, so watch it carefully and twist and adjust it as necessary. Keep it sucked out by passing a smaller tube down it, attached to a sucker. Use the same equipment to suck out the patient's mouth, and keep it beside his bed.

Tracheostomy. You may need to do a tracheostomy (52.2) if: (1) You cannot disimpact and reduce the fracture of the middle third of a patient's face. (2) You cannot control severe posterior bleeding. (3) He has oedema of his glottis, particularly following a neck injury. (4) He has a severe injury with much tissue loss. Tracheostomy will be difficult. Use ketamine, local anaesthesia and a cuffed tube.

CAUTION ! If his breathing is in danger and you have to refer him, he will be safer with a tracheostomy than with a suture through his tongue to pull it forward, which is the other alternative.

STOP BLEEDING Tie any large bleeding vessels. If there is troublesome oozing, apply an adrenaline soaked pack firmly to the bleeding surface. A postnasal pack (Chapter 24) will usually stop bleeding. If necessary, use large temporary haemostatic sutures (3.1), but take care not to strangle the tissues.

If a wound is deep, be prepared to pack it. Occasionally, you may have to tie a patient's external carotid artery (3.5).

A MAXILLOFACIAL INJURY

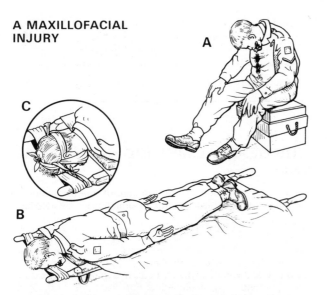

Fig. 62-4 A severe MAXILLOFACIAL INJURY. A, note that a conscious patient is likely to be more comfortable sitting forward. B, and C, if he has much tissue loss, transport him face down like this. *After Killey with kind permission.*

SHOCK is unusual. If a patient is shocked, suspect that he also has an abdominal or a thoracic injury.

THE HISTORY AND EXAMINATION OF A MAXILLOFACIAL INJURY

The patient is probably unable to talk, so enquire from observers if he lost consciousness and so might have a head injury (63.1).

Gently wash his face with warm water to remove caked blood. Look at it carefully for asymmetry. Compare one side with the other throughout the examination. Is his nose or his face flattened? If you suspect a fracture of his zygoma, look at it from above and below and use the two pencil test in Fig. 62-12.

BRUISING This is a useful guide to underlying injuries.

Zygomatic fractures There is always bruising round the patient's orbits, which develops rapidly as a uniform continuous sheet. It is limited peripherally by the attachments of his orbicularis muscle, and extends subconjunctivally towards his eye from the lateral side. Ask him to look inwards. You will see bruising extending back into his orbit without a posterior limit.

Look inside his mouth and examine his upper buccal sulcus for bruising, tenderness, and crepitation over his zygomatic buttresses.

Nasal fractures There is bruising round his orbits which is most severe medially.

Black eye This is the main differential diagnosis. Orbital bruising is most severe medially. It is subconjunctival, patchy, and bright red.

EYES Has either of the patient's eyes sunk inwards or downwards? Are they level? Displacement may indicate herniation of the contents of his orbit through its floor into his maxillary sinus, or a fracture at the fronto–zygomatic suture line.

Separate his eyelids, and test the sight of each of his eyes separately. If an eye is blind, its optic nerve may be injured. Ask him to follow your finger as you test for diplopia. This may be due to: (1) displacement of his orbit, (2) displacement of his globe, (3) a 6th nerve palsy, or (4) oedema. If his eye is unable to look upwards, its inferior rectus is trapped, and his orbital floor is probably fractured. Note the size of his pupils and their reaction to light.

If he has massive proptosis, he has a retrobulbar haemorrhage which may be compressing his optic nerve. Make a

TWO COMPLICATIONS

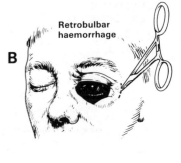

Fig. 62-5 TWO COMPLICATIONS OF A HEAD OR MAXILLOFACIAL INJURY. A, fractures of a patient's ethmoid may make his CSF leak. B, a fracture of the base of his skull may cause severe proptosis and compress his optic nerves. Drain the blood by making an incision near his outer canthus. *After Duke Elder.*

small incision at his outer canthus, take a haemostat and push this into the incision (B, Fig. 62-5); blood will squirt out. If you don't do this, his eye will become blind.

FRACTURES OF THE FACE AND SKULL Carefully feel all over the patient's head and face for tenderness, step deformities, irregularity, or crepitus. Feel his zygomatic bones, the edges of his orbits, his palate, and the bones of his nose. In a Le Fort Type Two or Three fracture you will feel many small bony fragments under the skin in his ethmoid region.

Hold the root of his nose between your finger and thumb. At the same time put two fingers from your other hand into his mouth. If you can move his facial skeleton on his skull, he has a Le Fort fracture. You may feel it move more easily if you hold his upper gum between your thumb and index finger.

Can he open and shut his mouth, bite normally, move his jaw from side to side and protrude it? Do his teeth meet normally? If his bite is abnormal, one or both of his jaws have been fractured. Failure to move his jaw normally may indicate a displaced fracture of his zygoma or his mandible.

Examine the mucosa of both his jaws for bruising, tenderness, irregularity, and crepitus.

NERVE INJURIES Test for anaesthesia of his cheeks (infraorbital nerves) and upper gums (superior dental nerves).

TOOTH INJURIES Feel his teeth and try to rock them. Individual teeth may move abnormally, so may several adjacent teeth. Mobile teeth can be caused by: (1) A fracture. (2) Exposure of their roots. (3) Periodontal disease.

Inspect his teeth with a mirror and probe. Tap them; if they give a 'cracked cup' sound, the bone above them may be fractured. If a piece of tooth is missing, X-ray the patient's chest in case he has inhaled it.

NOSE INJURIES Epistaxis is usually unilateral or absent in zygomatic fractures, and bilateral in nasal ones. Examine the patient's nasal septum with a speculum. This may be displaced in a nasal fracture. However, it is often asymmetrical in otherwise normal people. If he has a haematoma of the septum, it neeeds evacuating, goto 61.4

LEAKING CSF may be anterior or posterior, and is usually diagnosed after a few days when bleeding and oedema have subsided. The patient may complain of a salty taste in his mouth. If you are uncertain if a discharge is CSF or not, test it as in Section 63.12. CSF may leak in severe naso–ethmoidal fractures and in some Le Fort fractures.

OTHER INJURIES Look for these (51.3), and especially for a head injury (63.1), or an injury to the patient's cervical spine (64.3). These may be more serious than those of his face. A maxillofacial injury does not usually cause shock, so if he is shocked, suspect some other injury, especially an abdominal one, which may take priority.

X-RAYS are difficult to interpret, and involve turning the patient into a position which may obstruct his airway. Ask for: (1) An AP view of his mandible. (2) A Waters view of his skull in which you may be able to recognise: (a) filling of his maxillary antra, and (b) irregularities in the outlines of his orbits showing they have been fractured.

WOUND TOILET AND CLOSURE AFTER A MAXILLOFACIAL INJURY

This must be thorough, especially if sand or tar are ingrained in the patient's wounds. If you don't remove them, severe fibrosis and disfigurement will follow. You will find a sterile toothbrush useful.

Handle his tissues gently with skin hooks and fine forceps. Remove soiled tags of deeper tissues and mucosa with scissors. Trim only 1 or 2 mm of skin edge to provide non–bevelled uncontaminated skin edges which you can approximate accurately. Use a sharp No. 15 blade and ophthalmic scissors. Close his mucosa with 3/0 silk, or failing this with fine chromic catgut. Close his skin by primary suture after you have fixed any fractures. If necessary, you can undermine the skin of his face for 2 to 3 cm to assist closure.

If part of the patient's cheek is missing, refer him immediately for primary reconstruction. If this is impractical, stitch his buccal mucosa to his skin (61-4). If necessary, do the same with his nose.

If there are loose bone fragments, conserve them unless they are grossly soiled. You can sterilize detached fragments in boiling water and replace them as chip grafts.

CAUTION ! (1) Don't close his skin under tension. (2) Don't leave bone bare—try to cover all bony surfaces.

REDUCING FRACTURES AFTER A MAXILLOFACIAL INJURY

Reduce and, where necessary, fix any fractures of the patient's nose (62.4), zygoma (62.5), and mandible (62.7). These are not urgent operations, so resuscitate him first. For anaesthesia, see A 6.4, and A 16.10. You can do most operations on an injured jaw using pterygopalatine blocks, bilaterally if necessary.

CAUTION ! Always protect a patient's eyes when you operate on his face.

If he has a Le Fort fracture, or an orbital floor fracture, refer him. If you cannot refer him, the next section (62.2) describes some methods you may be able to use.

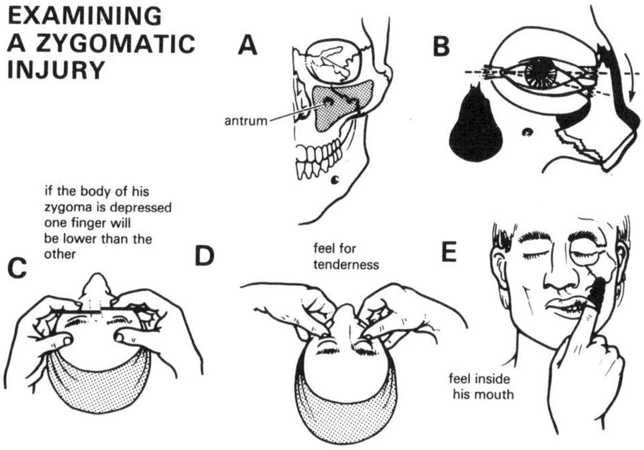

EXAMINING A ZYGOMATIC INJURY

antrum

if the body of his zygoma is depressed one finger will be lower than the other

feel for tenderness

feel inside his mouth

Fig. 62-6 EXAMINING A ZYGOMATIC INJURY. A, the zygoma forms the prominence of the cheek, and also the floor and lateral wall of the orbit. The maxillary antrum extends into it. B, if a fragment of the zygoma is displaced downwards, the patient's lateral canthus will also be displaced downwards, and his palpebral fissure will be oblique. C, press gently. If the body of his zygoma is depressed, one finger will be lower than the other. D, press gently on the lower border of his orbit, you may elicit tenderness and feel a fracture between his zygoma and his maxilla. E, feel inside his mouth for a fracture in the lateral wall of his maxillary antrum. See also Fig. 62-12. *After Watson Jones with kind permission.*

NURSING A MAXILLOFACIAL INJURY

If the patient is conscious, sit him well forward, so that his tongue falls forward, and blood and saliva can dribble out of his mouth. This will make him comfortable and also help him to breathe.

If he is unconscious, turn him onto his side into the recovery position (51-2), so that blood and saliva can run out of his nose and mouth. If other injuries prevent this, put a pillow under one shoulder, and turn his head to the other side.

FOOD AND FLUIDS If the patient is to be operated on, withhold these. Otherwise feed him through a tube.

CLEANING AND DISINFECTION is critically important for the healing of all wounds inside a patient's mouth. Ask him to rinse out his mouth after eating, using :(1) a rinse containing 10 ml of 0.5% chlorhexidine, or (2) 2% salt solution, or failing either of these, (3) plain water. As soon as possible, encourage him to clean his teeth regularly with a toothbrush or a clean chewing stick.

Coat his lips liberally with vaseline to stop them sticking together and interfering with his respiration.

DRUGS FOR A MAXILLOFACIAL INJURY

Give the patient amoxycillin, ampicillin, or fortified procaine penicillin for one week. Start immediately (2.7). This usually prevents bone infection, and is important if a fracture opens into his mouth.

If his CSF is leaking, give him 1 g of sulphadimidine 6 hourly until 48 hours after it has stopped. Most leaks stop spontaneously, except in severely comminuted fractures.

CAUTION ! Don't give him powerful analgesics, such as morphine, which will depress his cough reflex. If he is restless, give him paradelyde or diazepam.

Don't forget tetanus prophylaxis (54.11).

CHARTS Start a head injury chart (63-4) and a fluid balance chart (A 15-5).

FURTHER MANAGEMENT OF A MAXILLOFACIAL INJURY

If possible, refer all more serious injuries. Read on for injuries to a patient's teeth and alveoli (62.2), simpler methods for maxillary fractures (62.3), fractures of the patient's nose (62.4), fractures of his zygomatic complex (62.5), dislocation of his jaw (62.6), the general method for a dislocated lower jaw (62.7), fractured condyles (62.8), fractures of the ascending ramus of his mandible (62.9), fractures of the angle and body of his mandible (62.10), difficulties with mandibular fractures (62.11), and fixing mandibular fractures with acrylic resin (62.8).

TRANSPORT MAXILLOFACIAL INJURIES PRONE OR LYING ON THEIR SIDES

62.2 Injuries to the teeth and alveolus

The front of a patient's upper jaw is most at risk. In less severe injuries only his teeth are damaged, in more severe ones his alveolus may be fractured. Although injured teeth do not threaten life, they are acutely painful, especially when the pulp is hanging out. When a tooth is hit: (1) its crown may fracture, (2) its root may fracture, (3) the whole tooth may subluxate, (4) it may be impacted into the surrounding tissue, or, (5) it may be inhaled, and be followed by a lung abscess.

INJURIES TO THE TEETH AND ALVEOLUS

If the patient's oral mucosa is torn, suture it with fine 4/0 waxed silk or chromic catgut.

If the crown of a patient's tooth is missing, its exposed pulp will be visible as a pink spot on the root surface. It will

METHODS FOR LE FORT FRACTURES

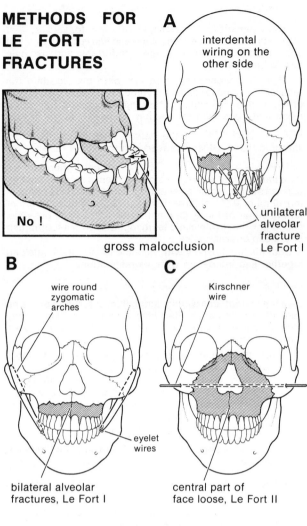

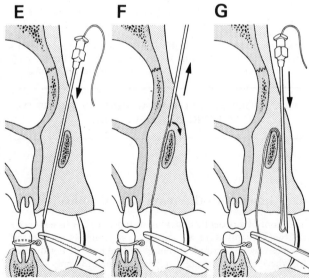

Fig. 62-8 SIMPLER METHODS FOR LE FORT FRACTURES. A, interdental wiring holding a unilateral fracture in place. B, wire round the patient's zygomatic arches holding a bilateral fracture in place. C, a Kirschner wire holding the central part of his face in place. D, this figure was drawn from a cast, and shows what can happen if you fail to reduce a severe maxillary injury. Note the gross malocclusion. The patient's jaws will have to be refractured and reset. Aligning them would have been much easier at the time of the injury. E, a lumbar puncture needle has been passed medial to his zygomatic arch into his upper buccal sulcus, and was passed down it. F, the needle has been withdrawn. G, the needle is being passed lateral to the zygomatic arch. *Kindly contributed by Susan Likimani and Andrew Curnock.*

be acutely painful, so touch it with phenol on a small piece of cotton wool. This will kill and anaesthetize the nerve. Take a chest X-ray in case he has inhaled the missing fragment. It will have to be removed by bronchoscopy.

If a tooth is only mildly subluxed, leave it in place; it will probably tighten up and live. Meanwhile splint it with a piece of lead foil or the top of a milk bottle moulded to the tooth and gum.

If a tooth is so loose that you can lift it up and down in its socket, remove it. A dentist may be able to splint it and re-implant it, if he sees it soon enough, so don't delay.

If there is an opening between a patient's antrum and his mouth, try to close it. If his antrum is already infected, leave it open and irrigate it daily. Don't pack it.

COMMINUTED FRACTURES OF THE ALVEOLUS If the bony fragment with its teeth is still attached to periosteum, leave it, and splint the patient's teeth as best as you can with an arch bar. If the fragment of alveolus is completely detached from the periosteum, dissect it out and remove it.

GAPS IN THE MAXILLARY SINUS Close these temporarily by packing them with gauze impregnated with bismuth, iodoform, and paraffin paste (BIPP), or with vaseline gauze. As soon as the patient's general condition is stabilized, close the gap with a flap of mucosa from his adjacent cheek. Suture it carefully, preferably with 3/0 black waxed silk sutures. Tell him not to blow his nose and to sneeze with his mouth open.

MISSING DENTURES A piece of denture can also be inhaled. It is unlikely to be radio-opaque, so a normal chest X-ray does not exclude inhalation.

62.3 Simpler methods for maxillary fractures

There are few easy methods for Le Fort fractures. If the patient is lucky enough to have an intact mandible, you can wire his broken maxilla to it. Packing his maxillary sinuses and repairing his orbital floor are beyond a district hospital.

Le Fort Type One fractures with an intact mandible Alveolar fractures are quite common, so to be able to do anything for them is useful. Although they are much easier to fix if the patient has an intact mandible, you may be able to fix a mandibular fracture with an arch bar, and then proceed as if his mandible were intact.

If he has a Le Fort Type One fracture on one side only, half his alveolus hangs loose on that side, as in A, Fig. 62-8. If his mandible is intact you can wire it to the intact half of his alveolus, so that it holds the fractured half reduced.

If his alveolus has fractured on both sides, and he has an intact mandible, you can wire his zygomatic arches on both sides to his mandible, as in B, Fig. 62-8.

Type Two Fractures In some Type Two fractures the zygomatic arches are intact, but the bones of the centre of the patient's face are displaced. You may be able to drill a Kirschner wire through one zygomatic arch, through the displaced central fragment of the face, and then out through the other arch.

WIRING THE ZYGOMATIC ARCH TO THE MANDIBLE

INDICATIONS Maxillary fractures with an intact mandible.

ANAESTHESIA Premedicate the patient well and use infiltration anaesthesia of his gums (A 6.3),

Fix wire eyelets to his teeth on both sides of his lower jaw as in Section 62.10.

Protect his eyes as in Section 62.4. Push a blunt aspiration needle or large lumbar puncture needle through his skin just above his zygomatic arch and posterior to his outer canthus. Push the needle downwards behind his zygomatic arch into his superior buccal sulcus, as in E, Fig. 62-8.

Thread wire through the needle and then remove the needle, leaving the wire in his tissues (F).

Now pass the needle up from his buccal sulcus, superficial

UNREDUCED NASAL FRACTURES

A blow from in front

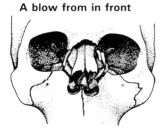

depressed bridge
of the nose

A blow from the side

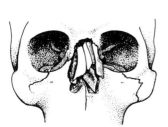

deviation of the nose

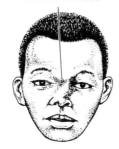

Fig. 62-9 UNREDUCED FRACTURES OF THE NOSE. If you don't reduce a patient's broken nose, these are some of the possible results. *After Killey, permission requested.*

ELEVATING A FRACTURED NOSE

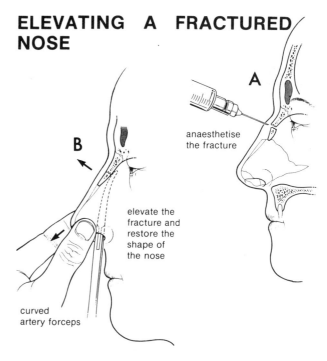

A

anaesthetise
the fracture

B

elevate the
fracture and
restore the
shape of
the nose

curved
artery forceps

Fig. 62-10 ELEVATING A FRACTURE OF THE NOSE. A, inflitrating the site of the fracture. B, raising the depressed bones with curved artery forceps. Always suspect a fracture after any blow on the nose. Swelling of the soft tissues can easily hide it. *Kindly contributed by Peter Bewes.*

---

to his zygomatic arch, under his skin, to come out of the same hole in his skin as the wire (G).

Pass the other end of wire through the needle so that it emerges in his buccal sulcus. Remove the needle. You will now have a loop of wire passing round his zygomatic arch with both ends emerging in his buccal sulcus.

Repeat the process on the other side, and then join the wire loops to the eyelets that you have previously fixed to his mandible.

62.4 Fractures of the nose

A patient's injured nose is displaced, swollen and bleeding. Sometimes the swelling hides his displaced bones underneath, so always suspect a fracture after any blow on the nose. He may have blood in his orbits and under the medial halves of both his conjunctivae.

A force applied to the side of the nose pushes it sideways. A force applied from in front squashes it and splays it outwards. If you don't treat these injuries, they produce the deformities shown in Fig. 62-9. If the force is severe enough, it can: (1) Fracture the frontal processes of a patient's maxillae. (2) Displace his nasal cartilages. (3) Dislodge his septal cartilage from its groove in his vomer. (4) Comminute his vomer. (5) Fracture his ethmoid bones so that CSF flows from his nose.

TREATING A BROKEN NOSE

See also Section 61.4.

CONTROLLING BLEEDING If this is severe, pack the patient's nose with ribbon gauze soaked in saline. Treat him as soon as possible without waiting for the swelling to go down.

EQUIPMENT If possible, use Walsham's forceps to reduce his nasal bones, and Ash's forceps to straighten his nasal septum. If you don't have them, you can use any stout clamp, but

don't close it tight. Walsham's forceps don't quite meet, and therefore don't crush tissue.

ANAESTHESIA (1) Pterygopalatine block (A 6.4). (2) Give the patient a general anaesthetic, and pass a tracheal tube (A 13.2). (3) Use local infiltration anaesthesia.

PROTECT THE PATIENT'S EYES Put squares of vaseline gauze over both his eyes to prevent plaster getting into them.

REDUCTION Clean the patient's face with cetrimide to remove grease. Examine his nose carefully with your fingers.

Cover one blade of Walsham's forceps, or some other suitable instrument, with rubber tube. Pass it into his nose and lever the fragments of his bridge into place. Then do the same on the other side.

If necessary, mould his comminuted lachrymal bones, and the medial walls of his orbits, so as to reconstitute the bridge of his nose.

CAUTION ! (1) Don't forget to protect his eyes. (2) Try hard to restore the full height of the bridge of his nose.

When you have done this, pass one blade of Asch's septal forceps, or any other suitable instrument, down each side of the patient's septum and straighten it, so that it lies in the midline. If necessary, grasp his septal cartilage, bring it forward, and replace it in its groove in his vomer.

Pass an instrument down each side of the nose to make sure he has a clear nasal airway. Pack both his nostril's with 1 cm selvedgeless gauze soaked in liquid paraffin.

SPLINTING If the fracture is mild, no splint is needed. If the fracture is severe, splint it, either with a plaster cast, or with lead splints.

A plaster cast Make eight thicknesses of plaster bandage into a T-shape. Wet this and put it on the patient's nose and forehead. If any plaster overlaps the lower end of his nose, turn it up like a brim. As it sets, mould it to his forehead and the sides of his nose. Strengthen the plaster over the bridge of his nose with two more layers of plaster bandage.

Remove the vaseline gauze squares from his eyes, and then wrap a crepe bandage round his head to hold the cast. Or, hold it in place with adhesive strapping. It will hold his nose in place by suction.

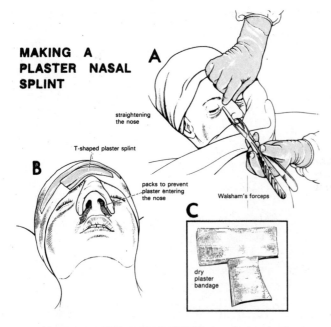

MAKING A PLASTER NASAL SPLINT

A straightening the nose

B T-shaped plaster splint

packs to prevent plaster entering the nose

Walsham's forceps

C dry plaster bandage

Fig. 62-11 A PLASTER NASAL SPLINT. A, reducing the fracture with Walsham's forceps. B, the splint in place. C, dry plaster bandage ready for preparing the splint. *Kindly contributed by Peter Bewes.*

CAUTION ! Don't fix the splint to a plaster headcap, because if this displaces, it will displace his broken nose.

When oedema has subsided in a few days, fit a fresh cast. Leave this for 2 weeks.

A lead splint If the fracture is too severely comminuted to be held in a plaster splint, hold it with two lead plates, one on each side of the patient's nose. You can use two or three layers of the lead backing from some intra–oral X-ray films. Pass a mattress suture of 0.35 mm soft stainless steel wire through his nose with a straight needle.

62.5 Fractures of the zygomatic complex

A blow to the side of a patient's face drives his zygoma inwards, usually on one side only. The zygomatic bones are so closely

TESTING FOR A FRACTURE OF THE ZYGOMA

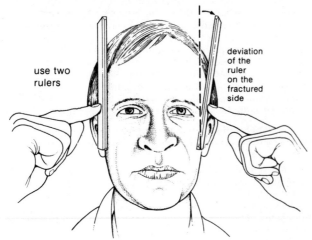

use two rulers

deviation of the ruler on the fractured side

Fig. 62-12 EXAMINING FOR A FRACTURE OF THE ZYGOMA. See also Figure 62-6. *Kindly contributed by Peter Bewes—it is a good likeness of him!.*

united to the frontal and temporal bones, that, when they fracture, the neighbouring parts of these other bones usually do so too. The zygomatic complex therefore usually fractures as a whole. The displaced zygomatic fragment can rotate clockwise, or anticlockwise, and its orbital rim can be inverted or everted. The floor of the orbit is always partly comminuted.

If you see a patient early enough, you may see that the side of his face is flattened. Oedema fills out this flattening within three hours, and it does not return for a week, after the oedema has subsided. If you are in doubt, there is a useful test for flattening of the zygoma. Put two pencils on either side of his face. They should lie parallel to one another. If the lower end of a pencil is tilted inwards, the patient's zygoma is flattened on that side, as in Fig. 62-12. The obviousness of this flattening depends greatly on whether he has a thin bony, face which accentuates the displacement, or a fat one, which hides it.

When a patient's zygoma is injured, his maxillary sinus fills with blood, so that his nose bleeds from that side. Injury to his infra–orbital nerve makes his cheek numb, and displacement of the lower part of his orbit pushes his eye downwards, and restricts its movements. Herniation of the fat in his orbit into his maxillary sinus may also make his eye sink inwards and downwards, and cause diplopia. This can also be caused by injuries of his 6th nerve, or his ocular muscles or their attachments. It can be temporary or permanent. If it is due to a fracture of his zygomatic complex, reducing this may correct it.

Fractures of the zygomatic arch Sometimes, only the arch of a patient's zygoma is fractured. There is a depression over it, and the movement of the coronoid process of his mandible is restricted. Although the depression may be obvious at the time of the injury, it may rapidly fill with oedema and become invisible. If his mouth was open when he was injured, he may be unable to close his jaw. Don't try to elevate the fragment, unless he has difficulty moving his jaw.

Reducing fractures of the zygomatic complex Fragments of the zygomatic arch are held by the zygomatic fascia, and although they may displace inwards, they don't move in other directions. The patient's temporalis fascia is attached to the superior border of his zygomatic arch, whereas his temporalis muscle is attached to his coronoid process. This enables you to pass an elevator between the fascia and the muscle, and lever his zygomatic arch outwards into place. Try to operate within the first 48 hours, when the replaced fragment is more likely to be stable and less likely to need wiring. After two weeks, the ends of the fragments will have softened and rounded, and you will probably need to wire them, after 4 weeks they will have united so that you cannot move them. After this length of time they will probably need open refracture, open reduction, and wiring.

The methods below do not include packing the maxillary sinus, and repairing the orbital floor. If the contents of a patient's orbit have prolapsed into his maxillary sinus, and you cannot refer him, he will have to live with his enophthalmos and wear an eye patch.

ELEVATING A FRACTURED ZYGOMA

INDICATIONS (1) Inability of the patient to open and close his jaw. (2) Diplopia. If you are inexperienced, and he can move his jaw normally and can see straight, disregard any deformity and don't operate.

The method described here is for the zygomatic arch. By a slight change in the position of the lever, you can also use it for fractures of the body of his zygoma and the adjacent part of his maxilla.

EQUIPMENT A general set with a Bristowe's elevator, or a McDonald's elevator, or a long secrewdriver.

ANAESTHESIA Give the patient a general anaesthetic and intubate him (13.2).

ELEVATING A DEPRESSED ZYGOMA

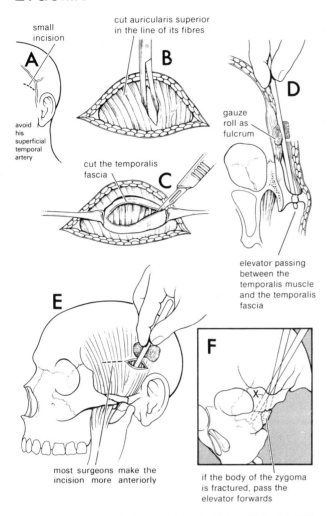

Fig. 62-13 ELEVATING A DEPRESSED FRACTURE OF THE ZYGOMATIC–MAXILLARY COMPLEX. A, the initial incision avoiding the superficial temporal vessels. B, dividing the auricularis superior. C, incising the temporalis fascia. D, passing an elevator. E, elevating the arch. F, elevating the body of the zygoma. *Kindly contributed by John M. Loré Jr.*

REDUCTION Be sure to protect the patient's eyes. Make a 2 cm antero-posterior incision in his temporal fossa, just above his hairline, as in A, Fig. 62-13.

Reflect his skin. Underneath the skin and the superficial fascia you will see his auricularis superior muscle. Cut in the line of its fibres (B). If his hairline is low, and the incision is lower, you may meet the fibres of auricularis anterior. These run more horizontally, so separate them in a horizontal plane. Underneath them lies his tough deep temporal fascia. Cut this to expose his temporalis muscle (C). The fascia may have two layers. If so, incise them both.

Pass a Bristow's elevator between his temporalis fascia, and the surface of his temporalis muscle. Push it down until its end lies between his zygomatic bone and his temporalis muscle (D). It should slip easily between the bone and the muscle.

Using a gauze roll as a fulcrum to protect the upper skin edge, gently lever his zygoma into a slightly overcorrected position (E).

If the body of a patient's zygoma is fractured, pass the elevator forwards, and lever it into position (F).

If the fragment is stable, no wiring is necessary.

If the fragment is unstable, wire its junctions with his frontal or maxillary bones, or with both of them, through separate small incisions.

WIRING A ZYGOMATIC–FRONTAL FRACTURE Expose the fracture line by blunt dissection through an incision in one of the wrinkles at the corner of the patient's eye. Take care to avoid the branches of his facial nerve supplying his orbicularis muscle. Drill small holes in the bone and fix the fragments in place with soft stainless steel wire.

WIRING A ZYGOMATIC–MAXILLARY FRACTURE Make a 1 cm incision just below the lower rim of the patient's orbit. Drill small holes and wire the fragments together.

ALTERNATIVELY, in some fractures you may be able to grasp the fragments through his skin with tenaculum forceps.

CLOSING THE WOUND Close his deep temporal fascia with a few monofilament sutures. Put a firm pressure pad over the skin incision.

62.6 Dislocation of the jaw

When a patient dislocates his jaw, his mandibular condyles slip forward in their sockets over the articular eminences of his temporomandibular joints. This can happen when he laughs or yawns, or is hit in the face with his mouth open. The mouth of a patient with a dislocated jaw remains permanently half open in an anterior open bite. Swallowing is difficult, so that saliva dribbles from the corners of his lips. When you examine him, you find a small depression over his temporomandibular joints. If his mandible dislocates one side only, it deviates away from the midline.

THERESA was cultivating her fields in Zaire when she yawned and dislocated her jaw. She had been told that patients had to pay at the Catholic hospital, and as she had no money, she had to wait some weeks to sell some produce before she could go there. The doctors there failed, because her dislocation was no longer recent, so she waited a few more weeks, sold some more produce, and tried the Protestants. Her dislocation was now even older, and they too failed, so she now walks about with her mouth permanently open. LESSONS Dislocations of the jaw are much easier to reduce if they are done early. The tragedy of this patient is that both hospitals would have treated her for free, if she had come early and told them she could not pay.

REDUCING A DISLOCATED JAW

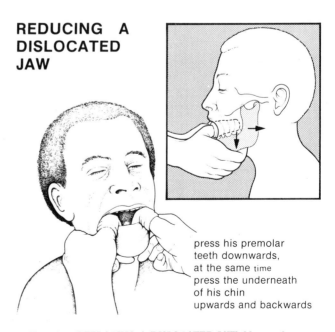

press his premolar teeth downwards, at the same time press the underneath of his chin upwards and backwards

Fig. 62-14 REPLACING A DISLOCATED JAW. Most patients don't need an anaesthetic. If necessary, give a patient pethidine or diazepam.

REPLACING A DISLOCATED JAW

RECENT DISLOCATIONS Most patients need no anaesthetic.

Sit the patient forward in a chair. Ask an assistant to stand behind him and hold his head. Put some gauze over his lower posterior teeth on each side. Press his premolar teeth downwards. At the same time press the underneath of his chin upwards and backwards.

If he opens his mouth too wide again, the dislocation may recur. So bandage his jaw to keep his mouth shut for 3 days. Allow him to open it just a little for eating.

OLD DISLOCATIONS Fix arch bars to each jaw (62.10). Cut an ordinary rubber eraser into two pieces, and put a piece between the patient's posterior molars on each side to act as a fulcrum. Fix strong rubber bands between the arch bars in front. During the following few days they will exert steady traction and close his anterior open bite. If this fails, refer him.

62.7 The general method for an injured lower jaw

A patient is hit on his jaw. One or more fractures tear the mucoperiosteum covering the body of his mandible. He dribbles bloody saliva, and can neither speak, swallow, nor close his teeth normally. Moving his injured jaw may be so painful that he holds it in his hands. If you move it gently for him, you may be able to feel crepitus.

Mandibular fractures can be unilateral or bilateral. The weak parts of the bone and the common sites for fractures are: (1) the neck of the condyles (B in Fig. 62-15), (2) the angles of the mandible (E, and F), and (3) the premolar region (G). Fractures of the angle and body of the mandible are open, but not those of the rami, condyles, or coronoid processes. Often, the patient has other injuries too, and the combination of a jaw injury and a head injury is common. But, provided there is no gross comminution or tissue loss, you should be able to treat most of these fractures successfully. The mandible remodels readily, even after a comminuted fracture, and left untreated, many fractures will heal themselves, but only with considerable disability.

PATTERNS OF MANDIBULAR FRACTURE

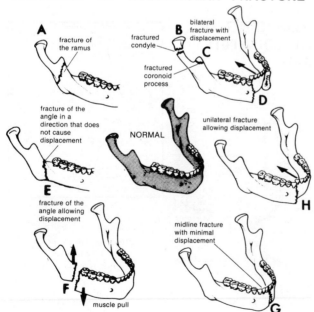

Fig. 62-15 PATTERNS OF MANDIBULAR FRACTURES. The principle of reducing these fractures is to make the patient's bite normal.

The purpose of the mandible is to bite, so *decide whether or not the patient has a normal bite. If he has not, think how best you can restore it.* The methods described below are for single fractures. You will have to adapt them for multiple ones.

THE GENERAL METHOD FOR AN INJURED LOWER JAW

This extends what has already been said in Section 62.1, on the care of a severe maxillofacial injury. If possible, consult a dentist early.

EXAMINATION Feel both the patient's condyles with the tips of your fingers, and then continue feeling downwards along the borders of his mandible. Feel for tenderness, step defects, alterations in contour, and crepitus.

Look inside his mouth with a good light. Gently swab away any clotted blood. Lift any loose pieces of tooth and alveolus out of his mouth.

Examine his buccal and lingual sulci. Bruising in his buccal sulcus does not necessarily indicate a fracture, but bruising in his lingual sulcus almost certainly does. Palpate his mandible down the whole length of each sulcus carefully. If you suspect a fracture, can you make the fragments move relative to one another?

Examine the patient's ears for bleeding. Put both your little fingers into them and compare the movement of his condyles. If you cannot feel a condyle moving, suspect a fracture.

BITE AND MOVEMENTS Examine the patient's bite. If he can cooperate, ask him to carry out a full range of mandibular movements, and note any pain and limitation of movement.

Test for anaesthesia of his mental nerve. Is he anaesthetic below his lower lip to one side of the midline?

X-RAYS Take antero–posterior, and right and left lateral oblique views to show his rami, condyles, and coronoid processes.

SOFT TISSUE INJURIES Do a careful wound toilet inside and outside his mouth. Remove any foreign bodies and all loose teeth in the line of the fracture, together with their roots. If there is loss of soft tissue, stitch his mucous membrane to the skin around the defect as best you can.

ANTIBIOTICS If a patient has an open fracture, give him an antibitoic, such as amoxycillin, ampicillin, or fortified procaine penicillin, daily for 5 days in the hope of preventing bone infection.

BANDAGES are usually unnecessary. If a patient needs one, apply a simple suspensory barrel bandage, not a four–tail bandage.

METHODS FOR PARTICULAR FRACTURES Apply the appropriate methods for fractured condyles (62.8), for fractures of the ramus (62.9), and for fractures of the body of the mandible (62.10). The coronoid processes (C, Fig. 62-15) can also be fractured, but the diagnosis is difficult. The treatment is active movements, so disregard this fracture.

62.8 Fractured mandibular condyles

These are the most common mandibular fractures (B, Fig. 62-15). They are often undiagnosed, and are often bilateral.

Unilateral condylar fractures The patient has pain, swelling, and tenderness over his temporomandibular joint on the injured side. He cannot move his jaw normally. Movement away from the injured side is particularly difficult. When he tries to move his jaw, it deviates towards the side of the fracture. His bite may or may not be normal and he occasionally bleeds from his ear.

Bilateral fractures All movements are painful and limited. Sometimes the patient's bite is normal, or he may have an anterior open bite. Often he has a midline fracture also.

The mandibular condyles are difficult to X-ray, and need special views, so it is fortunate that X-rays are not essential. Management depends on whether or not the patient has an anterior open bite. If you fail to correct this, his molar teeth may later have to be ground away, so that his incisors can meet. If he has no teeth, an anterior open bite is less important, because it can be corrected with dentures.

FRACTURES OF THE MANDIBULAR CONDYLES

If possible, refer the patient, because ankylosis and deviation of his jaw may follow unsuccessful treatment. If you cannot refer him, proceed as follows.

FRACTURES WITH A NORMAL BITE

All unilateral fractures have a normal bite (if there is no other associated fracture) and so do some bilateral ones.

Encourage the patient to move his jaw. Deviation of his mandible towards the injured side is usually due to muscle spasm, and soon improves, so that his bite becomes normal. Observe him to make sure that it does so.

CAUTION ! If you decide to immobilize his jaw because of pain, don't do so for more than 10 days, or he may later have so little movement that he will be unable to open his mouth normally.

FRACTURES WITH AN ANTERIOR OPEN BITE

All these patients have bilateral fractures, or fracture dislocations.

If the fragments are not impacted, you may be able to splint them using interdental wiring. If the patient has few teeth, you may need to use an arch bar.

If the fragments are impacted, splint his jaws so as to distract the ramus in the condylar region. Take an ordinary rubber. Cut two pieces from it 6 mm thick, and put them between his molar teeth on both sides. Then use adhesive tape traction or interdental wiring to make his incisors meet, as in treating an old dislocation (62.6). Maintain this splinting for 5 weeks.

DIFFICULTIES WITH FRACTURES OF THE MANDIBULAR CONDYLES

If the patient is a CHILD, no treatment is needed initially. But follow him up carefully, because the growth of his mandible may be arrested.

If a patient's BITE DOES NOT IMPROVE, refer him to a dentist. If serious malunion occurs condylectomy may be necessary.

FRACTURES OF THE CONDYLES ARE OFTEN MISSED

62.9 Fractures of the ascending ramus of the mandible

The ramus of the patient's injured mandible is tender, swollen, and bruised, both outside and inside his mouth (A, Fig. 62-15). The fracture does not open into his mouth and there is little displacement unless violence has been extreme, because the muscles attached to the ramus splint it so well. If there is no displacement, encourage him to move his jaw. If there is significant displacement, fix his mandible by interdental wiring as described below.

62.10 Fractures of the angle or body of the mandible

The angle of the mandible is one of its weak points, and is the next most common site for fractures after the condyles. The fragments may or may not be displaced, depending on the severity

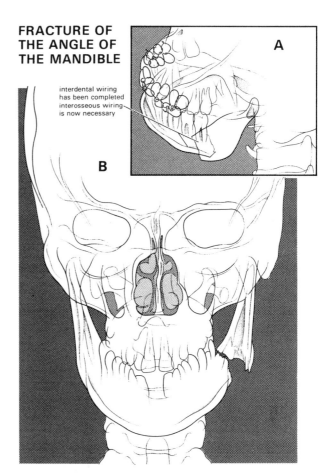

FRACTURE OF THE ANGLE OF THE MANDIBLE

interdental wiring has been completed interosseous wiring is now necessary

A

B

Fig. 62-16 A FRACTURE OF THE ANGLE OF THE MANDIBLE. A, shows the fracture after interdental wiring and before interosseous wiring. B, shows it before wiring. This is the patient whose mandible is being wired in Fig. 62-20. *John Maina's patient.*

of the injury and the direction of the fracture line (E, or F, in Fig. 62-15). If the fragments are displaced, the anterior one is pulled downwards by the muscles attached to it, while the posterior one is pulled upwards by the patient's masseter (F). Sometimes there is a tooth on the posterior fragment.

If the fragments are not displaced, as in A, Fig. 62-15, you can bandage the patient's jaws together, and need not wire them, although it is good practice to do so.

If the fragments are displaced, you will have to reduce and fix them. If they have enough teeth in them, you can use the patient's upper jaw as a splint and wire the teeth of both his jaws together (interdental eyelet wiring or intermaxillary fixation, IMF), or you can use an arch bar. Fortunately, most patients are young and have enough teeth to let you do this. Interdental eyelet wiring (occasionally with an arch bar) is thus all that is necessary in most cases. If you don't have an arch bar, you can use Risdon wiring, as in Fig. 62-19, which is as good if not better. Or you can make an improvised arch bar with paper clips or fencing wire. If you don't have the right kind of stainless steel wire, you can use ordinary brass wire, but it is not so strong.

If a patient does not have suitable teeth for interdental wiring, you can drill holes in the fragments and wire them together (interosseous wiring). Or, you can combine interdental and interosseous wiring. For example, if the anterior fragment has enough teeth to wire it to the maxilla, but the posterior fragment has not, you may be able to wire it to the anterior one. *Interosseous wiring is never enough by itself, and is only an adjunct to interdental wiring.*

Interosseous wiring is the most practical way of fixing those fractures in which there is no other way of controlling the

119

posterior fragment. The inferior alveolar nerve runs through the centre of the mandible, so always wire the mandible through its edges. You may need to wire it anywhere along its length. Wiring is easiest on the front of a patient's chin. There are two approaches: (1) You can wire the lower border of his mandible from outside his mouth. (2) It is possible to wire the upper border from inside it, but this is more difficult, so avoid it if you can. The patient is likely to be elderly and will probably tolerate his malocclusion.

If a patient wears a denture, you may be able to use this as a splint, You can wire a lower denture to his mandible by circumferential wiring, or you can suspend an upper denture from his zygomatic arches by an adaptation of method B, in Fig. 62-8.

Fractures of the ramus are open, and are easily infected by bacteria from the mouth. Osteomyelitis, sometimes with extensive fistulae, is thus an important complication, and may follow interosseous wiring. Fortunately, prophylactic antibiotics will usually prevent it.

If for any reason you cannot fix these fractures, remodelling will occur in those which involve the angle with upward and forward displacement of the posterior fragment, and in most comminuted fractures. It will not occur in fractures near the genial tubercles.

CAREFUL REGULAR ORAL HYGIENE IS ESSENTIAL TO PREVENT OSTEOMYELITIS

Anaesthesia is critical. If neither you nor your assistant is an anaesthetic expert, the patient is probably safest under local anaesthesia. The alternative is to give him a general anaesthetic, pass a nasotracheal tube, and pack his throat. The dangerous moment comes when you remove the pack before you finally close his jaws. While you are doing this, blood and saliva can collect in his pharynx. You cannot suck this out through wired jaws. So, when you do finally pull the tube out, he may inhale the collected blod and saliva, perhaps fatally, or he may have a severe inhalation pneumonia. Another moment of danger occurs as he recovers from the anaesthetic, when he may try to cough or vomit through closed jaws, so that you have to open them urgently. Local anaesthesia also reduces this risk. You can use ketamine, but it is not ideal.

MOST FRACTURES OF THE BODY OF THE MANDIBLE NEED FIXING

FRACTURES OF THE BODY OF THE MANDIBLE

FRACTURES WITHOUT DISPLACEMENT

If the patient's upper and lower teeth oppose one another, so that he bites normally, there is no displacement. Provided he is cooperative, there is no need to wire his fracture, although it is better practice to do so.

If the patient is cooperative, bandage his mandible to his maxilla, so that his teeth are firmly together. Use a crepe bandage, adhesive strapping, or a plaster bandage round his chin, his face, and his forehead. If you use a crepe bandage, rewrap it every day to maintain tension.

CAUTION ! A bandage can be detrimental if you apply it in a displaced fracture.

If a patient is uncooperative, he may remove his bandage, so you had better wire his fracture.

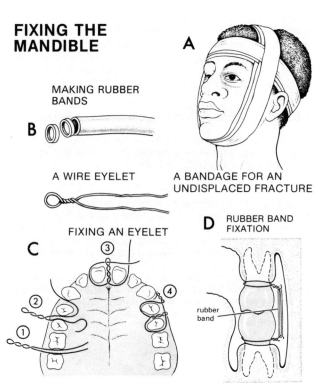

FIXING THE MANDIBLE

MAKING RUBBER BANDS

A WIRE EYELET

A BANDAGE FOR AN UNDISPLACED FRACTURE

FIXING AN EYELET

RUBBER BAND FIXATION

rubber band

INTERDENTAL EYELET WIRING

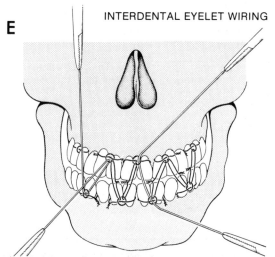

Fig. 62-17 FIXING THE MANDIBLE. A, this patient has an undisplaced fracture, so he only needs a bandage. B, keep rubber bands and eyelets ready in the theatre. C, the steps in making an eyelet. D, the eyelets made into hooks and held with a rubber band. E, passing wires between the eyelets. *With the kind permission of Michael Wood and Hugh Dudley.*

FRACTURES WITH DISPLACEMENT BUT NO TISSUE LOSS

If the fracture lies within the tooth bearing area, you have two choices.

(1) If the patient is cooperative, unlikely to take the wires off, and has plenty of teeth, use interdental eyelet wiring.

(2) If he is uncooperative, if he has few teeth, or if there is gross displacement, use arch bars or Risdon wiring.

If the fracture lies outside the tooth bearing area, use interosseous wiring combined with interdental wiring, or arch bars or Risdon wiring on the same criteria as (1) and (2) above.

If he has no teeth, refer him. If you cannot refer him, do your best with interosseous wiring.

If you have no suitable wire, do your best with a head bandage, as in Fig. 62-17.

If possible, operate during the first 24 hours, but if oedema is severe, you can wait up to a week to let it subside. If you are in any doubt about the patient's general condition, wait.

FRACTURES WITH SEVERE TISSUE LOSS
Usually, there is severe displacement also. Toilet the patient's wound, replace the bone and soft tissues as best you can, and fix the remains of his mandible to his maxilla by any suitable method. Close his wound, suture his skin to his mucous membrane, and refer him.

INTERDENTAL EYELET WIRING FOR MANDIBULAR FRACTURES

INDICATIONS Displaced fractures of the mandible with: (1) a sound maxillary arch, and (2) enough teeth opposite one another to take the wire.

CONTRAINDICATIONS If a patient is drunk and there is any danger of vomiting, don't wire his teeth until his stomach is empty.

ANAESTHESIA FOR EYELET WIRING OR ARCH BARS See above. There are several possibilities. (1) If displacement is mild and he is cooperative, use local anaesthesia only. Premedicate him with pethidine and diazepam (A 5.2). Use pterygopalatine (A 6.4) and mandibular (A 6.3) blocks, if necessary on both sides. Supplement these where required, by infiltrating the mucosa round his teeth (A 6.3). Alternatively, use infiltration anaesthesia only. If you are using local anaesthesia, sit him in a dental chair. (2) If his injuries are severe and you are an anaesthetist expert, induce him with ether or halothane (A 11.3), and intubate him through his nose (A 13.4). (3) Ketamine can be used.
    CAUTION ! Pass a nasogastric tube and aspirate his stomach before inducing him.

WORKING WITH WIRE Use soft 0.35 mm stainless steel wire, or any convenient soft wire. Stretch it before you use it, or it will become slack, but don't over-stretch it, or it will become hard and brittle.
    Making eyelets Cut the wire into 150 mm lengths, take hold of each end in a pair of artery forceps, and twist it round a 3 mm bar to make the eyelets shown in B, Fig. 62-17. Keep 20 of them ready in a box in the theatre.
    Twisting wire inside the mouth Twist it by holding its ends in a stout pair of artery forceps. Pull the ends taught from time to time, and rotate them in your fingers, as in Fig. 62-18. You will need to make many twists and this is much the quickest way of making them.
    Precautions with wire Whenever you work with wire, protect the patient's eyes, because a loose end can spring back and injure them. (1) Close them, and cover them with vaseline gauze and a dressing. (2) When you are not working with the free end of a piece of wire, anchor it with a pair of forceps.

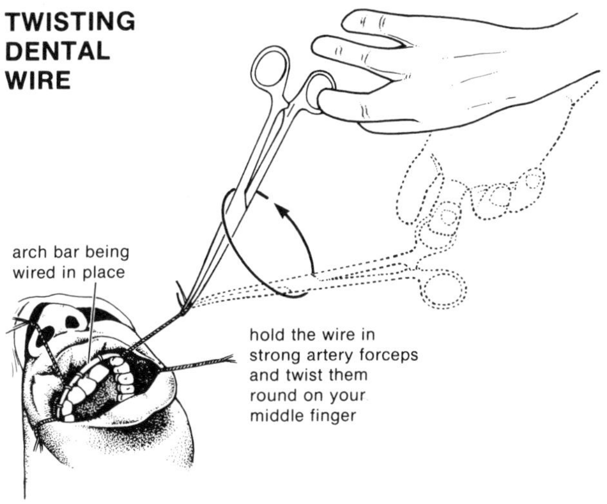

INSERTING THE EYELETS Look carefully at the facets on the patient's teeth and study the way his jaws fit together. If there is any abnormality in the way they occlude, allow for it when you immobilize the fragments.
    Push an eyelet well down between two teeth (1) as shown in C, Fig. 62-17, bring the ends of the wire back between two adjacent teeth (2), pass one end of the wire through the eye (3), twist both ends together, pulling tightly as you do so, and cut them off (4). Tuck the sharp ends between his teeth. Pull on the eye to bring it nearer to the occlusal surface and make sure it is secure.
    Fix about five eyelets in either jaw in suitable places, so that when they are joined by tie wires, these will run diagonally in both directions and brace his jaws together. Don't place the eyelets immediately above one another, or you will not be able to anchor the fragments.
    Alternatively, wire the teeth directly as in D, and E, Fig. 62-19. This is a quick temporary measure if you have many casualties, but the wires loosen more easily.

REDUCING A FRACTURED MANDIBLE If there are any loose teeth in the fracture line, this is the time to remove them. Bleeding sockets will not now obscure the wiring.
    CAUTION ! (1) Control bleeding. (2) If you have intubated the patient and his throat is packed, remove the pack before you wire his teeth. Leave his nasotracheal tube down. (3) Suck out his throat before you close his jaw.
    Reduce the fracture by closing his jaws. When the patient's teeth fit together properly, the fragments will be aligned. Place the tie wires loosely at first, and only tighten them after you have checked the occlusion. Tighten them little by little, first in the molar area on one side, then in the molar area on the other side, working round towards the incisors as you do so.
    CAUTION ! (1) If you tighten the wires firmly on one side only first, you will cause a crossover bite. (2) If you tighten the incisor wires first, you will cause a posterior open bite. (3) Don't twist the wire too tightly on a single rooted tooth, or you may pull it out. You can exert more tension on a multi-rooted one. (4) Make sure that you have not trapped his tongue.
    Finally, run your finger round his mouth to make sure that there are no loose wires which might injure his lips. Coat his lips and the inner surfaces of his cheeks with vaseline.

ALTERNATIVE METHOD OF EYELET WIRING USING HOOKS AND RUBBER BANDS

This is shown in D, Fig. 62-17. Use it when there is any danger of vomiting, or if a patient has to travel. You will need thicker wire than with eyelet wiring.
    Surround the neck of every second or third tooth with a loop of wire. Leave the two ends free towards the lips. Twist them a few times and then make a small hook with the free ends. Make sure they really are smooth.
    Pass short rubber bands diagonally over these wire hooks. If necessary, cut them from a suitable size of rubber tube as in B, in this figure.

RISDON WIRING FOR A FRACTURED MANDIBLE

INDICATIONS As an alternative to an arch bar for a fracture of the mandible that needs fixation. Some surgeons prefer a Risdon wire to an arch bar.

METHOD Take two pieces of soft 1 mm stainless steel wire about 25 cm long. In the middle of each piece twist a loop that will fit over one of the posterior teeth of the patient's broken lower jaw. Fit the loops over these teeth, and twist them secure. Then twist the ends of each wire double. Bring the twisted strands from each side together, reducing the fracture as you do so. Twist them together in the midline, so that they lie along the necks of the teeth. Cut the joined pieces of wire short. Fix the twisted wires to some individual teeth with 0.35 mm wire loops. Finally, wire the mandible to eyelets placed on the maxillae.

TWISTING DENTAL WIRE

arch bar being wired in place

hold the wire in strong artery forceps and twist them round on your middle finger

Fig. 62-18 TWISTING DENTAL WIRE. Use soft 0.35 mm stainless steel wire, or any convenient soft wire, and take care to protect a patient's eyes. *Kindly contributed by Frederick Onyango.*

MORE WIRING METHODS FOR THE TEETH

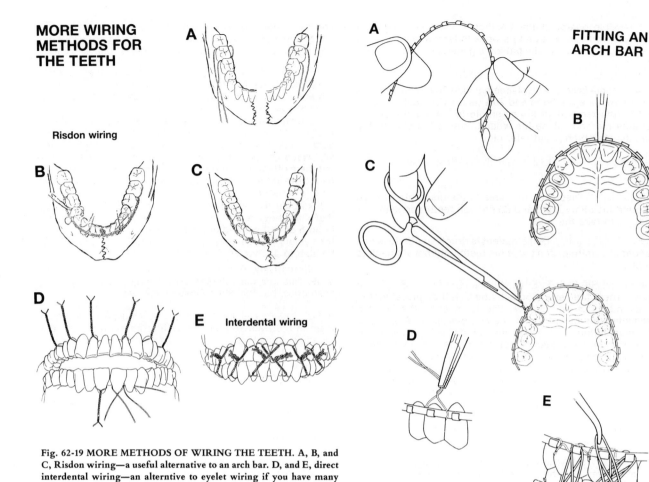

FITTING AN ARCH BAR

Risdon wiring

Interdental wiring

Fig. 62-19 MORE METHODS OF WIRING THE TEETH. A, B, and C, Risdon wiring—a useful alternative to an arch bar. D, and E, direct interdental wiring—an alterntive to eyelet wiring if you have many casualties; it is quicker, but not so secure as using eyelets. *After Killey, with kind permission.*

Fig. 62-19a FITTING AN ARCH BAR. A, bending it to shape. B, fitting it round the maxilla. C, wiring it to the maxilla. D, passing a wire round a tooth. E, fixing the rubber bands. *After R.O. Dingman and P. Navig 'Surgery of Facial Fractures' W.B. Saunders Co. Publishers, permission requested.*

FITTING ARCH BARS FOR MANDIBULAR FRACTURES

This is not as easy as it looks! Use a pair of heavy cutting pliers to cut the bars to the right length for each jaw; try to make them span as many teeth as possible; and leave them long enough for the end to be bent towards the posterior surface of the last available tooth. Bend them to shape along the necks of the teeth with the hooks facing towards one another. The patient's lower jaw will be displaced, so shape the arch bar for it to fit round his upper jaw, or fit it round the lower jaw of another person with the same size of arch.

Use 15 cm lengths of 0.35 mm wire to wire the arch bar to the teeth. It is usually best to start in the premolar region by wiring one tooth on each side. Pass the wires round the necks of the teeth and wire as many as you can. Because of their shape, incisor teeth are usually difficult to wire, so you may have to leave them. If the wire tends to slip off, be prepared to raise the gum with a periosteal elevator. Tuck the ends of the wires aside where they will not injure the lips. Fix the arch bars with rubber bands.

AN IMPROVISED ARCH BAR

Take some paper clips, open them, twist them together, make side hooks on them, point these upwards on the top teeth, and downwards on the bottom ones. Fix this improvised arch bar to the teeth with ordinary stainless steel wire, and pass rubber bands between the hooks.

LOWER BORDER INTEROSSEOUS WIRING FOR MANDIBULAR FRACTURES

INDICATIONS (1) Control of the posterior fragment when this has no teeth. (2) Control of both fragments when the patient has no teeth or insufficient teeth for interdental wiring. You will usually need interdental wiring or an arch bar also.

CONTRAINDICATIONS (1) Established infection of the fracture site. (2) Children in whom unerupted teeth may be injured.

ANAESTHESIA Endotracheal anaesthesia is essential (A 13.2).

METHOD Make a 3 cm incision over the fracture site in line with the patient's facial nerve, as in A, Fig. 62-20. The exact site of the incision will depend on where his fracture is. Reflect the skin. Under the incision you will find the superficial fascia and the platysma muscle.

Cut across the fibres of his platysma, and use blunt dissection to find his facial artery and his anterior facial vein. These pass diagonally upwards and forwards across the lower border of his mandible at the anterior edge of his masseter. Retract these vessels gently backwards or forwards away from the line of the fracture. If necessary, cut and tie them. Often, the fracture line will lie just posterior to the anterior edge of his masseter. If so, retract the vessels anteriorly.

Use a rongeur to strip his masseter and the periosteum away from the lower border of his mandible (B).

Define the fracture line. You will probably find that the posterior fragment lies deep to the anterior one and overlaps it. Disimpact the two fragments and remove any old blood clots and loose fragments of bone, which may prevent you aligning the two parts of his mandible.

Now pass your finger under the lower border of the patient's mandible (C), and separate it from the deep tissues of the floor

LOWER BORDER WIRING

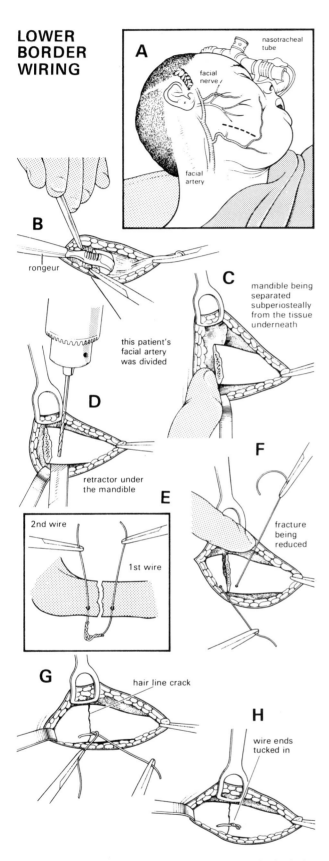

Fig. 62-20 LOWER BORDER WIRING. A, a nasotracheal tube has been passed and the patient's head turned to one side. B, the periosteum is being removed from around the fracture line with a rongeur. C, the undersurface of his mandible is being freed from the tissues under it. D, the first drill hole. E, the two pieces of wire joined to one another under the mandible. F, and G, the fracture being reduced. H, the wound ready for closure. *John Maina's patient.*

of his mouth. Replace your finger with a flat broad retractor in this position (D).

Drill a hole in each fragment about 3 mm from the fracture edge—be certain the holes pass through both cortical plates of the bone. You will feel the drill touch your retractor when this has happened.

CAUTION ! Don't make the holes in the middle of the patient's mandible, or you may injure his inferior alveolar nerve.

Keep the retractor blade in place deep to his mandible. Take two 15 cm lengths of wire. Pass the first wire through one of the holes in his mandible from the buccal to the lingual side. Secure it with artery forceps at both ends. Now take a second wire and twist a small eye onto one end. Pass this eye through the hole in the other fragment of his mandible from the buccal to the lingual side. Thread the deep end of the first wire through the loop and twist it round itself (E). Use it to pull the second wire through the first hole. Remove the 'eye' wire and twist the two ends of the first wire gently together to reduce the fracture until there is only a hair–line crack (F).

When you have secured the fracture (G), cut the twisted ends of the wire off short and tuck the cut end into one of the holes, so that it doesn't stick out into the soft tissues (H). Cut a very fine strip of rubber glove and insert this as a drain.

Close the wound in layers and bandage it with a light pressure bandage. Remove the drain after 24 hours.

UPPER BORDER INTEROSSEOUS WIRING FOR MANDIBULAR FRACTURES

INDICATIONS This is seldom necessary. In bilateral fractures insert an upper border wire to prevent the muscles pulling the anterior fragment downwards, and making the fracture line gape.

METHOD Wire the upper border before the lower one. Make an incision along the crest of the alveolus inside the patient's mouth. Drill small holes on either side of the fracture line, pass a piece of soft stainless steel wire through it, reduce the fragments, and twist the ends of the wire tight. Cut the ends short and tuck them into the nearest drill hole. Close the incision very carefully, because infection is common.

POSTOPERATIVE CARE FOR MANDIBULAR FRACTURES

Don't remove the patient's tracheal tube until anaesthesia is really light. If you have wired his teeth under general anaesthesia, send him back to the ward with a nasopharyngeal airway in place and his tongue held with a strong suture. Use a large cutting needle to insert it transversely through the dorsum of the back of his tongue. Lead its end between his teeth and hold them with haemostats. Some surgeons consider this is unnecessary. Lie the patient on his side and have a sucker ready, with a tube attached which you can pass down his nasopharyngeal tube.

If he has been starved preoperatively, any vomit will be watery and will pass between his wired teeth.

CAUTION ! Have wire cutters beside his bed or with the nurse, in charge. Be sure that the nurses know how to remove the wire, if he wants to vomit. Tell them to cut the closing wires, not the eyelets. Later, he will be more comfortable if you nurse him sitting up.

POST REDUCTION X-RAYS If these are not satisfactory, correct the malposition as soon as possible.

ANTIBIOTICS Give these as described earlier (A 62.7).

FEEDING A PATIENT WITH A CLOSED JAW Feed him frequently with liquid food through a rubber tube between his teeth. Let him suck between his teeth or round the back of his molars. Feeding will be easier if he has a few teeth missing. He will probably lose much weight. If he cannot swallow, feed him through a nasogastric tube.

Careful oral hygiene is essential to prevent osteomyelitis. Ask him to clean his teeth with a tooth-brush after every meal. Or, irrigate his mouth with saline or 0.5% chlorhexidine from a Higginson's syringe.

FOLLOW–UP FOR A MANDIBULAR FRACTURE If you send a patient home wired, tell him to keep a pair of pliers available, so that he can remove the wire if necessary. Ask him to reattend regularly, so that his wire can be tightened or renewed. Keep children wired for 4 weeks before you test for union, young adults for 5 weeks, and elderly ones for 7 weeks. If you immobilize a patient's jaw too long, it will ankylose.

TESTING FOR UNION Remove the tie wires and gently test for union across the fracture line. If the fragments seem firm, clean the patient's mouth and remove the eyelet wires. Leave interosseous wire in place unless it becomes infected.

DIFFICULTIES WITH MANDIBULAR FRACTURES

If a patient CANNOT OPEN HIS JAW, don't worry for the first week or two. It will open more easily after a few weeks of active use. If, however, he fails to reattend to have the wires removed, so that his jaw remains closed for too long, his jaw movements may be limited permanently. Encourage him to exercise his jaw regularly and to progressively insert a wooden cone between his teeth, so as to separate them a little more each day.

If his JAW HAS FAILED TO UNITE, encourage him to accept his disability. Non–union is rare. It may follow infection, or be the result of leaving a tooth in the fracture line.

If his MANDIBLE HAS BECOME INFECTED, give him antibiotics (2.7), clean up his jaw as much as possible, remove loose teeth in the fracture site and rewire his teeth. Osteomyelitis is an important complication and is more likely to occur if you fail to fix a fracture, so that the fragments are kept moving, of if you try to wire one which is already infected. Prevent it by always giving prophylactic antibiotics whenever the mucoperiosteum is torn.

If his LOWER LIP IS NUMB, it will probably recover. Warn him of the danger of burning his lower lip with hot drinks or cigarettes.

If his TEETH DO NOT MEET when the fixation is removed, his malocclusion will probably correct itself if it is mild. If it is more severe, his cusps can be ground away. If it is gross, refer him for refracture of his mandible, or the removal of selected teeth. If he adopts a bite of convenience across a partly healed fracture, it may cause a fibrous union, so refer him for a suitable denture.

If the patient is a CHILD, manage his fracture as if he were an adult, but remember the following differences: (1) Growth disturbances of his condyles may follow, particularly in condylar fractures. (2) Don't use interdental eyelet wiring unless he has a sufficient number of firm teeth, either deciduous or permanent. (3) Don't use interosseous wires, because you may damage his unerupted teeth. (4) Mild malocclusion will correct itself as his mandible grows and his deciduous teeth erupt. A bandage, as in A, Fig. 62-17, may be all he needs.

62.13 Fixing mandibular fractures with resins

You can use two types of synthetic resin to fix a patient's broken mandible, as an alternative to wiring it. The method is quick, easy, and non–traumatic. Fixing hooks with composite is easier than wiring them directly to his teeth, less traumatic, and more comfortable for him because there are no wire ends to scratch his mouth.

Cold curing quick setting acrylic resin is weaker than the composite material described below, but is cheap and widely available from dental supply houses or dental technicians. It will allow you to fix an arch bar to a mandible, but it is not strong enough to let you stick hooks to it.

Composite filling materials of the 'Adaptic' or 'Isopaste' type, together with a bonding agent are more expensive and less readily available than quick curing acrylic resin. A composite is supplied as two pastes which you mix together and which then set solid. It is usually used for filling cavities, but you can use it to make bridges between the teeth of a patient's upper and lower jaw, or you can use it to stick hooks to his teeth, and then pass rubber bands or wire over them as with interdental wiring (D, Fig. 62-17). To allow the composite to stick you will have to clean the surfaces of his teeth at each fixation point, wash them, etch them

with phosphoric acid, wash them again, dry them, coat them with a special bonding agent, and then press the composite onto them. This is not difficult, but it needs care. Be sure you follow the instructions exactly. If you use bridges of composite between a patient's jaws, one difficulty will be getting them into the right position and getting the composite into place simultaneously. Using hooks avoids this difficulty.

At present, proprietary dental resins are unnecessarily expensive, for example, proprietary compound filling material costs $75 for 100 g, whereas it only costs $6 to manufacture. Fortunately, cheaper 'generic' dental materials are now being made, and when they became available this method of fixing mandibular fractures will become more economically feasible.

ANOTHER METHOD OF FIXING THE MANDIBLE

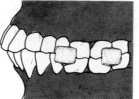

Bridges of compound material between the jaws

Hooks stuck on with compound material

Fig. 62-21 ANOTHER WAY OF FIXING THE MANDIBLE. A, using bridges of filling material. B, using hooks. *Kindly contributed by W.J. Bailey.*

FIXING THE MANDIBLE IN OTHER WAYS

ANAESTHESIA (1) Mandibular block (A 6-3). (2) Ketamine (A 8.1). (3) Diazepam (A 8.6). Atropinize the patient to dry his saliva.

USING ACRYLIC TO FIX AN ARCH BAR

MATERIALS Ordinary cold cure acrylic ('Simplex'),as used by dental technicians to repair broken dentures. This is supplied as a liquid monomer and a powdered polymer.

Put some of the powdered polymer into a small pot. Drop the liquid monomer onto it and stir it with a spatula until it is the consistency of putty.

METHOD Sit the patient up in a chair. Make an arch bar from several strands of thick (2 mm) stainless steel wire, and fashion it to fit the arch of his mandible, lingually, or buccally, or both.

To stop the resin sticking, lightly spread vaseline on the patient's lips, mucous membrane and tongue—but not his teeth.

Hold the arch bar in place with blobs or a continuous wad of cold cure acrylic. Lightly spread vaseline on your fingers (to stop the acrylic sticking) and press the acrylic into place over the arch bar. Press it firmly between the bases of the patient's teeth. If the arch bar is going to stay in place, the resin must go between the overhanging parts of his adjacent teeth. If he is older, and his gingival papillae have resorbed, or he has missing teeth, the resin will be able to pass between them and stick more firmly.

Hold the arch bar in place until the resin has set (in about 10 minutes).

USING COMPOUND FILLING MATERIAL TO STICK HOOKS ON

INDICATIONS (1) Conscious and cooperative patients. (2) This method is particularly suited to unilateral fractures. (3) Recent fractures that will be fairly easy to reduce.

CONTRAINDICATIONS Much bleeding which makes cleaning and drying the surfaces of a patient's teeth impractical.

MATERIALS Compound filling material, such as 'Adaptic' or 'Isopaste' and their special bonding compounds, or their generic equivalents. 50% phosphoric acid, 2 mm stainless steel wire. Rubber bands.

METHOD The patient will probably need about six hooks depending on the site of his fracture.

Sit him up in a chair. Clean the surfaces of his teeth at each fixation point carefully, and dry them free of saliva. Use spirit on a pledget of cotton wool, or a dental engine brush.

While his teeth are still dry, apply phosphoric acid on a paint brush for 60 seconds.

Wash his tooth for 30 seconds, and then dry it again.

Keep his teeth dry with suction, rolls of paper tissue, or cotton wool in his buccal sulcus.

Apply the bonding material to the dry, etched surface with a small brush or a wisp of cotton wool.

Mix a little of the the compound material and the catalyst with a spatula on a small paper pad, and immediately press it into place with lightly vaselined fingers over the prepared surfaces of his upper and lower teeth. While it is still soft, press a hook into it.

Join up the hooks with rubber bands or wire. Rubber will place less strain on the hooks. If you join them with wire, take care not to exert too much force, or you may displace them. After 6 weeks you can chip composite away quite easily. The last remaining pieces may have to be removed with a dental drill.

ALTERNATIVE NOT USING HOOKS Hold the patient's jaws together with bridges of filling material passing from one jaw to another. You will probably only need about 4 bridges. As they set, keep his jaws aligned and his teeth in occlusion.

63 Head injuries

63.1 The general method for head injuries

'No head injury is so severe as to be despaired of, nor so trivial as to be lightly ignored'—so wrote Hippocrates. This is still true. Unfortunately, seemingly trivial injuries are often ignored, and every patient who dies from one is an indictment of the hospital which failed to treat him. Although a patient's scalp can be wounded and his skull broken, it is the concussion, contusion, or compression of his brain that affects his consciousness.

Concussion prevents a patient reacting to stimuli for a few minutes after a head injury, but has no after effects.

Contusion resembles concussion except that: (1) A patient is unconscious for more than a few minutes. (2) He may have petechial bleeding in his brain. (3) Serious consequences may follow. These range from minor character changes to spastic hemiparesis.

Compression is the result of spreading oedema or an expanding blood clot which gradually damages the surrounding brain.

It is the relief of compression that makes the care of head injuries so rewarding. A timely burr hole to remove the blood clot which is compressing a patient's brain may save his life. This clot can take two forms: (1) The small veins under his dura may bleed and cause a subdural haematoma. (2) Less often, a fracture of the vault of his skull tears a branch of his middle meningeal artery and causes an extradural haematoma. Evacuating this will usually restore him to perfect health, because his brain is usually normal underneath it. Unfortunately, his brain is more likely to be injured under a subdural haematoma, so evacuating this is not so dramatically successful.

Making a burr hole is so comparatively simple that any doctor should be able to do it. If a patient dies, he will probably do so because his brain is hopelessly injured—or because you operated too late. So operate on the suspicion that a patient *might* have an expanding blood clot. If you fail to find one, you will have done him no harm. You will certainly not have time to refer him—*the commonest mistake is to do nothing!*

INTRACRANIAL HAEMORRHAGE

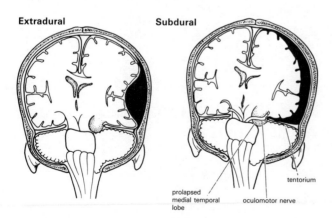

Fig. 63-1 INTRACRANIAL HAEMORRHAGE. A, an extradural haematoma. B, a subdural haematoma causing coning. *After Graham Martin.*

A patient with a head injury often has other injuries also, so make sure he has a clear airway, look for and treat any chest injuries, assess the state of his circulation, and look for injuries to his abdomen, spine, and limbs.

In practice, compression of the brain by a clot is uncommon, and a patient is more likely to be in coma because his brain is contused. So try to keep him alive until his natural healing processes have done what they can. This means good nursing care while he is unconscious, and especially the care of his airway to prevent him inhaling blood, vomit, or secretions. *A patient is more likely to die from these complications, than from any other cause, except irreversible injury to his brain.* Even a short period of respiratory obstruction can raise the carbon dioxide tension in his blood and cause irreversible cerebral oedema and death. So don't let a patient die from unnoticed airway obstruction in the ward. *Although craniotomy is the dramatic part of the care of a head injury, only a few patients need it. The careful nursing of coma is even more important than prompt surgery—it saves more lives than even the most expert surgeon—so make sure your nurses know this!*

JAQUES (10 years) was discharged following a minor head injury. He was brought back in again the following day deeply unconscious, with one fixed dilated pupil. He was rushed to the theatre, still in his out–door clothes. Within 20 minutes burr holes were being made. A large extradural clot was found and washed out. Next day he was up and walking. This is what we mean by a real emergency—rush these patients to the theatre, every minute matters!

● *BRACE, Hudson's, standard, 254 mm, one only.* This is the neurosurgical equivalent of a carpenter's brace. If you don't have one, you can use gouges and short taps from a heavy hammer.

● *PERFORATOR, Hudson's, with standard Hudson fittings, 12 mm, one only.* Use this to start making a hole in his skull that you will later continue with burrs.

● *BURRS, spherical, Hudson pattern, 11 mm, 13 mm, 16 mm, 19 mm, one only of each size.* Use these to enlarge the hole made by the perforator. Trephines were traditionally used for opening the skull, and some hospitals still have them, but burrs are easier to use and have now replaced them. Spherical burrs are less likely to suddenly plunge through the dura and enter the brain than are conical ones.

● *RONGEUR, (bone nibbler), Cairns, with fine angled on flat jaws and curved handles, 152 mm, one only.* When you have made a hole in the skull with a perforator and burrs, enlarge it with these bone nibblers.

● *RONGEUR, Sargent, or van Havre, double action, curved on flat, 229 mm, one only.* These are more powerful but more clumsy rongeurs than those of Cairns, listed above.

● *ELEVATOR, skull, Penfield, double ended, one only.* Use this to elevate depressed skull fragments.

● *TUBE, suction, fine, 4 mm diameter, one only.* This is used for sucking away injured brain. If it blocks, clear it with a stilette.

● *HOOK, dural, Cairns, sharp, 130 mm, one only.* Use this for lifting up the dura. If you don't have one, use a skin hook.

**CAREFUL NURSING MAKES ALL THE DIFFERENCE
A TRACHEAL TUBE MAY SAVE THE PATIENT'S LIFE**

NEUROSURGICAL EQUIPMENT

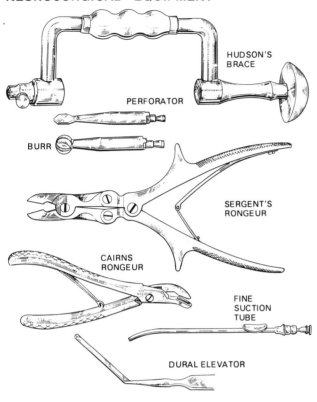

Fig. 63-2 THE ESSENTIAL NEUROSURGICAL EQUIPMENT. This should be in every hospital and every doctor should know how to use it. Hudson's brace is the neurosurgical equivalent of a carpenter's brace.

THE GENERAL METHOD FOR AN UNCONSCIOUS PATIENT WITH A HEAD INJURY

This extends Section 51.3 on the care of a severely injured patient. It applies to *all* patients who have lost consciousness after an injury, ever if their most obvious injury is a fractured femur.

CAUTION ! Admit all patients, especially children, who have been unconscious with a head injury even for a moment. Observe them carefully for 24 to 48 hours.

THE IMMEDIATE CARE OF A HEAD INJURY

AIRWAY This is critically important. (1) Place the patient in the recovery position (51-2). (2) Clear his mouth and pharynx. (3) Insert an oral airway.

If his consciousness is much impaired, so that he has no cough reflex, intubate him before you pass a stomach or a nasogastric tube. If his consciousness is not so deeply impaired, a tracheal tube is less essential. As soon as his consciousness improves he will reject a tracheal tube.

If he is deeply unconscious and intubation is impossible, or he fails to maintain an adequate airway, do a tracheostomy. He may need one if he is in coma for a long time.

EMPTY THE PATIENT'S STOMACH Many patients vomit and aspirate their stomach contents after admission to hospital. If a patient's stomach was full when he was injured, it will still be full now. If it is obviously distended, pass an oral stomach tube, and when it is empty, pass a nasogastric tube. Otherwise, pass a nasogastric tube to begin with.

CAUTION ! If you decide to pass a stomach tube do so: (1) After you have intubated a patient, or you may drown him in his own gastric contents. (2) Pass it while he is in the recovery position.

THE HISTORY OF A PATIENT WITH A HEAD INJURY

What exactly happened? As far as possible, try to assess the patient's level of consciousness, from the moment of his accident. Now, or later, enquire how much loss of memory he has for the events following the injury. The duration of pre- and post-traumatic amnesia are good indications of the severity of a head injury.

Question witnesses. Did the patient have a lucid interval (a period of consciousness before becoming comatose) following the injury?

THE EXAMINATION OF A HEAD INJURY

GENERAL EXAMINATION Look at the patient in a good light, examine his body and limbs first, and then his head and neck. Smell his breath for alcohol and acetone, and don't forget the other causes of coma, including epilepsy, diabetes, liver failure, meningitis, drugs, malaria, and trypanosomiasis.

CAUTION ! (1) However strongly he smells of alcohol, don't assume that this is the cause of his impaired consciousness. (2) Always admit an alcoholic who has sustained a head injury.

NEUROLOGICAL EXAMINATION If the patient is sufficiently conscious, test the motor power of all his four limbs. Look especially for signs of weakness on one side of his body. Recognizing this requires practice in a patient who is not fully cooperative.

If he is restless, observe how he moves each side of his body. Rub his chest over his sternum with your closed fist and see how he responds. Press firmly with your nail above his orbits. His grimace may be weaker on one side than the other. Lift his arms and legs, release them and see how they fall away.

See how his limbs respond when you pinch them firmly. The signs may only be minimal. For example, a child may not be able to move his limbs quite so well on one side as on the other.

Examine his knee and ankle jerks, and his abdominal and plantar reflexes. Test for neck stiffness, and examine for Kernig's sign.

PUPIL REACTIONS IN CEREBRAL COMPRESSION

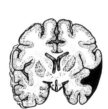

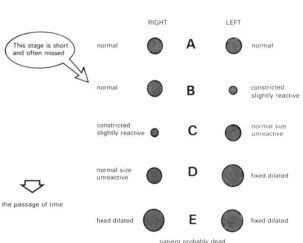

Fig. 63-3 PUPILLARY CHANGES AFTER A HEAD INJURY. Stage A, the pupil on the side of the lesion constricts first and then dilates. Stage B, constriction on the side of the lesion, usually lasts only a short time and is often missed. If you miss it, you will only see stages C, and D, a normal sized unreactive pupil, and then a fixed dilated pupil on the side of the lesion. Enlargement of the pupil is more important than its failure to react to light. *Kindly contributed by Peter Bewes and Gerishom Sande.*

CAUTION ! Don't do a diagnostic lumbar puncture early on, because it will give you no information that you cannot get more safely in other ways. If a patient's CSF pressure is raised, lowering it suddenly may kill him. However, if you suspect meningitis (63.13) or subarachnoid haemorrhage, proceed to do one.

EXAMINE THE PATIENT'S EYES Record the size and equality of his pupils, and whether they react to light. You may have to use a very bright light. Examine his eyes now before they are closed by swelling, and frequently later, even if they become severely swollen. Don't give him atropine, because this will destroy the great diagnostic value of a unilateral dilating pupil.

Examine his nervous system often, because unequal pupils and unequal reflexes are important signs as to which side of his brain is being compressed. The inequality may disappear later. If you don't examine a patient often this important information will be lost.

Look for papilloedema. It is a rare but certain sign of raised intracranial pressure.

A 'black eye' is the result of bleeding into the eyelids and is of little significance by itself. Conjunctival haemorrhages only indicate a fracture (usually of the orbital plate of the frontal bone) if: (1) They make the patient's conjunctiva oedematous. (2) They are so large that you cannot see their posterior limit in any position of his eye. (3) They displace or restrict the movement of his eye. Otherwise, they are merely signs of local bruising.

EXAMINE HIS SCALP AND SKULL (1) Look for cuts and bruises. This is especially important if the patient is drunk, and you are not sure if he also has a head injury. *Observe the site of the trauma accurately,* before it becomes enlarged and oedematous. It is also a useful indication of the site of an intracranial haematoma. (2) Feel for: (a) The edges of a depressed fracture; this is not an easy sign and swelling of the scalp with blood in the tissues can give a similar feeling and be very deceptive. (b) Extensive boggy swelling of the patient's scalp. (c) Thickening of his temporalis muscle. These are all signs of a fractured skull.

A pad and bandage will usually control bleeding from his scalp, but if it does not, sew it up temporarily. Don't attempt to explore it until you have taken him to the theatre!

ASSOCIATED SKULL FRACTURES Surprisingly, a patient seldom has a depressed skull fracture and a compressing intracranial lesion at the same time. A plain or simple depressed fracture is usually an urgency rather than an emergency. If he does have a depressed skull fracture, this can, if necessary, wait 12 hours or longer. A compressing intracranial lesion will probably reveal itself before this, and if it does, you can deal with both lesions together.

The only emergencies are compound depressed fractures with open brain. Explore these early and close the patient's skin before you refer him.

CAUTION ! Remember that the only time that a fracture alters the management of an unconscious patient with a head injury, is when it is depressed. Otherwise, you can proceed as if it was not there.

EARS AND NOSE A bleeding nose may indicate a fractured base, and a bleeding ear almost always does. If a patient's ear is bleeding, don't examine it for fear of introducing infection. If it is not bleeding, examine the drum because blood behind it confirms a fractured base. If you see it leave it.

Postmastoid bruising a few days after the injury also confirms a fractured base, but its absence does not exclude one.

Look also for leaking CSF.

INJURIES ELSEWHERE Look especially for injuries of a patient's neck and back that may indicate fractures of his cervical spine (64.3). Carefully roll him onto his side while maintaining gentle head traction (64-4). Palpate every spinous process. Look for even a small kyphus or an abrupt misalignment.

If you suspect a fracture of his cervical spine, fit him with a cervical collar. He may also be paraplegic (64.13). If he is, make sure that he does not develop bed sores.

CAUTION ! (1) If the patient is shocked, look for severe injuries in other places, especially in his thorax and abdomen.

By themselves head injuries seldom cause shock, unless bleeding is very severe. There are several special tests for abdominal injuries which may help you (66.1). (2) If a patient has any serious abdominal or thoracic injuries, these take precedence over his head injury.

RECORDS FOR HEAD INJURIES

Assess the patient's state of consciousness and start to fill in a coma chart (63-4). Careful notes are most important, especially if several people have to care for him. Note the exact times at which all observations are made.

X-RAYS FOR HEAD INJURIES

PLAIN X-RAYS are less important than regular assessment of the patient's clinical state. Poor films are useless. Even good ones are difficult to interpret and may fail to show serious fractures. If possible, take an AP and a lateral of the patient's cranial vault, especially if you suspect an extradural haematoma (impaired consciousness after a lucid interval). The position of the fracture line may tell you where to make your first burr hole. Most patients with an extradural haematoma have a fracture (but not vice versa). Fractures of the base are difficult or impossible to see on X-ray films. If litigation is no problem and films are scarce, keep them for more useful purposes.

If you X-ray the patient's skull, take a lateral view of his cervical spine at the same time and an AP view of his chest.

CAUTION ! While he is in the X-ray department his airway may obstruct, or he may vomit, or have a convulson, so send a responsible nurse to watch him.

If you have difficulty deciding what is a fracture and what is not, remember that:—

Fracture lines have clean cut edges, run in all directions, may cross arterial and suture lines, change direction abruptly, and branch irregularly.

Suture lines are fine or dentate, are in constant positions, and may be widened by trauma.

Grooves for the meningeal vessels run in known directions, branch dichotomously, and get smaller from below upwards.

Channels for the diploic veins run irregularly, and change course abruptly. They often start in lacunae near the superior sagittal sinus, and they vary in width.

Look carefully for a fracture line crossing a meningeal groove, and note which side it is, because it may indicate the site of an extradural haemorrhage. If you do see a fracture, make sure it does not date from a previous injury.

ARTERIOGRAMS Any X-ray machine that can take a skull X-ray can take an arteriogram. The only equipment you need is a 1.2 mm spinal needle. Arteriograms are usually not too difficult to interpret, and are very useful: (1) In an acute deteriorating head injury. (2) In the patient who is not improving after a week, and who may have a chronic clot.

NURSING A HEAD INJURY

POSITION Provided a patient has no other injuries which might prevent it, *nurse him in the recovery position (51-2)* and turn him 2 hourly. Raise the foot of his bed until his cough and swallowing reflexes have returned. This will raise his intracranial pressure, but his airway is more important.

If he is disturbed or violent and you have no proper cot in which to nurse him, put him on a mattress on the floor. This better than tying him to his bed, which may cause a wrist drop and other injuries. You may occasionally have to do this to prevent him soiling the dressings over his head wounds.

BED SORES Care for his skin from the start, as for paraplegia (64.13).

PAIN AND SEDATION If a patient is so violent on admission that he is a danger to himself and other people, give him chlorpromazine 25 to 50 mg, or diazepam 10 mg intramuscularly, or intravenously. Avoid stronger sedatives, especially morphine, because they interfere with the assessment of consciousness and depress his respiration.

Moderate restlessness is useful, because it is good physiotherapy for his lungs and prevents pressure sores. Make sure that his overactivity is not caused by a full bladder, or an uncomfortable position. If he is noisy, put him in a side ward.

TEMPERATURE If possible, take a patient's rectal temperature every hour during the first 12 hours. Watch for hyperthermia and start cooling him if it reaches 39°C.

CORNEA If his blinking or corneal reflexes are absent, take care that his cornea does not rub against his pillow, or the sheets, and ulcerate. If his eyes remain open, put adhesive strapping across his closed eyelids—this is critically important!

FOOD AND FLUIDS Start a fluid balance chart. While a patient is unconscious, give him fluids intravenously. At 24 to 48 hours, or earlier if his cough and swallowing reflexes return, give him food and fluids through a nasogastric tube. Pass a tube and start feeding him, even if his cough reflex has not returned at 24 to 48 hours, provided he has bowel sounds. He needs energy; about 12 MJ (3 000 kcal) in 3 litres of fluid (58.11). He may be unconscious for many days and eventually recover, so don't let him starve meanwhile.

BLADDER Examine this to make sure it does not distend, and catheterize a patient when necessary to prevent overflow.

Bed wetting may require an indwelling catheter in a female, a Paul's tube strapped to the penis of a male, or a polythene urinal in a child. If you pass a catheter, releasing it 4 hourly is better than letting it drain continuously.

OPEN HEAD INJURIES Give the patient benyzl penicillin and sulphadimidine intramuscularly, both 6 hourly.

ANTICONVULSANT THERAPY Give all patients phenobarbitone prophylactically while they are in hospital. 30 mg 8 hourly in an adult will not impair consciousness.

TETANUS PROPHYLAXIS Don't forget to give a patient tetanus toxoid (54.11).

OTHER INJURIES If a patient with a head injury has fractures elsewere, at least splint them temporarily in the reduced position, even if you cannot treat them definitively.

THE FURTHER MANAGEMENT OF A PATIENT WITH A HEAD INJURY

Read on for: methods of monitoring a patient's consciousness, pulse and blood pressure (63.2), patterns of head injury (63.3), the indications for burr holes (63.4), how to make a burr hole (63.5), open head wounds (63.6), fractures of the vault (63.7), ping–pong ball fractures in children (63.8), controlling bleeding (63.9), hyperthermia (63.10), convulsions (63.11), leaking CSF (63.12), meningitis (63.13), more difficulties with a head injury (63.14).

IF A PATIENT WITH A HEAD INJURY IS SHOCKED, LOOK FOR ANOTHER INJURY

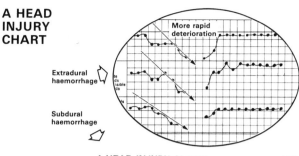

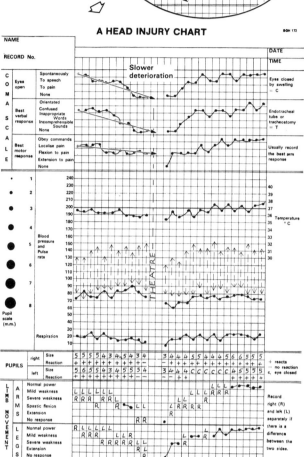

Fig. 63-4 CHARTS FOR A SUBDURAL AND EXTRADURAL HAEMATOMA. The changes are similar. The main difference is that the changes in an extradural haematoma develop faster. There is a blank copy of this chart on one of the endpapers so that you can photocopy it. *Kindly contributed by Gerishom Sande.*

63.2 Monitoring a patient with a head injury

The best indicator of the function of a patient's brain is his level of consciousness. If this is deteriorating he needs burr holes. Deterioration is a *trend* (for the worse), and is much more important than his *status* which is his state of consciousness at any one time. The idea that 'trend is more important than status' is the key to monitoring these patients. The only reliable way to monitor deterioration is to use a head injury chart, like that in Fig. 63-4. There is a blank full sized version of this on one of the end pages of the book. Have some photocopies made. All patients with a head injury need one, because even a mildly injured patient can deteriorate rapidly. When you assess consciousness, don't rely on subjective statements like 'fully conscious', or 'partly conscious'. Instead, record objectively what a patient can do. Use, and teach the nurses to use, expressions

which do not need description, such as 'alert but confused', or 'not speaking but obeys commands'. Show them how to fill in a head injury chart. If it is too complicated, teach them to fill in part of it. Encourage them to form their own base lines, so that they can say at any time if they think a patient is getting better, or worse.

Date the chart from the moment of a patient's injury, and enquire most carefully about his level of consciousness before admission. To begin with, make hourly, and later 2 hourly observations of his verbal responses, his motor activity, and his pupils. Record his systolic blood pressure and his pulse. Warn the nurses to expect rapid changes in the things you ask them to watch, and to report them urgently. For example, a blood pressure reading, which is obviously different from the previous one half an hour before, may be very important, but check it again before acting on it. Make sure they know how to examine a patient's pupils, and test their reactions to light. The easiest test for pain is to pinch him firmly with your finger nail. As with all charts,

TRENDS OF CONSCIOUSNESS

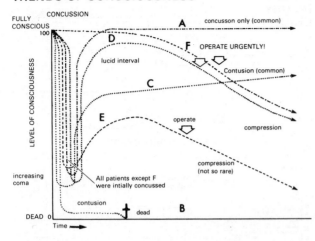

Fig. 63-5 LOSS OF CONSCIOUSNESS AFTER A HEAD INJURY. All patients, except F, were concussed to begin with. Patient A, was concussed, lost consciousness momentarily, and then became normal again (common). Patient B's brain was seriously contused, he became deeply unconscious and remained so (common). Patient C was concussed and contused, and became deeply unconscious, after which consciousness steadily improved (common). None of these patients is deteriorating, so they don't need burr holes.

The patients who have cerebral compression and need decompression are D, E, and F, all of whom are deteriorating. Patient D was concussed then had a lucid interval before becoming unconscious again (rare but important). Patient E was concussed, his consciousness improved and then deteriorated again (not so rare). Patient F did not lose consciousness at the time of the injury, but progressively lost it afterwards (rare). *Kindly contributed by Peter Bewes*

nobody is going to fill them in carefully, unless they understand them and see you look at them and act on them.

Assume that any deterioration of consciousness is caused by rising intracranial pressure, and needs burr holes, until you have proved otherwise. Here are some of the other causes.

Some major thoracic or abdominal injury causing severe blood loss, or impairing respiration and raising the carbon dioxide tension in the patient's blood. When this happens operate without delay, whatever his level of consciousness.

A major generalized or focal convulsion, especially in a child, can impair consciousness for several hours. Don't accept this as the cause, unless someone saw it happening. Prophylactic phenobarbitone should prevent it.

Fat embolism can cause rapid deterioration in consciousness, but usually only if the patient has long bone fractures of his legs, or severe soft tissue injuries (78.6). His consciousness can deteriorate before petechial haemorrhages appear. His pupils remain equal, and the characteristic pulse and blood pressure changes of cerebral compression are not seen.

ALL PATIENTS WITH A HEAD INJURY MUST HAVE A CHART

63.3 Patterns of head injury

Cerebral compression can be the result of bleeding in three places.

Extradural haemorrhage Bleeding outside the dura only occurs in about 2% of all head injuries. Some of these patients have a lucid interval (Patient D in Fig. 63-5) which is usually only a few hours, but it may be a week or more. Others have steadily deepening coma from time of the injury (Patient F).

If they do have a lucid interval, their important first symptom *is increasing headache,* so take a complaint of headache very seriously in any patient with a recent head injury. If he also has giddiness, mental confusion, or drowsiness, he is may be bleeding extradurally. As this gets worse his unconsciousness deepens, and he develops pyramidal signs on the opposite side.

Subdural haemorrhage Bleeding under the dura occurs in about 8% of head injuries, and can follow any of the patterns D, E, and F, in Fig. 63-5. Unfortunately, removing the clot is less dramatically beneficial than it is in extradural haemorrhage. In *acute* subdural haemorrhage the patient's unconsciousness deepens in a few hours, in the subacute form in a few days, but in the chronic form he may not become unconscious for months. The lucid interval before symptoms develop can thus be much longer than in extradural haemorrhage. In the *chronic* form the patient, who is usually elderly, suffers from repeated or increasingly severe headaches, drowsiness, apathy, or mental changes. The typical picture is that of a slowly developing cerebral crisis some time after a complete or partial recovery from a head injury, perhaps a very minor one, which the patient may not even remember.

Unfortunately, you can seldom diagnose whether bleeding is subdural or extradural until you operate. The only clue is the short lucid interval and rapid progression of extradural haemorrhage.

Intracerebral haemorrhage Sometimes, when you open a patient's skull expecting to find a subdural haemorrhage, you find that his brain is swollen and discoloured, due to bleeding inside it or to cerebral oedema.

63.3a The prognosis in head injuries

During the first few hours following an injury you can seldom forecast what is going to happen to a patient with a head injury. If he has fixed dilated pupils and does not respond to any stimuli, his prognosis is not good. If he is alert, he is going to live. But between these two extremes anything can happen. Children, especially, can recover remarkably from seemingly severe trauma.

You will find yourself caring for the following kinds of patient. Some will be children. Some of the adults will also be drunk. A few will have open head injuries.

The patients who are conscious, or are rapidly becoming so, when you first see them (Patients A, and C, in Fig. 63-5) Although a patient may seem normal after a head injury, he may not be fully aware of what has happened, or be fit to drive a car. Subdural or extradural haemorrhage may occur later, so warn him and his relatives that he must return immediately, if he becomes drowsy or his headache gets worse.

The 2% of patients who are unconscious when you first see them, but who have had a lucid interval at some time since the accident. An example is Patient D in Fig. 63-5 who is particularly precious, and whose life you may be able to save. Patient F, who did not lose consciousness at the time of the accident, but who has lost it since, is especially precious. If you remove his clot, his brain will probably recover completely.

The patients who are unconscious when you first see them, and who have never been conscious since the accident These patients are of three kinds. Patient B is comatose; he shows no signs of improvement and dies. Patient C is drowsy, or even comatose, but his coma is lightening and his trend is towards improvement. Carefully nursed, he will recover. Patient E is important: he is unconscious, but his unconsciousness is deepening. His trend is to get worse—operate on him.

MANJI One Christmas Day a missionary doctor was called 40 kilometres to see a patient who had been beaten over the head with an axe haft. By the time that the doctor arrived the patient had such a severe degree of cerebral compression that he appeared lifeless apart from his pulse. It seemed that each breath he took would be his last.

Unfortunately, the primitive operating theatre had collapsed, so the operation was done in a little laboratory barely 4 metres square, with unglazed win-

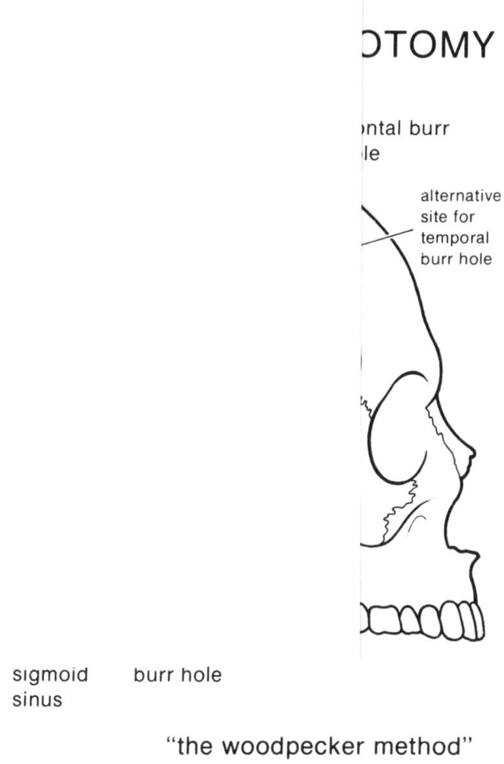

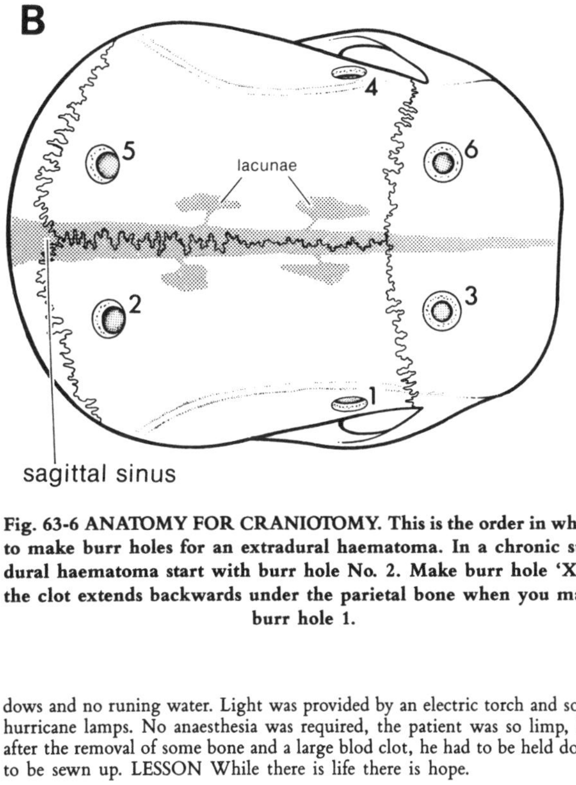

ntal burr
le

alternative
site for
temporal
burr hole

sigmoid   burr hole
sinus

"the woodpecker method"

B

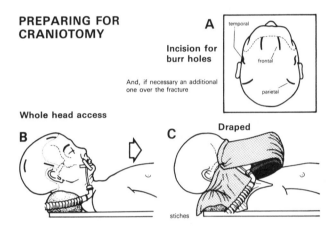

lacunae

5

4

6

2

3

1

sagittal sinus

Fig. 63-6 ANATOMY FOR CRANIOTOMY. This is the order in which to make burr holes for an extradural haematoma. In a chronic subdural haematoma start with burr hole No. 2. Make burr hole 'X' if the clot extends backwards under the parietal bone when you make burr hole 1.

dows and no runing water. Light was provided by an electric torch and some hurricane lamps. No anaesthesia was required, the patient was so limp, but after the removal of some bone and a large blod clot, he had to be held down to be sewn up. LESSON While there is life there is hope.

63.4 Should you make burr holes, and if so where?

The patients who are worth great efforts to save are those whose consciousness is deteriorating, especially if they were fully conscious a short time ago. In order of importance, the factors to help you to decide are: (1) Deterioration in a patient's level of consciousness. (2) The development of localizing signs, such as weakness on one side of his body. (3) Change in his pupils, as in Fig. 63-3. (4) A rise in his blood pressure. (5) A slowing of his pulse.

As cerebral compression develops, a patient's blood pressure

rises and his pulse becomes slow, full, and bounding. These signs are evidence of a physiological attempt to maintain the circulation to a patient's vital centres in the presence of cerebral compression. These signs are the reverse of those in internal haemorrhage, as from a ruptured spleen, for example, in which a patient's blood pressure falls and his pulse becomes rapid and weak. As with consciousness it is the *trends in his pulse and blood pressure which are important,* especially if he is a child, rather than any particular value.

Restlessness, and particularly a very severe headache, are useful additional signs of intracranial bleeding in a conscious patient. Another suggestive sign is boggy oedema of his scalp over the site of a fracture.

Don't depend on the presence of a fracture. The signs which do *not* in themselves indicate the need for urgent exploratory burr holes include: (1) Focal neurological signs in an alert patient. (2) A depressed skull fracture.

PREPARING FOR CRANIOTOMY

A

temporal

frontal

parietal

Incision for burr holes

And, if necessary an additional one over the fracture

Whole head access

B

C

Draped

stiches

Fig. 63-7 PREPARING FOR CRANIOTOMY. A, the sites of burr holes. You need to make an additional hole over the fracture. B, positioning the patient's head so that you can get at all of it. C, draping his head so as to expose his ears and zygomas. *After Graham Martin.*

WHICH SIDE TO MAKE THE FIRST BURR HOLE?

Here are the localizing signs in *decreasing* order of reliability.

If, as occasionally happens, the X-ray shows the fracture side crossing a vessel, make the first burr hole there.

If you don't have this useful localizing sign, make it on the side which: (1) Is bruised or lacerated. (2) Is stronger if one side of the body is weaker than the other. (3) Has a dilated pupil, or was the first to have one, if they are now both dilated. (If his pupil was dilated from the moment of the injury, and fails to react to light, he has an orbital injury, and the sign is not helpful.) (4) Shows less vigorous knee and ankle jerks, if these are unequal.

Rare localizing signs include focal epileptic fits, homonymous hemianopia which develops after the injury, and dysphasia.

WHERE TO MAKE THE FIRST BURR HOLE?

If the fracture crosses a vessel, make the hole there.

If a patient has an obvious scalp injury, make it in the centre of this.

If there is no fracture line or obvious scalp injury, make the first hole in the classical position in Fig. 63-9.

If the first hole is negative, make the next one in the parietal region, and then one in the frontal region.

If this too is negative, repeat the same three holes in the same order on the other side.

Occasionally, you will have to make six holes; only if they are all six negative can you be sure that there is no clot above a patient's tentorium. He may still have a clot in his posterior

AN URGENT CRANIOTOMY

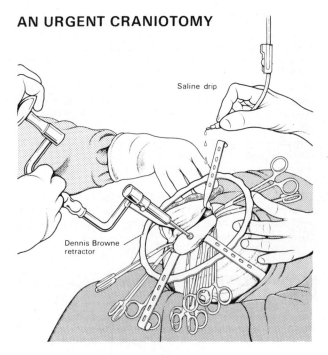

Fig. 63-8 AN URGENT CRANIOTOMY. Alternatively, apply saline with a 20 ml syringe and a 20 Ch catheter. Maintaining sterility may be easier this way. *Kindly contributed by Peter Bewes.*

fossa, but you have no practical way of diagnosing it. To begin with, each burr hole will take you an hour. Looking for a clot by this 'woodpecker method' may be tedious, and is certainly less elegant than doing a CAT scan, but it is not difficult. Only when you have reached the dura will you see if the bleeding is outside or inside it. The one place *not* to make a burr hole is over a major sinus!

THE PUPIL ON THE SIDE OF THE LESION DILATES FIRST

63.5 Making burr holes

Treatment is urgent. As soon as you have made the diagnosis tell the theatre staff that the patient is coming. He should be on the operating table within a few minutes of the diagnosis being made. If his respiration is failing, operation is very urgent indeed. There have been times when burr holes have had to be made without asepsis, before even the theatre could be reached. Don't try to raise flaps—they are not necessary for emergency surgery.

ALPHONSE (22 years) fell out of a truck. Six weeks later he went to a health unit complaining of a severe headache. Fortunately, the health unit had a radio, and the pilot from the local mission hospital was in the area, so he was able to call and pick up the patient. By the time the pilot arrived the patient was in coma, but a medical student who was doing his elective, and who met the plane, obtained the history that he had previously fallen out of a truck. The signs of cerebral compression were classical. He was on the operating table within 2 hours, burr holes were made, and he was sitting up conscious the following day. LESSON A chronic extradural haematoma can follow a head injury incurred weeks, or even months, before.

SUBDURAL AND EXTRADURAL BLEEDING

Be sure you are familiar with the methods of controlling bleeding in Section 63.9.

EQUIPMENT A general set (4.11), a self retaining mastoid or thyroid retractor such as Mallison's, a brace, a perforator, burrs, a curved dissector, a dural elevator, a dural hook or fine needle and holder, a wide bore cannula and stillette, a fine suction tube, and a large Volkmann's spoon or a small teaspoon. Horsley's bone wax to plug the bleeding diploe, and a sterile pointed match stick. A bottle of warm sterile saline and a drip set, or a bowl of warm saline and a bladder syringe.

ANAESTHESIA See *Primary Anaesthesia* Section A 16.8. General anaesthesia is best because you can hyperventilate the patient, which will make his brain contract. A method of local anaesthesia is described below.

CAUTION ! Keep his airway clear. The slightest obstruction will make his brain swell.

PREPARATION Work quickly; shave the patient's whole scalp so that you can operate on both sides if necessary. Take care not break his skin. Include his ears in the area you prepare.

MAKING A BURR HOLE

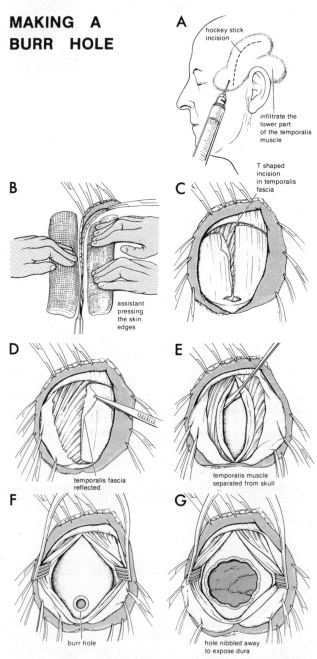

Fig. 63-9 MAKING A BURR HOLE. A, the line of the incision is being infiltrated. B, the incision with an assistant helping to press the skin edges. C, incising the temporalis fascia. D, reflecting it. E, separating the temporalis muscle from the skull. F, the burr hole. G, the edge of the burr hole nibbled away. *After Rowbotham with kind permission.*

Close his eyes, pad them and seal them with strapping, so that the fluid used for skin preparation or blood cannot drip into them.

Prepare one of his thighs so that you can take a fascial graft, if necessary, as in Fig. 63-17.

POSITION Position him yourself. Support the patient's head carefully with sandbags or a kidney dish, so that it projects over the end of the table, and does not move about when you operate. If you are using local anaesthesia, strap him to the table. After preparing him, scratch the sites of the burr holes, and inject local anaesthetic. If you don't do this, you may not know where you are when his nose and eyes are hidden under the drapes.

DRAPES Wet a towel with antiseptic and wrap it round the base of the patient's cranium. Stitch it to his head so that you can move his head with the towel attached. Expose his occiput, the tops of his ears, his zygomas, and the whole of his forehead, so that you can get at the whole of his head. If possible, lay the drapes from his face across to an overhead table, so that the anaesthetist can get at his face. Ideally, use the special frame made for the purpose.

Arrange to minimize venous bleeding by adjusting the slope of the table, so that the patient's head is above his heart. Make sure that nothing obstructs the veins of his neck.

SITING THE BURR HOLE

Site the burr hole according to the rules in Section 63.4. The classical position is as follows.

THE CLASSICAL POSITION Make the burr hole midway between the posterior margin of the patient's orbit and his external meatus 2 cm above his zygomatic arch, and 1 cm in front of his ear.

CAUTION ! The common mistake is to make the hole too high.

Make a hockey stick incision starting at the lower border of his zygoma 4 cm in front of his ear, and carry it upwards and backwards for 8 cm, as A, Fig. 63-19. Experts make a shorter incision.

If you are using local anaesthesia, infiltrate the line of the incision with anaesthetic solution. Also anaesthetize a line from the margin of the patient's orbit anteriorly to his mastoid posteriorly. Take care to anaesthetize the tissues above his ears.

Inject the anaesthetic solution at right angles to his skin in several places, so as to infiltrate the lower part of his temporalis muscle and block his deep temporal nerves as they turn upwards. Use a generous quantity of solution and make his whole temporalis fossa insensitive.

Control bleeding by asking your assistants to press the edges of the wound (B, Fig. 63-9). Pick up the edges of the patient's galea in haemostats and evert them. When you remove them at the end of the operation bleeding will have stopped. Make a T-shaped incision in his temporalis fascia (C), and turn it back as two short flaps (D). The small horizontal incision above his zygomatic arch makes access to the inferior surface of his brain easier.

Split the patient's temporalis muscle from top to bottom in the line of its fibres, and separate it from his skull with a curved dissector (E).

Insert a self-retaining retractor, to expose about 4 cms of his skull (F).

AN ALTERNATIVE PROCEDURE FOR A DESPERATE EMERGENCY

INCISION This is quicker, and many operators prefer it to the classical one in Fig. 63-9, especially if they are in a hurry in the middle of the night.

To minimize bleeding infiltrate the line of the incision with adrenaline in saline (or local anaesthetic solution). Make this incision over the temporal lines of the patient's skull (you can feel these) above the mid part of his zygomatic arch. Cut down through it right down to his pericranium in one quick deep incision. Quickly free the cut edges of his galea from his skull, pick them up with several haemostats, and turn them over to control bleeding.

USING A PERFORATOR AND BURRS

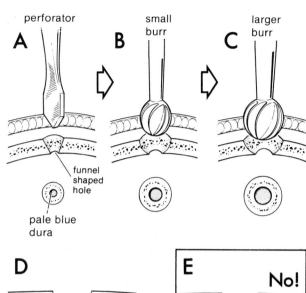

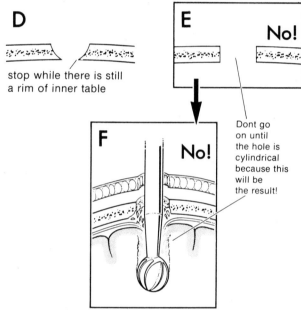

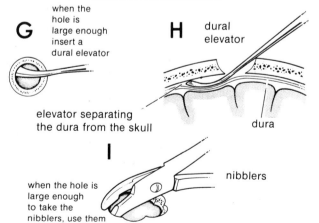

Fig. 63-10 USING A PERFORATOR AND BURRS. A, making a funnel shaped hole with the perforator. B, and C, enlarging it with a small and a large burr. D, stop at this stage—don't go on to stages E, and F. Insert the dural elevator (G, and H) and then nibble (I). *After Rowbotham.*

Make the burr hole in his upper temporal region at the edge of his temporalis muscle in the position in Fig. 63-6 marked 'alternative site for temporal burr hole'. Nibble downwards fast. Separate the dura, and insert a catheter down inside the patient's skull to drain the clot. Because you are not going through his temporalis muscle, you can be inside his skull much faster. You will leave a larger hole in his skull, but this is not important.

USING A PERFORATOR AND BURRS

Place the knob at the top of the brace in the palm of your left hand; take its handle in your right hand. With the perforator in position, make a funnel shaped hole in the bone as in A, Fig. 63-10, until you just see the pale blue of the normal dura, or the dark purple of an extradural clot, then stop!

CAUTION ! (1) Don't go on any further, because you may pierce the patient's dura and lacerate his cortex. This is *very* easily done. (2) The squamous temporal bone is often thin so don't press too hard.

Replace the perforator with a burr (B) and enlarge the hole. Avoid the smaller burrs and choose one which is large enough to rest on the edges of the hole. A small burr can easily go through into the brain. Use a certain amount of force, but lock your shoulder muscles, so that the brace is under control, if the bone gives way. The burr must not suddenly go thorugh the skull into the brain, as in F!

Stop turning when the bite on the burr increases suddenly, because this shows that it is now through to the inner table. Stop while there is still a rim of inner table round the edge of the burr hole, as in D, Fig. 63-10. Don't go on until you have made a parallel sided hole E, or the burr will certainly go through into the brain. You should be able to make a large enough hole with a single burr. If not, replace it with a larger one one, until the hole is just large enough to let you put in the nibblers.

Nibbling should not be necessary in the first instance because most subdural haematomas can be drained through an ordinary sized burr hole. Only nibble if you need more room. Push the dura gently away from the inner table with a dural elevator (G, and H), so that it is not torn when you insert the nibbler to enlarge the edge of the hole (I).

The cut edges of the bone will bleed. Suck away the blood and don't apply wax until you are about to close the wound.

WHAT DO YOU SEE THROUGH THE BURR HOLE?

Make sure you have a good light. The normal brain and dura should pulsate; if they do not, suspect that there is something abnormal underneath. If you don't see anything, enlarge the burr hole a little. This is why it is best to make burr holes away from the line of the middle meningeal artery, not over it.

If a meningeal artery spurts at you as soon as you make the burr hole, you probably cut it with your instruments, and an extradural haematoma is not present.

If there is clot immediately under the hole, the patient has an extradural haematoma, so see below. You will not see the dura or the middle meningeal artery because these will have been displaced inwards by the clot.

If the patient's dura looks abnormally purple, he has a subdural haemorrhage, or occasionally an intracerebral one, so deal with it as described below. This is more common than extradural bleeding.

If his dura is its normal pinkish white and swollen, the brain underneath is swollen. Open his dura, to make sure that the swelling is due to his brain and not to a subdural clot, then make another burr hole.

If his dura is normal in colour and not swollen, explore the hole for 5 cm in all directions with the dural elevator. There may be clot close to the hole which the elevator may reveal. If you find blood, nibble towards it, or make a new hole.

If thorough exploration reveals no clot, make more burr holes, in the order shown in Fig. 63-6.

EXTRADURAL HAEMORRHAGE

You made a burr hole and found clot immediately under it. Nibble the hole in the patient's skull to make it larger. If necessary, lengthen the skin incision upwards and backwards, and extend the split in his temporalis muscle. Retract the tissues widely, so that you get a good look into the hole. If you are able to turn back a small flap, do so. This is quicker than enlarging a burr hole by nibbling.

Nibble away the bone in the direction of the clot; this is usually towards the base of the skull. The common error is to remove too little bone. If necessary, nibble away ruthlessly to get the access you need. A cranioplasty can be done later if he survives to need it. It is seldom necessary. The hole should be at least 7 cm in its maximum diameter. With a low temporal haematoma, remove bone well down to and including the pterion, which is the outer end of the sphenoid ridge. This is the only way you can remove clot lying low under the temporal lobe. Use a curved dissector to separate the patient's dura from his skull each time you nibble more bone.

After you have removed bone, wait a few minutes to allow the circulation in the patient's brain to adjust itself to the new conditions.

CAUTION ! (1) Don't disturb the clot until you are in a position to control bleeding. (2) Don't put your finger into the wound to try to remove the clots, because the extra compression may kill him. Instead, remove the clot, a little at a time with a teaspoon or a curved dissector, or suck it out, or syringe it away forcibly with warm saline.

Watch for further bleeding, and if necessary, nibble towards it—this is very important; don't worry about how much bone you remove.

If there is no further bleeding, after you have removed the clot, don't hunt for the injured artery, instead close the wound. The patient's dura will probably be slack showing that there is no significant brain swelling. Pull up his dura to the bone with black silk stitches through the surrounding pericranium and temporalis muscle. You may have to make a small incision in the dura to do so. This is good practice anyway, because you may find some removable subdural clot. If you don't do this, clot will reaccumulate. Usually, the brain does not expand rapidly, unless air or saline gets underneath it.

If the bleeding is arterial and floods up into the wound as you remove the clot, it is certainly coming from his middle meningeal artery, so try to find it. Syringing with warm saline may help. The best way may be to make a hole in the dura beside the bleeder, and catch it with a haemostat. Or, pick it up with a sharp hook and pass a needle round it, so that you do not mistakenly damage any cortical veins. When you have controlled bleeding you can coagulate the vessel with diathermy or tie it. Immediate coagulation with diathermy usually results in the vessel 'burning back' and continuing to bleed.

If the bleeding is venous, it is either coming from the veins which accompany his meningeal artery, or from the veins of his dura. If it is very severe it may be coming from a tear in his saggittal sinus, or its lacunae. Try to find the bleeding point and stop it as described in Section 63.9. In about 10% of cases the blood is coming from a sinus, so raise the patient's head and insert a pack as described below. If there is a venous ooze from everywhere, insert a suction drain.

If you have secured the main bleeding point, but there is much persistant bleeding, don't hurry. Leave a pack in place. Go away and wait for 10 minutes. It will probably settle spontaneously over the next hour, and allow you to close the wound. Provided you are able to replace the blood that is lost, you can afford to wait. Don't forget to remove the pack!

If the clot extends backwards under the patient's parietal bone, the posterior branch of his middle meningeal artery has probably been torn. You cannot tie this from your present incision. So try to tie its main trunk. If this is impossible make another burr hole 4 cm above and behind his ear. This is the burr hole marked 'X' in Fig. 63-6. Fortunately, it is rarely needed.

If the vessels in a bone groove or tunnel are bleeding, apply Horsley's bone wax, or plug them with a sterile pointed match stick. Do the same if his diploic veins are bleeding. Some surgeons say that match sticks don't work and that these vessels are better plugged with muscle.

If arterial bleeding comes from the under surface of the patient's brain, his middle meningeal artery may have ruptured at or close to his foramen spinosum. Retract his brain and the dura so as to expose it, and plug it with bone wax, or a sterile pointed match stick. Fortunately this is rarely necessarily.

If you cannot find the bleeding vessel, pack pieces of haemostatic gauze, or temporalis muscle, between the patient's dura and the bone where the bleeding is coming from. Hold them in place by stitching the dura to the pericranium over the edges of the hole in his skull, as in Figure 63-19. Insert a suction drain and raise the patient's head.

If bleeding is uncontrollable, it is probably coming from a torn sagittal sinus. Raise the patient's head. Leave the wound open for a few hours, or even until the next day. Pack it lightly with gauze towards the bleeding point, keep it covered with sterile dressings, and transfuse him with several units of fresh blood. Give him calcium gluconate. Severe bleeding of this kind is also rare, which is lucky because it is often fatal.

SUBDURAL HAEMORRHAGE AFTER A HEAD INJURY

You have found purple clot under the patient's dura. Extend the skin incision, and enlarge the hole with nibblers, if necessary, which it usually is not. Hold up his dura on a hook. Use a No. 11 blade on a holder to make a cross-shaped incision in it. Interpreting what you find may be difficult. His brain may be contused and lacerated, with some clot and blood in the subdural space. This is not in itself a significant compressing lesion. He will only benefit if you can remove a subdural clot about 1.5 cm thick or more. Remove it in the same way as for an extradural haemorrhage.

If moderate bleeding is still taking place, enlarge the burr hole in the direction of the bleeding, and then try to seal it with diathermy, or by one of the methods in Section 63.9.

If there is a venous ooze from everywhere, which is impossible to control, leave it and insert a drain, preferably a mild suction drain.

If torrential bleeding occurs from a tear in a large venous sinus or from deep in the patient's brain, its source may be impossible to find, or repair. Try to control it as in Section 63.9. This type of bleeding is seen in acute subdural haemorrhage; his outlook is bad.

If you have controlled all bleeding, close the dura without a drain. Otherwise, leave a rubber drain in when you close the wound. Stitch it to the skin, take great care with asepsis and remove it after 24 hours. Some surgeons consider that a Paul's tube rubber drain is useless.

BLEEDING INTO THE BRAIN AFTER A HEAD INJURY

You have made a burr hole; the dura under it is purple and bulges into the incision. Insert a wide bore cannula, or a Tuohy needle, into the swollen area and remove the stilette. Purple fluid may exude. If it does not, gently aspirate 2 or 3 times in various directions. If this fails, widen the hole in the skull, incise the cerebral cortex and suck out the clot, or syringe it away.

FURTHER BURR HOLES WHEN THESE ARE NECESSARY

EXTRADURAL HAEMORRHAGE is rarely bilateral. So if you find extradural bleeding, and the patient is recovering, and the X-ray shows no fracture on the other side, there is no need to make any more holes.

SUBDURAL BLEEDING. In 20% of cases bleeding is bilateral, so never make less than 4 holes.

When you make more holes, do so in the order shown in Fig. 63-6. Make the parietal holes through a separate longitudinal incision over the point of maximum convexity of the patient's skull, above and behind his ear. If this is unsuccessful, make a frontal burr hole in the line of his pupil 2 cm behind his hair line. If you find nothing here, make the same three burr holes on the other side.

Unless you find extradural bleeding, *always make at least one hole on the other side,* and don't stop operating, even if the patient is dying. The relief of his cerebral compression is his only chance of living. You can cut more burr holes very quickly. Incise the skin and periosteum with a single cut, quickly elevate the periosteum, insert a retractor, and then apply the perforator.

In subdural bleeding you will usually find clots through temporal burr holes when the patient's history is less than 2 weeks, and through frontal or parietal ones in more chronic cases. Sometimes, there is no clot, only pale yellow fluid under tension, but treatment is the same.

CLOSING THE WOUND AFTER MAKING BURR HOLES

SUBDURAL HAEMORRHAGE There is no need to suture the patient's dura, or to insert a drain routinely. Most wounds will drain quite satisfactorily into his temporalis muscle. Only insert a drain if you have been unable to control bleeding. If you do insert one, be sure to remove it in 24 hours.

Occasionally, you may need to close a gap in his dura with fascia lata (63-17).

EXTRADURAL HAEMORRHAGE If you can, insert an extradural suction drain. Some surgeons don't insert one if they have been able to draw the patient's dura up well.

ALL PATIENTS Stop bleeding from the cut edges of the patient's skull by pressing Horsley's bone wax into it all round. Use fine monofilament sutures on curved needles to bring the edges of his temporalis muscle together.

If the patient's brain bulges into the wound, and makes it difficult to close his dura, close it with a fascia lata graft, while hyperventilating him. Give him mannitol and frusemide as described below.

Suture his temporalis fascia. It contracts during the operation, so you will probably only be able to sew up its lower half. Careful closure will diminish the evidence of a bony defect in his skull.

Close his galea with buried sutures of monofilament or chromic catgut, cut the sutures close to the knot, or their ends may project from the wound, prevent healing, and encourage infection. If closing the wound is difficult, close it with monofilament, as in Fig. 63-14.

DIFFICULTIES WITH BURR HOLES

If you DON'T HAVE A BRACE AND BURRS, use a hammer and gouges and control them carefully. Small taps with a large hammer are better than large taps with a small one. Or, borrow a drill from a garage.

Some hospitals have trephines instead of burrs. If you use a trephine, start with a small one and hold it in a handle, or a brace. Put the locating pin in the trephine and start to make the hole with this. It will be hard work! As soon as the trephine

IF YOU DONT HAVE A BRACE AND BURRS

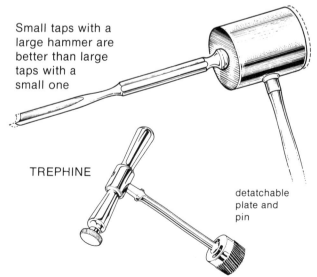

Small taps with a large hammer are better than large taps with a small one

TREPHINE

detatchable plate and pin

Fig. 63-11 IF YOU DON'T HAVE A BRACE AND BURRS use a hammer and gouges and control them carefully. *Kindly contributed by Peter Bewes.*

has started to bite, remove the pin. It must not go through the dura.

If a CHILD needs burr holes, fit the perforator into the handle for it, and open his skull with this. Then go straight to the nibbler, without using burrs. A child's skull is thin with no distinct inner and outer table, so a brace and burrs, and especially a drill, can be dangerous. You may be able to remove the blood from a haematoma in a baby with a large needle without using a perforator.

If a BURR GOES STRAIGHT THROUGH the patient's dura into his brain, this is not as dangerous as you might suppose, and he will probably recover. It should never happen, but when it does happen, as in F, Figure 63-10, it usually does so in a child.

If BRAIN OOZES LIKE TOOTHPASTE from an open hole in a patient's skull, pass a tracheal tube, and hyperventilate him. His brain will suck itself in, and he may recover. If his intracranial pressure is high enough, his brain can ooze from a burr hole, or from an open wound in his skull.

If, after hyperventilation and a thorough search for bleeding, the patient's BRAIN BULGES THROUGH THE WOUND, there is either deep intracerebral bleeding or oedema. There is nothing you can do for deep intracerebral bleeding, but you can reduce oedema with mannitol. Give him 500 ml of 10% mannitol (50 g) over 30 to 60 minutes. Repeat this every 6 to 8 hours if his consciousness improves, but don't exceed 200 g in 24 hours. Drain his bladder with a catheter because he should have a marked diuresis. From the second day onwards for 3 or 4 days give him frusemide 40 to 80 mg intravenously daily. Steroids are useless.

63.6 Open head wounds

The first principle in an open head wound is that what may look like a simple scalp wound may have a tear in the dura underneath it. The dura forms an excellent barrier to infection, so that wounds which go through it are much more serious than those which do not. Even the most seemingly trivial head

wound is potentially dangerous. If you neglect a wound of the dura, meningitis, a brain abscess or osteomyelitis may follow. X-rays are useful—much more so than in fractures of the base. So X-ray all but the most trivial open head injuries in search of: (1) An open fracture under a penetrating wound. (2) A depressed fracture needing elevation. (3) A spicule of bone going through the dura which needs to be removed. (4) A foreign body. If you suspect that any of these four things might be present, explore the patient's scalp right down to the bone.

ARE YOU SURE THERE IS NO PENETRATING SKULL WOUND?

OPEN HEAD WOUNDS

If the patient has more serious wounds elsewhere, his head wound can usually wait 12 or 18 hours. Before you operate, study the control of bleeding in Section 63.9.

X-RAYS If a patient has anything more than the most trivial wound, X-ray the vault of his skull.

THEATRE Unless a patient's wound is very superficial, take him to the theatre, because it may be deeper than it looks. Torrential bleeding can occur, so you may need the full facilities of the theatre in a hurry. Examine his wound on a tipping table, not in a chair. He may bleed severely, or become shocked.

ANAESTHESIA Do a ring block of the scalp as described in A 6.6.

WOUND TOILET Shave the patient's whole scalp, and clean it with detergent. Be prepared to use several razor blades, because any grit in his scalp will blunt them. Protect his wound meanwhile with a sterile swab or towel.

If his wound is clean–cut, and its edges are healthy and bleeding, don't excise them.

If it is dirty and ragged, as in C, Fig. 63-19 excise the skin edges all round it in one clean sweep right down to his pericranium. Take care not to cut away more scalp than is necessary, or there will be so much bare skull that his wound will be difficult to close.

Put in a self retaining retractor, and explore his wound cautiously with your gloved finger. This is safer and provides more information than a metal probe. Remove all debris and dead tissue, and syringe it out with saline.

If you feel any sharp bony edges, expose the surface of his skull widely, and goto Section 63.7.

STITCHING A wound which only cuts a patient's skin does not gape, but one which cuts his galea gapes widely. Close it with big square vertical mattress sutures of stout monofilament, as in Fig. 63-14. Put them through his skin and his galea. Unless you catch the skin edges in the suture, they will dive inwards, and you will not know if you have closed his wound properly or not. Put most of the sutures in place before you start to tie them.

LOSS OF SCALP Try to bring the skin edges together without too much tension, or his scalp may necrose. Follow the methods for flaps in Section 57.11. Don't leave bare bone exposed, or it will slough.

(1) If there is comparatively little loss of scalp, you may be able to free it from his pericranium round the wound, so as to mobilize it over the subgaleal space. Mobilize his scalp in the layer between his galea and his pericranium, as in Fig. 63-12.

(2) You may be able to elongate the ends of the wound in a long curved 'S'. Move the skin at the edges of these flaps, so that it closes the incisions, as in Fig. 63-13.

(3) You may be able to cut the flaps shown in Fig. 63-13, or Fig. 63-15. Cut them big. If possible, design them round one of the arteries supplying his scalp. If there is a dog ear at the

SOME SURGICAL ANATOMY

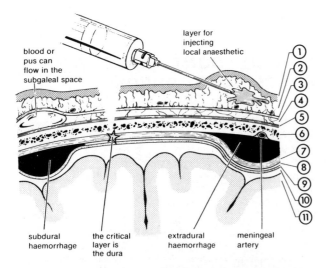

Fig. 63-12 THE ANATOMY OF THE SCALP AND SOME IMPORTANT LESIONS. A patient's epidermis (1) is separated by a fibro–fatty layer of dermis (2), from his strong fibrous galea (3). These three layers are firmly united to one another to form his scalp. Under his galea there is a potential space, his subgaleal space (4), which enables his scalp to slide over his pericranium (5). Under his pericranium lies his skull (6), his dura (7), his subdural space (8), his arachnoid (9) his subarachnoid space (10), and his brain (11). When you anaesthetize a patient's scalp, inject the solution into the fibro–fatty layer, not under his galea. Blood or pus sometimes collects in the subgaleal space and spread through it. An extradural haematoma forms between the skull and dura, and a subdural one between the dura and the arachnoid.

CLOSING A DEFECT IN THE SCALP

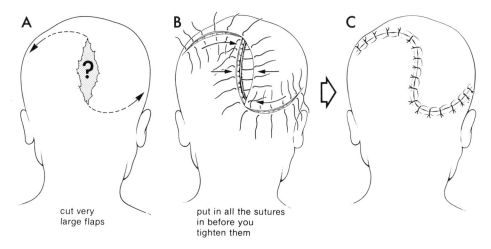

cut very
large flaps

put in all the sutures
in before you
tighten them

Fig. 63-13 CLOSING A SCALP WOUND WITH FLAPS. Try to bring
the skin edges together without too much tension, or the patient's scalp
may necrose. Follow the methods for flaps in Section 57.11. *With the
kind permission of Hugh Dudley*

end of the flap, disregard it, or close it with a small incision
at right angles to the main one, as in Fig. 57-16.

DIFFICULTIES WITH OPEN HEAD WOUNDS

If BLOOD COLLECTS UNDER A PATIENT'S GALEA, don't
drain the swelling, or you may infect it. The haematoma will
subside spontaneously, just as a cephalhaematoma does in
a newborn child.

**If he has a head wound, you have NO X-RAYS and you don't
know if he has a penetrating wound involving his dura or not,**
explore and toilet his wound. If you are in doubt, do a burr
hole close beside it, insert the nibblers, and work towards the
fracture.

If you CANNOT CLOSE A SCALP WOUND even with flaps,
don't leave the bare bone of the outer table of his skull at the
bottom of the wound, for it will take months to granulate over.
(1) See again if you can cover the bone with any of the flaps
in Fig. 63-15. If necessary, graft the area from which you
mobilized the flap. (2) If his exposed skull is covered by
epicranium, graft it immediately (57.2). (3) If his epicranium
has been stripped off, so that bare bone is exposed, gouge
away the outer cortex of his skull. The exposed area of bone
will granulate rapidly, and you will soon be able to graft it.

**If a patient's SCALP HAS BEEN PARTLY TORN OFF and
hangs loose from his head,** transfuse him, trim his scalp, wash
it with an antiseptic, such as hydrogen peroxide, and suture
it back. Its excellent blood supply, which caused it to bleed
so much, will probably keep it alive, provided it is attached

CLOSING   THE SCALP

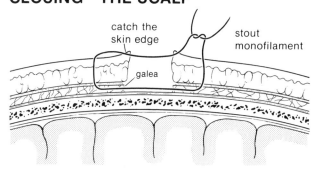

catch the
skin edge

stout
monofilament

galea

Fig. 63-14 AN EASY WAY OF CLOSING SCALP WOUNDS. If you
don't catch the edges of the scalp like this, they will dive inwards. *Kindly
contributed by Peter Bewes.*

to his head by a reasonably broad base. If any exposed skull
is still covered by pericranium, graft it immediately. If his
pericranium has been removed, gouge the surface of his skull,
let it granulate and graft it, as above.

63.7 Fractures of the vault of the skull

When you suspect that a patient has fractured the vault of his
skull, ask yourself these questions: (1) Are the fragments
depressed? Provided that his dura is not torn, you can leave most
depressed fractures, which will be safer than trying to raise them.
(2) Does he have an overlying skin wound? If he has, toilet it.
(3) Has his dura been torn? If it has, repair it. (4) Are there
any foreign bodies in the wound and particularly in his brain?
If so, remove all foreign bodies from the wound. You may
sometimes have to leave a bullet, or a large bony fragment deep
in his brain. (5) Has his underlying brain been damaged? If it
has, there is unfortunately little you can do.

Try to repair a patient's torn dura. Sometimes his X-ray shows
a fracture which has obviously torn it, or it may show air in
his subdural space. Often, the diagnosis is far from obvious, so
don't hesitate to explore a wound if: (1) There might be a dural
tear. (2) There might be a bony fragment piercing the patient's
dura. If necessary, enlarge his scalp wound, and feel and look
at his skull. You may find any of these things :—

A fissured fracture should be left alone, unless it is filled
with dirt or leaking CSF. CSF seldom leaks from fractures of
the vault, and more often does so from basal fractures which
involve a patient's nose or ears.

If a wound in the skull is leaking CSF from a fissured fracture, make a burr hole and then nibble away the patient's skull
towards the tear, so as to expose enough of his dura to allow
you to repair the tear.

A depressed fracture with fairly small skull fragments
can be fatal if you try to elevate them. So, base your decision
to operate on the indications given below. If you need to elevate
a depressed fracture, make a burr hole in the nearby normal skull,
enlarge the hole with nibblers, insert a bone elevator, and lever
up the depressed fragment(s). Often, you cannot do this because
they are jammed up against one another, so you have to remove
them. Then, if necessary, repair the dura.

A large, closed, depressed fracture is caused by a blow
from a large blunt object, and involves wide areas of the skull.
A child's skull merely bends, and the result is the 'ping – pong
ball fracture' in Section 63.8. In an adult the fragments may

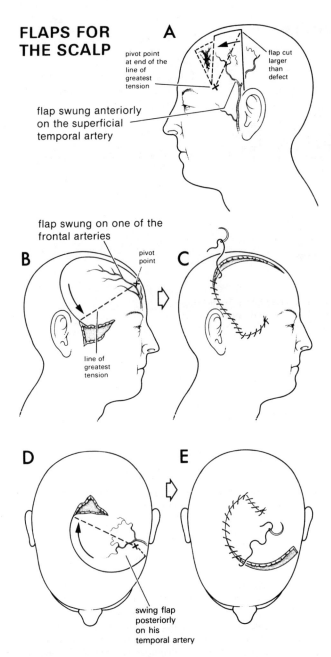

FLAPS FOR THE SCALP

A

pivot point at end of the line of greatest tension

flap cut larger than defect

flap swung anteriorly on the superficial temporal artery

B

flap swung on one of the frontal arteries

pivot point

line of greatest tension

C

D

E

swing flap posteriorly on his temporal artery

Fig. 63-15 MORE SCALP FLAPS. If necessary, graft the area from which you mobilized the flap. *A Rowbotham.*

be comminuted, and those at the apex of the fracture may tear the dura and enter the brain. Fragments of the inner table displace more than those of the outer table, so an injury may be worse than it looks. Even with a large depressed fracture, a patient may be conscious and have no neurological signs.

Raising large pieces of bone is difficult, and you may not be able to do it through a trephine hole. So, if possible, leave them. Don't operate merely because a fracture is depressed. If a patient has neurological signs, or a marked depression, or an obviously torn dura, refer him.

A serious consequence of an infected wound of the vault is 'brain fungus'. The patient's brain becomes infected, swells through the gap in his skull and dura, and forms a stinking, fungating swelling on the surface of his head. Once this has happened, there is nothing anyone can do. It is the result of: (1) infection, (2) foreign bodies including bone fragments in his brain, and (3) a raised intracranial pressure. It used to be thought that the important step in preventing brain fungus was to close the dura. This is now thought to be much less important than a careful wound toilet and the removal of all foreign bodies.

If you have to leave a gap in the dura, close it with an absorbable sponge ('Sterispon') or fascia lata from the patient's thigh. This will lie between his brain and his scalp, both of which are highly vascular, so it will readily take and fuse with the surrounding dura. You may be able to replace the pieces of his skull, as described below, but if you cannot, this is not important.

JULIUS was walking about quite fit, smiling and gesticulating, but quite unable to speak since the previous week when he had been hit on the head in a fight. Palpation showed him to have a depressed fracture of his skull. As this was being elevated under local anaesthesia a sepulchral voice from under the drapes called out "Shikamoo" ("I am holding your feet", a local term of subservience and indebtedness). The patient went home talking volubly and everyone was happy. LESSON Aphasia is one of the indications for raising a depressed fracture.

FILIMON'S scalp was split and torn, his brains were pouring out of his head and dripping slowly to the ground. This is the literal truth. A tree had fallen on it, smashing it like an egg. On the operating table it became clear that his skull was in five pieces. As these were manoeuvred into position more brain kept oozing out. At last the jigsaw was complete and his scalp was sewn up. To everyone's suprise he made a quick recovery and walked home. He did seem to have a rather simple and euphoric personality, but his family said that he had always been like that. LESSON Few patients are so severely injured that they must be given up as hopeless. Both these accounts are from Leader Stirling's 'Tanzanian Doctor', William Heinemann, London.

DON'T HESITATE TO EXPLORE A HEAD WOUND
ALWAYS CLOSE THE DURA
IF NECESSARY, GRAFT IT

ELEVATING A FRACTURE

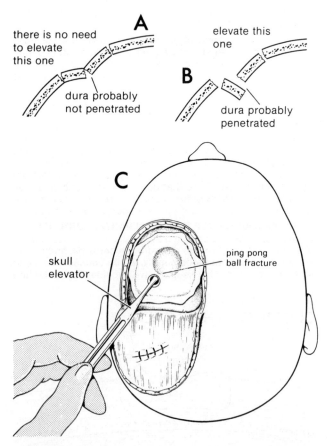

A

there is no need to elevate this one

dura probably not penetrated

B

elevate this one

dura probably penetrated

C

skull elevator

ping pong ball fracture

Fig. 63-16 DEPRESSED FRACTURES. A, a fracture which has probably not penetrated the dura. B, one which probably has penetrated it. Occasionally, you will need to elevate a ping pong ball fracture in a child, as in C. The base of this flap should face downwards (caudally) not as shown here. In an adult, you will seldom be able to do this and you are more likely to have to remove the fragments one by one, as in Fig. 63-18. *Kindly contributed by Peter Bewes and Gerishom Sande*

FRACTURES OF THE VAULT

Be sure you are familiar with the methods of controlling bleeding in Section 63.9.

INDICATIONS FOR RAISING DEPRESSED FRACTURES IN ADULTS (1) Coma, or other signs of cerebral compression. (2) Local neurological signs such as hemiplegia or aphasia. (3) A depressed fracture over the patient's motor cortex. (4) Fragments of bone or foreign bodies in his brain. (5) Penetration of his dura. (6) Leaking CSF. (7) If a fragment is depressed by more than the thickness of his skull, say 5 mm, most expert surgeons would raise it, even if there are no other indications for doing so. If it is causing the patient no symptoms, you, who are less expert, would be wise to leave it. (8) If a fracture is open, this is a strong indication for raising it, and, if necessary, removing the fragments which may promote infection.

CONTRAINDICATIONS (1) Depressed fractures over a sinus (63.9) without neurological signs. (2) Very large closed depressed fractures. Most experts would operate on these.

WHEN TO OPERATE? If a patient has more serious injuries elsewhere, you can, if absolutely necessary, leave his depressed fracture for up to 24 hours or longer. This is provided you toilet and close his scalp wound and provided his dura is not damaged.

X-RAYS Look carefully at these to see if the patient's sagittal or lateral sinuses are in danger. If they are, expect severe bleeding.

PREPARATION Shave all the hair from his scalp.

ANTIBIOTICS In the hope of preventing infection, give the patient an antibiotic which will enter his CSF, such as suphadiazine 2 g followed by 1 g 4 hourly, or chloramphenicol. Also, give him penicillin; start immediately, and don't continue antibiotics beyond 5 days.

EQUIPMENT A general set, preferably two general sets, so that you can use the second one when you are inside his skull. Hudson's brace, a perforator, and burrs. A fine suction tube. A malleable copper retractor. A bottle of warm sterile saline and a drip set arranged so that you can irrigate the wound to wash away blood and damaged brain.

ANAESTHESIA If possible, give the patient a general anaesthetic (A 16.8).

Local anaesthesia is also possible. The skull, the dura, and the brain are insensitive to pain, so you need only anaesthetize the patient's skin. Before you inject the anaesthetic, test the mobility of his scalp, and plan carefully

TAKING A GRAFT OF FASCIA LATA

fascia lata and the minimum amount of muscle

flap reflected

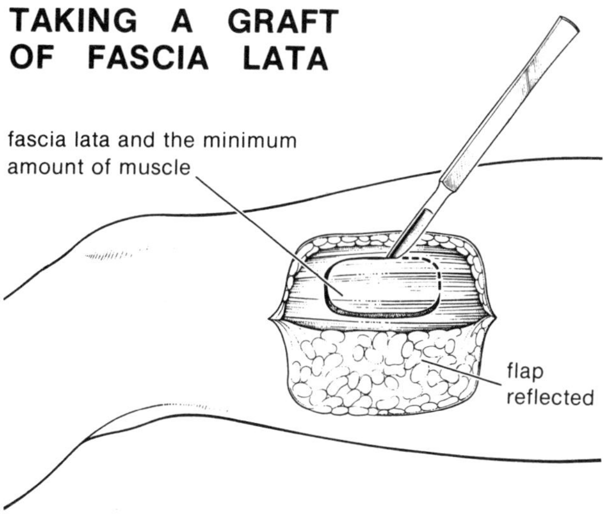

Fig. 63-17 TAKING A GRAFT OF FASCIA LATA. **Always prepare and towel the lateral aspect of a patient's thigh, so that you can quickly take a piece of his fascia lata to repair a torn sinus or a gap in his dura.** *Kindly contributed by Peter Bewes.*

how you can best cover his wound subsequently. You may need to swing flaps to close the incision. Add adrenaline to the anaesthetic solution to control the bleeding. Inject it well beyond the edges of his wound, wherever you expect to incise.

Arrange to minimize venous bleeding by adjusting the slope of the table, and carefully positioning the patient's head and neck as in Section 63.9.

PREPARING THE PATIENT'S OUTER THIGH Always prepare and towel the lateral aspect of his thigh, so that you can quickly take a piece of his fascia lata to repair a torn sinus or a gap in his dura. Take it as in Fig. 63-17. Be sure to take it from the lateral aspect—there is little fascia anteriorly.

THE SCALP INJURY Toilet and explore this to remove all visible dirt as described in Section 63.7.

If the patient's scalp wound is small, excise any very ragged edges, sew it up, and turn down a separate U–shaped flap with its base facing downwards. Make this flap carefully and use the methods in Section 63.9 to prevent excessive bleeding.

If there is a gap in his scalp, you may be able to close it by using one of the sliding flap methods (Fig. 63-15).

Explore the surface of his skull thoroughly. If you find a fissured fracture, leave it, unless it is leaking CSF, or is filled with dirt. Remove all dirt and contaminated periosteum.

RAISING A DEPRESSED SKULL FRACTURE

Discard the instruments you have used for the skin, and take a fresh set.

Insert a self retaining retractor, to improve the exposure. Strip the patient's pericranium away from the depressed bone, starting at the edge of the depression. Then strip it off the surrounding bone, as far as the edges of the wound. Make a burr hole in sound bone of his intact skull, close to the edge of the depressed area. If there is a choice, make it over a silent area in his brain. Start with a perforator, and use the brace and burrs as in Fig. 63-10.

CAUTION ! Don't make the burr hole in the depressed fragment. It may be loose and go straight into his brain with the burr.

Enlarge the hole with bone nibblers. Before you insert them, push his dura away from the inner table with a dural separator.

Occasionally, you will be able to insert a bone elevator and lever up the depressed fragments, as in Fig. 63-16. More often, you will have to remove them piece by piece as in Fig. 63-18. Remove all loose or grossly contaminated fragments. If they are clean, lay them back on the surface of the dura. They will act as a graft, and help to close the bony defect.

If the fragments are locked, you may have to make a second burr hole to unlock them.

If the fragments are very large, expose the fracture widely with large skin flaps which must have an adequate base. Lift up the fragments, and suture them in position with stitches through the pericranium.

If a clean fragment remains attached to the patient's pericranium, leave it.

If the surrounding edges of the patient's skull are dirty, nibble them away.

CAUTION ! If there are any fragments in or near a venous sinus, leave them. It may bleed torrentially if you try to remove them.

THE DURA IN A FRACTURE OF THE VAULT OF THE SKULL

If the patient's dura is intact, leave it, remove any extradural haematoma present, and close the wound.

If his dura is blood stained or CSF oozes from the burr hole, his dura has been torn. Expose the whole tear by nibbling away more bone to expose 2 cm of intact dura all round it. This will allow you to see any laceration in his cortex.

If the tear in his dura has ragged edges, cut them away. If necessary, enlarge the tear. The bony fragments responsible for the tear are usually near the surface of the brain. Remove them.

If his brain is uninjured, close his dura with interrupted stitches of fine monofilament and close the wound.

REMOVING BONY FRAGMENTS

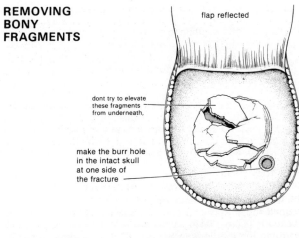

flap reflected

dont try to elevate these fragments from underneath,

make the burr hole in the intact skull at one side of the fracture

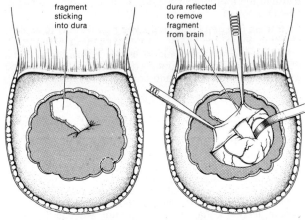

fragment sticking into dura

dura reflected to remove fragment from brain

Fig. 63-18 REMOVING BONY FRAGMENTS IN A DEPRESSED FRACTURE. Where possible, try to pick up the fragments from above. The normal dura is rather light in colour. *After Rowbotham.*

If part of the patient's dura has been lost, you cannot close it by simple suture, so sew a piece of pericranium or fascia lata in place with fine monofilament. For small gaps use pericranium, for large ones use fascia lata. Trim the edges of the dura, then trim the patch to fit the gap exactly, and sew it in place edge to edge.

If his dura is purple and bulging, stroke its surface with the point of a No. 11 scalpel blade. As soon as it is opened, enlarge the opening with fine scissors, to expose the blood clot.

THE BRAIN IN A FRACTURE OF THE VAULT OF THE SKULL

If necessary, get a better view of a patient's brain by nibbling away more of his skull and opening his dura wider. Handle his brain gently. Remove all the dead tissue, clot, bone fragments, and foreign bodies that you can reach.

Remove any damaged brain tissue with a jet of warm saline from a syringe or by suction. Fix a rubber catheter on the end of the sucker and gently suck out any blood clots or purple damaged brain. Provided the nozzle of the sucker is not too wide, it will suck away soft injured brain safely, without injuring normal brain. Foot suction is usually safe. Stroke the surface of his brain with a fine suction tube until you get to healthy tissue. If you are not sure how much brain to remove, take away too much rather than too little.

When the toilet is complete, there should be a clean hole in his brain. It will close up and become smaller.

If there might be a foreign body in the patient's brain, insert brain retractors, suck and look. If you know where it is because you can see it on an X-ray, explore very gently with fine dissecting forceps. You can usually find and remove it quite easily. Or, you may be able to remove it on the end of a sucker. Don't try to feel it with your finger, you may push it further in. If you cannot remove it easily, leave it. You may

have to leave a deeply embedded bullet, but try to remove a large deep bony fragment.

CAUTION ! Keep the patient's exposed brain wet with saline.

Control bleeding by the methods in Section 63.9.

CLOSING THE DURA IN A FRACTURE OF THE VAULT OF THE SKULL

When you have controlled all bleeding inside the patient's dura, close it, if closure is easy. Otherwise graft it. If necessary, hitch the dura to the pericranium as in Fig. 63-19.

The wound should be perfectly dry before you close a patient's skull, especially after an extradural haemorrhage, and when his brain has not completely expanded. If it is not dry, a clot will form postoperatively, and bleeding will not stop until the tension in it raises sufficiently to cause undesirable pressure on his brain.

CLOSING THE WOUND IN A FRACTURE OF THE VAULT OF THE SKULL

Ask an assistant to close the patient's thigh wound, while you close his head. Most scalp wounds heal by first intention, and delayed primary suture is seldom necessary. Close them with the stitiches in Fig. 63-14.

CAUTION ! Accurate closure of the skin wound without tension is most important. If necessary cut flaps (Fig. 63-15).

Continue penicillin, sulphadiazine, and chloramphenicol for 5 days.

DIFFICULTIES WITH A FRACTURE OF THE VAULT OF THE SKULL

If a WOUND HAS LEFT A GAP IN A PATIENT'S SKULL suggest that he wears a helmet if his occupation is such that his head might be injured. If his skull defect is over a prominent convexity, repair may be necessary.

If you DON'T HAVE A BONE NIBBLER and the patient has a fissured fracture which is leaking CSF, do a careful wound toilet and close his skin. Or, you can plug a fissured fracture with a piece of his temporalis muscle to prevent his CSF leaking out. If there is enough space for CSF to leak out, there will be enough space for you to push some muscle in. So explore and toilet his scalp wound. Take a piece of his temporalis muscle, crush it and force it into the fissure. Then close his skin wound, and give him antibiotics.

If he has a BULLET WOUND toilet the entry and the exit wounds, and suck out the clot together with any pulped brain. If the wound is deep, pass a rubber catheter along its path. Control bleeding with hydrogen peroxide packs.

If the bullet comes out easily, extract it together with any foreign bodies or pieces of bone that you can remove without too much difficulty with fine dissecting forceps. But, if the bullet is difficult to remove, toilet the superficial parts of the wound carefully, and leave it where it is. Close the wound (Fig. 63-14), and give the patient antibiotics. A bullet makes a smaller wound on entering the skull than on leaving it, and fractures the inner table more severely than the outer one. Remove any bony fragments in the brain; these must come out, the bullet need not.

CAUTION ! 20 vols hydrogen peroxide produces 20 times its volume of oxygen, so make sure that there is a space for the oxygen to come out, or it may compresss the brain. Inexpert surgeons would be wiser not to use it.

If a FRACTURE HAS ENTERED HIS FRONTAL OR ETHMOID SINUSES, do nothing if the posterior wall of the sinus is intact. But if it is fragmented and torn, so that he has rhinorrhoea, he is in danger of meningitis, a brain abscess, or a pneumatocoele. Treat him conservatively with antibiotics, and he will probably recover. If a pneumatocoele develops, or CSF continues to leak for more than two weeks, refer him.

If a patient has a penetrating injury and PRESENTS LATE WITH MOTOR WEAKNESS ON THE OPPOSITE SIDE, he has escaped the immediate danger of meningitis, and he probably now has a cerebral abscess. Refer him if you possibly can. If you cannot refer him, all you can do is to explore the wound, and open his dura and his brain. Syringe out the abscess cavity with a jet of saline, and close his wound as above.

63.8 Ping–pong ball skull fractures in children

A blunt object, which causes a large depressed fracture in an adult, causes a ping–pong ball fracture in a child, whose skull is soft and dents instead of fracturing. The indications for not operating on a child are even stronger than in an adult, because these fractures rarely cause trouble. If a child has a single fit, disregard it. The dent will disappear as he grows.

ELEVATING A PING PONG BALL FRACTURE If you decide to raise the fracture, try first with a vacuum extractor. Apply one of the vacuum cups, as you would during delivery. Pull, and hold the surrounding skull with your other hand. If this fails, make a hole with a perforator at the edge of the depression and elevate the fracture with a skull elevator, as in Fig. 63-16. Make the hole for it with a perforator and nibblers and *don't use burrs.*

63.9 Controlling bleeding in head injuries

The scalp has an excellent blood supply from: (1) The temporal arteries ascending in front of the ears. (2) The supraorbital arteries which ascend over a patient's forehead from the medial ends of his eyebrows. (3) The occipital arteries behind his mastoid processes. This excellent blood supply helps wounds to heal quickly, and maintains the circulation in skin flaps with a small base, but it does mean that a patient can quickly lose much blood from a scalp wound. Minimize this bleeding by making incisions from above downwards parallel to the main vessels, rather than across them, or round his head.

Controlling bleeding in head injuries can be difficult, and there are some useful special methods. You must have a sucker, and you will find diathermy useful. If you don't have it, you will have to use a muscle patch to control venous bleeding. Don't use diathermy superficial to the galea, and especially not on skin edges, or the small areas of necrosis it causes will prevent the skin healing by first intention. For the same reason, when you are operating deep to the galea, don't let the diathermy electrode accidentally touch the haemostats on the skin edges.

CONTROLLING BLEEDING IN HEAD INJURIES

From without inwards, control a bleeding head injury like this:

BLEEDING FROM THE SCALP
Bleeding scalp vessels are difficult to pick up in haemostats, because they are held by the fibro-fatty tissue. Instead, use stitches, and control bleeding like this:

(1) Ask one, or even two assistants, to press on the patient's scalp close to the edges of the wound.

(2) Pick up the cut edge of his galea with haemostats 1 cm apart along the incision. Then evert them so that they compress the bleeding vessels in the edge of his scalp. Keep them together in bundles with rubber bands round their handles, out the way of the operation.

(3) Add adrenaline to the local anaesthetic solution. If the patient is having a general anaesthetic, infiltrate his scalp and temporalis muscle with adrenaline and saline.

Try to control all bleeding before you stitch up his scalp. If you don't, a large haematoma may form under it, become infected, and need opening later.

BLEEDING VEINS AND VENOUS SINUSES
When you operate, prevent venous bleeding by taking the following precautions before you start:

(1) Use methods of anaesthesia which minimize bleeding. It will be worse if the patient strains. Ideally, give him a general anaesthetic, intubate him under relaxants, and hyperventilate him. This will reduce his intracranial pressure and minimize bleeding. If general anaesthesia is unlikely to be perfect, local anaesthesia may be better.

(2) Make sure that nothing obstructs the veins of the patient's neck. If necessary, raise his shoulders on sandbags.

(3) Reduce the venous pressure in his wound. Arrange the position of his head so that his wound lies uppermost. Give the table just enough head up tilt, about 10°, to raise his head above his heart and minimize venous bleeding. Don't raise it too much because air may be sucked in and cause an air embolus. The first sign of this will be sudden weakening of his pulse and an increase in its rate. Embolism will be less likely if there is fluid over the surface of his wound, so keep syringing it with saline.

Elevating the head of the table will also help to control bleeding from his dura or his brain, but is less useful on the more superficial tissues.

If a sinus bleeds during an intracranial operation, apply the above measures. But:

Don't: (1) Apply haemostats to the patient's bleeding sinus, because they will tear out and make bleeding worse. (2) Don't try to sew up a torn sinus. This can increase bleeding, especially if you cannot get at it adequately.

Instead: (1) Tie any smaller sinuses on either side of the tear, or fix them with a silver clip. (2) Push muscle grafts or pieces of surgical gauze between his dura and his skull. Then keep them in place by passing a few interrupted sutures between his epicranium and his dura over the nibbled edge of the bone. These sutures will hitch up his dura, and help to keep the muscle grafts in place. (3) Plug his bleeding sinus with a piece of muscle. If necessary, hold it in place with a deep suture passed under the sinus with a big curved needle.

If blood pours out as a dark venous stream from his sagittal sinus, controlling it can be very difficult. This sinus runs in the midline on the inner surface of the skull from the forehead to the occiput. Several irregular venous spaces (lacunae) join it on the top of the head (63-6). Fortunately, it is rarely injured, because the skull is more often hit from the side than directly from on top. The transverse sinuses in the occipital region are still less vulnerable, but when they are injured, bleeding is even harder to control.

Plug the patient's torn sagittal sinus with haemostatic gauze. Suture his scalp over it, apply a tight bandage, and refer him. If you don't have any haemostatic gauze, or cannot refer him, use ordinary gauze and remove it cautiously in the theatre 48 hours later. If necessary, replace it with a muscle graft or a patch. Or, cover the gap with a thin piece of bone wax, and close his scalp over this. You can safely obstruct the superior saggital sinus in the first quarter of its length. Obstructing it further back will probably kill him.

Often, a sinus does not bleed until you begin raising a depressed fracture near it—don't!—treat it conservatively! These fractures are for real experts.

BLEEDING FROM THE BRANCHES OF THE MIDDLE MENINGEAL ARTERY
These vessels lie between the dura and the inner table of the skull. Underrun them with silk or cotton on a fine curved needle. This is easier than trying to coagulate them with diathermy.

BLEEDING FROM THE DIPLOE
Push Horsley's bone wax into the bleeding cut surface of the patient's skull. Or, use Bismuth and iodoform paste BPC. Or, use autoclaved beeswax or paraffin (candle) wax. If an artery spurts from the bone, push the sharpened point of a sterile match stick into it.

BLEEDING FROM THE VESSELS OF THE DURA
These tear so easily that you cannot grasp them with haemostats and tie them in the usual way. Instead, control bleeding like this.

(1) Place the wound uppermost, as described above.

(2) Press gently on the patient's injured sinus for about a minute. When you let go, the bleeding will probably have stopped. Pressing too hard may injure the smaller veins joining the sinus and make bleeding worse.

(3) Grasp the bleeding vessels with fine dissecting forceps and touch these with the diathermy electrode.

(4) Grasp the bleeding vessel with fine dissecting forceps,

ask your assistant to hold them very still, while you under-run the vessel with 3/0 silk on a small curved atraumatic needle. When the suture is complete, apply a muscle patch, as described below.

(5) USING A MUSCLE PATCH If a piece of some suitable material is pressed over the bleeding area for a few minutes, blood will clot around it and seal it. Synthetic absorbable gauze is best, but if you don't have that, use a piece of muscle, or muscle and fascia squeezed flat. The temporalis muscle is close at hand, so use it. Although these patches will not stop an obviously bleeding vessel, they will stop a steady ooze.

Take a piece of the patient's temporalis muscle, and squeeze it flat between artery forceps until it is a thin sheet, the size of a postage stamp. The muscle will now be dead, but it will readily promote clotting. Press it onto the bleeding vessel, cover it with moist gauze, hold it in place with the sucker and drip saline onto it. The saline will keep the surrounding brain wet, and you will see through the gauze when bleeding has stopped. Leave it for five minutes.

If the flap you have reflected does not contain temporalis muscle, extend it so that you can take some. If you have already prepared the patient's thigh, you can take some muscle from that.

Alternatively, scrape off a piece of the patient's epicranium exposed by the wound, or take a piece from his mastoid process and hammer this flat to make the patch.

BLEEDING FROM THE BRAIN

Diathermy or silver clips will usually stop venous or arterial bleeding from any size of vessel. Use the lowest diathermy current that will cause coagulation, and the finest forceps. If don't have diathermy, or silver clips, avoid using haemostats, because the bleeding vessel too easily pulls out of the brain. Instead, apply a muscle patch, as described above, or soak a pad of cotton wool in hydrogen peroxide and put this on the patient's bleeding brain.

If his brain is bleeding, a warm pack will almost always control it. If necessary, put a piece of haemostatic gauze between his brain and his dura before closing it, and then place more gauze outside this. Don't pack or plug head wounds with ordinary gauze.

ALWAYS OPERATE WITH THE PATIENT'S HEAD
ABOVE HIS HEART

63.10 Hyperthermia after a head injury

Injuries to the heat regulating centres in a patient's brain may cause hyperthermia, especially during the first 12 hours after an injury. When he is first admitted his temperature is usually low, and any rise over 39°C is a grave sign. During the first few days a temperature fluctuation of a degree or so is unimportant, but a rise after a day or two is serious, because it may indicate renewed subarachnoid bleeding, pneumonia, or meningitis. Hyperthermia can kill a patient with a head injury who might survive otherwise, so monitor his temperature carefully, and treat him promptly. It can rise very suddenly: it may be 38°C one moment and 42°C half an hour later.

HYPERTHERMIA Take the patient's temperature regularly. During times of crisis take it every 10 or 25 minutes. If his temperature rises above 39°C, take off his pyjamas, cover him with a wet sheet, and turn a fan on him. Bring his temperature down to 40°C or below, and keep it there. If necessary give him chlorpromazine 50 mg 6 hourly, intramuscularly or by stomach tube.

63.11 Convulsions after a head injury

These can occur following a head injury at any time, and can be of almost infinite variety, either focal or general. They are usually associated with sudden deterioration of consciousness. Prevent them with phenobarbitone. Treat them promptly in the hope of preventing status epilepticus, which may be fatal.

CONVULSIONS Make sure the patient has a good airway. This may stop them.

If improving his airway fails, give him diazepam (A 2-4) intravenously for its immediate effect. Follow this with phenytoin sodium ('Epanutin'), first 250 mg intramuscularly, and then 50 mg, 6 hourly by mouth or tube. Phenytoin causes very little depression of consciousness, so it will not mask the signs of clot compression.

If these fail to stop convulsions, give him paraldehyde into the outer side of his thigh. Give infants under 6 months 1 to 2 ml, older children 2 to 4 ml, adults 7 to 10 ml.

If even these methods fail, give the patient 10% paraldehyde in 0.9% saline (50 ml in 500 ml of saline) by

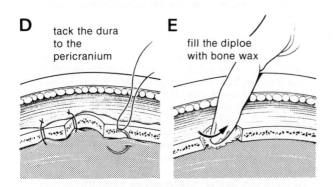

SOME WAYS TO CONTROL BLEEDING IN A HEAD INJURY

A
press
evert the scalp

B
muscle patch

C
multiple haemostats evert the scalp

ragged wound being excised

assistants pressing on the edges of the scalp

D
tack the dura to the pericranium

E
fill the diploe with bone wax

Fig. 63-19 WAYS TO CONTROL BLEEDING IN A HEAD INJURY. A, evert the edges of the patient's scalp with haemostats, or press on them. B, press a flattened muscle patch on his bleeding brain, cover it with gauze, drip saline onto it, and suck. C, when you excise a ragged head wound ask your assistants to press on its edge. D, tack the patient's pericranium to his dura. E, fill his diploe with bone wax. *By kind permission of Hugh Dudley and Gerishom Sande.*

intravenous drip slowly, as necessary. You can supplement this with phenytoin sodium 250 mg intramuscualrly, or by slow intravenous injection.

Sedate the patient with phenobarbitone for a month after discharge. You may need to sedate him permanently. Reduce the dose gradually. Never halve it at any one time, instead, cut it by a quarter. The difference between a half and a quarter of a tablet may be critical.

Alternatively, maintain him on phenytoin to control convulsions.

63.12 When CSF leaks from the patient's nose or ears

This is the result of a fracture of the base of a patient's skull, which puts his arachnoid space in communication with his nose or ears. If you are not sure if the fluid is CSF, or merely nasal discharge, test some fresh fluid for glucose with a urine test strip. Only CSF contains glucose. Mop his nose or ears clean, but don't plug them. Don't lumbar puncture him, because this will lower his CSF pressure, and may assist organisms to enter his meninges.

LEAKING CSF FOLLOWING A HEAD INJURY

If the patient's airway and level of consciousness permit, lower his CSF pressure in the wound by nursing him sitting up.

ANTIBIOTICS Give him co-trimoxazole 960 mg 8-12 hourly, or sulphadimidine 2 g initially followed by 1 g 6 hourly. Also give him chloramphenicol 50 mg/kg/24 hrs in 6 hourly doses.

NOSE A leak of CSF from a patient's nose is much more common than a leak from his ears, and rarely lasts more than a few days. Note which nostril the CSF escapes from. Don't let him blow his nose, because this may blow bacteria through the crack in his skull into his meninges.

If CSF leaks from his nose for more than 10 days, refer him for repair of his dura.

EARS A leak from the ears is less significant than a leak from the nose. If CSF leaks from a patient's ears for more than 3 days, he is probably bleeding intracranially and needs burr holes.

63.13 Meningitis follows a head injury

A stiff neck soon after an injury can be caused by meningeal bleeding, by a fracture of the patient's cervical spine, or by soft tissue injuries, so it is not of great significance early on. Some days later a stiff neck is more serious. So do a lumbar puncture if: (1) His neck becomes stiff some days after the injury. (2) He has a positive Kernig's sign at any time.

MENINGITIS AFTER A HEAD INJURY

If the organisms have entered from the patient's nose, they are probably pneumococci, and are usually sensitive to penicillin. Give him penicillin 2 megaunits immediately, and then 1 megaunit 6 hourly.

Also, give him intrathecal penicillin 20 000 units immediately, and then 10 000 units daily for 5 days. Give it in a dilution of 2 000 units per ml in water for injection because stronger solutions, or larger doses, can cause severe meningeal reactions. Withdraw an equivalent quantity of CSF before you inject. At the same time give him chloramphenicol 50 to 100 mg/kg/day. Or give him sulphadiazine or sulphadimidine orally or by tube, 3 g initially, followed by 1.5 g 4 hourly, together with plenty of fluid.

If the organism is insensitive to penicillin, give him streptomycin 1 g intramuscularly, and 50 mg in 1 ml intrathecally.

63.14 More difficulties with a head injury

We have described most of the difficulties you are likely to meet, but here are a few more. They are not common.

MORE DIFFICULTIES WITH A HEAD INJURY

If a patient has CRANIAL NERVE PALSIES, they are usually the result of fractures of the base of his skull. There is no specific treatment for them.

If he CAN MOVE HIS HEAD AFTER A HEAD INJURY, BUT NOT THE REST OF HIS BODY, he is quadriplegic as the result of a fracture of his cervical spine. When a patient's head is injured, his broken neck is often missed.

If he STARTS TO SNEEZE he almost certainly has a pneumatocele. This is the slow development of an air filled cavity in his brain connecting with one of his sinuses, usually his frontal sinus. His skull may be resonant to percussion, and an X-ray may show an air filled cavity. He is in great danger of meningitis. Refer him for neurosurgery immediately.

FEW HEAD INJURIES ARE SO SEVERE AS TO BE HOPELESS
NO HEAD INJURY IS SO TRIVIAL AS TO BE TAKEN LIGHTLY

---

64 The spine

64.1 Introduction

A fracture of the spine, like a fracture of the skull, is less important than the injury to the nervous system inside it. In a district hospital your main responsibilities are: (1) To see that patients with spinal injuries are not made worse unnecessarily. (2) To diagnose stable fractures of the cervical spine and put them into some kind of collar. (3) To apply neck traction to the occasional patient who has an unstable fracture of his cervical spine, with a normal or nearly normal cord. (4) To care for all injuries of the thoracic and lumbar spines conservatively. (5) To care for paraplegics in the manner we describe.

Unfortunately, there is almost nothing you or anyone else can do for a patient who is already totally quadriplegic (64.13). There are no indications for operations on spinal injuries in a district hospital, and few for referring a patient for them. Manipulation, whether under anaesthesia or not, is also contraindicated, because it is very dangerous, even in in the hands of most experts.

The common error is *to fail to fit a collar when this is indicated*. The only special equipment you will need is Gardner Wells tongs. If you don't have them you can apply Hoen's traction using a brace and burrs.

• *TRACTION TONGS, Gardner Wells, one only.* These expensive tongs are the most practical way of applying traction to an unstable fracture of the cervical spine. The alternative, Crutchfield tongs, is less satisfactory, but they are easy to apply and will hold for about 6 weeks. Alternatively, you can make the halo in Fig. 64-12. Better still, these halos can be made centrally and distributed to all the district hospitals of a country. When you need a halo, you will need it urgently, and there will not be time to make it, so make one now.

64.2 Syndromes of spinal injury

The spinal cord, the bones, and the soft tissues of a patient's spine can be injured by accidents which compress, hinge, or shear them. Occasionally, in a hyperextension injury, his vertebrae only sublux momentarily at the time of the accident and then return to their normal places, so that a severe cord lesion can be combined with a normal X-ray, especially in the neck. The opposite is also true, and a patient with a gross bony injury can have a normal spinal cord. Luckily, most patients who injure their spines don't injure their cords. But if they do, this dominates their treatment, and their prognosis.

A patient's spinal injury can be stable or unstable. If his injury is stable, his spine was able to protect his cord from the forces of the original accident, and it will still be able to protect his cord from being harmed by ordinary movement. But if his injury is unstable, his spine cannot now protect his cord from the bony displacement that may follow normal movement. So, be safe and assume that: *(1) any spinal injury is unstable, until you have proved it otherwise,* and (2) make sure that a patient is moved with the greatest care, from the moment of his injury until you are sure, either that his spine is normal, or that its injury is stable. He has already received one injury, it would be tragic for him to receive another from careless mishandling. *Any wrong movement may prevent the recovery that might otherwise have occurred.* If a patient's spine is unstable, it must be protected from any movement, from the moment of the accident until it has stabilized several months later.

Serious spinal injuries can harm: (1) the cells of the spinal cord, (2) the tracts passing up and down it, and (3) the spinal nerve roots. Some or all of these can be injured, either completely or partly, at any level. The critical diagnostic steps are: (1) to find the patient's sensory level (to pinprick) and his motor level, (2) to find the bony level of his lesion, then (3) to compare these. If the bony level is below the sensory one, take more X-rays higher up his spine. You have probably missed a second injury there.

Here are some of the more common patterns of spinal injury. The further an injury is down the cord, the better the chances of the patient is being able to walk, but the worse the outlook for his bladder control.

Injuries above the level of T10 The important injury here is the complete or incomplete division of the tracts passing up and down the patient's spinal cord, destroying sensation and causing an upper motor type of paralysis. Great force is needed to fracture the thoracic spine, so that if it does fracture, the cord inside it is either normal, or completely transected. Lesions elsewhere are more often incomplete.

If a patient's cord injury is incomplete, as is common in the cervical region, some sensation and muscular power usually returns slowly over many months.

If a patient's cord injury is complete, it remains so. There is immediate flaccid paralysis in the lower part of his body, and he has no sensation whatever. If his anal or penile reflexes remain when he is like this, it is a further indication that transection is complete and he is unlikely to recover. Later, the reflex activity of his spinal cord below the lesion may recover, so that his bladder and bowel reflexes return. His knee and ankle jerks recover

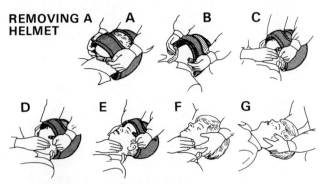

Fig. 64-1 REMOVING A HELMET. If you don't do this properly, you can aggravate a cervical spine injury after a motorcycle accident. Find an assistant. A, apply traction in the line of the patient's cervical spine. B, loosen the straps while maintaining traction. C, ask an assistant to hold the patient's neck and exert traction. D, remove his helmet. It is egg shaped, so expand it to clear his ears. E, your assistant keeps the patient's head still. F, take over traction from your assistant. G, continue to exert traction until you can support the patient's head as in Fig. 64-5. *Kindly contributed by Nancy Caroline.*

THE DERMATOMES

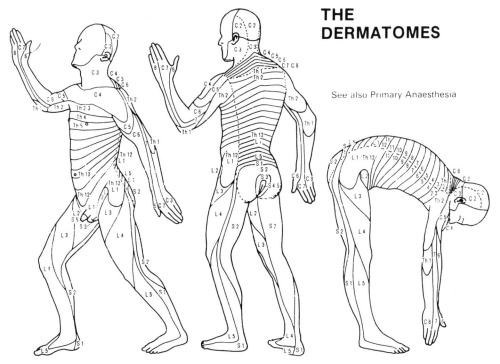

See also Primary Anaesthesia

Fig. 64-2 THE DERMATATOMES. If a patient is paraplegic, test his sensation with a pin from below upwards and use this chart to find the neurological level of his lesion. *From Ciba – Geigy, with kind permission.*

LEVELS OF SPINAL INJURY

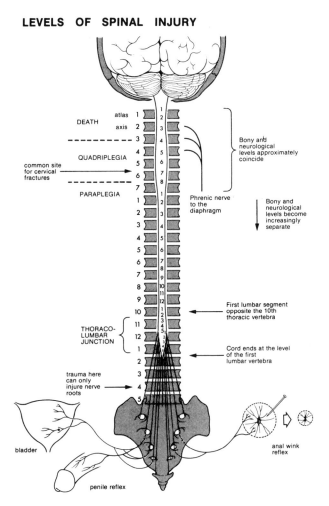

Fig 64-3 LEVELS OF SPINAL INJURY. Note that the cord ends opposite vertebrae T12–L1. A fracture dislocation of these vertebrae causes a neurological lesion at this level—unless some roots escape injury. The only importance of distinguishing between cord and veretebral levels is when the cord has been damaged, and some roots escape.

and then become exaggerated; his muscles become spastic and he may have severe spasms. If his bladder or bowel reflexes return without any sensation or motor power, this is an almost certain sign that his cord injury is complete.

Any lesion above C5 causes quadriplegia. At C5–T1 it causes quadriparesis. A common site of injury is the C5–C6 region. This may paralyse his hands, his intercostal muscles, and partly paralyse his diaphragm. Cord injuries at C3 or above may paralyse his respiration completely and kill him.

Injuries at the thoracolumbar junction (T10-L1) As Fig. 64-3 shows, an adult's first lumbar segment is at the level his tenth thoracic vertebra, and the end of his cord is at the lower border of his first lumbar vertebra. Trauma in this region can injure the nerve cells of his lumbar enlargement or the nerve roots of his cauda equina, or both. A severe fracture with marked displacement will sever his conus and his spinal nerve roots down to T10, so that the fracture level and the dermatome level are not the same. Occasionally (especially at T12–L1) his nerve roots escape and his only conus is injured ('root escape').

An injury to a patient's spinal cord in this region makes his lower sacral segments anaesthetic (saddle anaesthesia) and destroys his central bladder reflex. It may however spare just enough of the nerve roots supplying his legs to allow him to walk. Apart from pain, which suggests a root rather than a cord injury, there is no way of telling which of the two have been injured. This is unimportant because the treatment of both is the same.

Injuries below the level of the first lumbar vertebra Trauma here can only injure the lumbar and sacral nerve roots of a patient's cauda equina. If they have only been bruised they recover slowly, so his prognosis is good. But if they have been cut, they isolate his bladder from the reflex centre in his cord, so that his bladder control is less satisfactory than it would be if his cord had been severed higher up. His paralysed legs remain permanently flaccid.

DOES THE PATIENT HAVE MORE THAN ONE SPINAL INJURY?

64.3 Caring for a spinal injury

Spinal injuries are often missed for two reasons:

(1) An injured patient may be unable to say that he has lost the feeling in part of his body. His other injuries may be so much more visible than his fractured spine that, *unless you routinely exclude a spinal injury in all severely injured patients, you can easily miss one.* You may save a patient's life by removing his spleen only to find bed sores developing because he is also paraplegic. A routine check is very quick. Can he move his legs? If you pinch one, does he move it away? If he cannot move his arms or legs, his cord is almost certainly injured.

(2) A patient with an unstable injury of his cervical spine may walk into hospital after a seemingly minor injury. So *beware of anyone who complains of a painful neck after an accident.* Immediately fit him with a soft collar and X-ray his neck. He may only have a minor soft tissue injury, or he may have an unstable fracture and be in danger of instant paralysis.

A spinal injury is terrifying for a patient because he may be completely paralysed and yet fully conscious. His prognosis and management are determined by the following facts: (1) If his injury is severe enough to cause immediate total paraplegia, or quadriplegia, his spinal cord is almost certainly damaged beyond repair, and no treatment, surgical or otherwise, is going to make it recover. (2) If any function remains immediately after the injury, his prognosis is completely unpredictable. He may make a substantial recovery or he may make none at all. So one of your first aims in examining him should be to see if any function still remains. (3) If he shows any signs of recovery during the first few days, his outlook is much better, *so don't give any prognosis for several days.* The earlier and the more rapid his early recovery is, the more hope he has.

Should you refer a patient with a spinal injury? You will have to compare the care you can give him with the care he is likely to get in a referral hospital (1.8). Your care may be better—he is in much greater need of devoted nursing than of skilled surgery. There is seldom any advantage in referring a patient with a serious spinal injury immediately, because you can probably do as much for him, or more, than a referral hospital. Injured nerve cells cannot regenerate, so there is little to be gained by trying to decompress his spine in the hope that they will regenerate. Immediate laminectomy may do more harm than good. Some weeks later an operation to fuse an unstable spine may occasionally be useful. The only procedure that is practical in the acute phase is cervical traction. But although this needs only simple equipment, it needs great skill.

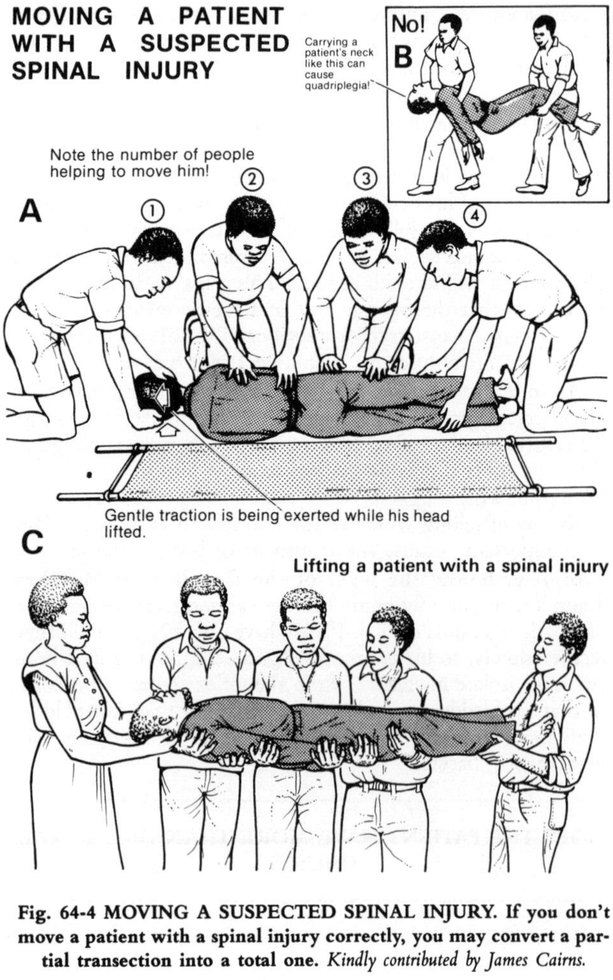

THE GENERAL METHOD FOR A SPINAL INJURY

This extends what has already been said about caring for a patient with multiple injuries in Section 51.3.

MOVING AND UNDRESSING A PATIENT When you move or turn a patient with a suspected spinal injury you will need *at least 2 helpers,* and preferably 4. Try to move him 'in one piece'. Minimize the movement of his spine, especially its cervical region.

If he is on the ground, carefully turn him onto one side as you roll him onto a stretcher, or a stretched blanket, as in Fig. 64-4. As you turn him, take the opportunity to examine his back and his spine, as described below.

If you suspect that a patient has a neck injury, place one hand under his chin and the other under his occiput, as in A, Fig. 64-5, expert gentle traction on his neck, and lift and turn his head while you turn his body—don't let his head drop to one side. *Holding his head is the task for the most skilled person in the team.* When you have finished turning him onto his back, wedge his head between sandbags, or rolled up sheets or blankets, as in B, Fig. 64-5, or fit him with a collar as in C, in this figure.

CAUTION ! (1) Keep his spine stretched and as straight as possible. Don't move his head. Keep it in a neutral position at all times. Never let anyone carry an injured patient with his head hanging down as in B, Fig. 64-4. Unfortunately people often do. (2) If there is any possibility of a spinal injury, especially a cervical one, this careful handling must go on until you have made sure the patient's spine is radiologically stable. (3) Fit him with a temporary cervical collar as soon as possible and never transport him anywhere without one. Failure to do so may: (a) convert a patient with a normal cord into a quadriplegic, (b) convert a partial transection into a total one, or (c) deprive a partially quadriplegic patient of a few critically useful segments.

SUPPORTING AN INJURED CERVICAL SPINE

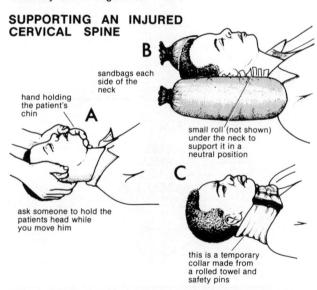

Fig. 64-5 SUPPORTING AN INJURED CERVICAL SPINE. A, holding a patient's head is the task for the most skilled person in the team. B, when you have finished turning him onto his back, wedge his head between sandbags, or rolled up sheets or blankets. C, or fit him with a collar. *Adapted from de Palma with kind permission.*

MOVING A PATIENT WITH A SUSPECTED SPINAL INJURY

Carrying a patient's neck like this can cause quadriplegia!

No!

Note the number of people helping to move him!

Gentle traction is being exerted while his head lifted.

Lifting a patient with a spinal injury

Fig. 64-4 MOVING A SUSPECTED SPINAL INJURY. If you don't move a patient with a spinal injury correctly, you may convert a partial transection into a total one. *Kindly contributed by James Cairns.*

If you suspect that a patient has an injury of his thoracic or lumbar spine, transport him prone with a pillow under his shoulders and pelvis to hyperextend his spine at the site of the injury, unless he has multiple injuries or his airway is in doubt. If it is in doubt, transport him supine.

THE HISTORY AND EXAMINATION OF A SPINAL INJURY

Leave the patient on his stretcher until you have examined him. Enquire carefully about the circumstances of the accident. This will tell you what type of injury to suspect.

If he is conscious, ask him "Where is the pain?" He may be able to say that he has a pain in his back, pains round his body, or that his body feels dead below a certain level. Signs of injury on his face and skull may help you to decide the kind of force responsible.

SPINE Carefully slide your hand underneath the patient's back, or turn him very carefully while an assistant holds his head. (1) Feel for any local bruising, swelling, and tenderness along his spine. Examine his spinous processes systematically from his neck to his sacrum. (2) Look for any break in the line. (3) Feel for any soft 'doughy' areas between his spinous processes into which your fingers can sink. You may feel a palpable gap. These last two signs indicate an unstable fracture.

CAUTION ! Don't test the movements of his spine!

DON'T FORGET TO EXAMINE HIS BACK

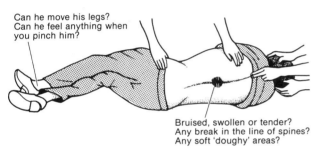

Can he move his legs?
Can he feel anything when you pinch him?

Bruised, swollen or tender?
Any break in the line of spines?
Any soft 'doughy' areas?

Fig. 64-6 EXAMINING A SPINAL INJURY. Feel for any local bruising, swelling, or tenderness along the patient's spine. Examine his spinous processes systematically from his neck to his sacrum. Look for a break in the line. Feel for any soft 'doughy' areas. *Kindly contributed by Ronald Huckstep.*

NEUROLOGICAL EXAMINATION This has two stages, and if a patient has an associated head injury, interpreting either of them may be difficult.

A rapid test to exclude a spinal injury Use this to exclude quickly a spinal injury in any severely injured patient (50.4). Can he move his legs? Are they equally strong? Can he feel anything when you pinch them?

A more extensive examination if you suspect a spinal injury. Test the sensation on the patient's trunk with a pin, starting from below and working upwards. Find the sensory level, using the dermatome chart in Fig. 64-3. Can he recognize movements of his feet or knees? Test his knee and ankle jerks and his plantar responses. Test to find out if his sacral segments have been spared by pricking the skin beside his anus with a pin.

If the patient has severe continuous pain radiating from his neck to both occipital regions, suspect a fracture dislocation of his atlas on his axis.

Assess the level of a fracture dislocation like this: Dislocations between C1 and C2 cause severe continuous pain radiating from the neck to the occiput. Dislocations between C3 and C5 cause quadriplegia. If C5 is dislocated on C6, a patient's biceps is weak or paralysed. If C6 is dislocated on C7, his biceps is normal. In dislocations above C7 and T1 Horner's syndrome (ptosis, a constricted pupil, anhydrosis on the affected side of his face, and enophthalmos) may be present.

The lumbar nerve roots supply: (1) sensation to a patient's legs, except that supplied by his sacral segments, (2) the

muscles of his hip and knee, (3) his cremasteric reflexes, his knee and his ankle jerks. Lumbar or sacral root pain suggests a root rather than a cord injury.

The sacral nerve roots supply: (1) sensation in his saddle area and a strip down the back of his leg and thigh, (2) the muscles controlling his ankle and foot, (3) his ankle and plantar responses, (4) his anal and cremasteric reflexes, (5) micturition.

The penile reflex Squeeze his glans penis, and feel his bulbocavernosus muscles. If they contract, the reflex is positive.

The anal wink reflex Scratch the skin round his anus. If his anus contracts and wrinkles, the reflex is positive. If either of these reflexes is positive immediately after the accident in the absence of sensation in his legs, they indicate transection of his cord and are a poor prognostic sign.

X-RAYS Don't send him for an immediate X-ray. Find the level of the lesion first. Some patients present with leg problems, but have an upper thoracic fracture, so examine his spine with care before you decide which part of it to X-ray. If you have enough film, X-ray his entire spine routinely, because spinal fractures are sometimes multiple. Otherwise, X-ray the relevant area only. See him onto the X-ray table yourself.

IS THE PATIENT'S FRACTURE STABLE? This decision is partly clinical and partly radiological. Make it by the criteria in Sections 64.4 and 64.5.

ASSOCIATED INJURIES About a third of patients have other severe injuries, particularly of the head (63.1) and abdomen (66.1), so look for them—this is critically important.

IMMEDIATE PROGNOSIS If a patient is paralysed with a sharp line of anaesthesia, no reflexes, and no bladder control, and with his anal and penile reflexes present, his cord is probably transected completely. Priapism (persistent, painful erection of the penis) is another bad sign.

Firmly hyperextend his big toe. Test his toes, heels, and perineum with a pin. If he is paralysed but can feel any of these things, his cord is probably only shocked, and its function will improve.

PROGNOSIS AT 24 HOURS If at this time he still has no perianal sensation, no voluntary control of his toe flexors, or rectal sphincters, he has a 90% chance of having a permanent paraplegia or quadriplegia. If any of these things are spared, or he shows any improvement in the first 48 hours, significant recovery is possible. If there have been no signs of improvement at 4 weeks, further recovery is very unlikely.

THE IMMEDIATE TREATMENT OF A FRACTURED SPINE

This varies with the level of the lesion.

Cervical spine Apply traction to all patients with: (1) any unstable fracture or any dislocation, (2) any patient with incomplete paralysis or impending paralysis, whatever the X-ray findings. Use a halo or Gardner Wells tongs (5 to 7 kg), or a halter (3 to 4 kg), loosened periodically, to prevent the skin of his chin necrosing; a patient can only stand a halter for a few hours.

Lumbar and sacral spine Lie him in his most comfortable position.

THE INITIAL TREATMENT OF PARAPLEGIA AND QUADRIPLEGIA

If a patient is paraplegic, immediately start 2 hourly turning to prevent bed sores. They can start in the first few hours after the accident only too easily. Don't let his bladder fill up, start intermittent sterile catheterization, if you have the staff and committment to manage it (64.16).

If he is quadriplegic, also pass a nasogastric tube and remove his stomach contents, so as to prevent them being aspirated.

Transection of his cord interrupts his sympathetic pathways and causes immediate hypotension. His blood pressure will not return to normal for several days, so set up a drip meanwhile.

Watch for abdominal distension and absent bowel sounds

A NORMAL NECK

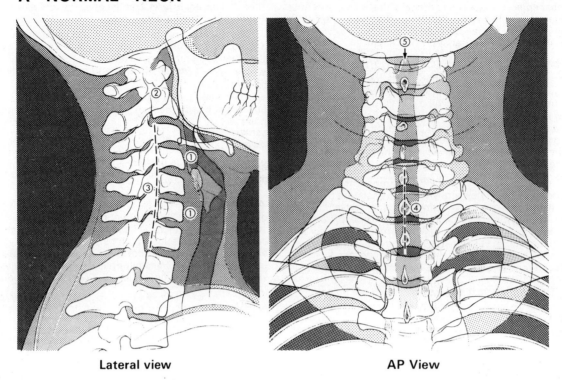

Lateral view   AP View

Fig. 64-7 A NORMAL CERVICAL SPINE. Note: (1) The normal soft tissue shadow in front of the patient's cervical vertebrae. (2) The relation of his odontoid process to the rest of C2. (3) The posterior margins of his vertebral bodies form a smooth curve. (4) His spinous processes are in line. (5) His normal odontoid. *Kindly contributed by John Stewart.*

caused by ileus. This is a common complication of a spinal cord injury and of a lumbar spine injury, even if there is no cord lesion. So give him only intravenous fluids, or sips of fluid by mouth, until you can hear persistalsis. On the fifth to seventh day he will need an enema, or manual removal of his faeces.

SHOULD YOU APPLY TRACTION YOURSELF, IF HE NEEDS IT, OR SHOULD YOU REFER HIM?

Transporting a patient with a spinal injury is never easy, even by air. If the roads are bad, the journey long, and the quality of care at the other end uncertain, he will probably be safer with you, especially in the earlier stages. If you decide to refer him (and you may be wise not to), start his initial care (see above) before he goes. Fit him with an efficient collar, and send a competent medical assistant or nurse with him, who must understand that his neck must be kept straight, and not flexed, extended, or rotated.

IF YOU SUSPECT A NECK INJURY, APPLY TRACTION OR FIT A TEMPORARY COLLAR IMMEDIATELY

64.4 Interpreting the X-rays

The important question in managing a patient's injured spine, and particularly his injured neck, is to decide if his injury is stable or not. One of the criteria for deciding this is his X-rays. Dislocations should always be considered unstable, so should bending or twisting injuries of the posterior elements of his spine. These include its pedicles, laminae, facets, and ligaments. *It is injuries to these posterior elements that make an injury unstable.* Compression injuries of a vertebral body are usually stable. In a flexion injury the posterior ligament is particularly liable to be ruptured, and in an extension injury, the anterior one. Both types of injury can damage the intervertebral discs.

The films should be good ones; those from a portable machine are usually useless. Even radiologists have difficulty interpreting X-rays of the spine, so you will probably have difficulty too.

The standard views in acute injuries are AP and lateral ones with the patient's head in its normal position. If these views are normal, take flexion and extension views *yourself* with the greatest care. They may show one vertebra moving abnormally on another when the standard films are normal. Finally, remember that a normal X-ray does not necessarily mean a normal spine.

IS A SPINAL INJURY UNSTABLE?

Take the patient to the X-ray room yourself. If possible X-ray him without moving him. If he has to be moved, supervise how this is done. An inexperienced X-ray assistant can make a partial cord lesion into a complete one.

Take one good AP view and two lateral views with the patient lying, one lateral view centred over his vertebral bodies at the site of maximal pain and tenderness, and another over his spinous processes at this level. Also take an open mouth view. You must see his whole cervical spine, so make sure his shoulders are well pulled down. Lesions at C6–C7 and C7–T1 are often missed. Don't try to take oblique views; they are difficult to take and interpret.

If possible, take a 'swimmers view'; this requires considerable experience and ability. Count the vertebrae in the lateral view to make sure that you have not missed C7. If necessary, take another view with traction to the patient's arm. You will see C7 and perhaps the upper border of T1.

As always with difficult films, sit down and look at them on a viewing box, or with an electric light bulb, while you have no other distractions. Start at the extreme edges of the film, and work in towards the middle. It is quite common for the injury to be at the edge of the film. Use the signs which follow and Fig. 64-8 as a check list.

AP VIEWS OF AN INJURED CERVICAL SPINE

In the following section the numbers in brackets refer to Fig. 64-8.

Are any vertebral bodies displaced (1)? If they are, the injury may be unstable.

Are any spinous processes out of line (2)? A rotational injury can twist them out of line, especially in the cervical

148

spine, even though the vertebral bodies themselves are still in line. If they are out of line, the injury is probably unstable.

Are the pedicles on either side of the spinal canal displaced laterally out of the line, compared with those above or below (3)? If they are, the injury is probably unstable. The vertebral arch forms a ring, so if part of the ring is to displace, it has to fracture in two places. Either both pedicles are displaced, or neither of them.

Are the transverse processes of the patient's lumbar vertebrae broken (4)? If they are, they make no difference to his spine, but suspect that his abdominal organs may be injured, especially his kidneys, and that he may have a retroperitoneal haemorrhage.

LATERAL VIEWS OF AN INJURED CERVICAL SPINE

Take a good lateral film at the level of the lesion. Examine the vertebral bodies from top to bottom, they should have a normal box–like appearance.

Is the body of a vertebra wedge shaped? (5) If so, the patient has a compression fracture. These fractures are usually stable, so, if there are no other signs which indicate instability, diagnose a stable injury confidently.

Has the body of a vertebra broken into many fragments (6)? If so, he has a burst fracture. This is more likely to be unstable and to have injured his spinal cord than a wedge fracture.

Has one vertebra slipped forwards on another (7)? This is a serious sign of instability, particularly in the cervical region. It usually shows that the posterior longitudinal ligament has ruptured, perhaps with dislocation of the articular facets, or with fractures of the laminae and pedicles. The patient's posterior intervertebral joints may have subluxed or dislocated on one or both sides.

If displacement is equal to half the vertebral body, one intervertebral joint has probably dislocated.

Do the posterior margins of all the vertebral bodies form a smooth curve? They should be smooth and continuous. Any abrupt change or step is a sign of subluxation and instability. Regard the odontoid as a vertebral body.

FRACTURES OF THE SPINE

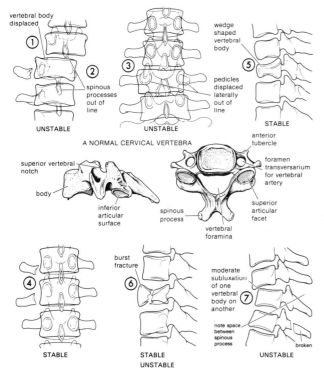

Fig. 64-8 FRACTURES OF THE SPINE. (1) Displacement of the vertebral bodies. (2) Spinous processes out of line. (3) Pedicles displaced. (4) Transverse processes broken off. (5) Wedge fracture. (6) Burst fracture. (7) Forward displacement of a vertebra. *Kindly contributed by John Stewart and James Cairns.*

Is the space between the vertebral spines unequal? They may be widely separated at the site of the injury. If so, the injury is probably unstable.

Have any of the spinous process broken at the base, so that they are lying free? Have any of the articular facets fractured? These are difficult to see, and both indicate instability.

If there is a sharp angulation with widening of the spinous processes, this suggests an unstable injury.

Does a facet on an upper vertebra lie in front of the facet of a lower one? If it does, the facets are locked. Unilateral locked facets are difficult to be certain about, they are easier when they are bilateral. They are very rare indeed outside the cervical region. Locked facets, especially if they are bilateral, are not necessarily unstable.

Are the articular facets displaced? The first two facets in the cervical region are easily seen, but the third needs a very good X-ray.

Special signs in the lateral view in the cervical region. Examine the gap between the back of the patient's pharynx and the front of his vertebral bodies. Soft tissue swelling here suggests that he may have a spinal injury, probably an unstable one. Study every lateral view of the cervical spine you see carefully, so that you know what the normal soft tissue shadow looks like.

Look carefully at the base of the patient's odontoid, and at the arch of his atlas.

OTHER FINDINGS
Fractures of the spinous and transverse processes are unimportant—they are essentially muscle injuries.

LATERAL VIEWS IN FLEXION AND EXTENSION

INDICATIONS These views are only indicated if you suspect a high fracture of a patient's neck, and the standard AP and lateral views, and an AP view through his mouth are normal. Some surgeons consider these much too difficult for most of our readers.

CAUTION ! (1) The manoeuvres necessary to take these views may be dangerous in acute lesions. (2) The patient must be conscious. (3) Always be present yourself when these views are taken, do them gently, and stop immediately if he has arm or leg symptoms.

Carefully flex his neck and take a film, then carefully extend his neck and take another one. Look for abnormal movement of one vertebra on another. In a flexion view look for the vertebral bodies slipping forwards over one another. In an extension view look for an abnormal gap between the front of two vertebral bodies, or for a posterior dislocation.

ATLAS AND AXIS See Section 64.8.

DIAGNOSTIC DIFFICULTIES WITH INJURIES OF THE CERVICAL SPINE

If you SUSPECT AN INJURY CLINICALLY BUT CANNOT SEE ONE IN THE FILMS, take more films higher up the spine. This is especially important if there are signs that the cord has been injured.

A NORMAL X-RAY DOES NOT NECESSARILY MEAN A STABLE SPINE

64.5 Managing injuries of the cervical spine

If a patient has injured his spine, the important factor in caring for him is whether his injury is stable or not. The diagnosis of stability is partly clinical and partly radiological, and is critically important in his neck. *An injury of any part of the spine is unstable if any of the following conditions hold:*

(1) The patient has any neurological signs (the only exception is an acute extension injury of his neck, as in Section 64.9.)

(2) He has any signs of instability on clinical examination. These are: (a) some break in the continuous line of spinous processes from his neck to his sacrum, or (b) any soft doughy areas between his spinous processes into which your finger can sink.

Such an area shows that the ligaments between the spines of his vertebrae have been ruptured, and that his spine is unstable at this point.

(3) He has X-ray signs of instability, in normal or flexion and extension views. Don't be misled by a normal X-ray, because his bones may have moved out of place at the time of the injury, and now be back in place again. *So, if a routine X-ray is normal, he can still have an unstable spine.* You may need flexion and extension views to show instability.

If a patient has had no neurological signs at any time, no clinical signs of instability, and his X-rays are normal, treatment depends on his pain and stiffness. If this is mild, persuade him to ignore his injury and move his neck. If pain and stiffness are severe, put him to bed. If you cannot X-ray him or interpret his films, be safe and fit him with a collar.

If he has a stable injury radiologically and no neurological signs, fit a collar. Stable injuries are: (1) all anterior wedge fractures, (2) minor burst fractures (major ones are unstable), (3) fractures in which there is an anterior gap between two vertebral bodies in an extension film.

If he has an unstable injury and no neurological signs, put him in cuirasse. Traction is a preferable alternative, but if you are not expert and nursing care is less than perfect, he may be safer in a cuirasse. These injuries include all dislocations. These are rare precious patients.

If a patient has or has had neurological signs, his injury must be unstable, even if his X-ray looks normal. Treatment depends on their severity. If his neurological signs have now gone, give him a cuirasse, or better, apply traction. If his quadriplegia is only partial, apply traction. If his quadriplegia is complete, apply traction for a week. If it shows no sign of improving in a week, there is no point in continuing it, because it will hinder nursing care. Complete or partial recovery is more likely to occur with cervical than with thoraco–lumbar injuries.

If you are in doubt as to what to do, treat the injury as if it is unstable. Overtreat an injury of the cervical spine rather than undertreat it. This is the reverse of the advice for the lumbar spine. For example, if a patient has a painful neck after an injury, and you are not sure what to do, fit a collar. If you think traction might help, apply it.

PARTICULAR CERVICAL SPINE INJURIES **Wedge fractures** Ignore these, but fit the patient with a collar for comfort.

Burst fractures If he has no neurological signs, apply traction for 6 weeks, followed by a collar for 12 weeks.

Extension injuries don't usually cause fractures, but they may injure the anterior longitudinal ligament. Fit a collar for 2 to 3 months.

If he has a collar and if there are no other reasons for keeping him in bed, encourage him to get up.

IF IN DOUBT, OVERTREAT AN INJURED NECK

64.6 Collars and traction tongs

If an ambulant patient has an unstable or doubtfully stable fracture, there are several ways you can prevent the sudden sharp movements his neck that might injure his cord. In order of decreasing convenience but increasing security they are: (1) A home made collar. (2) A proper orthopaedic collar. (3) A plaster cuirasse, as in Fig. 64-10. (4) A Minerva cast.

A Minerva cast extends to a patient's iliac crests, and is sometimes advised, but it uses more plaster than a cuirasse and it is more difficult to apply. It is also very uncomfortable, especially in a hot climate, and it is totally contraindicated if he has any sensory defect, because it will cause ulcers. The marginally greater security of a Minerva cast is outweighed by all these disadvantages, so it is not described further here.

You can apply traction with: (1) Gardner Wells tongs, (2) Hoen's traction, (3) a halo, or (4) a halter. If you don't have

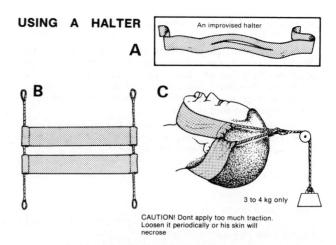

USING A HALTER

A

An improvised halter

B **C**

3 to 4 kg only

CAUTION! Dont apply too much traction. Loosen it periodically or his skin will necrose

Fig. 64-9 USING A HALTER. This is suitable for temporary traction only (less than 24 hours). Loosen it periodically and don't apply too much weight.

tongs you can make a halo locally. A halter like that in Fig. 64-9 is useful *for temporary traction only*. It does not apply enough traction to reduce a dislocation, and it becomes very uncomfortable after a few hours. If you apply too much traction with a halter for too long, it can cause pressure sores. Use a halter to reduce muscle spasm until you can apply cervical traction or a cuirasse. You are unlikely to have a turning frame for paraplegic patients. The next best is a foam mattress.

• *COLLAR orthopaedic, Zimmer pattern, two only of each of the three standard sizes.* These are not expensive and should be standard equipment.

APPLIANCES FOR NECK INJURIES

A COLLAR MADE WITH TOWELS Fold a bath towel lengthwise so that it is 10 cm wide. Wrap it round the patient's neck, and pin its loose ends together, as in C, Fig. 64-5. If necessary, strengthen it with a few a turns of plaster.

A CARDBOARD COLLAR Take a length of stiff cardboard, cut two curves in it as in Fig. 64-10, wind it round the patient's neck, cut it to fit, damp it where necessary to mould it to shape, pad it appropriately, and keep it together with adhesive strapping. If necessary, strengthen it with a few plaster bandages. It will work, but it will not be beautiful.

Or, take the top of a plastic bucket, if you can spare one, and cut it to shape to make a plastic collar.

A CUIRASSE Use this for: (1) Stable fractures without neurological signs. (2) Unstable fractures after a period in traction. Some surgeons use a collar for both these indications. (3) Unstable fractures if you do not feel competent to apply traction.

Apply a layer of stockinette and pad the bony points over the patient's lower jaw, occiput, and clavicle. Apply a broad slab down the front of his neck from his chin to his upper sternum, and another down the back of his neck. Bind these slabs in place with circular plaster bandages. Let the cuirasse set with his chin up as in Fig. 64-10. Finally trim it to shape, turn over the edges of the stockinette and bind them in place.

A HALTER Use this for temporary traction only. Don't apply a halter for longer than 24 hours. Make one from canvas and cord, as in Fig. 64-9. Don't apply more than 4.5 kg, and remove it at least every 4 to 6 hours to rest his skin.

A LOCALLY MADE HALO Any good machine shop can make this from 15×4 mm mild steel strip. Draw some 20 mm squares on paper, and copy the pattern in Fig. 64-12 onto them. Give this to the mechanic. The halo will fit any head except a very small one. The space between the head and the halo is not critical, provided the halo is not actually pressing on the patient's skull. The type of hollow point shown will not penetrate the inner table. If the mechanic cannot turn a hollow point, a conical one will do. If he has no stainless steel rod

A COLLAR AND A PLASTER CUIRASSE

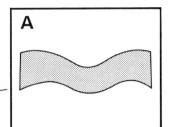

piece of cardboard cut this shape to fit round his neck, pad it well

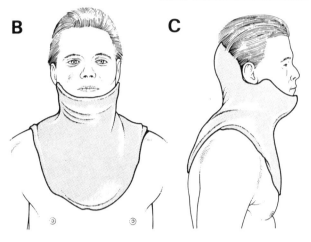

Fig. 64-10 A CARDBOARD COLLAR AND A PLASTER CUIRASSE. A, shows how you can make a cardboard collar by cutting a strip of card with two curves. B, a cuirasse is more comfortable than a Minerva cast. *Kindly contributed by John Stewart.*

to make the 6×50 mm screws, give him two Steinmann pins. Or, he can use mild steel screws and inset a small piece of stainless steel into the tips.

IF A PATIENT'S CERVICAL SPINE MIGHT BE INJURED, FIT A TEMPORARY CERVICAL COLLAR IMMEDIATELY

64.7 Skeletal traction

This is the best treatment for an unstable fracture of a patient's cervical spine. Surgeons differ in the method they like. Some like Hoen's traction, in which wires are passed through burr holes, while others prefer Gardner Wells tongs or a halo. The trouble with a halo is that it is difficult to align and may slip off, which is why Hoen's traction is gaining in popularity. This allows a patient to move his head freely, and you can leave it in position for months if necessary. It takes slightly longer than applying tongs, but is much more reliable. You will have to learn to make burr holes for head injuries anyway (63.4), so this is an additional use for them.

Traction is the surest way of stabilizing an unstable fracture or fracture dislocation, or occasionally of releasing locked facets. Be prepared to apply it yourself because: (1) patients with injured cervical spines travel badly, especially over bumpy roads, (2) the equipment is simple, (3) it may be the only way to prevent severe disability, (4) it can be used effectively. But it is not easy to apply and it requires expert nursing, so the indications we give for it differ from those of the experts. They always apply traction if a patient has a normal cord, because it is the best way of preserving it. But, if you are not expert and your nursing is less than perfect, a patient *may* be safer in a cuirasse. There is little point in anyone applying cervical traction if a patient is already quadriplegic.

If a patient has a fracture dislocation, traction will draw the fragments of his spine apart, restore the diameter of his cervical

canal, and reduce the danger of pressure on his cord. When you apply traction, aim to draw the fragments apart with steadily increasing traction over a few hours, then maintain traction with a smaller weight for several weeks. Finally, protect the patient's neck with a cast or collar, so that his spine can heal and become stable in about 8 weeks. To be on the safe side it is desirable to protect it for 6 months.

If a patient has bilateral locked facets of his cervical spine (rare), they are usually associated with complete permanent quadriplegia. If so, traction is pointless. In the unlikely event that he has no neurological lesion, immobilization in a cuirasse or an efficient collar is a possible alternative to trying to unlock them, which is difficult.

When you apply traction to a fracture dislocation, apply only just enough weight to reduce it. If you apply too much too suddenly, you may increase the patient's soft tissue injury, and harm his cord. Adjust the traction to his build and don't exceed what is advised below.

SKELETAL TRACTION FOR THE CERVICAL SPINE

INDICATIONS (1) Unstable fractures or fracture dislocations of a patient's cervical spine, with partial quadriplegia, or early (within a few days) complete quadriplegia, in whom there is still some hope of improvement. (3) Rupture of the posterior ligaments. (4) As a temporary splint for cervical fractures while a patient is being treated for his other injuries.

In more expert hands the most important indication for traction is an unstable fracture with no neurological signs. If you are less expert, he *may* be safer in a cuirasse.

CONTRAINDICATIONS (1) Complete permanent quadriplegia in which traction is almost pointless. (2) Unstable fractures in which there have been neurological signs, but in which

CERVICAL TRACTION WITH GARDNER WELLS TONGS

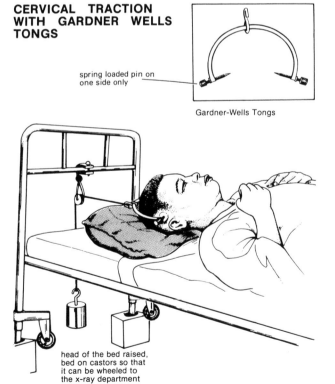

spring loaded pin on one side only

Gardner-Wells Tongs

head of the bed raised, bed on castors so that it can be wheeled to the x-ray department

Fig. 64-11 CERVICAL TRACTION WITH GARDNER WELLS TONGS. When you apply traction to a fracture dislocation, apply only just enough weight to reduce it. If you apply too much too suddenly, you may increase the patient's soft tissue injury, and harm his cord. *Adapted from de Palma with kind permission.*

these have now gone (fit a cuirasse). (3) Stable fractures in which traction is unnecessary (fit a collar). (4) Signs of instability which are only present in flexion and extension views (fit a cuirasse). (5) Locked facets, unilateral or bilateral, with or without neurological signs. Experts would apply traction. If you cannot refer the patient, fit a cuirasse.

CAUTION ! You must be able to take bedside X-rays. If you cannot do this, don't try to apply traction—fit him with a collar or cuirasse.

HALTER Fit the patient with a halter temporarily while you are organizing the traction device.

THE BED Apply traction on a bed with fracture boards (or a door) covered with at least 10 cm of foam rubber, and large castors. You should be able to adjust the height of the pulley vertically.

NURSING Turn the patient 2 hourly—left side, supine, right side. Alternate periods in which he is turned completely left and right with periods in which he is turned partly left and right. Take great care to move his head 'in one piece' with the rest of his body. You will need 3 nurses while you do this, with one to look after his head and neck. At 6 weeks, when traction is replaced with a cervical collar, add the prone position when he is turned. Rub his pressure areas 2 hourly.

X-RAYS Either apply traction in the X-ray department, or wheel him there in traction for films to be taken.

SEDATION Give the patient diazepam with pethidine. Don't give him a general anaesthetic. Intubating him may be difficult and dangerous.

CAUTION ! (1) Monitor his neurological state carefully. If you apply too much traction too suddenly, you may injure his spinal cord or his medulla. (2) Never apply more traction than the maximum indicated. (3) If at any time there are signs that his neurological state is getting worse, reduce traction immediately. (4) If you are in doubt as to what to do, be safe and reduce the traction or take it down.

GARDNER WELLS TONGS FOR CERVICAL TRACTION

These grip a patient's skull a finger's breadth above his ears in the line of his mastoid processes. Fit them in the ward. Apply them symmetrically without shaving his scalp. The pins should enter his skull just caudal to its maximum diameter, so that they don't slip. Sterilize the points. Dab iodine on the place where you want them to go, raise a wheal of lignocaine and anaesthetize his scalp right down to his periosteum. Apply iodine to the points of the screws.

One screw is spring loaded, so that as the tension is increased a small nipple protrudes. When it protrudes about 1 mm the tension is correct. Twist the screws so that their points go through his anaesthetized skin, and grip the outer table of his skull. Tighten them until the small nipple in one of the screws protrudes 1 mm from its hole, then tighten the lock nut.

A HALO FOR CERVICAL TRACTION

Fit this in the ward. Support the patient's head off the bed, try the halo for fit, and decide which screw holes to use. Shaving the skin in the areas where the pins will go is optional. Anaesthetize his skin, and apply the halo in the same way as for Gardner Wells tongs. Tighten the screws alternately, so that the halo is not pulled to one side. Tighten them as securely as you can, using only your thumb and three fingers on the screwdriver: more force is dangerous. After tightening, secure each pin with lock nuts on either side of the halo.

Thread cords through four of its unused holes, bring the cords together into two slings, and tie the main traction cord to them. Adjust them to determine the flexion and extension of his head.

CAUTION ! With both forms of traction device: (1) Make sure the points of the screws are needle sharp. (2) Try to keep them still, because this will minimize the risk of infection. (3) Tighten up the screws several times during the first 24 hours, then don't tighten them any more. Don't tighten them unnecessarily, or they may perforate his inner table. (4) If the traction sites become infected, move the pins on the halo.

HOEN'S SKULL TRACTION

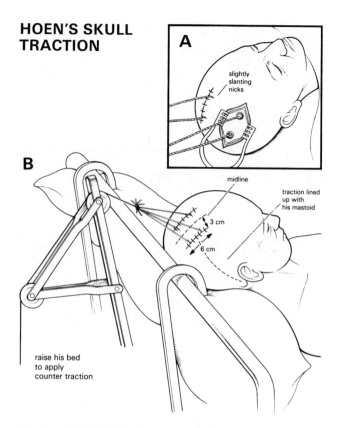

Fig. 64.11a HOEN'S TRACTION. Wires are passed through burr holes. Traction is easier to align by this method than with a halo, and cannot slip off; a patient can move his head freely, and you can leave him in traction for months if necessary. *Kindly contributed by Laurence Levy*

HOEN'S TRACTION FOR CERVICAL TRACTION

ANAESTHESIA (1) If anaesthetic skills are good, consider general anaesthesia with intubation, taking due care of the patient's spine. (2) Or, use local anaesthesia, with intravenous diazepam if he is restless.

METHOD Make two linear 5 cm incisions in the parasagittal plane centred on the patient's mastoid processes and 3 to 4 cm from the midline. Place these so as to straddle the desired line of pull, which is usually in line with his cervical spine.

Reflect the skin and make two burr holes (63.4) 3 cm apart, with a 2 cm bridge of bone between them.

Loop a pice of stainless steel wire into 4 or more strands, depending on its strength. Pass the blunt looped ends from one burr hole to another. You may need the help of the guide of a Gigli saw, or the the blunt end of a long slightly curved needle, with the wire in its eye.

CAUTION ! (1) Position the incisions and the burr holes away from the mid line, so as to avoid the patient's sagittal sinus. (2) Separate his dura very carefully, because infection may follow if you pierce it.

Pull the wires through until they are equal in length. When you have done the same thing on the other side, tension all four wires together to provide equal tension on all four.

Close the incisions. As you do so, make four slightly slanting nicks to prevent the medially slanting wires from pressing on the skin edges, where they would be uncomfortable, cause necrosis, and so promote infection. The wound will soon heal and a dressing is rarely needed.

Connect the wires to a rope passing over a pulley, apply a weight, and raise the patient's bed to apply counter traction.

APPLYING TRACTION FOR CERVICAL SPINE INJURIES

HOW MUCH TRACTION? This depends on: (1) The type of traction. With a halter 4 to 5 kg is the maximum, but with skeletal traction you will need 5 to 15 kg. (2) The build of the

A LOCALLY MADE HALO

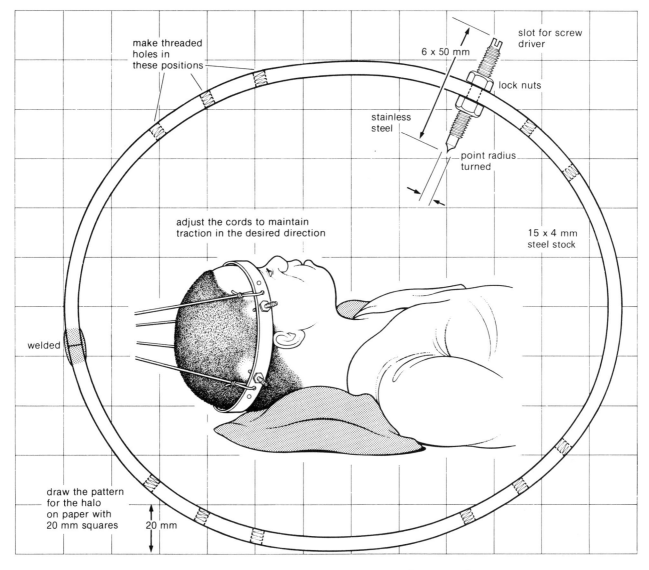

make threaded holes in these positions

slot for screw driver

6 x 50 mm

lock nuts

stainless steel

point radius turned

adjust the cords to maintain traction in the desired direction

15 x 4 mm steel stock

welded

draw the pattern for the halo on paper with 20 mm squares

20 mm

Fig. 64-12 A LOCALLY MADE HALO. A garage mechanic can make this if you give him some stainless steel Steinmann pins. *Kindly contributed by Alan Workman*

patient; large men need more than small women. (3) What you are trying to do. To begin with you may need 15 kg to reduce a dislocation. Later, you may only need 3 to 5 kg to maintain traction. (4) The position of the injury. Higher up the spine less traction is required (2 to 5 kg), than with the common C5 C6 injuries (5 to 15 kg).

Here is a rough guide, C1 2.5 to 5 kg, C2 3 to 5 kg, C3 4 to 7 kg, C4 5 to 10 kg, C5 and 6, 7 to 15 kg. Apply the weights over a pulley. Raise the head of the bed about 4 cm for each kilo, as for a fracture of the femur.

TRACTION FOR A FRACTURE DISLOCATION

The weights which follow apply to a large adult with a hyperflexion injury in his C4-C6 region, as A, Fig. 64-13. With other injuries adjust the weight appropriately. His X-ray may show: (1) a flattening, reversal, or distortion of the normal spinal curve, (2) displacement of the body of a vertebra forwards on the one below, (3) a compression fracture, (4) fracture of the pedicles.

Apply traction in a straight line, avoid flexion, extension or, rotation and start with 7 kg. Cautiously add 2 kg every 15 minutes, checking constantly for neurological changes.

When you have applied 15 kg for 30 minutes, x-ray him. The facets may begin to disengage (B), but you may have to wait longer.

If there is no disengagement, leave him with 15 kg traction for a maximum of 12 to 48 hours, taking X-rays every 6 to 12 hours.

As soon as: (1) the articular processes are completely disengaged, (2) overriding is corrected, and (3) the distance between the fragments of the pedicles is narrowed, reduce the weights and keep the patient's neck in a straight line. Usually, the facets will come into line.

At 2 to 3 weeks you can reduce traction to 3 to 5 kg. Take weekly lateral check X-rays for the first month, or after you have altered the weights.

At 6 weeks replace traction by a cuirasse or a collar (64.6). Leave this on for another 6 weeks. If immobilization is going to stabilise his spine, 3 months will do it.

At 3 months remove his cuirasse or collar. Take AP and lateral X-rays. If these still show reduction, take flexion and extension views.

If the patient's vertebrae show no signs of slipping in normal or in flexion or extension views, advise him to increase the movements of his neck gradually, to avoid sudden movements, and to restrict his outdoor activities.

If he still has a painful unstable neck after 3 months, (6 weeks in traction followed by 6 weeks in a collar or cuirasse), refer him. This is rare. Fusion of his cervical spine may be indicated. If you cannot refer him, fit him with a collar.

If his injury is mainly bony, the fragments will probably fuse and his injury will become stable.

If his injury mainly involves the ligaments, stable union may not be achieved. He should be watchful for up to a year in case late displacement occurs.

DIFFICULTIES WITH CERVICAL TRACTION

If you have MADE THE DIAGNOSIS LATE, the patient's fracture may or may not be stable. Fit him with a collar for 3 months. If this does not relieve his symptoms in 2 weeks, apply traction for 2 weeks and then replace his collar.

If a patient with a recent cervical injury has OTHER SERIOUS INJURIES which make cervical traction impossible, fit him with a cervical collar.

If a FRACTURE REDISPLACES, immediately traction is reduced, or later, or if a dislocation of the articular facets recurs as traction is reduced, reapply it, especially if nerve root symptoms recur. You may need more weight (up to 17 kg). The danger of quadriplegia is great, so refer him if you can.

FOLLOW UP THE PATIENT CAREFULLY

64.8 Fractures of the atlas and axis

Some injuries of of the first two cervical vertebrae are instantly fatal. If a patient survives he complains of a stiff painful neck

REDUCING A FRACTURE DISLOCATION

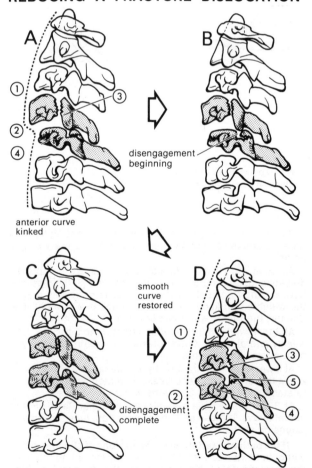

Fig. 64-13 REDUCING A FRACTURE DISLOCATION. A, before applying traction. B, disengagement beginning. C, disengagement complete. D, the smooth anterior curvature of the patient's spine restored. Unfortunately, reduction is rarely as easy as it looks here, and often fails. *After de Palma with kind permission*

following an injury, often a head injury. He supports his head in his hands and has difficulty turning it. Although he may have no neurological symptoms, if he jerks his neck suddenly, he is in danger of serious paralysis. He may have fractured his atlas, or the odontoid process of his axis.

The atlas is seldom injured, except by downward blows on the skull, or in severe hyperextension. No treatment is required except immobilization in a soft collar and bed rest for comfort.

The odontoid process of the axis is its most vulnerable part, and is usually injured by a direct blow to the front of the patient's skull, which extends it sharply. So look for a fractured odontoid if a patient has had a severe hyperextension injury after a fall, or a car accident. As his skull moves backwards, it carries his atlas and his odontoid process backwards also. Either his odontoid process fractures, or, more seriously, the transverse ligament that retains it tears and allows his odontoid to press on his cord and kill him instantly. If he survives, his injury is probably stable enough to be treated in a cuirasse until there is bony or firm fibrous union.

The X-rays of most fractures of the upper cervical region are difficult to interpret. You should, however, be able to recognize a fracture of the odontoid. If you are in doubt, fit a patient with a collar, or preferably a cuirasse.

FRACTURES OF THE ATLAS AND AXIS

X-RAYS You need special views. If the films are bad, try again. You cannot make the diagnosis from poor films.

An AP view Take this through the patient's open mouth to avoid his teeth. Place a cork or a card between his teeth to hold them open while you do so. Place his head in moderate extension, so that the edge of his upper teeth falls in line with the base of his skull as it joins his cervical vertebrae. You will need an exact AP view, so that his palate does not obscure his atlas and axis.

Look for a fracture of his odontoid, especially a step at its base. The odontoid ossifies from a separate centre, so in a young person don't interpret the normal growth line as a fracture. This growth line sometimes persists into adult life.

If the lateral masses of the patient's atlas have spread significantly, he has a burst fracture, which has torn the transverse ligament.

Lateral view Focus the tube on the lobe of his ear which overlies his odontoid. A visible prominence of the soft tissues at the back of the pharynx suggest an injury to his cervical spine.

If you cannot refer a patient, treat him as follows.

FRACTURES OF THE ODONTOID PROCESS OF THE AXIS
The patient survived the original injury, so his chances of final recovery are good. Take a good AP view through his mouth and lateral views; diagnosis may be difficult.

If there is a neurological defect, use traction as for other fractures and dislocations of the cervial spine.

If there is no neurological defect, traction is best. It gives better stability and prevents backward displacement and angulation. An efficient collar or cuirasse for 12 weeks is a possible alternative, but is less reliable.

BURST FRACTURES OF THE RING OF THE ATLAS The ring bursts at its weakest point where its posterior and lateral masses join. The X-rays are particularly difficult to interpret. If you cannot refer the patient, fit him with a collar.

IF AN INJURED PATIENT IS SITTING UP HOLDING HIS NECK, FIT HIM WITH A COLLAR

64.9 Cervical hyperextension injury ('porter's neck')

This is a common spinal injury in places where people carry large loads on their heads. Fortunately, the cord is not often

154

FRACTURES OF THE ATLAS AND AXIS

a force applied to the top
of the patient's skull
compresses his atlas

atlas splayed out by
a compression force

transverse
odontoid
ligament

A

B

BACKWARD DISPLACEMENT
OF THE ODONTOID

FORWARD DISPLACEMENT
OF THE ODONTOID

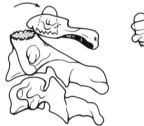 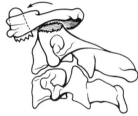

**Fig. 64-14 FRACTURES OF ATLAS AND AXIS. If a patient complains
of a stiff neck after an injury, he may have one of these fractures.** *Adapted
from de Palma with kind permission.*

injured, and even if it is, there is some hope of recovery. The
patient, who is usually a woman, stumbles and falls. The heavy
load she is carrying falls backwards and extends or rotates her
head violently. In hospital she is found to have a quadriparesis.
X-rays may show no fracture. If she has narrowing of her cervical discs and osteoarthritic overgrowth, they are probably not
responsible for her symptoms which are due to a sudden infolding
of her ligamentum flavum pressing on her cord. The prognosis
with this kind of paraplegia is usually good. Fit her with a soft
collar, and care for her quadriparesis until she recovers.

64.10 Torticollis at birth

This is the end result of the birth injury known as 'Sternomastoid
tumour'. Make every effort to try to turn the child's head the
opposite way to his deformity. For example, if his head turns
to the right, have him nursed on the left. If the condition lasts
more than 2 months, refer him for possible lengthening of his
sternomastoid. This is an operation for the expert, because part
of the sternomastoid is inserted behind the clavicle and is very
close to the great vessels.

64.11 Torticollis in older children

A child's head may turn to one side, or slip forwards onto his
chest, due to the softening of his transverse ligament, which
normally holds his atlas to his odontoid (this ligament is shown
in B, Fig. 64-14). Torticollis can follow a variety of neck or throat
infections, such as peritonsillar abscesses, or it can follow an
injury. Measure the distance between the child's odontoid peg
and the back of the anterior arch of his axis. If this is more than

FORMS OF NECK INJURY

**ACUTE
TORTICOLLIS**

**CERVICAL HYPEREXTENSION
INJURY**

the child's head is
locked in this position

X-ray probably
normal

quadriparesis

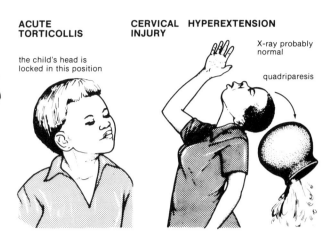

**Fig. 64-15 TWO COMPARATIVELY BENIGN FORMS OF INJURY
TO THE CERVICAL SPINE. A, acute torticollis in older children. B,
spinal hyperextension injury in people who carry loads on their heads.**
Kindly contributed by John Stewart.

3 mm in adults or 4.5 mm in children, his transverse ligament
has been stretched and the ring of his atlas has slipped forward.
Atlanto–axial subluxation is serious, because paraplegia may
follow, and because of the torticollis which may last weeks, or
occasionally permanently, if you don't treat it. The differential
diagnosis includes tuberculosis, but here collapse is much more
usual than subluxation.

ATLANTO–AXIAL SUBLUXATION Exclude tuberculosis. If
necessary, treat the child's respiratory infection.
    Treat him in gentle halter traction for 2 weeks, and then
apply a soft collar, with his head turned slightly in the corrected position. Maintain this position by wrapping a few turns
of plaster round the collar. Many patients will recover with
this treatment, but not all of them.

64.12 Fractures of the thoracic and lumbar
spine

The spinal cord ends at L1. A patient with a fracture at or above
this level is usually either grossly injured and paraplegic, or has
a stable fracture. Below this level he can have an unstable fracture and a normal cauda equina. If a patient has no cord injury,
you can easily miss these fractures, especially if he has severe
injuries elsewhere, or is unconscious. His spine can be injured
by a force which compresses or flexes it, usually at T7–T8, the
apex of his thoracic kyposis, at T12–L1, the thoraco–lumbar
junction, or at L4–L5. The result can be a wedge fracture, a
burst fracture, or a fracture dislocation.
    *If a patient has a fracture, especially a wedge fracture, after only
a minor injury,* suspect that it may be pathological, and the result
of a secondary tumour or osteoporosis. If all you can see is a
widened disc space, count his spinous processes, and see if they
match his vertebral bodies. The widened disc space may be all
that remains of a vertebral body.
    If his fracture is stable by the criteria (1), (2), and (3) in Section
64.5, the active movements regime described below will give
better results than a plaster cast and be cheaper.
    If his fracture is unstable his accompanying paraplegia dominates
his management. Fixation with interspinous plates is not
established as better than conservative management which almost
always leads to stable union in 6 to 10 weeks. The position in
which the fracture unites is unimportant. He will probably be
no better off in a referral hospital than in your hands.

FRACTURES OF THE THORACIC AND LUMBAR SPINE

Assess whether the patient's fracture is stable or not by the criteria already described (64.5). If you are in doubt, treat his injury as unstable.

STABLE FRACTURES Treat wedge fractures, minor burst fractures, and laminar fractures in the same way. Treat the patient in bed with fracture boards under a 10 cm foam rubber mattress. Put a pillow between his legs and a pillow under his back when he is lying on his side.

Keep him in bed until he can arch his back sufficiently for you to be able to put your hand underneath it, and until he is sufficiently pain–free to walk, if necessary, with crutches. He can get up when pain allows him to, usually in about 3 weeks.

UNSTABLE FRACTURES are usually fractures of the posterior elements with subluxation.

If the patient is not paraplegic, keep him in bed. Turn him 2 hourly in one piece, using at least 3 people. Use his right and left sides, the supine, the lateral, and the prone positions. At about 3 weeks he can start to turn himself using a balkan beam and a handle.

When pain at rest has gone and light bouncing with a clenched fist causes little pain, usually at 6 to 10 weeks, mobilize him, at first with someone either side of him, and then using crutches.

If he is paraplegic, concentrate on his morale, his skin, his bladder, and his bowels, rather than on his fracture. Turn him 2 hourly and care for his skin as in Section 64.15.

When you turn him, put blocks of foam rubber underneath him, so as to minimize displacement of his spine. For example, put a block under the fracture when he lies on his back. This will encourage moderate extension and reduce the tendency of his spine to collapse. Change and adjust these blocks each time you turn him.

If you cannot get foam rubber blocks, or if adjusting them each time you turn him takes too long, forget about them and nurse him on a thick rubber mattress.

After 6 to 8 weeks in bed, when his spine is no longer painful or tender, mobilize him as effectively as his paraplegia will permit.

CAUTION ! Never apply a cast if he is paraplegic. It will rapidly cause ulcers in his anaesthetic skin.

IF IN DOUBT, UNDERTREAT A FRACTURED LUMBAR OR THORACIC SPINE

64.13 Paraplegia

The arrival of a paraplegic patient is bad news in a district hospital because it means that a bed will be filled for a very long time. Can he be saved from bedsores, contractures, a small contracted bladder, and all the other miseries that are only too common? The answer most certainly is yes! There are some very simply equipped hospitals, with very dedicated workers, who can turn their patients every 2 hours, so that they do not get bedsores. So it can be done and it has been done! It is, however, so demanding that the care of paraplegia is perhaps the ultimate test of the real quality of a hospital, and of the morale and dedication of everyone in it. In paraplegia your aim must be—(1) no bedsores, (2) no contractures, (3) an uninfected bladder, with the early onset of reflex micturition in upper motor neurone lesions, and (4) the patient's ability to support himself with a craft. Ultimately, most paraplegics die from the uraemia that follows chronic urinary infection, but they may live many years.

The consequences of not managing paraplegia properly can be even worse than the patient shown in Fig. 64-16. Thus one patient was seen who had been admitted in quadriparesis (not quadriplegia) one year earlier in fairly good shape. In hospital

HOW A PARAPLEGIC SHOULD NOT BE TREATED

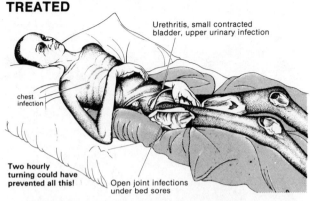

Urethritis, small contracted
bladder, upper urinary infection

chest
infection

Two hourly
turning could have
prevented all this!

Open joint infections
under bed sores

Fig. 64-16 HOW PARAPLEGICS SHOULD NOT BE TREATED. They can be saved from bedsores, contractures, and small contracted bladders, even in simply equipped hospitals, if their staff are sufficiently dedicated and can turn their patients every 2 hours. This is, however, so demanding that it is the ultimate test of the real quality of a hospital. *Kindly contributed by Peter Bewes—not one of his patients!*

he developed pressure sores over his sacrum, both hips, both knees, and both ankles. The joints under all these lesions were open and suppurating. He had more sores on his back and forearms, and flexion contractures of both his hips and knees. He had a urinary infection, a small contracted bladder, an indwelling catheter, and chronic urethritis. Mercifully he soon died.

Although quadriplegics should never reach this state, their outlook is much worse than for paraplegia, and is always hopeless in the end. However devoted your care, they will almost certainly develop severe pressure sores, hypostatic pneumonia, and die. Although you may be tempted to reproach yourself, you should not try to set yourself impossible targets. Paraplegics, on the other hand, are very well worth fighting for.

The key to success is to prepare your staff psychologically. Make the first patient you care for your top priority, and that of your ward team. The most critical days are the first ones, especially the first and second weeks of admission. The whole battle may be lost by careless treatment then. Leaving a patient unturned for only four hours may start a bed sore that leads to osteomyelitis, dislocation of a hip, contractures, and a series of surgical operations lasting years. Should he get a bed sore, you may be unable to refer him because no hospital will accept him.

THE FIRST 24 HOURS ARE CRITICAL

64.14 A paraplegic's morale

A severe spinal injury is so horrible that doctors and nurses are often too embarrassed to discuss it with the patient. Nevertheless, he is usually completely conscious and aware, and needs to be treated as a human being. He needs reassuring that his condition has been diagnosed, and is being urgently and carefully treated. He needs to be told that he has a serious injury, and that the people who care for him understand he is paralysed. If he asks whether his injury is going to be permanent, don't be too dogmatic too early.

During the entire course of treatment, keep his morale uppermost in your mind. Don't just pass by the foot of his bed saying."Ah, yes, the paraplegic. . .", and then pass on. Talk to him often. Manage him always with encouragement and hope, not necessarily hope that his cord will eventually recover, but hope that he will one day rejoin society, and find there a place for himself. His relatives need encouragement too. It is tragic for him when they stop coming, so make sure that someone explains your plans for him to them. Meanwhile, make his life as comfortable as possible. If he can read, make sure he has a reading board and something to read. If he ever stops eating from the effects of misery and chronic infection, his death is near. So make sure he is adequately fed, and watch for anaemia.

NEVER PASS BY WITHOUT SAYING SOMETHING TO THE PARAPLEGIC

64.15 A paraplegic's skin

Bedsores occur in sensory paraplegia and occasionally in any very sick or very old patient who is left in the same position too long without being moved. You can prevent them completely, even in complete paraplegia and quadriplegia, *but, only provided you turn a patient every 2 hours day and night.*

The cause of bedsores is clear. The pressure of the body on any part of the skin and subcutaneous tissue causes temporary ischaemia. In a normal person this causes mild discomfort, so that he turns about every 15 minutes to let another part of his anatomy bear his weight. Because a paraplegic patient cannot feel discomfort, or move, he cannot vary the skin on which he lies, so it remains ischaemic for hours at a time, it becomes necrotic, breaks down, and causes a bedsore. If only you can interrupt this period of ischaemia, you can prevent a sore forming. Explain the pathology of bedsores carefully to all your nurses, and to everybody who looks after paraplegic patients. Later, explain it to the patient too, so that he can play his part in preven-

MAKE A PARAPLEGIC'S LIFE COMFORTABLE

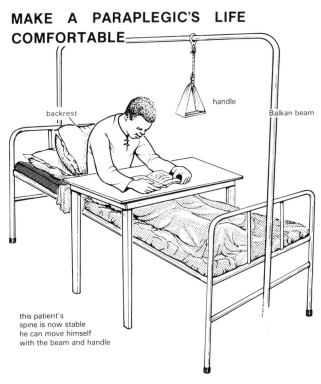

backrest
handle
Balkan beam

this patient's spine is now stable he can move himself with the beam and handle

Fig. 64-17 MAKE A PARAPLEGIC'S LIFE AS COMFORTABLE AS POSSIBLE. If he can read, make sure he has a reading board and something to read. If he ever stops eating from the effects of misery and chronic infection, his death is near. *Kindly contributed by Peter Bewes.*

ting them. They are particularly likely to occur immediately after the injury, and during an intercurrent infection later.

TURN A PARAPLEGIC EVERY 2 HOURS AND CHART THAT YOU HAVE DONE SO

Bedsores can only be prevented *if prevention has a high priority in the surgical ward.* So, put a chart at the foot of a patient's bed, with the time marked on it every 2 hours. Ask the nurses to *sign this chart each time they turn him,* and to record the side onto which they have turned him—left side, back, front, etc. At least 2 people are needed, and three are better. During the night the nurse on duty will need help, any help, even that of a relative, a watchman, a porter, or another patient. Show them how to turn him gently, so that they don't twist the patient's injured spine and injure it further. This is especially important if his fracture is unstable, when he must be 'moved in one piece'. Happily, nurses very rarely injure a patient's cord when they turn him.

ENORMOUS PRESSURE SORES CAN DEVELOP IN A FEW HOURS

The discipline of absolutely invariable 2 hourly turning is difficult to introduce because most nurses have seen paraplegics develop bedsores. Gloom and hopelessness thus pervades them all. So take the initiative yourself. Turn a patient yourself the first time, and next time, and perhaps the time after that. Ask a nurse to help you. If you show yourself prepared to get up a few times at 4 a.m. and help turn him (as some doctors have done), your nurses will play their part. Come early into the ward the next morning and inspect the pressure areas. If you find no redness (in a Caucasian) or blistering, congratulate the nurses, and help them with their plans for turning him during the rest of that day. Even offer to help them to turn him at night, if staff are short. If you are called, appear delighted, and conceal your distress!

Inspect the pressure areas on every ward round, and if they are healthy, congratulate the staff. At the slightest sign of redness or blistering, help the nurses to prepare an alternative routine of turning that will spare the red areas from pressure for a few days.

If any important person visits the hospital, show him the paraplegics. If he asks the inevitable question, ''Why are there no bedsores?'' ask him to ask the nurses. They will be only too ready to explain that it is because they are turning the patient every 2 hours. They will soon realize that they are becoming experts in this exacting field.

After a month or two, the patient and his relative between them can begin to work out their own routine for turning him, and plan how to manage him at home. After a few months it becomes almost reflex for him to be turning himself in bed at home. Once he is able to do this himself, he need only be readmitted to be turned by the nurses if he has an intercurrent infection, such as pneumonia.

Try to get him into a wheel chair or calipers quickly. When he is in them, teach him how to avoid getting pressure sores, as described below.

If he is only partly paraplegic and wears calipers, he must inspect where they press, so that he does not get pressure sores there. Let him see other patients with bedsores, so that he knows what he is trying to avoid.

Dr NICKEL took over a chronic care hospital in California with the worst of reputations for poor nursing care. He made it a rule that at the begining of each shift, the new shift examined the back of each patient for pressure sores. If a bedsore developed, the senior nurse on the shift was dismissed. His hospital became a showplace. LESSON Good discipline can prevent pressure sores.

SKIN CARE FOR PARAPLEGIA

Turn a paraplegic patient every 2 hours. *This is by far the most important treatment.* Each time you turn him, put his joints through a full range of passive movement, concentrating on hip and knee extension and dorsiflexion of his ankles.

BED Place a door on an ordinary hospital bed. On it place two 10 cm foam mattresses covered with mattress ticking. Put soft pillows or foam rubber cushions between the patient's legs and under his back.

If you have only a hard mattress, pad the pressure points with cotton wool, gauze, or pieces of fleece. Keep them in place with adhesive strapping, but watch these pads carefully. Don't allow them to become creased. Remove them at least once a day and check the skin under them.

Try to keep the patient's bottom sheet tight, dry, and free from creases, crumbs, and bits of food.

If his heels show any sign of pressure sores, put a pad under his ankles, or a ring pad around his heels.

PRESSURE POINTS Don't pad pressure points—*pad round them.* Watch the skin over his sacrum, his iliac crests, his hips, the sides of his knees, his heels, and his malleoli, and his penis if a condom catheter is applied.

INCIPIENT SORES The first sign of a sore is redness of the skin. Treat any red areas by careful massage and then apply one of these solutions: (1) soap and water followed by careful drying and powder, (2) hypochlorite('Eusol'),(3) borax in spirit, (4) 1% formaldehyde.

ESTABLISHED SORES Keep pressure off a sore until it has healed. Try to keep it clean. Use saline dressings or paraffin gauze. Honey and the fruit of the papaya (paw-paw) have also been used successfully. Small sores may heal slowly, if you keep them clean and protected.

If a skin lesion is obviously necrotic, toilet it and remove the necrotic tissue. You may find a much larger lesion under the surface. Large sores may need transposition, rotation, or myocutaneous flaps.

Keep the patient's haemoglobin above 12 g/dl.

TURNING A PARAPLEGIC NEEDS THREE PEOPLE

64.16 Paraplegic's bladder

If a patient has any significant degree of paraplegia, he will be unable to urinate voluntarily from the moment of the injury. His bladder will fill up slowly and will be full by about midnight on the day of admission. If you leave it, it will overflow, so anticipate this and prevent it. The best way of treating him is to use regular intermittent sterile catheterization. Infection is rare with this method. It imitates the natural cycle in which the bladder fills and empties. By leaving it almost empty for a significant period, this method relieves the pressure on its walls, both pressure of urine and pressure from the the balloon of a Foley catheter. This is important, because distension or pressure of any kind reduces the ability of the bladder to resist infection. It is also good training for student nurses. The disadvantage of this method is that it requires more nursing care, and if the patient is to do it himself, as described below, he must be cooperative. Some consultant surgeons in teaching hospitals say they cannot use this method, because they don't have the staff, and wonder that it can ever be done in smaller ones. In fact, some smaller hospitals can do it excellently. Don't use: (1) an indwelling catheter if you can possibly avoid doing so because infection is so common, or, (2) continuous suprapubic drainage, because it produces a small contracted bladder.

INTERMITTENT STERILE CATHETERIZATION Use a 14 Ch soft rubber Jacques catheter. Boil it and use gloved hands or sterile forceps. Pass it every 4 to 6 hours from the moment of the patient's injury. Later it can be every 6 to 8 hours. Empty

TWO REGIMES FOR A PARAPLEGIC BLADDER

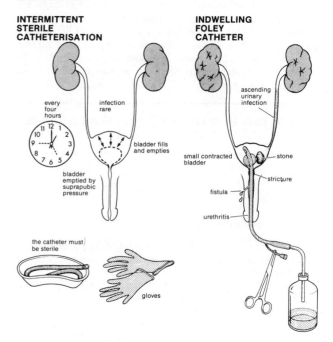

Fig. 64-18 TWO REGIMES FOR A PARAPLEGIC BLADDER. A, intermittent catheterization. Early on this is done in a sterile manner by the ward staff. Later, it can be done in a clean but non–sterile manner by the patient himself. B, an indwelling Foley catheter is much less satisfactory—avoid it if you can. *Kindly contributed by Peter Bewes.*

the patient's bladder completely by suprapubic pressure and then remove the catheter. Repeat the process 6 hours later, and again and again, four times a day. Record that catheterisation has been done on the chart which is used to record when he is turned.

CAUTION ! When you make rounds, check his bladder from time to time to make sure that it really is being emptied.

Continue, either until his cord recovers, or until an automatic bladder develops, usually in 2 to 3 months.

CATHETERIZE THE PATIENT WITH FULL STERILE PRECAUTIONS

Automatic bladder If a patient's spinal injury is above his lumbar enlargement, his bladder will eventually develop its own micturition reflex. After 2 to 8 weeks of intermittent catheterization he may discover a method of starting micturition himself. Fit him with a condom catheter or a Paul's tube and encourage him to try. He may be able to do this by stroking the side of his thigh, or his penis, or by pressing suprapubically. Such training may take a long time, it is not easy, and the nurses will require considerable persistence. Although training him may be difficult, it will save time in the end. When he has found a method which works, encourage him to use it more and more. Let him do this before he is catheterized. Don't stop catheterising him until his residual urine on catheterization after micturition has fallen to 75 ml, or less. Even when it has fallen to this volume, catheterize him once a week to make sure that he is not partly retaining his urine. If you find that his residual urine is more than 75 ml, consider referring him for resection or division of the external sphincter of his prostatic urethra (external sphincterotomy).

Intermittent clean but non–sterile self catheterization If a paraplegic's bladder is isolated from spinal control, emptying depends on a local reflex which is much less effective than a reflex arc via his cord. He does not develop an automatic bladder, and he has to catheterize himself. He can either boil up a catheter each time and try to pass it in a sterile manner, or he can catheterize himself regularly and cleanly, but without using sterile precautions.

Suprisingly, non—sterile self catheterization has many advantages. Because a patient does not need to boil up the catheter each time, he can catheterize himself more often, and does not allow his bladder to fill up. This reduces the incidence of infection, and in practice he is infected less often than if he waits and tries to sterilize a catheter. But for this method to succeed, *he must empty his bladder as completely as possible with the help of suprapubic pressure continued until the moment that he pulls the catheter out.* A bladder that is not emptied after catheterization will contain some organisms, but a bladder that is completely emptied will contain very few.

Many patients easily learn this method which has many advantages. For example, a patient can go to a football match, cheer widely, and in the interval go to the toilet, catheterize himself, and then return to the match! A patient who has been told to use sterile catheterization will either not be able to go to any such matches ever, or he will be inhibited from catheterizing himself in the toilet, so allowing pressure to build up in his bladder and running the risk of a urinary infection.

Some surgeons in the developing world say that they have never succeeded with this method; others are enthusiastic about it.

INTERMITTENT NON—STERILE SELF CATHETERIZATION

Give a man a Jacques rubber catheter. If he has difficulty, give him one with a small beak, such as an oliviary tipped Tieman catheter, or a coude catheter. Teach him which way to point the beak. Give a woman a small handbag mirror to help her find her urethral meatus.

Encourage the patient to catheterize himself *cleanly.* (1) He must keep the catheter clean. (2) He should if possible wash his hands and the tip of his meatus.

CAUTION ! Make sure he knows how important it is to empty his bladder completely.

INFECTION If his urine becomes infected and he has symptoms:

(1) Encourage him to catheterize himself at more frequent intervals. Usually, the reason for the infection is that he has not been catheterizing himself often enough.

(2) Give him an appropriate antibiotic. He has not been on a prophylactic antibiotic, so his infection is usually easy to treat; sulphonamides may be enough. Don't try to prevent infection by giving antibiotics routinely.

(3) If the first two methods fail, admit him to hospital for continued, intermittent, non—sterile catheterization under supervision, together with bladder wash-outs.

64.17 A paraplegic's bowels

If a patient's bladder fills up after a spinal injury, so will his bowel, which quickly becomes loaded with brick—like faeces. Distension may become so severe that his sigmoid colon presses on his left iliac vein and may make it thrombose.

Give him an enema three times a week until his bowel function has returned, usually in 3 to 6 weeks. Glycerine suppositories later on may help him to develop a defaecation reflex. He may be able to start this reflex himself by inserting a suppository and sitting on the lavatory 15 minutes later. Even so, faecal impaction is always a danger, and either he or his relatives must be taught how to remove his faeces manually. This is so important that it should be part of the routine teaching of everyone who cares for paraplegics. Occasionally, remove them manually yourself and encourage the nurses to follow your example. Make sure that a patient has a high residue diet and give him laxatives if necessary.

64.18 The muscles and joints in paraplegia

From the very beginning of a patient's illness, ask some concerned person to move all his paralysed joints passively through a full range of movements several times a day. This will become more difficult as he becomes more spastic. If he is neglected, his hips, knees, and ankles will roll up like a hibernating hedgehog. Established contractures are a sign of total failure because they are readily preventable. Where possible, sit a patient up out of bed. Although physiotherapists are useful, they are not essential. Any doctor, nurse, or relative can be taught to put a patient's knees, ankles, and hips through a full range of movements every day, and so prevent contractures. Avoid force, because this may damage a joint. Encourage him to move his non—paralysed joints as much as he can, using his own muscles.

The hips of a paraplegic patient have a tendency to flex. Prevent this by following the regime below. If his hips have already started to flex, he will ask for a pillow to be put under his groins, so as to let them flex, even when he is lying on his front. This may be kind when you are starting to cure a hip deformity, but make the pillow thinner and thinner each day until there is no pillow at all. If, however, a patient has no deformity to start with, don't give him a pillow when he is lying on his face.

TURNING REGIMES FOR PARAPLEGIA

CERVICAL SPINE Start by turning a patient 2 hourly: left side—supine—right side—supine. When his fracture is relatively stable, usually at about 6 weeks when traction is replaced by a collar, add a period in the prone position. Later increase the time in this position to reduce the tendency to develop flexion contractures in his hip and knee.

THORACO—LUMBAR SPINE Turn him 2 hourly: left side—supine—right side—prone. Later, increase time in the prone position as above.

LET THE NURSES DO THE PHYSIOTHERAPY

64.19 Mobilizing and rehabilitating the paraplegic

If you don't interest yourself in what happens to a paraplegic after discharge, he is only too likely to die and waste all the

REHABILITATING A PARAPLEGIC

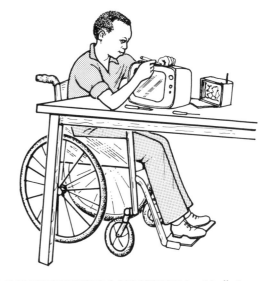

Fig. 64-19 REHABILITATING A PARAPLEGIC is critically important. Failure to rehabilitate paraplegics is one of the things that kills them after discharge. *Kindly contributed by Peter Bewes.*

159

care and attention he may have received while in hospital. This is especially likely to happen in the rural areas. So visit the patient's home, and try to make sure that he has a suitable bed and toilet. Often, money will be the major factor. If a patient was injured at work, the workmen's compensation fund may be able to support him.

Start to mobilize a patient when his fracture is reasonably stable and it is clear that his paralysis will be permanent. Stand him up regularly when his arms are strong enough to hold crutches. Use gutter plaster splints or walking calipers to support his knees and ankles.

Involve his whole family in rehabilitating him. He is going to need a wheel chair, and perhaps calipers and crutches to take home. Start thinking early about how to finance these. The first week of his illness is not too early for this. Early on during his stay in hospital, encourage him to develop extraordinary strength in the unparalysed parts of his body. Let him pull himself up with a Balkan beam, or give him weights to lift with his arms, so that they are strong enough to support him when he uses crutches or a wheel chair. Calipers may help him to keep his knees straight and his feet in neutral. Teach him some skill with his hands, such as making articles for sale, by basket making, weaving, or leather work. Encourage him to find markets for the things he is able to make, so that he can later earn his own living.

Aim for a date of discharge 4 or 5 months after his admission. Some caring member of the hospital staff should visit his home with a relative, to see if it is suitable for a paraplegic to live in. Is the floor flat, so that it can take a wheel chair? Are there any steps that cannot be managed with crutches? Sometimes, parallel bars can be put up outside his house so that he can exercise himself, as he did in the hospital. If his home is not like this, and many homes are not, his outlook is grim.

He may have to live in a sheltered home and be found work in a sheltered workshop. Such workshops have been set up in many parts of the world, and it is a very uncaring community that cannot make some provision for its own handicapped.

Success in rehabilitating paraplegia is one of the best indicators of high quality care. Where it fails, a district hospital accumulates 3 or 4 paraplegics, and a provincial one perhaps 12, each with an average stay of perhaps 10 years, with all that this means for unnecessary expense, and for the other patients who might have been treated in their beds.

FURTHER CARE FOR PARAPLEGIA

WHEEL CHAIRS **Start a patient in a wheel chair slowly, 2 hours once a day to begin with, then 2 hours twice a day. Teach him to lift up his buttocks a few times every 15 minutes. Sit him on two foam rubber cushions, or sit him on the blown up inner tube of the kind of motor cycle that has small wheels and big tyres. Cover this with a foam pad.**

Give him a washable rubber bag for the time his bladder works unexpectedly.

If he develops skin sores or a urinary infection, he must return to the hospital rapidly.

AMPUTATION If a patient has grossly infected lower legs, there may be a case for amputating both of them above his knees. He can then move and be moved more easily, and some possible sites of bed sores will have gone, but he will have difficulty sitting. If you decide to amputate, don't remove both legs on the same occasion.

PARAPLEGIA CAN BE TREATED IN A DISTRICT HOSPITAL

---

65 Thoracic injuries

65.1 The general method for a thoracic injury

A severe chest injury is terrifying for a conscious patient. You can usually save the patient's life, but you must have a logical approach worked out in advance. His injury can be a blunt one from a road accident, or a penetrating one from a bullet, a spear, or an arrow. Often, his chest injury is only one of several other injuries. The procedure that he is likely to need most urgently is to have blood and air drained from a pleural cavity—rapidly and, if necessary, on both sides. *This is the critical procedure in thoracic surgery, and is often not done when it should be.* A patient may have any of the following chest injuries:

(1) Broken ribs. A thoracic injury usually breaks the ribs of an older patient. But if a patient is young, his ribs may be so elastic that he can have severe internal injuries without breaking them. By themselves broken ribs are not important and soon heal.

(2) A haemothorax. The blood in a patient's pleural cavity can come from his chest wall, or from his lungs.

(3) A pneumothorax. Air in a pleural cavity usually comes from a patient's lungs, but it can come from his trachea, his bronchi, or his chest wall. A small pneumothorax is usually harmless and resolves spontaneously.

(4) A haemopneumothorax. He may have both blood and air in a pleural cavity.

(5) A tension pneumothorax. The air in a patient's pleural cavity may be under pressure when a wound of his lung, or (rarely) an open chest wound, acts as a valve and allows air to get in but not out. More air is trapped each time he breathes. The lung on the injured side collapses, his mediastinum moves towards the normal side, and restricts the movement of that lung too. His bronchi may kink and make his breathing even more difficult. Unless you rapidly let out the air, he dies.

(6) A flail chest. Multiple fractures of a patient's ribs can cause a large part of his chest wall to move independently of the rest of it, or allow it to be pushed inwards (stove–in chest). The danger of a flail chest is that the loose piece, which should be moving outwards during inspiration, may be sucked inwards (paradoxical movement), and greatly impede his breathing. His mediastinum can also move paradoxically as he breathes. The result is that air, which should be replaced with each respiration, merely moves from one lung to the other (paradoxical breathing).

(7) A sucking chest wound allows a pleural cavity to communicate with the outside air, with the result that the lung on the injured side collapses, the patient's mediastinum moves paradoxically, and he has paradoxical breathing. Closing his open wound may save his life.

(8) Surgical emphysema is the result of air escaping into the tissues, usually under the skin. Air in the mediastinum is much more serious and may indicate the rupture of a bronchus.

(9) Shocked lung is the result of contusion by a shock wave. This is common and causes haemoptysis.

(10) Other injuries in a patient's thorax or abdomen include injuries to his aorta, his diaphragm, his heart, his liver, his spleen, or his thoracic spine. Aortic tears are a common cause of death in road accidents.

Here are some of the ways you can help a patient. The purpose of most of them is to make sure that his lungs are normally ventilated: (1) You can secure his airway, and encourage him to cough and clear it. It is easily obstructed, especially if he is a child, and he can only too easily inhale blood, secretions, or the contents of his stomach. He may need bronchoscopy, suction, tracheal intubation, or occasionally tracheostomy. This will reduce his dead space and make a tracheal toilet easier. (2) You can remove air from the top of his pleural cavities or blood from the bottom using a drain with an underwater seal. (3) You can close his open chest wound, particularly a sucking one. (4) You can stabilize his flail chest. (5) You can assist his ventilation with a self–inflating bag. (6) You can transfuse him. (7) You can prevent infection. (8) You can relieve cardiac tamponade by aspirating blood from his pericardial cavity. Last and certainly not least, you can provide physiotherapy which will help him to cough. The great danger with all chest injuries is that retained secretions will cause infection, collapse of a lung, and death. Only active physiotherapy will prevent this.

In more severe injuries a patient's chest must be opened and the organs inside it repaired (thoracotomy). This major procedure is beyond our scope here, but fortunately only about 5% of the chest injuries which need a drain need a thoracotomy. Ideally, if a patient has anything but the mildest degree of flail chest, he should be connected to an intermittent positive pressure respirator (IPPR), and have his blood gases monitored. This too is unlikely to be possible.

If you don't have a respirator, you can keep a patient inflated with a self inflating bag while you refer him. If this is impossible, we describe other ways of treating a flail chest (65.6).

Don't be too optimistic. Chest injuries can be as deceptive as abdominal ones—although a patient may seem to be in fair condition to start with, he can deteriorate rapidly.

ABDULLA (41) was hit in the left flank by a passing car. He had a cold nose, a fast weak pulse, and a normal blood pressure. His left flank and lower left ribs were tender. An X-ray film showed gut in his chest. He was in the theatre in 20 minutes, by which time two intravenous drips had improved him considerably. A right upper paramedian incision was made and a hand passed up to his diaphragm. This revealed a hole. The skin incision was therefore extended up into his eighth left intercostal space. It was now seen that his spleen, although not actively bleeding, had been badly bruised. Splenectomy was easy through the enlarged incision. His diaphragm was repaired with interrupted figure–of–eight sutures in one layer, and his chest closed with two layers of continuous monofilament. He recovered. LESSONS (1) Opening the chest, when you have to, may make surgery much easier. (2) It will also be easier if you do it early.

THE GENERAL METHOD FOR A CHEST INJURY

This extends Section 51.3 on the care of a severely injured patient.

THE RAPID ASSESSMENT OF A CHEST INJURY

If a patient's airway is blocked, clear it as in Section 52.1.

If air is going in and out, but his breathing is distressed, he may have multiple fractured ribs or severe abdominal pain.

If he is making great respiratory efforts, but is still hungry for air, think of a flail chest or a pneumothorax.

A SEVERE CHEST INJURY

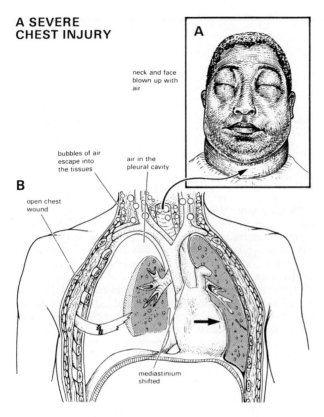

neck and face blown up with air

A

bubbles of air escape into the tissues

air in the pleural cavity

B

open chest wound

mediastinium shifted

Fig. 65-1 A SEVERE CHEST INJURY. A, this patient has surgical emphysema—in spite of his alarming appearance, this part of his injury is benign. B, a broken rib has punctured his lung, air has collected under pressure in his right pleural cavity, compressed his right lung, and forced his mediastinum over to the left, impairing the ventilation of his left lung. Air has also escaped into his mediastinum and tracked up into his neck and face. *Adapted from an original illustration by Frank H. Netter, M.D. from the CIBA collection of medical illustrations, copyright by CIBA Pharmaceutical Company, Division of CIBA–GEIGY Corporation.*

If he is cyanosed in the presence of an adequate airway, he may have a badly damaged lung, a flail chest, or a pneumothorax. Give him oxygen.

Many patients with chest injuries breathe much more easily as soon as they are intubated.

THE HISTORY OF A CHEST INJURY

Assess the force of the patient's injury carefully. The greater the force, the greater the chances that he has a severe injury.

THE EXAMINATION OF A CHEST INJURY

If a patient is conscious, and is now breathing easily, strip him to the waist, and ask him to describe the pain and show you exactly where it is. If unconscious, remove his clothes and examine his chest carefully.

INSPECTION Assess the rate and depth of the patient's breathing, while he is breathing normally. Ask him to take a deep breath. If his ribs are broken, his attempts to do so will soon be stopped by sharp pain.

Mediastinal shift Is his apex beat in its normal place? Feel in his suprasternal notch to find out if his trachea is displaced.

Do both sides of his chest expand equally?

Look carefully for any areas of diminished chest movement. This may be in one area only, or involve the whole of one side. Look at him from the sides and from the top and bottom of the trolley.

CAUTION ! Look carefully for paradoxical movement. Look at the movement of a normal area, then compare this with the possibily abnormal one. Paradoxical movement may be difficult to see when a patient is shocked and his respiratory movements are small; it may only come on later, when he is

resuscitated. Don't be confused by the indrawing of his lower costal margin that is common in mild respiratory obstruction, especially in children.

Are his intercostal spaces distended on one side compared with the other? (tension pneumothorax).

Is he cyanosed? Look at his mucous membranes and his finger nails.

CAUTION ! Anaemic patients do not become cyanosed, and may die of anoxia without showing it. There must be 5 g/dl of reduced haemoglobin in a patient's circulation before you can observe cyanosis.

Look carefully for any bruises on his chest caused by a steering wheel or a safety belt, or by the imprint of his clothes.

Are the patient's jugular veins abnormally distended? (anything which impedes the venous return to the heart, a tension pneumothorax, mediastinal shift, and especially cardiac tamponade).

PALPATION If a patient is conscious, start by feeling a pain–free area, and then move towards the injured one. Feel for: (1) Tenderness. (2) Crepitus when fractured ribs move with respiration. (3) The crackly feeling of surgical emphysema.

Feel his abdomen for rigidity, tenderness, and distension.

PERCUSSION Do this gently. Don't fail to turn him or sit him up so that you can examine his back. Dullness may indicate blood or the collapse of a lung, and hyper–resonance may be caused by a tension pneumothorax.

ASCULTATION Can you hear the patient's breath sounds all over his chest, or are they diminished? Note especially: (1) Clicking sounds from fractured ribs. (2) The coarse crepitations of surgical emphysema. (3) Reduced or absent breath sounds on one side indicating fluid, or air in a pleural cavity, or the collapse of a lung. Listen for this sign while he is supine, as in Fig. 65-7. (4) High pitched breath sounds suggesting a tension pneumothorax.

The two coin test Place a coin on the patient's chest and tap it with another coin. A bell–like note (combined with other signs) suggests a tension pneumothorax.

OTHER SIGNS OF A CHEST INJURY

ABDOMEN Examine this carefully. Note any tenderness, rigidity or distension. If a patient's lower left ribs are fractured posteriorly, think of a ruptured spleen. If he is tender in his right upper abdomen, suspect a ruptured liver. Fractures of the lower 6 ribs can cause abdominal tenderness without there being any injured abdominal viscera.

FRACTURED RIBS If a patient is not too ill, *gently* spring his chest from front to back, or from side to side, between your hands. If this causes severe pain he has probably broken some ribs. Feel for the tender fracture sites. They will be easier to feel than to see on an X-ray.

PULSE Is this stronger on inspiration than on expiration? Is his jugular venous pressure raised? These are both signs of cardiac tamponade (65.9).

X-RAY all patients you suspect of having a serious chest injury. X-rays are not necessary to diagnose fractured ribs (which are difficult to see), but are a useful way of making sure that a patient's lungs and pleural cavities are normal. Unless other injuries prevent it, try to take an erect x-ray. If he cannot stand, you may be able to support him sitting up on a trolley for the very short period that is necessary for a film to be taken.

Examine the films systematically noting first his rib cage and other bones, then his trachea and lungs, and finally his heart and mediastinum. Look for rib fractures by holding the film obliquely, and looking along each rib.

If you have to X-ray him lying flat on a trolley, try to give the table a slight head up tilt. The films may show a large pneumothorax or a haemothorax, fractured ribs, or surgical emphysema. They will not show a small pneumothorax, or a fluid level in a haemopneumothorax.

Haemothorax A diffuse opacity in a lower lung field, which is more easily seen in an erect film. *A haemothorax may not be easy to diagnose radiologically, so rely on your stethoscope.*

DRAINING AIR AND FLUID FROM THE CHEST

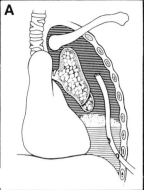

if you use one tube, insert it like this ⇨

tube as near the top of the pleural cavity as possible

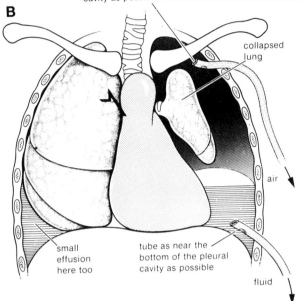

collapsed lung

air

small effusion here too

tube as near the bottom of the pleural cavity as possible

fluid

Fig. 65-2 DRAINING AIR AND BLOOD FROM THE CHEST is much the most valuable procedure in chest injuries, and all that most patients need. A, two drains are better than one drain, but, if you do use one drain, leave a sufficiently long length of tube inside the chest with holes near the entry of the tube through the chest wall. B, two tubes, upper and lower are better than one. The bottom tube must be low in the chest if blood is to drain properly. *Kindly contributed by James Cairns.*

Pneumothorax (1) The lung markings do not reach all the way out to the edge of the thoracic cage. (2) You can see the pleura as a faint line. (3) The apices look different.

Contusion of the lung Diffuse mottling with dense patches in places. These intensify in the next few days and then clear.

Aortic injury If the patient's mediastinum is significantly widened, check the pulses in each of his arms and in each side of his neck. He may have injured his aorta or the great vessels at the root of his neck.

Cardiac tamponade A wide heart shadow.

THREE MAJOR DIFFERENTIAL DIAGNOSES IN A CHEST INJURY

If a patient has a large haemothorax, he will be sweaty and clammy, have a rapid, thready pulse, collapsed neck veins, an apex beat in its normal place, and *a chest which is stony dull to percussion.* Sometimes even a large haemothorax causes very few signs.

If a patient has a tension pneumothorax, he will have increasing difficulty breathing, a rapid pulse which may be of good volume, perhaps slightly distended neck veins, *an apex beat and trachea displaced to the other side,* and a tympanitic note on percussion.

If he has cardiac tamponade, he will be severely distressed and shocked, he will have a rapid weak pulse, *grossly distended neck veins,* an apex beat you can neither feel nor see, and a normal percussion note.

PHYSIOTHERAPY is very important to prevent collapse of a lung. There are these possibilities; (2) and (3) are not suitable for patients with severe rib injuries. (1) Try deep breathing and coughing every 2 to 4 hours, accompanied by suction if necessary. (2) Vibration to the chest wall. (3) Slapping the chest wall.

PARTICULAR INJURIES Read on for methods of draining a patient's chest (65.2), managing uncomplicated fractures of his ribs and sternum (65.3), and treating a haemothorax (65.4), a pneumothorax (65.5), a flail chest (63.5), open chest injuries (65.7), and stab wounds (65.8).

If you are in doubt how to manage a patient, admit him and observe him. A haemothorax may take some days to form.

DON'T OVERLOOK A HAEMOTHORAX

65.2 Draining the pleural cavity

Drainage is all that a patient with a chest injury usually needs. Remove air by putting a tube into the top of his pleural cavity, usually in his third intercostal space just lateral to his midclavicular line. Drain blood, fluid, or pus from the bottom, usually through his eighth or ninth space in his posterior axillary line. The easiest way to prevent air entering his chest is to lead the tubes from it under the surface of the water in a large bottle (Tudor–Edwards bottle). The principle of this is shown in A, Fig. 65-5. Air from his chest will bubble up from under the surface of the water, without allowing more air to enter. Any fluid in his chest will drip down the tube into the water. Provided the bottle is always well below the patient's bed, water from it cannot enter his chest. If he has both air and fluid in his pleural cavity, some surgeons would put one tube low in his chest and allow air and fluid to bubble out together as froth. Wiser ones insert two tubes.

Here is the equipment for a chest drain set. The life of one medical student was saved after an elephant had punctured his lung, because a tiny clinic had a chest drain set ready. Here is the equipment for it. Have it instantly ready, you will need it in a hurry.

• *NEEDLES, hypodermic, large for chest aspiration, 1.6×100 mm, 'Luer–lok' mount each, five only.* This mount fits the three way stopcock listed below, and is a useful aspirating and exploring needle.

• *STOPCOCK, for chest aspiration, 'Luer–lok' male to 'Luer–lok' female, with side arm for tubing, two only.* Use this for aspirating the chest.

• *SYRINGES, 5 ml and 20 ml, both 'Luer–lok'.* These fit the stopcock.

• *BOTTLE, Tudor–Edwards, 3 litres, chest drainage, including rubber bung and tubes, one only.* This provides an underwater seal for closed drainage of the chest.

• *CONNECTOR, for Tudor–Edwards chest drain, five only.* This completes the equipment for an underwater chest drain.

• *Alternatively, CHEST DRAIN SET, plastic, disposable, sterile, in packet complete, five only.* You will not use a chest drain set very often, so the modest expense of a disposable one may be justified.

YOU WILL NEED A CHEST DRAINAGE SET IN A HURRY

SOME URGENT METHODS FOR CHEST INJURIES

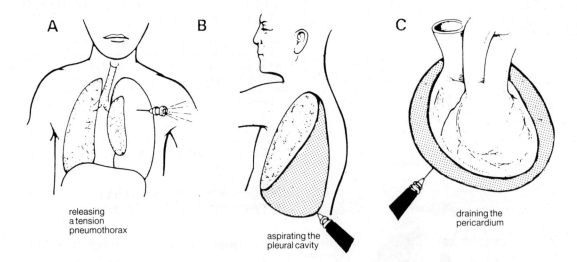

Fig. 65-3 SOME URGENT METHODS FOR CHEST INJURIES. A, releasing air from a tension pneumothorax (uncommon). B, aspirating blood from a pleural cavity (common). C, aspirating the pericardium (rare). *After Naclerio with the kind permission of Grune and Stratton.*

A CHEST SET

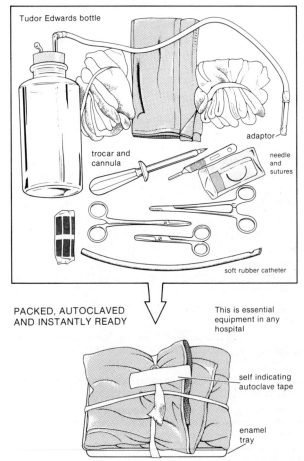

Fig. 65-4 A CHEST SET. You will need this in a hurry, so always keep a chest drain set ready. *As assembled by Sam Smith*

The first step is usually a diagnostic aspiration to make sure that a patient really does have fluid in his chest. After this, there are various ways you can put a tube in the chest. The easiest one is to push a large trocar and cannula between his ribs to remove the trocar, and then to push a plastic or rubber tube down the cannula. The cannula is then removed leaving the tube in place. If you don't have a suitable cannula, you can stab his chest wall with a scalpel and then use artery forceps to push a tube through an intercostal space. Always: (1) Take the strictest aseptic precautions. It is tragic to convert a haemothorax to pyohaemothorax, or to introduce new strains of bacteria into an empyema. (2) Prevent more than the minimum amount of air entering his pleural cavity.

The alternatives described below do not include the use of a drip set to drain the chest, because: (1) the tube of a drip set is too narrow so that it is easily blocked, and (2) the needle is usually too short to reach the fluid.

DRAINING BLOOD OR AIR FROM THE CHEST

DIAGNOSTIC ASPIRATION

EQUIPMENT A 10 or 20 ml 'Luer–lok' syringe and a 1.6 mm short bevel 'Luer–lok' needle. A 5 ml syringe, a fine needle, a No.11 scalpel blade, and some local anaesthetic.

METHOD FOR BLOOD Find an assistant. Sedate the patient, sit him up, and lean him forwards over a bed table or a pile of pillows.

Sit on a stool beside his bed, and percuss his chest to find the area of maximum dullness. This is usually over his sixth, seventh, or eighth rib in his posterior axillary line.

Use a fine needle to infiltrate a little local anaesthetic into the tissues at the site of the aspiration. Nick his skin with a scalpel blade parallel to his ribs. Push a large needle on the end of a 10 or 20 ml syringe slowly into his chest wall through the nick, pulling back the plunger as you do so.

Remove the syringe as soon as it fills with blood or fluid, and put a swab on the hole. Record your findings and the site of the puncture accurately in his notes.

DRAINING FLUID FROM THE CHEST

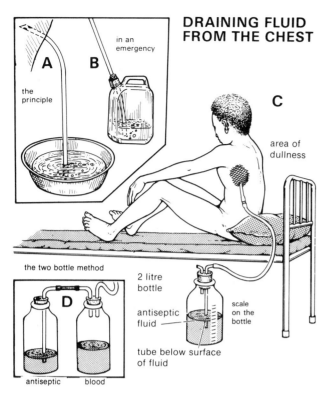

Fig. 65-5 DRAINING FLUID FROM THE CHEST. A, shows the principle, which is merely to lead a tube from the patient underwater. B, if you don't have the proper equipment, use any suitable bottle. C, the one bottle method. D, the two bottle method. *Kindly contributed by Peter Bewes and James Cairns.*

INSERTING A CLOSED INTERCOSTAL DRAIN

A CHEST SET consists of: (1) A large trocar and cannula 8.3 mm (25 Ch). (2) A 24 to 30 Ch Malecot or de Pezzer catheter which just fits through the trocar. (3) A metre of 8 mm (24 Ch) plastic or rubber tube to join the catheter to the bottle, using a connector. If you don't have a suitable catheter, you can push the end of this tube through the trocar into the chest. If you do, the tube must be thick and stiff enough not to collapse when it goes through the chest. If convenient, you can use a thinner tube (5 mm, 16 Ch) for draining air. (4) A drainage bottle (Tudor–Edwards) complete with a cork and two tubes. Adjust the size of the bottle to the size of the patient. A child needs only a small bottle. (5) A needle holder. (6) Stout artery forceps to clamp the tube. (7) A No. 4 scalpel with a No. 23 blade. (8) Some No.1 monofilament. (9) Ordinary stitch scissors. (10) Gauze swabs and a gallipot.

Wrap all this equipment together in a green towel, put it in a tray, tie it up with bandages, and autoclave it. Have it always ready sterile, as in Fig. 65-4.

USING A TROCAR AND CANNULA Position the patient, and find the point of maximum dullness as for aspiration.

Infiltrate the place where the tube is to go with anaesthetic solution as in A, Fig. 65-6. Push the needle down to the rib infiltrating as you go. Inject the solution in 1 ml portions, aspirating between each injection. Try to anaesthetize the patient's pleura without entering his pleural cavity. If necessary, anaesthetize one space above and one below the site of insertion of the tube.

Alternatively, block the intercostal nerve (A 6.7) 1 cm proximal to where you intend to introduce your cannula.

Apply the first pair of artery forceps some way up the tube (B, Fig. 65-6). It will both clamp the tube, and serve as a gauge as to how much tube there is inside the chest. There must be at least 2 cm (for the free end of the tube in the pleural cavity), plus one chest wall thickness (which will vary with the patient's build), plus the length of the cannula, plus 4 cm spare.

Apply the second forceps to the distal end of the tube.

Nick the patient's skin with the scalpel blade (C), push the trocar and cannula through the infiltrated area into his pleural cavity (D).

Pull out the trocar (E) and quickly push the tube down the cannula (F). Then pull out the cannula up as far as the first forceps, leaving the tube in his chest. The first pair of artery forceps ensures that the depth of tube inside his chest is just right. Apply the second pair of artery forceps close to his chest wall (G) and remove the cannula from the tube. Ask your assistant to connect the tube to an underwater seal drain as described below.

Release the artery forceps. Anchor the tube to his chest wall with a safety pin and adhesive strapping, or, better with a stitch. Alternatively, use strapping as in Fig. 65-8.

Connect the catheter to an underwater seal drain.

INSERTING A CLOSED INTERCOSTAL DRAIN

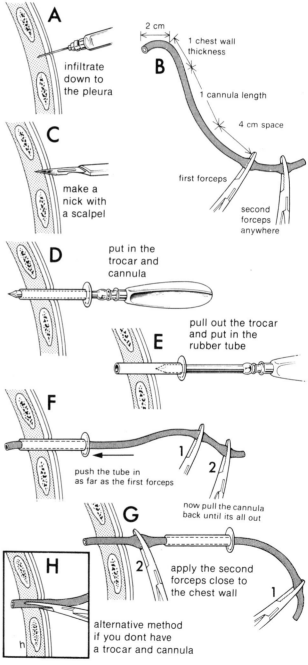

Fig. 65-6 INSERTING AN INTERCOSTAL DRAIN. You can also use a Malecot or de Pezzer catheter on an introducer. *Kindly contributed by Peter Bewes.*

CAUTION ! Don't let air get into his chest through the tube. Apply the artery forceps as above, and don't release them until the tube is connected to the underwater seal. If there is any delay in putting the tube into the cannula, plug it with your finger.

ALTERNATIVE USING A SCALPEL, ARTERY FORCEPS, AND A CATHETER

Use a scalpel with a No. 11 blade to make a 1 cm incision down to the upper edge of the rib and then through the intercostal space for about 3 mm. Avoid its lower edge, because the intercostal vessels run there. Push a pair of artery forceps or scissors down the incision, and by blunt dissection open up a track down to the pleura. Try not to enter it with the scalpel.

Clamp the catheter with artery forceps, hold the other end of it with another pair of artery forceps, and push it down the track into the pleura, as in H, Fig. 65-6. Alternatively, you can insert a Malecot or de Pezzer catheter on an introducer.

DRAINING AIR FROM THE PLEURAL CAVITY

Using any of the methods above, puncture the patient's third intercostal space well outside his midclavicular line, and lead the tube into an underwater seal drain.

MAKING AN UNDERWATER SEAL DRAIN FOR A CHEST INJURY

Take a 3 to 5 litre glass bottle with a large top, and a cork with two holes. Put a litre of water or dilute antiseptic into the bottle. Pass two glass tubes through cork and let one tube go down 5 cm below the level of the fluid. Connect the top end of the long glass tube to the rubber tube draining the patient's chest. Make sure the fit is airtight. The rubber tube must be long enough so that, if he moves about, he does not detach it from the bottle or raise it above the water level.

Ask him to cough. Blood or bubbles should come out of the tube.

Keep a pair of artery forceps near by, so that the rubber tube can be clamped if it becomes detached from the bottle. Fix a piece of strapping to the bottle, and mark the upper level of the fluid on it, so that you can measure how much blood or exudate is discharged.

When the bottle is changed, clamp the rubber tube with the forceps, and release them only when the bottle has been reconnected.

If necessary, you can join the tubes from the top and bottom of the patient's chest with a Y-connector and drain them into one bottle.

Measure the volume of blood that drains and transfuse the patient as necessary.

CAUTION ! (1) The end of the tube must be 5 cm below the level of the water so that if the pressure in the chest rises above this, air or fluid will be blown off. It is an *underwater* seal. (2) Make sure that the nurses understand what the bottle is for and that nobody disturbs it. If anybody raises it above the level of the patient's chest, the water and antiseptic in the bottle may go into his pleural cavity!

Alternatively, arrange 2 bottles, as in D, Fig. 65-5. This will allow you to collect the exudate separately from the fluid.

DIFFICULTIES DRAINING THE CHEST

If you have NO SPECIAL BOTTLE, use any large bottle such as the plastic bottle in B, Fig. 65-5 and lead the tubing under the surface of the water. Hold it in place with adhesive strapping. If you want to see the water moving in the tube, fix a piece of glass tubing into the end of the plastic tube. You can use the narrow tube from a drip set, but this is not nearly so effective.

THE TUBE MUST NOT COME OUT ACCIDENTLLY

65.3 Uncomplicated fractures of the ribs and sternum

Fractured ribs are not important unless many are fractured, or unless there are serious injuries inside the patient's chest. The first three ribs are protected by the shoulder girdle in all but the most serious injuries, so it is usually the middle or lower ones that break. When many of a patient's ribs have been broken, the organs inside his chest are sure to have been injured also.

X-rays show only about half of the fractures that exist. They are not really necessary, if you are sure there is no pneumothorax, or least not a large one.

If there are no complications, fractures of the ribs need no treatment except for pain. Local anaesthesia properly done, especially with bupivacaine (A 6.7), can be very effective in relieving this.

Fracture of the sternum is another steering wheel injury. A patient's sternum fractures at the junction of its manubrium and body. Or, it can fracture in an acute flexion injury of his spine. Pain is severe and may interfere with breathing. Treatment is straightforward. Lie him flat in bed for 10 days, unless this interferes with breathing.

Sometimes, a patient's ribs break all round his sternum, so as to produce a 'flail sternum'. This is merely a variety of flail chest.

BROKEN RIBS AFTER A CHEST INJURY

LOCAL ANAESTHESIA FOR BROKEN RIBS Carefully feel the tender areas that indicate the patient's fractures. Mark them on his skin. Inject each fractured rib with 3 ml of 1.5% bupivacaine, or 1% lignocaine, making sure the tip of the needle is down on the rib in the subperiosteal space close to the fracture site. Often, pain relief lasts days, much longer than would be expected after a single dose of anaesthetic solution. The patient will be very grateful.

MANAGEMENT depends on how many ribs are broken and where they are broken.

If only a few of a patient's ribs are broken, (less than 4 fractures are visible on an X-ray, if you take one), and if there are no pulmonary signs, management depends on his age and activity. If he is young, treat him as an out-patient.

The main risk is infection in the underlying injured lung, especially in a frail old person, and particularly in a heavy smoker, who is not physically active. Keep him moving, give him analgesics, and *encourage deep breathing exercises.* Warn him that pain may take 3 months to go away.

If a patient's sternum is fractured, lie him flat in bed for a few days, unless this interferes with his breathing.

If he has signs of a haemothorax or pneumothorax, admit him.

If his lower ribs are broken, consider the possibility of a rupture of his liver (66.7) or spleen (66.6).

65.4 Haemothorax and haemopneumothorax

Blood, or blood and air in a patient's pleural cavity, is the commonest complication of a chest injury. *Bleeding can occur slowly over several days, so it is often overlooked,* especially if a patient has multiple injuries. Detect it by: (1) Dullness to percussion. (2) Reduced breath sounds. Listen for these by sliding a flat stethoscope under his chest while he is lying down. (3) A diffuse opacity in an X-ray, which is more clearly seen in an erect film. If there has been much bleeding, he will have all the usual signs of internal bleeding (53.2). He may also be cyanosed. If you don't remove blood urgently, it will clot, organize, and prevent his lung re-expanding. When this happens, it can only be made to expand again by decorticating it at thoracotomy. So make sure you diagnose haemothoraces, drain them immediately, and keep a patient's injured pleura drained. Removing blood also removes the danger of leaving a fluid medium in his chest, which may become infected.

HAEMOTHORAX AND HAEMOPNEUMOTHORAX

HAEMOTHORAX Aspirate a patient's chest on the suspicion that there *might* be blood in it. If necessary, aspirate on both sides. If you find blood, insert an intercostal drain with an underwater seal bottle (65.2), on both sides if necessary. Leave the tube in until bleeding stops.

Replace the blood that he loses by transfusing an equal volume.

Examine his lungs several times daily. If drainage is successful, his breath sounds will gradually reappear and increase in strength. His pulse rate should fall and his blood pressure should rise.

If a patient's intercostal drain becomes blocked, reinsert it.

If his lungs fail to expand, refer him for decortication as soon as possible. The earlier you do this the easier the operation will be. If possible, refer him within 3 days.

HAEMOPNEUMOTHORAX Blood and air form a froth in the pleural cavity. Some blood will drain through a catheter inserted high up anteriorly. But you will usually need to insert a second one for blood lower down posteriorly. One tube may be enough; two tubes are better. If you decide to rely on a single tube, cut side holes in it and push it well up inside the pleural cavity.

DIFFICULTIES WITH BLOOD OR AIR IN THE CHEST

If EARLY ASPIRATION FAILS TO WITHDRAW BLOOD, don't be put off. If you think blood is present, insert a drain. Sometimes the blood clots in the first few hours, after which the clot liquifies again before it finally organises a few days later. If the haemothorax is a large one, and clots continually block the tube, a thoracotomy may be necessary, so refer the patient rapidly.

If this is impractical, try resecting a rib and inserting an open drain (6.1).

If a patient has a severe chest injury and FAILS TO IMPROVE, (his pulse does not fall and his blood pressure does not rise), consider these possibilities:

(1) Has he any other injuries? X-ray him. You may see: (a) Broadening of his mediastinum suggesting an injury to his aorta. (b) The contents of his abdomen in his pleural cavity. (c) Patchy consolidation in one or both lung fields ('wet lung').

(2) Does he have an abdominal injury? Try peritoneal lavage (66.1). It will not interfere with treatment of his chest injury. If you are in any doubt, don't postpone laparotomy.

If BLOOD CONTINUES TO DRAIN from his pleural cavity, a large vessel has probably been injured, perhaps in his lung. Fortunately, this is rare. Replace blood as it is lost. If more than 500 ml drains during the second hour, thoracotomy is indicated. This is fortunately only necessary in about 5% of cases. If you can refer him for a thoracotomy, do so early.

If his HAEMOTHORAX BECOMES infected, treat it as an empyema (6.1).

DRAIN HAEMOTHORACES EARLY AND, IF NECESSARY, REPEATEDLY

65.5 Pneumothorax

A little air in a patient's pleural cavity causes no symptoms. It is slowly absorbed and needs no treatment. Larger

A HAEMOPNEUMOTHORAX

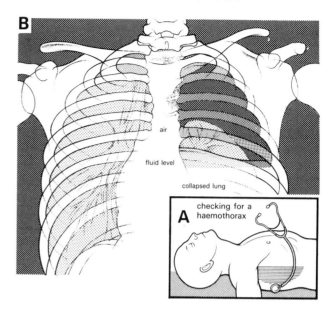

air

fluid level

collapsed lung

checking for a haemothorax

A

Fig. 65-7 HAEMOPNEUMOTHORAX. A, when you examine for a haemothorax, slide your stethoscope under the patient while he is lying down, and listen for reduced air entry. B, this patient's lung has collapsed and he has a fluid level in his pleural cavity. C, if you drain a haemopneumothorax with a single tube, cut side holes in it and push it well up inside the pleural cavity. *Kindly contributed by James Cairns and Peter Bewes.*

pneumothoraces may cause his lung to collapse permanently, so you must drain them. If air enters through a valve—like injury, the pressure in his pleural cavity rises, displaces his mediastinum, and impairs both his respiration and his circulation. If he has dyspnoea, treatment is urgent, and life—saving. Mediastinal shift makes the diagnosis easy—provided you remember to look for it!

You can easily miss pneumothoraces if a patient has multiple injuries, and they can be fatal if you try to anaesthetize him without diagnosing them. So if there is any doubt, X-ray him first.

A pneumothorax can occasionally occur spontaneously, and complicate tuberculosis.

PNEUMOTHORAX

SIMPLE PNEUMOTHORAX

There is no need to insert an intercostal drain unless: (1) The patient is dyspnoeic. Or, (2) there is enough air in his pleural cavity to lower the apex of his lung about 3 cm below the top of his pleural cavity.

TENSION PNEUMOTHORAX

DIAGNOSIS The patient has severe chest pain, severe and increasing dyspnoea, and sometimes cyanosis. His chest on the side of the lesion is hyper—resonant with poor respiratory movements, and absent breath sounds. His trachea and apex beat are deviated to the other side. Sometimes he has severe abdominal pain which may confuse the diagnosis.

X-RAYS are characteristic, but you have no time to look for them. On the affected side there is: (1) collapse of the lung, (2) the absence of lung markings, (3) flattening of the patient's diaphragm, and (4) widening of his intercostal spaces.

EMERGENCY TREATMENT ANYWHERE Let out the air with a large needle, or with any convenient instrument. This may be life—saving, so don't wait for an X-ray. Take the largest needle you can find; in a real emergency there may not be time

167

SOME MORE METHODS

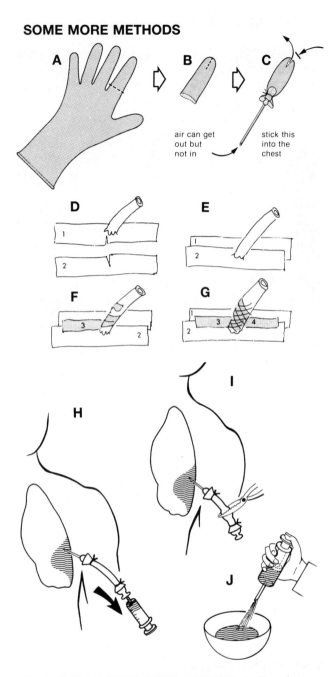

Fig. 65-8 SOME MORE CHEST METHODS. A, B, and C, an emergency one way valve made from the finger of an old glove. D, to G, a method of making sure a chest drain is not pulled out. Cut nicks in two pieces of strapping, lay them round the tube, and overlap them. Stick two narrower pieces of strapping on top of them and twist these round the tube. H, to J, if you don't have a 3–way tap, drain the chest like this. Tie a piece of tube to two needles, aspirate the chest, and clamp the tube while you discharge the syringe. *Kindly contributed by Peter Bewes and James Cairns.*

to sterilize it. Push it through the patient's third intercostal space in his midclavicular line.

The air will hiss out of the needle, his trachea will return to the midline, and he will immediately breathe more easily. He will now live and you can move him. Sometimes this is the only treatment he needs. He usually needs an underwater seal drain.

LATER TREATMENT Follow this emergency treatment by connecting the needle to an underwater seal drain. If none is available, make a valve. Cut the finger off a rubber glove, make a slit in it, and fix it over the adaptor of the needle, as in Fig.

65-8. This valve will let air out, but not in. Don't use it if there is blood in the patient's chest, because it may become blocked. As soon as possible, insert an underwater seal drain.

If there is blood in the pleural cavity, drain this with a second tube through a lower intercostal space posteriorly, as for a haemothorax (65.2).

Deep breathing exercises will help the air to be absorbed.

DIFFICULTIES WITH A PNEUMOTHORAX

If AIR CONTINUES TO BUBBLE OUT OF THE UNDER-WATER SEAL, it may be coming from the patient's lungs, his trachea or his bronchi. X-rays may show that his lung is partly or totally collapsed. Bronchoscopy may show a blood clot in a bronchus and no lumen behind it. If air continues to bubble out of the underwater seal after 5 days, attach a high volume low pressure suction pump to the chest tube. This may expand his lung and bring it up against his chest wall where it may seal itself. Adjust the pressure to produce bubbling only in expiration. If this fails, refer him for thoracotomy and repair of the tear.

If the patient's LUNG HAS STILL NOT EXPANDED weeks or months after the injury he may have an undiagnosed tear in his bronchus. If possible, refer him for bronchoscopy followed by repair of the tear, or lung resection.

IF YOU SUSPECT A TENSION PNEUMOTHORAX,
DON'T WAIT FOR AN X-RAY

65.6 Flail chest

This is one of the really grave emergencies. If a patient is thrown forcefully onto the steering wheel of his car, it may push in part of his rib cage, and break several of his ribs at the front and the back. These fractures may be so aligned with one another that they isolate part of his chest wall. When he inspires, this part of his chest wall moves inwards also (paradoxical movement). He breathes with difficulty, because air can now move from one lung to another, instead of being exhaled. The result is dyspnoea, hypoxia, cyanosis, and carbon dioxide retention, which are especially dangerous if he is older or bronchitic. Multiple fractured ribs cause such great pain and muscle spasm that he tries

THE MECHANISM OF A FLAIL CHEST

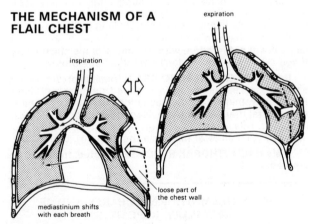

Fig. 65-9 THE MECHANISM OF A FLAIL CHEST. When the patient inspires and his chest expands, the flail section sinks in, and his mediastinum moves towards the normal side. When he expires, the flail section moves out and his mediastinum moves to the other side. The dotted lines show some air moving uselessly from one lung to the other. All this greatly impairs his ability to ventilate his lungs. *Adapted from an original painting by Frank H. Netter, M.D. from THE CIBA COLLECTION OF MEDICAL ILLUSTRATIONS. Copyright by CIBA Pharmaceutical Company, Division of CIBA–GEIGY Corporation.*

not to cough. This encourages fluid to collect in his lungs and further spoils their function. Tragically, paradoxical respiration is often overlooked.

A patient's fractured ribs may be anywhere. Sometimes, the whole front or side of his chest moves paradoxically. Or, he may have extensive fractures on either side of his spine, which allow a large part of his chest wall to be pulled downwards by his diaphragm. Paradoxical movement is less severe when he has fractures at the apex of his rib cage, or under his scapulae, because his shoulder girdle can splint his broken ribs.

Many broken ribs bleed severely, and cause a large haemopneumothorax. Sometimes, a patient's underyling lung is injured so that he has a pneumothorax, perhaps under tension.

The best way of treating the paradoxical movement caused by a flail chest is to use internal pneumatic fixation with IPPR, intubation, and tracheostomy. This has to be continued for several weeks while a patient's ribs unite. IPPR has the added difficulty that it should be combined with careful monitoring of his blood gases. Even if he is skillfully nursed on a respirator, the results of treatment are not good. If IPPR is impractical, you have two alternatives:

(1) You can intubate a patient and control his respiration with a self–inflating bag, while you transfer him to a larger hospital, which has a ventilator.

(2) You can try to fix the floating segment of his chest wall by applying some form of traction for several weeks. Bilateral flail chest is usually fatal without IPPR. But you may be able to treat a patient with a unilateral flail chest, provided he has no serious injures inside his thorax. Unfortunately, most of these patients die. But, if a patient does survive the immediate injury, his outlook is good. Even a permanent dent in his rib cage is unlikely to be important.

A tracheostomy sometimes helps.

FLAIL CHEST

FIRST AID Make sure the patient has a clear airway.

If he now breathes adequately, no further first aid is necessary.

If he is not breathing adequately, try the following methods of keeping the flail segment still until you find one which works.

(1) Gently press it with your hand.

(2) Turn the patient on to his side. This will: (a) keep the flail segment still, (b) keep his uninjured lung uppermost, and (c) prevent blood from his injured lung draining downwards into it.

(3) Support him with strapping or sandbags.

CAUTION ! Don't apply a pad or bandage, because this will only hide the abnormal movement, without stopping it. If necessary intubate him and inflate him with a self–inflating bag.

If possible, refer him.

If you cannot refer him, he will certainly need a chest drain and an underwater seal.

Treat his pain. Intercostal blocks (A 6.7) will help him. A single intravenous morphine injection may make a mildly blue, anoxic, sweating patient quiet and pink. Give it cautiously and don't give more than is necessary.

PREVENTING PARADOXICAL MOVEMENT IN A FLAIL CHEST

Under local anaesthesia, use any of the following methods to apply traction to one, two, or more points on the floating part of the patient's rib cage.

(1) Grip his flail ribs or sternum with several towel clips, or suitable forceps, and then tie these together with string. The clips or forceps must have a ratchet so that they remain closed.

(2) Pass wire or strong sutures under his ribs or sternum.

(3) Screw some sterile cup hooks into his ribs or sternum.

(4) Pass a Steinmann pin under his pectoral muscles close to his ribs, as in B, and C, Fig. 65-10.

Attach cords to any of these traction points, pass them over pulleys, and then tie weights to the cords. Usually, about 500 g per traction point is enough. You may need up to about 5 kg on either side. Fix the pulleys to a frame (70.9), as for fractures.

MANAGEMENT Pay great attention to the patient's breathing. Encourage him to cough and clear his respiratory tract. If loud rhonchi show that fluid is accumulating, consider doing a tracheostomy (52.2).

If the patient's breathing is 'rattly' and he cannot cough. suck out his pharynx. If this fails to clear his airway adequately, try bronchoscopic suction.

If his breathing becomes very weak and shallow, resuscitate him with a self–inflating bag (A 13.1), especially during the first 24 hours.

If he is still bleeding after 24 hours, he needs a thoracotomy to find the bleeding point.

Continue traction until his chest moves as one piece when the weights are temporarily lifted.

DIFFICULTIES WITH A FLAIL CHEST

If a patient has a FLAIL STERNUM, this is particularly serious. He is in great pain and cannot cough, so he retains

TRACTION FOR A FLAIL CHEST

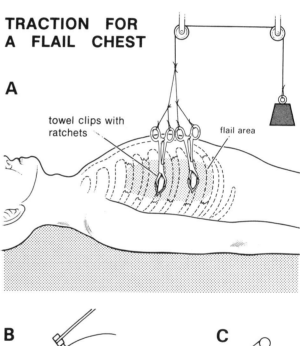

A

towel clips with ratchets

flail area

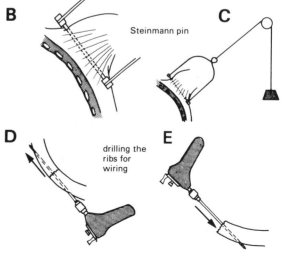

B

Steinmann pin

C

D

drilling the ribs for wiring

E

Fig. 65-10 TRACTION FOR A FLAIL CHEST. Towel clips (A) are usually the most convenient way to apply traction. Or, you can apply it with a Steinmann pin and a stirrup (B and C). If the patient has a severe open injury and is still alive, you can drill his ribs and pass a Kirschner wire through them (D and E). *After de Palma and Peter Bewes.*

his bronchial secretions, and his lungs become oedematous. If you don't have an Abrams pin, use any of the above methods to exert traction on his sternum. Cup hooks are useful.

If he is VERY FAT or muscular traction will be difficult. You may need to expose his ribs and apply it to them directly.

65.7 Open chest wounds

If a patient has an open chest wound, his injured pleural cavity fills with air (sometimes under tension), his lung collapses, he is in great respiratory distress, and he may die. There may be a sucking noise each time he breathes, or froth from his injured lung may come out of the hole in his chest—a sucking chest wound is an extreme emergency.

Teach your ambulance driver to put an occlusive dressing on open chest wounds. These need a surgical toilet, just like any other wound, but the patient's pleural cavity must be closed. Sucking wounds of the chest, including most gunshot wounds, need a thoracotomy. If you cannot refer a patient, you may be able to treat him, as described below.

MIHAIL (47) sustained a severe open chest injury with multiple fractured ribs and a haemopneumothorax. The consultant told his house surgeon to "get on with it". With the help of the anaesthetist he closed the patient's open wound, transfused him, and intubated and anaesthetized him. The house surgeon had never seen a thoracotomy. Even so, he enlarged the chest wound, and toileted it. The anaesthetist was able to get some air into the collapsed lung. The patient's ribs were brought together with Kirschner wire, his chest closed with continuous sutures, and drained with an underwater seal, after which he recovered completely.

OPEN CHEST WOUNDS

Can you hear air being sucked into the patient's pleural cavity each time he breathes? Is his trachea or apex beat displaced? If so he has a sucking chest wound. He may also have a tension pneumothorax.

EMERGENCY TREATMENT Block the hole with a pad made of several thicknesses of vaseline gauze and dry gauze. Keep it in place with adhesive strapping. If this is not available, use anything convenient.

ANAESTHESIA For large injuries intubate the patient and give him trichlorethylene or a ketamine drip with relaxants (A 8.4). For small injuries use intercostal blocks.

OPERATION Clean the patient's wound, and tie off any bleeding vessels. If you decide to probe, do so cautiously. Do a careful wound toilet. You will be wise to leave most foreign bodies where they are. Remove broken fragments of rib and muscle.

Close the patient's pleura. If possible, try to close his wound by suture. If this is not possible, close it with flaps of near by skin and muscle. If necessary, use Kirschner wire to thread together the ends of any fractured ribs.

If the patient's wound is heavily contaminated, close his pleura, but leave his skin wound open for delayed primary closure.

Insert two intercostal drains, one just below his clavicle to remove air, on one just above his diaphragm posteriorly to remove fluid (65.2). If you suture his skin without inserting a drain he may get massive surgical emphysema.

65.8 Stab wounds of the chest

You may have great difficulty deciding how deep a stab wound is, or which organs in a patient's chest or abdomen have been pierced or are bleeding. If there is air or blood in his pleural cavity, drain them. He will need a thoracotomy: (1) If blood continues to drain from his chest, because it may be coming from his lung, or some other organ inside his thorax. (2) If the stab wound is over his heart or the great vessels at the root of his neck. (3) When an underwater seal drain has failed to slow the loss of blood.

ASPIRATING THE PERICARDIUM

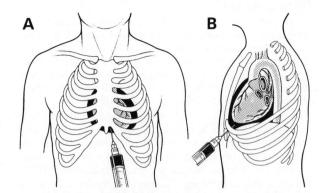

Fig. 65-11 ASPIRATING A PATIENT'S PERICARDIUM from under his xiphoid process. *After Naclerio, with kind permission.*

If there is the slightest possibility that the stab wound might have gone through a patient's diaphragm, explore his abdomen, and repair any injured abdominal organs. You do not want to find faeces coming out of a chest tube!

MANY ABDOMINAL ORGANS LIE UNDER THE RIBS!

65.9 Cardiac tamponade

This rare, treatable emergency usually follows a penetrating chest injury, or occasionally a blunt one, which causes bleeding into the patient's pericardial cavity. This prevents his heart filling normally, which: (1) raises his jugular venous pressure, (2) makes his heart sounds faint, (3) causes pulsus paradoxus. Normally, the peripheral pulse becomes stronger on inspiration, because the lower intrathoracic pressure increases the venous return. In pulsus paradoxus the peripheral pulse is *stronger on expiration*. (4) When there is blood in the pericardial cavity, X-rays show a widening of the heart shadow, especially in the cardiophrenic angle. Screening shows diminished excursion of the borders of the heart. If you can aspirate blood from a patient's pericardial cavity, you may save his life.

CARDIAC TAMPONADE Insert a needle into the patient's pericardial cavity from just under his xiphoid. Alternatively, and less satisfactorily, approach it through his fourth left intercostal space 5 cm from the midline, so as to avoid his internal mammary vessels. Refer him for thoracotomy urgently.

65.10 Other difficulties with a chest injury

There are three important difficulties, the collapse of a lung, traumatic asphyxia, and surgical oedema. Collapse is much the most common; traumatic asphyxia and surgical emphysema are alarming rather than serious.

OTHER DIFFICULTIES WITH A CHEST INJURY

If a whole lobe of a patient's LUNG FAILS TO EXPAND when you insert an underwater seal drain, he is suffering from PULMONARY COLLAPSE. This is partly due to retained secretions, which is why trying to get a patient with a chest injury to cough is so important, painful although this may be. If he will not cough out retained secretions, aspirate them.

If you have failed to prevent collapse, first try physiotherapy (65.1). Encourage him to breathe deeply and cough. If this fails, bronchoscope him within an hour. If you cannot do this, pass a sterile rubber catheter or bougie into his unanaesthetized larynx to start him coughing. If he has to be bronchoscoped more than twice, do a tracheostomy, so that you can aspirate secretions regularly with a fine catheter. Oxygen and antibiotics are only of minor value. Collapse of a lung is common and can complicate any severe chest injury.

If a patient's whole head and arms are COVERED WITH PETECHIAE, he is suffering from TRAUMATIC ASPHYXIA. In this rare syndrome violent compression of his chest forces blood into the veins of his head, neck, and arms. Small blood vessels burst and cover his skin with petechiae. He may also have retinal and conjunctival haemorrhages, and become unconscious. Provided he recovers from any other injuries he may have, traumatic asphyxia is not in itself serious. Sit him up in bed and give him oxygen.

If his FACE SWELLS ALARMINGLY, as in Fig. 65-1, and there is a crepitant swelling under the skin and muscles of his neck, he is suffering from SURGICAL EMPHYSEMA. This is common, but it is seldom serious in itself, and soon disappears. He may swell from his pelvis to his forehead. If his eyelids are swollen and he has difficulty seeing, show him how he can milk the air out of them. Where necessary, treat the underlying cause. This may be a leak from a lung that requires an underwater seal. You can remove small quantities of air by massaging it into a few pockets, and then aspirating it with a syringe and needle. If surgical emphysema spreads or threatens his life, do a tracheostomy. This abolishes coughing and the large rises in intrathoracic pressure it causes.

If air escapes into his mediastinium and pleura from tears in his trachea, oesophagus, or bronchi, it may press on the veins at the base of his neck and congest the veins of his head. Insert an underwater drain and seal and remove the air trapped in his pleura. This may cure him.

66 The abdomen

66.1 The general method for an abdominal injury

The organs in a patient's abdomen can be injured by a stab from a sharp object, or a blow from a blunt one. As Hippocrates knew, the gut can be ruptured, even if there is no visible mark on the abdominal wall. A patient can die from bleeding into his peritoneal cavity, especially from rupture of his spleen or liver, or from a leaking gut. Your main tasks are: (1) to diagnose that a patient has an abdominal injury, (2) to stop it bleeding, (3) to suture his injured small gut. Occasionally, (4) you will need to exteriorize his injured large gut. He has at least a 50% chance of having at least one other severe injury, so you will have to treat that too.

Blunt injuries are particularly difficult because: (1) A patient may give no clear history that he has had an abdominal injury, especially if he is a frightened child. His injury may be so mild that you have to question him carefully, and he may even walk into hospital. (2) His other more obvious injuries, such as a fractured femur, may distract your attention. (3) He may be drunk, or unconscious from a head injury and unable to tell you his symptoms. If you anaesthetize him to treat his other injuries, he cannot complain of increasing abdominal pain. (4) For the first few hours after a blunt injury his abdomen may be deceptively normal. Although a haemoperitoneum usually causes pain, tenderness, guarding, and absent bowel sounds, it occasionally causes none of these things, especially in children. (5) Distinguishing between muscle pain and peritoneal irritation can

be very difficult. (6) Some injuries may not show themselves for several days, especially a subcapsular haematoma of the spleen, or a retroperitoneal injury of the pancreas or duodenum.

For all these reasons, abdominal injuries need particular judgement, care, and skill. So, be vigilant and suspicious. You will need a watchful eye, a light touch, and a sympathetic ear. Don't let a patient go home if there is even a slight possibility that he might have injured his abdomen. If you are in any doubt, observe him carefully and use the special methods described below. They will be particularly useful if he also has a head injury, and may indeed save his life. The decision to operate will be much more difficult if you have already anaesthetized him to reduce a fracture, and he is already on traction or in a cast. If he is going to need a laparotomy, try to do it early.

MURAVULAL was a sailor who fell on to a crate. In the casualty department no injuries were found and his blood pressure was normal. However, the casualty officer was worried about the possibility of an abdominal injury, because there was an abrasion on his epigastrium, so she admitted him. When the registrar saw him in the ward half an hour later he was severely shocked. Urgent laparotomy revealed a ruptured spleen.

MOHAN (25) had been kicked in the abdomen during a fight. His abdomen was bruised and abraded, but he did not look as if he had been seriously injured. The medical assistant who saw him gave him aspirin and sent him home. Three days later he was admitted with severe peritonitis. A quantity of pus and intestinal contents were removed from his abdomen, but he died soon afterwards. LESSONS (1) Any abdominal abrasion after a blunt injury should make you suspect an internal injury. (2) A young adult can maintain his blood pressure for some hours after an injury, and it may even rise before it falls catastrophically.

A CLOSED INJURY CAN EXIST WITHOUT ANY EXTERNAL SIGNS

GENERAL METHOD FOR ABDOMINAL INJURIES

This extends Section 51.3 on the care of a severely injured patient. It is mainly concerned with blunt injuries. For penetrating ones goto Section 66.2.

HISTORY Most abdominal injuries are the results of car accidents, but some follow falls from a height, especially in children.

What object struck the patient's abdomen? Where did it strike him? For example, an injury to his spleen is much more likely after a blow to his left lower chest. How much force was used?

PAIN after an abdominal injury is always important. It is usually present, but a patient may not complain of it if he has even more painful injuries elsewhere.

Where is the pain? What kind of pain is it? Is it getting better or worse? If pain is getting worse after an abdominal injury, it probably means continued bleeding, or a leaking gut.

Has the patient got pain at the tips of either of his shoulders? (make sure that this is not caused by an injured shoulder). Shoulder tip pain is caused by irritation of his diaphragm, usually by blood. It is a particularly useful sign of injury to the liver (right shoulder) or the spleen (left

A SEVERE ABDOMINAL INJURY

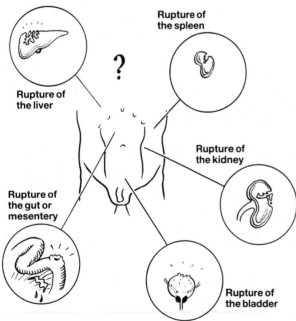

Fig. 66-1 AN ABDOMINAL INJURY can injure a patient's spleen, his liver, his gut, his kidneys, or his bladder. *Kindly contributed by Peter Bewes.*

shoulder), especially if tilting the patient's head down makes it worse.

CAUTION ! Almost all patients with abdominal lesions after a blunt injury have persistant pain, and vomit. So these are very important signs. To begin with they may be almost the only ones.

THE EXAMINATION OF AN ABDOMINAL INJURY

If the patient is bleeding, he is likely to be pale, anxious, and still, with cold extremities. Completely uncover his chest and abdomen and sit beside him.

How is he breathing? Shallow, irregular, or grunting respiration is typical of an abdominal injury.

Look for bruises and abrasions. They will show you where he was hit.

Feel for tenderness. This is less marked with a haemoperitoneum than it is with septic peritonitis. Its position may guide you as to which organ has been injured. Increasing tenderness usually requires a laparotomy.

Rebound tendernesss is unreliable and is easily confused with muscle bruising. Pain on coughing and on percussion with your finger tips is much more reliable.

Feel for guarding and rigidity. Guarding progressing to rigidity is a reliable sign of peritonitis. Percuss the patient's flanks for the dullness that may indicate a haemoperitoneum. Test for shifting dullness.

CAUTION ! Even minimal tenderness and guarding are significant.

Listen for bowel sounds for 2 minutes. If you hear them, they mean nothing. When you first examine a patient, his abdomen will probably not have had time to become silent. However, an abdomen which is silent, or becomes silent later, is a useful sign of peritonitis.

Has the patient any signs of fractured ribs (65.1)? If his lower left ribs are fractured, suspect a ruptured spleen. Thoraco–abdominal injuries are common. Cyanosis is a dangerous sign.

Examine him rectally. If the patient is a woman, examine her vaginally while she is lying on her back, then examine her rectally. Look also for blood on your glove. Fullness or tenderness in the recto–vaginal pouch in a woman or the recto–vesical pouch in a man may indicate a haemoperitoneum. Look for wounds of the perineum or buttocks at the same time.

CAUTION ! The rectum is completely out of sight at laparotomy. To begin with its injuries may cause no symptoms. If necessary, pass a sigmoidoscope.

Aspirate the patient's stomach and empty his bladder. If you aspirate blood, his stomach may have been injured. Leave the nasogastric tube down. You will want it later when he goes to the theatre.

HAS HE LOST MORE BLOOD THAN CAN BE ACCOUNTED FOR BY HIS KNOWN INJURIES? This is good evidence for abdominal (or thoracic) bleeding. Assess it by the methods in Section 53.2.

SHOULD YOU ADMIT THE PATIENT?

Admit and observe him if you think he *might* have an abdominal injury. Half the patients you admit will not have one, but you may save the lives of the other half. If his nose is cold (53.2), be sure to admit him.

SPECIAL METHODS FOR ABDOMINAL INJURIES

These are for doubtful or difficult cases only. Where there are signs that indicate the need for a laparotomy, these methods are quite unnecessary. A positive result in any of them is an indication for an abdominal injury.

TEST FOR ORTHOSTATIC HYPOTENSION This may be useful if a patient has no other obvious cause of blood loss.

Take his pulse and blood pressure while he is lying flat. Then take it again when he is sitting up. While he is lying flat, his circulation may seem to be compensated. But sitting him up may produce a sharp fall in blood pressure, and an increase in his pulse rate. This shows that his blood volume is depleted.

TWO TESTS FOR AN ABDOMINAL INJURY

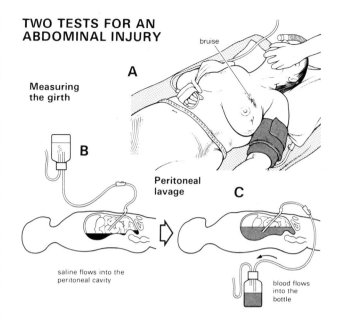

Fig. 66-2 TWO TESTS FOR AN ABDOMINAL INJURY. A, the patient's abdominal girth is being measured. She is being given oxygen. Note the bruise on her chest, the drip, and the sphygmomanometer. B, and C, peritoneal lavage. Saline is being introduced into her peritoneal cavity (B), and returns, blood stained, under gravity (C). *Partly from 'Techniques elementaire pour Medecins isolés', with kind permission.*

TEST FOR INCREASING GIRTH Note any initial distension and measure the patient's abdomen with a tape measure at his umbilicus. An increase in his girth will be a useful sign of the paralytic ileus that follows peritonitis or haemoperitoneum. So take a base line measurement now. An increase of only 2 or 3 cm indicates a large amount of abdominal fluid or gas. This test only works if: (1) You always measure his girth at the same place (mark it on his skin with a pen). (2) He has a nasogastric tube down. Without a nasogastric tube, swallowed air in his stomach can cause a false positive result. It will also prevent acute gastric dilatation, which may mimic a more serious lesion.

DIAGNOSTIC PARACENTESIS ('Four quadrant tap') This is a useful rapid test. Some surgeons omit it and proceed immediately with peritoneal lavage.

Take a syringe and a 1.4 mm needle. Under local anaesthesia, or no anaesthesia at all, and using an aseptic no–touch technique, tap all four quadrants of the patient's abdomen as in Fig. 66-3. Push the needle through his abdominal wall until the sudden give shows that you are just inside his peritoneal cavity, then aspirate.

If aspiration is negative, take the needle out, roll him towards the side of the suspected injury, and repeat the test.

If aspiration is still negative, repeat it in an hour or two, or try lavage as described below.

CAUTION ! (1) Although the blood from a haemoperitoneum is usually defibrinated and does not clot, there is always a chance that it may do so. A negative result does not exclude an abdominal injury. If necessary, repeat the tap in an hour or two.

This test is useful on other occasions (6.2). You may occasionally aspirate urine (from a ruptured bladder), cloudy or bile stained fluid (from a perforated gut or peptic ulcer), or pus (in primary peritonitis). If you are in doubt, examine a Gram film, and look for bacteria, leucocytes, or food.

PERITONEAL LAVAGE Many surgeons would say that if lavage is necessary, you should explore a patient's abdomen anyway. An unnecessary lavage wastes time. Lavage is useful if you are in doubt whether a laparotomy is necessary or not, especially if: (1) A patient is unconscious and cannot complain of pain. (2) He has multiple injuries and you want to assess priorities. (3) You have to take him to the theatre to

DIAGNOSTIC PARACENTESIS

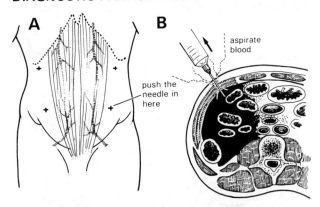

Fig. 66-3 THE FOUR QUADRANT TAP. A negative result does not exclude an abdominal injury. *Origin unknown.*

anaesthetize him for some other procedure, and if there is any suspicion that he might have an abdominal injury.

Catheterize his bladder. Prepare and drape his abdomen. Use lignocaine to infiltrate an area in the midline 2.5 cm below his umbilicus down to his peritoneum.

Use a scalpel to make a small nick down to his peritoneum. Using turning movements, push a trocar and cannula into his abdominal wall. You will feel a sudden 'give' as it goes into his abdomen.

Ideally, push a peritoneal dialysis catheter through the cannula and then withdraw the cannula. Or, use the tubing from an infusion set with a few extra side holes cut near its tip.

If blood flows up through the tube, you have confirmed a haemoperitoneum.

If nothing happens, connect the cannula or tube to a drip set and infuse 500 ml of warm saline into his peritoneal cavity for 10 minutes. While this is going in, tilt him up and down and from side to side to spread the saline round his abdominal cavity.

Lower the infusion bottle to the floor before it is completely empty, so that some saline syphons back. If blood or bile comes back in the fluid, he has an abdominal injury. The test is a little oversensitive: a trace of blood in the saline is unimportant. But, if you cannot read newsprint through the clear plastic tubing, he needs a laparotomy.

CAUTION ! A negative result does not exclude an abdominal injury.

CULDOCENTESIS is one of the most useful and accurate ways of confirming intraperitoneal bleeding in a woman (Fig. 16-4). If you aspirate more than 1 or 2 ml of blood which does not clot, she has a haemoperitoneum.

OTHER TESTS IN AN ABDOMINAL INJURY

URINE Examine this for blood from a bruised kidney or a ruptured bladder.

WHITE CELL COUNT A leucocytosis of 15,000 or more is common with a haemoperitoneum. The rupture of a hollow viscus does not usually raise the white count so high. A leucocytosis is more useful than a low haemoglobin or haematocrit. A patient will not become anaemic until there has been time for his blood to dilute.

X-RAYS Take erect films of a patient's chest and abdomen. If he cannot sit up, take a lateral film while he is lying on his side. Another good X-ray is to turn the patient on his left side and take an AP view of his liver area.

Look for: (1) His stomach and splenic flexure pushed medially. (2) Herniated viscera in his pleural cavities due to rupture of his diaphragm. (3) Fractures of his lower ribs, suggesting a crush injury to his spleen or liver. (4) Gas under his diaphragm, as in Fig. 66-4, indicating rupture of his gut. (5) Peritoneal effusions. (6) Bullets or foreign bodies. (7) Fluid (or fluid and air) in his pleural cavities. These are signs of a

GAS IN THE ABDOMINAL CAVITY

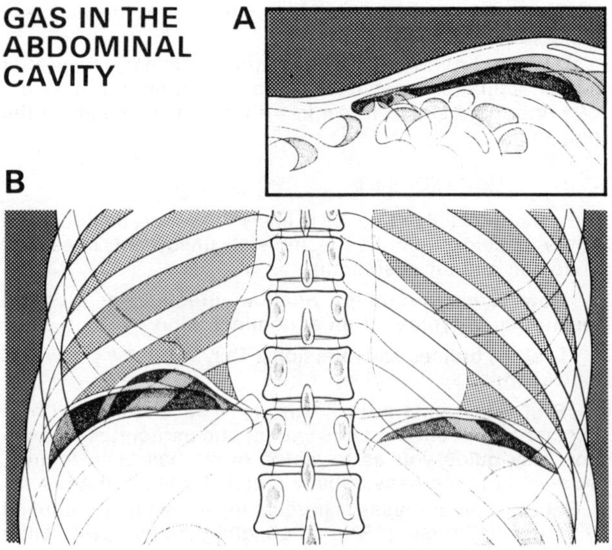

Fig. 66-4 GAS IN THE ABDOMINAL CAVITY. A, a supine lateral film showing gas under a patient's abdominal wall. B, an erect PA film showing gas under his diaphragm.

thoracic injury. If you suspect he has ruptured his bladder or urethra, X-ray his pelvis. (8) A grey 'ground glass' appearance between loops of small gut may be the first sign of a haemoperitoneum.

Ruptured spleen Signs include: (1) A raised left hemidiaphragm. (2) Indentation of his stomach. (3) An opacity in his left hypochondrium. (4) His transverse colon displaced downwards. (5) Displacement of his gastric gas shadow.

Always review X-ray films in the light of what subsequently happened. Next time you will recognize the signs in time.

THE MANAGEMENT OF ABDOMINAL INJURIES

The critical question is, should you do a laparotomy or not? Close observation and repeated examination is the main way to decide this. If you decide to do one, goto Section 66.2 for a penetrating injury, and to 66.3 for a blunt one.

Examine the patient every half hour. Watch for a rising pulse, restlessness, an increase in his girth, and deterioration in his general condition. It may be stable for a long time and then deteriorate rapidly. Don't wait too long, because the difference between the results of the best and the worst surgery is much less than that between early and late surgery.

CAUTION ! (1) If you do decide to operate, do so immediately. Don't delay longer than is necessary to organize the theatre and cross match more blood. (2) If you are in doubt as to whether to operate or not, be safe—operate.

REFERRAL Either refer the patient immediately, so that he can be operated on in a few hours, or operate yourself.

THE FURTHER MANAGEMENT OF ABDOMINAL INJURIES

Read on for: penetrating abdominal injuries (66.2), laparotomy (66.3), rupture of a patient's abdominal wall (66.4), rupture of his diaphragm (66.5), rupture of his spleen (66.6), rupture of his liver (66.7), stomach injuries (66.8), small gut injuries (66.9), injuries to his mesentery (66.10), large gut injuries (66.11), injuries of his caecum (66.12), injuries of his right colon (66.13), injuries of his transverse and descending colon (66.14), rectal injuries (66.15), duodenal injuries (66.16), pancreatic injuries (66.17), gall bladder injuries (66.18), other difficulties with an abdominal injury (66.19).

If a patient is unconscious, the diagnosis of abdominal bleeding will be difficult. Look for: abdominal distension, fluid in his abdomen as shown by shifting dullness, absent bowel sounds, a positive test on paracentesis, a fall in blood pressure, an unaccountable loss of blood (53.2), and the development of oliguria. These are all gross signs when well developed, so watch for them in their earliest stages.

If he develops an ileus or acute intestinal obstruction a few days after admission, operate, he may have an intestinal injury and be developing peritonitis.

For more difficulties, goto Section 66.19.

66.2 Penetrating abdominal injuries

If a patient has an abdominal skin wound the important questions to decide are: (1) Has it entered his peritoneal cavity? (2) Has it done any damage which requires surgery? Knives, bullets, or the horn of an animal can all penetrate the abdomen. It is the depth of a wound that matters, not its length. More severe injuries are often multiple and may penetrate a patient's thorax as well as his abdomen, as with the arrow in Fig. 66-6. Stab wounds and bullet wounds differ.

Stab wounds from knives and daggers follow a predictable path; only the organs through which the weapon passes are injured, and a laparotomy may not be necessary.

Bullets may follow an unpredictable path, may change direction, and cause widespread damage. The higher their velocity the worse this is. Bullets almost always cause serious visceral injuries, so operate on *all* bullet wounds.

If you select patients with penetrating wounds wisely, *and observe them all carefully,* about a third of them will not need a laparotomy. Be guided by the nature of the injury and the force used. If you try to treat a patient conservatively, monitor him carefully. Increasing pain, shock, and signs of peritonitis will tell you when to operate. Time is critical. Few patients survive if peritonitis has been developing for 16 hours, but most will live if you can operate in the first 6 hours.

Before starting to operate on a patient with a bullet wound, think carefully about the structures that it may have injured in its path between entering and leaving the abdomen. If it remains inside, see where it is in at least two X-rays taken from different directions. A patient may be grateful for the time you spend reviewing his anatomy.

AMOS (6 years) was playing on a child's slide. He went down on his front, feet first, and subsequently complained of abdominal pain. There was a small lacerated wound on his abdominal wall near his umbilicus. The signs of general peritonitis developed and laparotomy showed a splinter of wood 15 cm long and 3 cm wide, which had entered his abdomen and penetrated the anterior wall of his stomach. This was removed and he recovered.

PENETRATING ABDOMINAL INJURIES

This extends the general method for abdominal injuries in Section 66.1. Much of the section on blunt injuries (66.3), and eviscerating injuries (66.4), also applies.

If a knife, or any other penetrating object, is still in place, leave it there until you reach the theatre, as in Figs. 66-5 and 66-6.

Work out the track of the wound. Wounds can enter a patient's abdomen from his back, his chest, his buttocks, or his thigh.

If he might have a thoraco–abdominal injury, examine him for a haemothorax, or a haemopneumothorax (65.4).

Look for blood in the patient's urine and gastric aspirate. If he has haematuria, do an intravenous pyelogram.

THE CONSERVATIVE TREATMENT OF PENETRATING ABDOMINAL INJURIES

In the absence of any of the indications for laparotomy listed in Section 66.3, you may be able to manage a patient with a stab wound conservatively.

Record his pulse and blood pressure half hourly. Watch him closely. Operate if he shows signs of bleeding or peritoneal irritation.

A PENETRATING ABDOMINAL INJURY

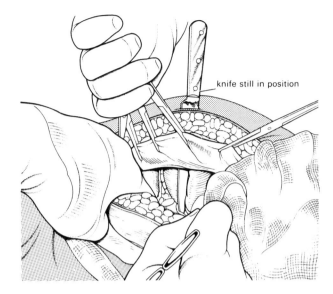

knife still in position

Fig. 66-5 A PENETRATING ABDOMINAL INJURY, illustrating the value of making a separate incision which enables you to see the track of the knife. Note that the knife was left in place until the patient reached the theatre. *Kindly contributed by Peter Bewes.*

THE OPERATIVE TREATMENT OF PENETRATING ABDOMINAL INJURIES

LOCAL TREATMENT When you operate, explore the patient's stab wound in the theatre and excise it down to his peritoneum. Open up the plane between his transversus and his peritoneum over a reasonable area and look at it.

If his peritoneum is intact, close his wound by immediate or delayed primary suture.

If his peritoneum has been opened, do a laparotomy, through a standard incision, and examine any organ which might have been injured.

If a plug of omentum protrudes through the wound, enlarge it, explore it, and make sure there are no injured viscera underneath.

If you have to get into his abdomen in a hurry, make a long midline or paramedian incision.

CAUTION ! As a general rule, don't try to explore the abdomen by extending the wound from the original injury. You will run into anatomical difficulties. Make a separate laparotomy incision.

Continue as with a laparotomy for a blunt injury, as described in the next section.

Always try to close the patient's peritoneum. Close the muscle layers as best you can. If necessary, you can close them as a single layer. If the skin wound of the original injury was contaminated, leave it open for delayed primary suture.

If you cannot close the peritoneum, goto Section 66.4.

66.3 Laparotomy for abdominal injuries

If you suspect that a patient might have an abdominal injury, don't be afraid to do a laparotomy, and don't delay. An occasional negative laparotomy is better than always waiting for some obvious indication of an abdominal injury. He will not die from a big incision, but he will die if you overlook a serious injury. If necessary, watch him carefully for at least 24 hours. The commonest causes of a haemoperitoneum are injuries to a patient's spleen, liver, and mesentery. So search for them in that order. Even if you find no free blood or intestinal contents, he may still have a small perforation, which is temporarily sealed off. So search his abdominal organs carefully.

Try to find and treat *all* the patient's injuries. Don't try to do this through an incision which is much too small. Although he may only have a tiny bullet hole in his abdominal wall, you will probably need a long incision to find all the harm it has done. Adequate exposure may save your time and his life.

Severe haemorrhage can be difficult to control. The secret is to control it temporarily with pressure, packing, and patience—especially patience. Then, slowly and carefully try to find the bleeding site. This is much better than frantic efforts to clamp bleeding points, regardless of the blood that is being lost while you try to do this. If bleeding is so severe that blood wells up in the wound, try packing, and pressure, if necessary on a major vessel. Be patient, and find another assistant to help you. Good relaxation will make the bleeding site easier to find; so will packing away the viscera, extending your incision, and tilting the table.

FIND AND TREAT ALL INJURIES
'PRESSURE, PACKING AND PATIENCE'

LAPAROTOMY FOR AN ABDOMINAL INJURY

Here are the common steps in any abdominal injury. Read on for the care of particular injuries. If the patient has a penetrating injury, consult Section 66.2 first.

INDICATIONS FOR LAPAROTOMY Always do an early laparotomy for: (1) Signs of internal bleeding, as shown by a rising pulse rate, restlessness, and pallor. (2) Increasing guarding, tenderness (including rebound tenderness) or rigidity (regardless of the bowel sounds). (3) All bullet and grenade wounds. (4) Herniation of a patient's viscera through his diaphragm, or his abdominal wall, even if there is only a tag of omentum protruding. (5) Thoraco–abdominal wounds. (6) Haematemesis, blood in his gastric aspirate (provided this is not obviously from his mouth or nose), or rectal bleeding. (7) Penetrating anal or vaginal injuries. (8) Positive findings on paracentesis or gastric lavage, or an increasing girth.

Many stab wounds don't need a laparotomy (66.2).

CAUTION ! (1) More harm is done by not exploring than by doing so. (2) You will not know the extent of an abdominal injury until you get inside the patient's abdomen, so, if referral is possible, you may be wise to resuscitate a patient with fluid and blood and refer him.

A PENETRATING THORACID-ABDOMINAL INJURY

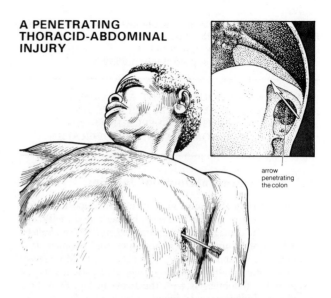

arrow penetrating the colon

Fig. 66-6 A PENETRATING THORACO–ABDOMINAL INJURY. Note that the arrow only appears to have gone into the patient's chest, but has in fact entered his stomach. *Kindly contributed by Peter Bewes.*

RESUSCITATION Set up a really good intravenous drip (A 15.2). Cross–match several units of blood. If this is scarce, and the patient's condition allows it, don't give it until you have clamped the bleeding vessel. Meanwhile give him Ringer's lactate or saline; if necessary, give him 3 or 4 litres of fluid over an hour or two as in Section 53.2.

CAUTION ! Operate as soon as you have got the maximum benefit from resuscitation. But if bleeding exceeds all your efforts at blood replacment, operate urgently to control it.

EQUIPMENT A general set (4.11). Use long instruments to enable you to work deep in the patient's abdominal cavity. Have the equipment for autotransfusion ready (16.11). Effective suction is essential.

Find a strong assistant to help with traction.

GASTRIC ASPIRATION If you have not already aspirated the patient's stomach, do so and leave the tube in. An empty stomach will make splenectomy easier. In bladder injuries, pass a Foley catheter and leave that in too.

PERIOPERATIVE ANTIBIOTICS If the patient's peritoneal cavity does become infected, Gram negative bacilli and

EXPLORING THE ABDOMEN — ONE

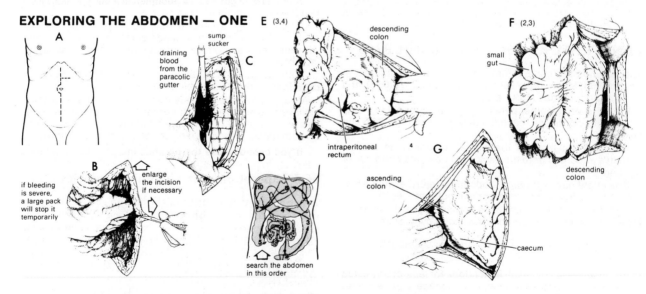

Fig 66-7 EXPLORING THE ABDOMEN—ONE. A, median incision, extended if necessary. B, control severe bleeding temporarily with a pack. C, suck blood out of the patient's left paracolic gutter. D, follow this plan to search his abdomen. E, his rectum, sigmoid, and ascending colon. F, explore his splenic flexure and his transverse colon. G, explore his caecum. *With the kind permission of Hugh Dudley*

anaerobes will probably be responsible—see Section 2.7. *Timing is critical.* Give him chloramphenicol with metronidazole. Give these intravenously *as soon as you suspect contamination of his peritoneal cavity from rupture of his gut.* Give them with the premedication.

If laparotomy shows no contamination, stop them immediately.

If contamination of the peritoneum occurs during surgery, but is not going to continue, as with resection of the colon, stop the patient's antibiotics after 12 hours.

If there is established infection, as with a perforation of 6 hours duration or more, continue antibiotics for 5 days.

CAUTION ! (1) It is much more important to start antibiotics early than to continue for long. Starting them after the patient returns to the ward is certainly too late. (2) This perioperative regime is always indicated if the operative field is, or will be, significantly contaminated. (3) Avoid gentamicin because it interferes with the reversal of some relaxants (A 14.3).

ANAESTHESIA The patient's stomach may be full of food and drink. You will need good muscular relaxation. So a combination of ketamine, suxamethonium, cricoid pressure, intubation, gallamine, and ether or trichlorothylene is probably best (A 14.3). Don't give him a relaxant until you are ready to open his abdomen and tie the bleeding vessel. The relaxant may promote bleeding by destroying the splinting effect of his muscles.

If a patient is drowsy from a head injury, and needs a laparotomy, don't be deterred from giving him a general anaesthetic.

If a patient's respiration is embarrassed because there is much blood in his pleural cavity, drain it under local anaesthesia, before you anaesthetize him. If an intercostal drain does not improve his respiration adequately, he should, ideally, have a thoracotomy before his laparotomy.

If he is so weak that he will not withstand a general anaesthetic, you may have to operate under local anaesthesia.

OTHER WOUNDS If a patient has serious wounds on his back explore these first. The problem if you leave them until last, is that he may not tolerate lying on his front after a long abdominal operation.

INCISIONS FOR BLUNT INJURIES Aim to get inside the patient's abdomen fast; you can tie bleeding vessels in his abdominal wall later. In general, make a midline or right rectus retracting or rectus splitting incision. Vertical extensions to an incision are easier to close than horizontal ones. So, if necessary, extend a vertical incision from a patient's xiphoid to his pubis. If you want even more exposure, make a T–shaped incision into either flank.

If the injury is in the patient's lower left chest, and the signs indicate a ruptured spleen, make a left upper paramedian incision. If exposure is inadequate, extend it towards his left costal margin.

If necessary, with any incision, tilt the table to make access easier.

INSIDE AN INJURED ABDOMEN

Have the sucker ready as you get inside the patient's abdomen. Watch for a puff of gas as you open it. This indicates an injury of his gut. If the gas smells faecal, he has injured his colon.

If there is blood in his left hypochondrium, you can be almost sure that he has ruptured his spleen.

If there is blood in his right hypochondrium, his liver is probably ruptured.

If there is blood in the middle of his abdomen, his mesentery may have been injured.

If there is bile in his peritoneal cavity (66.18), examine his gall bladder, his duodenum, the rest of his upper small gut, his cystic duct, his common bile duct, and his hepatic ducts.

If there is blood, intestinal juice, and bile in his peritonal cavity, he has probably torn his small gut.

Quickly suck away any free blood and intestinal contents. If you are going to use the blood for autotransfusion, see Section 16.11.

CAUTION ! If the blood in his peritoneal cavity is contaminated by bile or intestinal or pancreatic secretions, don't use it for autotransfusion.

CONTROL BLEEDING Do this before you examine the patient's viscera. If necessary: (1) Grasp or put a clamp across his splenic pedicle. (2) Clamp his mesentery. (3) Pinch the vessels in the free edge of his lesser omentum with your finger in his epiploic foramen.

Suck out the blood from his abdomen.

EXAMINING THE VISCERA IN AN ABDOMINAL INJURY

Examine the patient's abdominal organs systematically. Diagram D in Fig. 66-7 shows one pathway for doing so. Most surgeons have their own routine. Whatever routine you choose, be sure to examine everything.

Unless you find some major bleeding, such as from a ruptured spleen, complete your examination before starting to do any repairs. If you find an injury to the patient's small gut or mesentery, clamp it with a soft intestinal clamp, so that you can easily find it, making sure that it does not leak while you continue your search.

If there is any possibility of an injury to the posterior wall of the patient's stomach or the peritoneum behind it, detach his omentum from the anterior surface of his colon. It has almost no blood vessels. Open his lesser sac, and look at the back of his stomach, the back of his transverse colon, and the front of his pancreas.

If you have reason to suspect that the second part of his duodenum might be injured, (for example, you might see a retroperitoneal haematoma) incise the parietal peritoneum lateral to it, elevate his duodenum, and inspect its posterior wall.

Look for retroperitoneal bruising over the patient's ascending and descending colon.

If necessary, you can reflect his ascending or descending colon by making incisions in his paracolic gutters, and reflecting part of his colon forwards, as in K, and L, Fig. 66-8.

If necessary, you can reflect his duodenum forwards, as in M, Fig. 66-8.

CAUTION ! Don't be content with finding only one injury. He may have many, especially if he has a gunshot injury.

RETROPERITONEAL INJURIES Management depends on the site of the injury.

If the patient has a retroperitoneal haematoma in his flank, it is probably coming from his kidney (67.1). If possible, leave it. Don't open any retroperitoneal haematoma, unless you are obliged to.

If he has a haematoma near his duodenum or colon, these organs are probably injured retroperitoneally and need to be explored, if possible without contaminating the adjacent peritoneal cavity.

For haematomas of the mesentery and pelvic mesocolon, goto Section 66.10.

GUNSHOT WOUNDS Search meticulously for entry and exit wounds in anything that might have been injured. Small bullet wounds in the gut may seal themselves off temporarily. Bullet holes in the colon may be covered with a sheet of omentum which you must lift to find them.

INJURIES TO PARTICULAR VISCERA A a blunt injury is likely to have injured these organs in order of decreasing frequency: the spleen (66.6), the liver (66.7), the mesentery (66.10), the small gut (66.9), the colon (66.11), the kidneys (67.1), or the duodenum and pancreas (66.16 and 66.17).

CLOSING THE ABDOMEN AFTER A LAPAROTOMY

The danger of peritonitis will be reduced if you remove as much pus, intestinal contents, faeces, and blood as you can. So irrigate the patient's peritoneal cavity with *warm* saline before you close it. See Section 6.2. If you don't have any warm saline, mop it out as best you can.

CAUTION ! Bleeding *must* be completely controlled.

When you have closed the patient's peritoneum, irrigate the structures of his abdominal wall thoroughly, and close it with tension sutures of monofilament or stainless steel. If necessary, close it in a single layer.

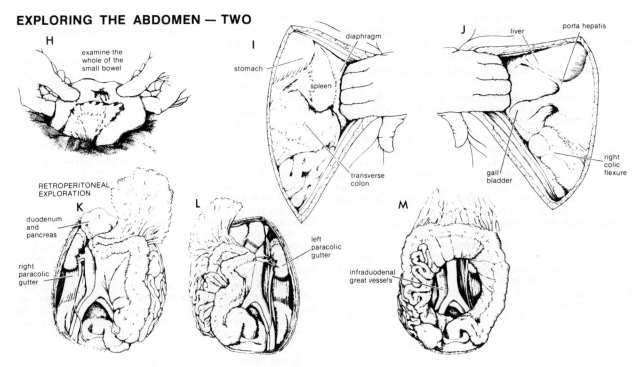

Fig. 66-8 EXPLORING THE ABDOMEN—TWO. H, examine the whole of the patient's small gut from one end to the other. I, draw his colon downwards to expose his left hemidiaphragm, his stomach, and his spleen. J, examine his porta hepatis, duodenum, and right hemidiaphragm. K, if necessary, explore his right paracolic gutter. L, if necessary, explore his left paracolic gutter. M, inspect the back of his abdomen. Note, these are artist's impressions, an injured abdomen never looks as good as this! *With the kind permission of Hugh Dudley.*

If there is much infection, and you expect the wound to disrupt, close the muscles of his abdominal wall with interrupted stainless steel wire or deep tension sutures, and his skin by delayed primary closure, as in Section 9.7.

If infection is present, or you expect it to develop, insert one or more drains through separate incisions. Use wide bore tubes, such as 30 Ch catheters and lead them into sterile bags or bottles (9.7).

RECORDS Sign the patient's notes to the effect that you have examined, and either dealt with or found normal, his diaphragm, stomach, spleen, liver (both surfaces), large gut (including his splenic and hepatic flexures), entire small gut, rectum, bladder, pancreas, kidneys, ureters, and a woman's gynaecological organs. Many surgeons prefer this order of examination to that in Fig. 66-7, and some have a rubber stamp made to this effect.

POSTOPERATIVE CARE Monitor the patient's haemoglobin, and correct his anaemia by transfusion. Continue intravenous fluids and nasogastric suction until bowel function is restablished. His bowel may be paralysed for many days, so monitor his fluid and electrolyte balance carefully. Watch for pelvic and subphrenic abscesses (6.3).

EXPLORE THE ABDOMEN IN A LOGICAL WAY

66.4 Rupture of the abdominal wall (evisceration of the gut)

How are you going to treat a patient who has been gored by a buffalo so severely that gut prolapses through his wounded abdomen? Fortunately, the treatment of this alarming injury is usually straightforward. To begin with he may not be very shocked. Later, loop(s) of gut may strangulate and cause severe shock. Sometimes his injured gut leaks.

EVISCERATED GUT AFTER AN ABDOMINAL INJURY
Resuscitate the patient, pass a nasogastric tube. Cover the exposed loops of gut with a warm saline pack or a towel.

If the patient's gut is strangulating, immediately enlarge his wound under local infiltration anaesthesia (A 5.4) to relieve it.

If his gut is injured and leaking, you can, if necessary, close it temporarily with a non-crushing clamp, or resect it before anaesthetizing him. Gut is insensitive, so he will feel nothing. This will prevent later soiling of the wound.

Anaesthetize him—you will need good muscular relaxation. Paint his abdomen with some gentle antiseptic, such as chlorhexidine, and irrigate the exposed loops of his gut with quantities of saline.

Enlarge his wound in the most appropriate direction to make an incision which most nearly approximates to one of

RUPTURE OF THE DIAPHRAGM

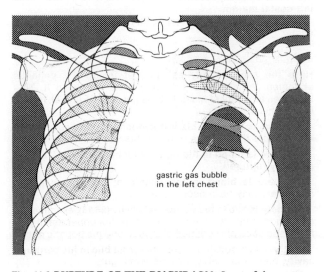

Fig. 66-9 RUPTURE OF THE DIAPHRAGM. Some of the contents of the patient's abdomen are now in his chest, including his stomach, which may contain a gas bubble.

the standard ones, or do a separate standard laparotomy, taking care to miss nothing. You may find several other injuries.

If necessary, revise the emergency closures that you did earlier. To do so, empty the injured section of gut, and apply soft clamps across its base to prevent it filling. Then undo any temporary sutures, freshen the edges of his gut, excise any damaged areas, and do a formal closure or resection, as in Section 9.3.

Always try to close a patient's peritoneum. Close the muscle layers as best you can, and leave his skin open for delayed primary suture. Excise the margins of the original wound.

If returning his viscera to his abdomen and closing it is difficult, try decompressing his small gut. Milk its contents proximally into his stomach, and keep aspirating all the time with a nasogastric tube.

If you cannot close his peritoneum (very unusual), try making long relieving incisions on the sides of his abdomen so that you can close his skin and subcutaneous tissues. Later, refer him for the repair of the muscles of his abdominal wall.

Alternatively: (1) Cover the wound with moist packs. The organs which present in it will granulate, and you can graft them about the fifth day. Refer him for a formal repair later.

ANATOMY FOR SPLENECTOMY

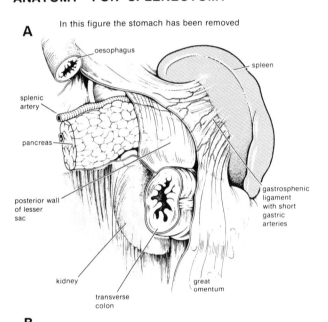

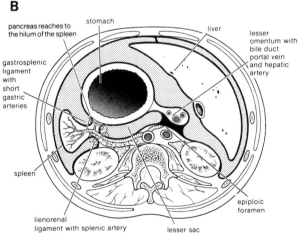

Fig. 66-10 ANATOMY FOR SPLENECTOMY. When you operate you will find a large friable, bloody mass–it will not look quite like this! A, shows the left recess of the patient's lesser sac extending to his spleen. B, shows the vessels that you will have to tie–his splenic artery and his short gastric arteries. When you tie his splenic artery, don't put your ligature round the tail of his pancreas. *After Maingot and Gray, with kind permission.*

Or, (2) make an artificial peritoneum with strong, sterile cloth heavily coated with sterile vaseline, sewn to the margin of the defect. Granulations will slowly grow over it from the edges. Leave the cloth prosthesis in for several days and repeat the procedure as necessary. Graft the granulations with split skin, pending a formal repair.

66.5 Rupture of the diaphragm

A patient's diaphragm more commonly ruptures on the left, so that his viscera herniate into his left chest. This is fortunate, because injuries on the left are more easily repaired. Sometimes his injury is so severe that he can hardly breathe, or it can be so mild that it may not be discovered for several weeks. Exclude rupture of the diaphragm by taking a routine chest X-ray. There are sure to be other injuries also.

RUPTURE OF THE DIAPHRAGM

This is not an easy operation, refer the patient if you can.

If the patient is severely dyspnoeic, try emptying his stomach with a nasogastric tube.

ANAESTHESIA Insert an intercostal drain and anchor it securely to the patient's chest. Give him a general anaesthetic, intubate him, and if possible give him a long–acting relaxant. Avoid distending his stomach.

LAPAROTOMY Divide the left triangular ligament of the patient's liver and draw its left lobe downwards and to the right. Pull his abdominal viscera out of his chest.

Retract the torn margins of his diaphragm downwards, and repair it with heavy interrupted non–absorbable sutures. Use the long ends of each stitch for gentle traction, until you insert the next one. The tear usually extends to his oesophageal hiatus. Repair this with special care.

Connect his chest drain to an underwater seal bottle (65.2), and remove it at 48 hours.

66.6 Injuries of the spleen

Rupture of a patient's spleen gives you one of your best chances of saving his life, and is the major indication for splenectomy in a district hospital. Big malarial spleens rupture readily, but big schistosomal spleens do not.

If a patient ruptures his spleen, you will not have time to refer him. To succeed, you will need to make the diagnosis promptly, resuscitate him vigorously, operate immediately, and expose his spleen adequately. Emergency splenectomy can be difficult, especially when his spleen has stuck to his diaphragm by dense vascular adhesions which bleed briskly.

Usually, a patient's spleen is only torn, but it may be shattered, pulped, or completely avulsed from its pedicle. Symptoms usually develop rapidly, but they may occasionally be delayed for a few hours. Rarely, a haematoma seals off bleeding to begin with, and then suddenly bursts. When this happens, symptoms may be delayed several days or even weeks.

The common mistake is to delay making the diagnosis until too late. Maintain the patient's blood volume. First, give him saline or Ringer's lactate. Then, when you have controlled his bleeding splenic pedicle, give him blood (53.2). Operate urgently.

DELAY IS THE COMMONEST ERROR, EVERY MINUTE MATTERS

The splenic pedicle is in two parts: (1) A fold of peritoneum, the lienorenal ligament, stretches across from its hilum towards the surface of the kidney. In it run the splenic artery and vein, and often the tail of the pancreas also. (2) A second fold of peritoneum, the gastrosplenic ligament, joins the hilum of the spleen to the greater curvature of the stomach. In it run the short gastric arteries. These two ligaments unite to form the pedicle of the spleen. Between them lies the extreme left edge

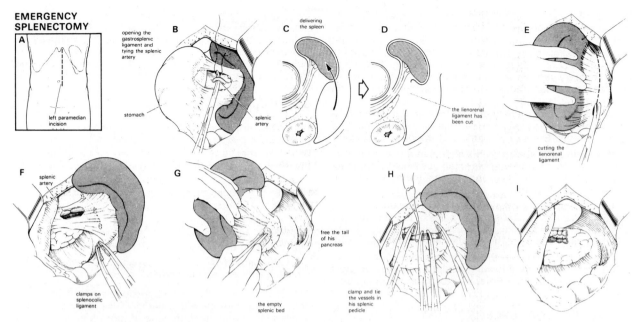

Fig 66-11 EMERGENCY SPLENECTOMY. A, make a left paramedian incision. B, open the patient's gastrosplenic ligament and tie his splenic artery. C, deliver his spleen. D, and E, cut his lienorenal ligament. F, divide his splenocolic ligament. G, reflect his spleen medially and use blunt dissection to separate the tail of the pancreas. H, clamp and tie the vessels in his splenic pedicle individual, so as not to damage the tail of his pancreas by clamping it in a wide pedicle. I, tie his splenic artery again.

of the lesser sac. You can compress the vessels in the splenic pedicle between two fingers, and so stop a spleen bleeding.

Controlling bleeding is the main difficulty. It will be easier if you have good exposure. If you find a huge haematoma, tying off the patient's whole splenic pedicle without first identifying the vessels may be life–saving. But there is a danger that you may tie the tail of his pancreas, or even a fold of his stomach or colon, as you do so. The ligatures are also more likely to slip.

The spleen is not quite the disposable organ that it was once thought to be. The risks of removing it include overwhelming infection, and reduced immunity to malaria, particularly in children. The easiest way of conserving some splenic tissues is to put a few slices under a covering of peritoneum below the left costal margin.

In the following method we advise you to start by opening the gastrosplenic ligament, then tying the splenic artery before rotating the spleen medially, and tying and dividing the vessels in its pedicle individually. In desperation you can start by putting a ligature round the entire splenic pedicle.

RUPTURED SPLEEN

For earlier steps in the operation see Section 66.3. Make sure the patient has a nasogastric tube in his stomach, and a free flowing drip in a big vein.

ANAESTHESIA Good relaxation is necessary. (1) A ketamine drip with a relaxant. (2) Ketamine induction followed by ether with a relaxant. In a grave emergency, when a patient is desperately ill, you may have to remove his spleen under local anaesthesia.

POSITION Lie the patient on his back with his left arm drawn over to his right and his forearm supported on a pad or arm rest. It is sometimes helpful to rotate his thorax to the right with a sandbag under his left chest and pelvis.

INCISION If you are sure that a patient's spleen has ruptured, make a left paramedian, rectus split, or upper midline incision. Otherwise, make a right paramedian or a midline incision.

CONFIRM THAT THE SPLEEN HAS BEEN INJURED
Fresh blood or clots in a patient's left hypochondrium nearly always mean that his spleen has ruptured. Confirm this by

feeling its surface. It should have a smooth surface facing his diaphragm, and a notch on its anterior border. The injury may have torn any of its surfaces, or pulled it off its pedicle. If it is damaged in any way, remove it. If you are not sure if it has been injured or not, extend the incision.

Control bleeding temporarily by compressing his splenic pedicle between the thumb and fingers of your left hand. Save as much blood as you can for autotransfusion (16.11). Keep holding the pedicle until the anaesthetist confirms that the patient is in a satisfactory condition to proceed.

First get at his injured spleen: (1) Tilt him on to his right side. (2) Pack his stomach and his transerve colon out of the way. Ask a strong assistant with a large left hand to draw the patient's stomach and colon downwards, and retract his left costal margin upwards. (3) If necessary, and especially if there are dense adhesions between the spleen and the diaphragm or abdominal wall, extend the incision. Extend a midline incision laterally, by cutting his left rectus through one of its tendinous insertions. If necessary, cut beyond its outer borders.

If you cannot find a tear, look elsewhere in the patient's abdomen. If you still cannot find a tear, return to his spleen, and examine it with more care.

TIE THE SPLENIC PEDICLE

If you are inexperienced and bleeding is severe, deliver the patient's spleen, rotate it forwards, and to the right. Put a thick ligature right round the entire splenic pedicle. This is safer than trying to grasp it with a large clamp. As you do so, try not to damage his stomach, and to cause the least possible damage to his pancreas. When you have controlled bleeding, proceed to tie the vessels individually.

If you are more experienced, use blunt scissors to open up a window in his gastrosplenic ligament, as in B, Fig. 66-11. This will let you into his lesser sac. Feel for his splenic artery along the upper border of his pancreas. Incise the peritoneum over it, pass a haemostat underneath it, and tie it.

Don't divide his splenic artery yet; his splenic vein lies under it—avoid injuring this. Clamp, cut, and tie his short gastric vessels passing from his spleen to the greater curvature of his stomach. Tie them individually using small artery forceps. If you tear them, oversew the wall of his stomach with atraumatic sutures.

CAUTION ! Don't include an area of stomach wall with your ligatures, especially at the upper margin of the spleen.

FREE THE PATIENT'S SPLEEN Feel for his spleen by putting your hand under his diaphragm, and breaking down any light adhesions.

If adhesions are dense, cut them with long curved Metzenbaum scissors, or incise the peritoneum and separate his spleen from his diaphragm extraperitoneally.

Rotate his spleen gently downwards and medially (C). Incise his splenorenal ligament (D). Put your finger into the peritoneal opening and gently free its margin. You can now bring his spleen well outside his abdomen (E).

Divide his splenocolic ligament between curved clamps, taking care to avoid clamping his colon (F).

Reflect his spleen medially and use blunt dissection to separate the tail of his pancreas from his splenic vessels (G). Tie them at the splenic pedicle just before they divide.

Clamp the vessels in his splenic pedicle (H). Pass ligatures of No. 1 linen thread or silk under the vessels of the pedicle, and tie them securely.

For extra security apply a second set of ligatures at the same point.

CAUTION ! Make sure your assistant releases the haemostats *gently and steadily*, as you tighten the ligature, without a sudden click. If the cut vessel drops off and is lost in a pool of blood, you may never find it again.

Bleeding vessels on the diaphragm are small, very persistent, and almost impossible to tie. If possible, use diathermy. Absolute haemostasis is essential.

Put a big dry pack over the patient's splenic bed. Leave it there for a few minutes. Remove it and look for any bleeding vessels, and tie them off.

Look for other abdominal injuries before you close his abdomen.

AUTOTRANSPLANTATION Use a large scalpel to cut two large thin 2 mm slices from the patient's spleen. Incise his parietal peritoneum under his left costal margin, slip the slices in, tie them flat against his intercostal muscles, and sew up the peritoneum over them.

If, 4 weeks later, he has no Howell Jolly bodies, and no target cells in his peripheral blood film, and his platelet count is normal, transplantation has probably succeeded.

DRAINS If: (1) the operative site is absolutely dry, and (2) you are sure you have not injured the tail of the pancreas, there is no need for a drain. Otherwise, place a large corrugated or tube drain down to the tail of the pancreas, and close the wound.

DIFFICULTIES WITH EMERGENCY SPLENECTOMY

If OOZING IS UNCONTROLLABLE, insert a large pack and remove it 48 hours later.

TRANSPLANTING THE SPLEEN

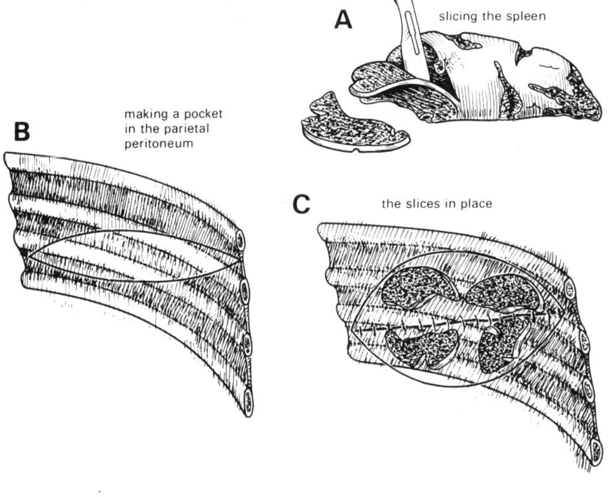

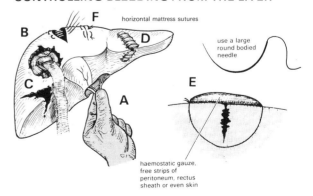

Fig. 66-12 TRANSPLANTING SLICES OF A RUPTURED SPLEEN. A, cutting slices from the injured spleen. B, opening up a window in the parietal peritoneum C, the slices in place. *Kindly contributed by Mervin Hawe.*

If a PATIENT SUDDENLY DETERIORATES postoperatively, a ligature has probably slipped. Operate immediately.

If a SEROUS EFFUSION DEVELOPS in his splenic bed it may resemble a subphrenic abscess; but it usually resolves slowly and spontaneously. If X-rays show that his stomach continues to be displaced, the effusion may need draining.

If VENOUS THROMBOSES OCCUR, they may involve any vein, but they won't be disastrous unless they involve his portal vein. The platelet count always rises after splenectomy and then usually falls without reaching dangerous levels. If possible, check his platelet count at 4 and 8 days. If there are more than 750,000 platelets mm³, give him heparin (5,000 units every 4 hours intravenously depending on his size and his associated injuries).

If his WOUND SLOUGHS and there is a fluid discharge, the tail of his pancreas may have been injured. Reopen the wound and do a suture ligation of his damaged pancreas. Insert a suction drain (9.7).

66.7 Liver injuries

Injuries to a patient's liver resemble those of his spleen with one critical difference—you can remove his entire spleen, but not his liver. Either massive bleeding kills him quickly, despite all you can do to resuscitate him, or signs of an intra–abdominal disaster develop more slowly. If blood immediately floods his whole peritoneal cavity, the signs are general; if bleeding is less severe, the signs are mostly on the right. Pain at the tip of his shoulder is less common than with rupture of his spleen.

The right lobe of the liver is injured more often than the left. You may find: (1) A minor tear, usually without serious bleeding. Most stab wounds are like this. (2) Ragged lacerations with severe bleeding. (3) Tears of the patient's hepatic artery, his portal vein, or his hepatic veins or their major branches. Controlling haemorrhage from these vessels is desperately difficult, and most patients die even in expert hands. If his hepatic veins have been injured, a tape has to be passed round his vena cava above and below their point of entry. They then have to be exposed and sutured—a difficult task.

Happily, not all liver injuries are impossibly difficult. The easier ways of controlling a bleeding liver are: (1) To pinch the vessels in the free edge of the patient's lesser omentum between your fingers temporarily. (2) To pack the tears with gauze for 24 to 36 hours. The main risk of doing this is that severe sepsis may follow. (3) To bind tears together with deep mattress sutures. (4) To use absorbable haemostatic gauze. Experts can excise large parts of the liver, or tie its arteries, relying on the fact that it has two blood supplies—arterial and portal. Even so, their results are usually bad.

The complications, particularly infection, are grave, but a live patient with complications is better than a dead one. The main

CONTROLLING BLEEDING FROM THE LIVER

Fig. 66-13 CONTROLLING BLEEDING FROM THE LIVER. You can pinch the vessels in the free edge of a patient's lesser sac (A), pack his liver (B), or suture a tear (C, D, and E). You can also use horizontal mattress sutures (F).

way to prevent infection is to insert really adequate sump drains (4 to 6 Ch), so that as few clots as possible remain in the patient's abdomen to become infected.

RUPTURED LIVER

For earlier steps in the operation, see Section 66.3.

Blood in the patient's right hypochrondrium is probably coming from his liver. If you have difficulty exposing it, make a T–shaped extension to the right of a median or paramedian incision.

If the patient's liver has stopped bleeding, when you examine it, leave it well alone, and merely drain it.

If his liver is bleeding severely, control it by pinching the free end of his lesser omentum, with your finger in his epiploic foramen (foramen of Winslow). Put your left index through the foramen behind his lesser omentum leaving your thumb in front of it. Pinch his portal vein, his hepatic artery (and his bile ducts) between your fingers. You have 15 minutes to enlarge the incision and get better access to the tear. If necessary, ask an assistant to hold the vessels while you operate.

CAUTION ! The liver can withstand 15 minutes of such ischaemia—not more.

Run your right hand over the dome of the right lobe of the patient's liver and feel for tears, puncture wounds, ragged lacerations, and major blow–outs. Pass your hand as far back as it will go behind the right lobe of his liver, as far as the coronary ligament. Then move it to the left and explore the upper and lower surfaces of the left lobe of his liver in the same way.

SMALL LACERATIONS OF THE LIVER CAPSULE Drain them and leave them.

MINOR TEARS When you first feel a tear, pack it with gauze for 2 or 3 minutes. When you remove it, you can: (1) pick up the bleeding vessels, or (2) coagulate and tie them, or (3) occlude them with through–and–through mattress sutures.

RAGGED LACERATIONS If you are confident in your ability, use your finger and thumb to pinch off any unhealthy, ragged, discoloured pieces of liver. If you leave them they may encourage secondary haemorrhage and sepsis. Small blood vessels and bile ducts will be left behind when you pinch off the liver from around them, so tie or cauterize these. Having done this, you can use either mattress sutures or packs. If you can suture the capsule adequately, it will probably contain the haematoma inside. Don't try to cauterize large areas with diathermy.

If you are less confident, suture the tear, or pack it without doing too much exploring.

A SUBCAPSULAR HAEMATOMA Empty this and oversew it to control bleeding.

SPECIAL METHODS FOR AN INJURED LIVER

Through–and–through mattress sutures are not easy. Use a *large*, semicircular, round bodied needle with No. 1 chromic catgut. Ideally, this should be a special liver needle with a blunt end. Make large through–and–through sutures, to join the edges of the tear together, as in D, and E, Fig. 66-13. Set the stitches back about 1 cm or more from the edge of the tear, and if necessary overlap them. If they cut through the patient's liver, tie them over pieces of haemostatic gauze, or free strips of peritoneum, his rectus sheath, or even pieces of his skin. If possible, pack a piece of haemostatic gauze into a laceration before you suture it.

Packing is a very useful and easy method. Make the pack from a roll of sterile dry, wide gauze. Pack the gauze in one long length into the cavity, and bring the end out through the patient's abdominal wall (B). If you have to use more than one roll, knot them together, so that when you pull out one pack, the other will come out too. Remove the pack very carefully in the theatre 48 hours later. If you are lucky, there will be no significant bleeding.

Except for the smallest wounds insert a large drain to carry away blood and bile from the wound. Don't insert a drain into the bile duct.

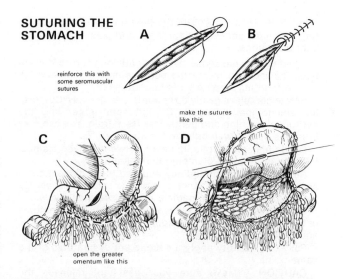

Fig. 66-14 SUTURING A STOMACH WOUND. A, and B, show the method of suturing. C, shows the wound in the anterior wall of the stomach, and D, the wound in its posterior wall. The edges of wound are being held in stay sutures, ready for repair. *With the kind permission of Peter London.*

DIFFICULTIES WITH LIVER INJURIES

If the patient's WOUND DISCHARGES BILE, he has a biliary fistula. This will take a long time to heal, so be patient. See Section 66.18.

If he becomes JAUNDICED, he will probably live, provided he has no other complications. Postoperative jaundice is common in major liver injuries, and usually resolves in about 2 weeks.

If there is a HUGE TEAR in the right lobe of his liver, and its inside feel like porridge, gently scoop it out and remove any broken bits with your fingers. Then put in a huge dry gauze pack. You will need several metres of 10 cm bandages. Alternatively line the cavity with a piece of sterile plastic sheet and fill this with packs. Remove the packs (and the sheet) later. He may live after recovering from many complications, both early and late, including a subphrenic abscess.

66.8 Stomach injuries

The stomach can be penetrated by a missile or by a stab wound. It is very vascular, and its mucosa readily bleeds, so suture it with a continuous suture which compresses the whole length of its mucosal edge.

STOMACH INJURIES

Examine both surfaces of the patient's stomach by opening his lesser sac through his gastrocolic omentum as in C, Fig. 66-14, and turning his stomach upwards so that you can inspect its posterior wall.

First trim the hole, to make sure you are suturing viable mucosa with clean cut edges.

Use 2/0 chromic catgut to close the wound in two layers. Make the first layer an all coats, continuous inverting suture. Make the second layer of continuous Lembert seromuscular sutures (9.3). Close the wound as if you were closing the small gut, except that there is no need for the closure to be transverse to the stomach.

Alternatively, insert a catgut stitch at one end of the hole, and tie it. Now put a running stitch in and out of the stomach all round the hole, closing it as you do so. Put your thumb into the hole to invert the mucosa as you pull up the stitches (this kind of suture does not invert automatically). If possible, try to get all the mucosa inside the stomach. When you have tied the knot, you have closed the hole. Hide the all coats layer of sutures with an extra layer of Lembert sutures (9.3).

PENETRATING SMALL GUT INJURIES - ONE

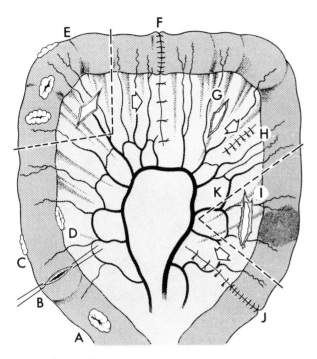

Suturing a laceration

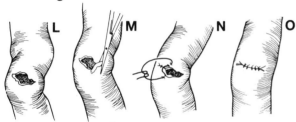

Fig. 66-15 PENETRATING INJURIES OF THE GUT AND MESENTERY may be bullet holes (A) with a similar wound on the other side of the patient's gut. The mucosa protrudes through the wound and there may be little leakage. Close wounds transversely (B) to avoid stenosis. If the wound is on the edge of the gut (C) there may be only one wound. Wounds close to the mesenteric border (D) may be easily missed. If several injuries occur together, or the omentum is injured, excise the injured segment, and anastomose the gut (F). You can suture small tears in the mesentery (G), especially if they run in the direction of the vessels perpendicular to the gut. If the tear is near the edge of the mesentery the circulation to the gut may be impaired (I), so resect the segment (J). The anastomotic arterial arcades (K) are some distance from the gut. Beyond them the arteries are end arteries, so that injuring them may kill the gut they supply. This is a composite diagram. If all these injuries occurred in the same loop, most surgeons would excise the loop altogether.

The lower diagram shows the method of repairing a laceration (L), trimming it (M), inserting the sutures (N), and finally sewing it up transverse to the axis of the gut (O).

66.9 Small gut injuries

Penetrating injuries from bullets or knives can make holes in a patient's small gut and its mesentery. Blunt injuries either tear or burst it by pressing it against his spine.

A patient's abdomen becomes tender after an abdominal injury. You may have difficulty deciding how much of this tenderness is caused by bruising of his abdominal wall, and how much by peritonitis from a ruptured gut. If you are in doubt, the decision *not* to operate is much more dangerous.

Provided the small gut is viable, it has remarkable powers of

repair. Although it may look very deformed and constricted at the end of the operation, it may be quite normal some months later. Although resecting gut does not increase mortality in skilled hands, it does so in less skilled ones. The main danger is a leak, because of poor technique, or sloughing of its wall. If you have a choice, repairing gut is safer than resecting it.

IF IN DOUBT OPERATE

SMALL GUT INJURIES

For earlier steps in the operation, see Section 66.3. For methods of resecting gut, see Section 9.3.

If, when you open the abdomen, there is a moderate amount of blood mixed with bile and intestinal juices, the patient's small gut has been perforated.

If there is no free fluid in his peritoneal cavity, his gut may still have been perforated, so search it carefully. In early cases ileus may minimize the leak.

Search the patient's small gut from end to end. Feel for its upper end, deliver it into the wound, search it carefully on both sides, and return it to his abdomen. Do the same with succeeding loops, until you reach his iliocaecal junction. Look carefully at his proximal jejunum, and his terminal ileum, because they are particularly likely to be injured. *Be prepared to find several holes!*

When you find a rupture, take care not to lose it again, while you search for others. Wrap it in an abdominal pack, and hold it aside in a light clamp. To see if a clamp is light, try it on your little finger. If it crushes this, it is not light.

Gut is normally sewn in two layers as in Section 9.3, the buried one to control bleeding, and the superficial serosal one to hold the gut together. However, these wounds rarely bleed by the time you see them, so you can use one layer, if you wish.

Tiny holes Use a purse string suture, and oversew this with Lembert sutures.

Larger holes Use 2/0 chromic catgut on atraumatic needles to make a double layer of inverting sutures, in the transverse axis of the gut, as in Section 9.3.

Large ragged tears, dead or dying gut, or multiple adjacent perforations Resect through healthy gut and anastomose it end-to-end. Suture the mesentery accurately, and avoid injuring its blood vessels.

Small areas of bruising without perforations Infold these with Lembert sutures (9.3), or cover them with omentum. Don't detach this, leave it with its own blood supply.

If mesentery is injured, goto the next Section.

Drain the patient's peritoneal cavity, and complete the laparotomy.

IF GUT IS DOUBTFULLY VIABLE, EXCISE IT

66.10 Injuries to the mesentery

An injured mesentery can bleed profusely after an open or a closed injury, and bleeding has little tendency to stop. The mesentery is usually injured near its relatively fixed top and bottom ends. When you examine it you may find a tear or a haematoma.

Short tears are not serious, especially if they are perpendicular to the patient's gut, as in G, Fig. 66-15. The danger in sewing a tear is that you may include the vessels supplying the gut in your sutures, and so impair its blood supply. Vessels approach the gut from the mesentery. Because there is very little circulation along the length of the gut, tears close to its mesenteric border and parallel to it are particularly dangerous.

Some haematomas limit themselves, and don't need treatment. Others expand, compress the vessels in the mesentery, and impair the blood supply to the gut. The difficulty is knowing what

CLOSING IN THE MESENTERY

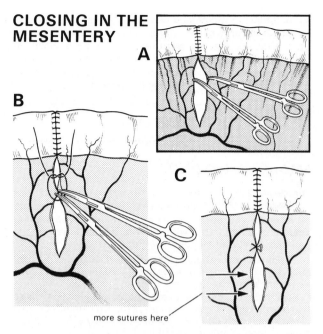

Fig. 66-16 CLOSING TEARS IN THE MESENTERY. Pick up the edges of the tear in haemostats (A), taking care to avoid any blood vessels. Bring these haemostats together and pass a ligature round their tips (B, and C). This is Hamilton Bailey's safe technique.

they are going to do. Opening a haematoma and trying to find the bleeding vessel increases blood loss, and risks damaging the vessel. Some surgeons leave haematomas alone. Others explore them to find the bleeding vessels, particularly if a haematoma is expanding. If the blood supply to a patient's gut is impaired, you will have to explore the bleeding vessel and, if necessary, resect his gut.

TEARS AND HAEMATOMAS OF THE MESENTERY

For the earlier steps in the operation, see Section 66.3. Suspect rupture of the mesentery if there is free bleeding in the centre of the patient's abdomen.

Assess the viability of his gut by the methods in Section 10.5. If gut is not viable, resect it.

TEARS IN THE MESENTERY

To avoid the danger of internal hernias, close all tears by the method in Fig. 66-16. Take great care to avoid blood vessels, especially those close to the border of the gut.

If a tear is close to the gut, parallel to it, and more than 3 or 4 cm long, resect the neighbouring gut.

If part of the gut looks non–viable, resect it.

If you are in doubt about the viability of a piece of gut, make a shallow incision through its antimesenteric border, opposite the centre of the tear. If it bleeds actively, it is viable, so control bleeding and leave it. If it does not bleed, resect it.

CAUTION ! (1) Don't clamp, or tie off, or include in your sutures, any vessels which might impair the blood supply to the gut. (2) Don't try to bunch the mesentery together to tie it.

HAEMATOMAS OF THE MESENTERY

There are two common sites, the mesentery of the small gut and that of the sigmoid colon.

IN THE MESENTERY OF THE SMALL GUT, management depends on whether or not the haematoma shows signs of spreading.

If the injury was several hours ago, and the haematoma has well defined edges, and looks as if it is not going to spread, leave it alone.

If the haematoma shows any sign of spreading, control bleeding by pinching the bleeding vessel between your finger and thumb. Open the haematoma, remove the clot, and swab

PENETRATING SMALL GUT INJURIES - TWO

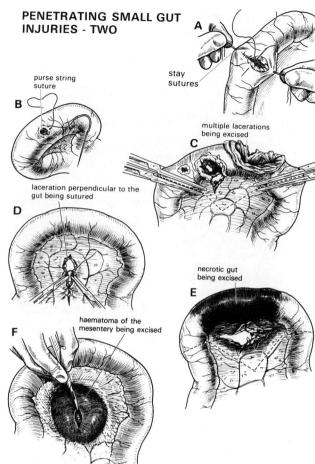

Fig. 66-17 MORE PENETRATING INJURIES OF THE SMALL GUT. A, suturing a transverse laceration. B, a purse string repair for a small laceration. C, extensive multiple wounds are being resected. D, a tear in the mesentery is being sutured. E, a longitudinal tear and the adjacent gangrenous gut are being excised. F, a haematoma is being incised.
Adapted from an original painting by Frank H. Netter, M.D. from The CIBA collection of medical illustrations, copyright by the CIBA Pharmaceutical Company, Division of CIBA–GEIGY Corporation. With kind permission.

it free of blood with a swab. Then momentarily release your finger and thumb, and find and tie the bleeding vessel.

If a haematoma bleeds and the gut is viable, insert some haemostatic sutures and wait 10 minutes. If it is still viable when you return, leave it. If it is not, resect it.

If the gut is not viable, resect it.

IN THE MESENTERY OF THE SIGMOID COLON, large haematomas are common after fractures of the pelvis. Sometimes the pelvic cavity is obliterated by bulging peritoneum filled with clot. Leave a haematoma unless it pulsates and enlarges showing that a major artery is torn and needs tying or repairing.

DIFFICULTIES WITH A GUT INJURY

If a patient BLEEDS PER RECTUM postoperatively, watch him. All patients with a gut injury pass some blood in their stools. If he has no signs of peritonitis, there is probably no need to reoperate. But, if bleeding is continuous or signs of peritonitis develop, do another laparotomy.

66.11 Large gut injuries

Most injuries of the large gut are caused by penetrating wounds, but blunt injuries can also damage it. These injuries are particularly difficult to treat, because: (1) The peritonitis which follows them is more serious than that which follows injuries to the small gut. Caecal peritonitis is particularly deadly. Even a small suture line can leak, and its consequences are only partly prevented by a drain. (2) Retroperitoneal infection from the ascending and descending colon is at least as dangerous as peritonitis. (3) There may be a large area of bruising around the tear, especially if this is caused by a high veolocity missile. (4) The patient's gut will not have been prepared for anastomosis. (5) He will probably have a haemoperitoneum which can readily become infected. All these factors make end–to–end anastomosis particularly dangerous. For all these reasons it is a good principle never to suture and close any but the smallest wounds of the large gut.

If you are not experienced, aim to: (1) Bring the wound outside the patient's abdomen as a loop colostomy, as described in Section 9.5. Or, (2) resect the injury and bring the ends of his gut out as a double barrelled colostomy. How best you can do this depends on how mobile the particular part of his injured large gut is. Two other factors are also important. (a) How large his injury is. (b) How old it is. Operate early, if possible within three hours. The larger and older the wound, the more important is it to exteriorize it. Later, when he has recovered, you can refer him to have his colostomy closed, or close it yourself. The closure of a colostomy is a major procedure and carries the risk of any large gut anastomosis. Refer him if you can.

If you are experienced, and his right colon is injured, you have the option of doing a right hemicolectomy and an end–to–side anastomosis, as in Fig. 9-7. Leaking ileal contents are less dangerous than those of the large gut, so a skillful ileocaecal anastomosis is acceptable.

MAKING A CAECOSTOMY

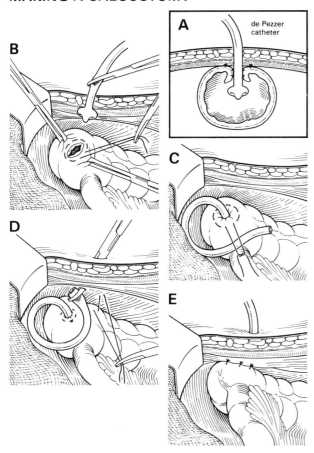

Fig. 66-18 MAKING A CAECOSTOMY WITH A DE PEZZER CATHETER. A, shows the final result with a de Pezzer catheter invaginated into the patient's caecum which is sutured to his abdominal wall. B, the opening in his caecum being closed with a purse string suture. C, the catheter in place and the purse string about to be closed. D, the catheter being drawn through a separate stab wound. The first suture to hold the caecum is loosely in place. E, the final caecostomy.
After Maingot with kind permission.

It is a good principle in all colonic surgery to dilate the patient's anus by Lord's procedure (21.5). This will help faeces to trickle out of it, instead of building up at the suture line, and threatening the anastomosis. His sphincters will recover in a few days, by which time the tear should have healed.

TRY TO BRING INJURED LARGE GUT OUTSIDE THE ABDOMEN

INJURIES OF THE LARGE GUT For the earliest steps see Section 66.3. Be sure to give the patient the perioperative antibiotics described in that section.

If there is an obvious wound in his large gut, cobble it up temporarily, or clamp it, before doing anything else, to prevent faeces spilling. Cover the wound with a pack.

If there is no obvious wound, start with his caecum and check the whole of his colon for tears, perforations, bruises, and blow outs. If a bullet or small missile fragment is responsible, look for tiny perforations which may be obscured by omentum.

If he has a bullet wound of his large gut, avoid suturing it if you can; the surrounding tissues are injured and the wound will break down. If you do decide to suture it, be sure to do a proximal colostomy.

CAUTION ! (1) Where possible, avoid bringing a colostomy out through his laparotomy wound, or it will probably become infected. (2) Try to avoid contaminating his laparotomy wound, or any missile wound, with faeces from his colostomy. (3) Beware of retroperitoneal bruises, because they may indicate hidden wounds. If necessary, mobilize his ascending or descending colon and look behind them. (3) Always complete the operation by doing Lord's procedure.

LORD'S PROCEDURE Do this in all cases. Dilate the patient's rectal sphincters so much by Lords procedure (21.5) that they are paralysed. They will recover in a few days, by which time the tear should have healed.

66.12 Injuries of the caecum

These are particularly difficult because the contents of a patient's caecum are fluid, leak easily, and irritate his skin, so you cannot make a surface caecostomy as if it were a colostomy. A proximal defunctioning caecostomy is also impractical. The alternatives are: (1) To insert a caecostomy tube into his caecum to prevent soiling of his skin, as in A, Fig. 66-18. This is useful for small bullet wounds and stab wounds of the caecum, but it will not defunction the rest of his large gut. (2) A right hemicolectomy, with an ileostomy and colostomy, if you are less skilled (as in C, Fig. 66-19), or with an end–to–side anastomosis (as in D in this figure), or with a side–to–side anastomosis (terminal ileum to transverse colon), if you are more skilled. Don't try to exteriorize the caecum. If a caecostomy is impractical, a right hemicolectomy will be safer.

The method below tells you how to make a caecostomy with a large de Pezzer catheter which is easier to manage than a Paul's tube. This is held in place with inverting purse string sutures, after which the caecum is anchored to the abdominal wall (Stamm's procedure).

CAECOSTOMY

INDICATIONS An injury of the caecum which leaves most of it intact.

METHOD If possible, make the caecostomy in the original wound in the patient's caecum. Otherwise, close this with two layers of sutures, and make a fresh incision for the caecostomy.

Apply a curved non-crushing clamp to prevent the contents of the patient's gut coming out of the hole, and cover this with a swab. Clamp a large self-retaining de Pezzer catheter, and

WOUNDS OF THE CAECUM AND ASCENDING COLON

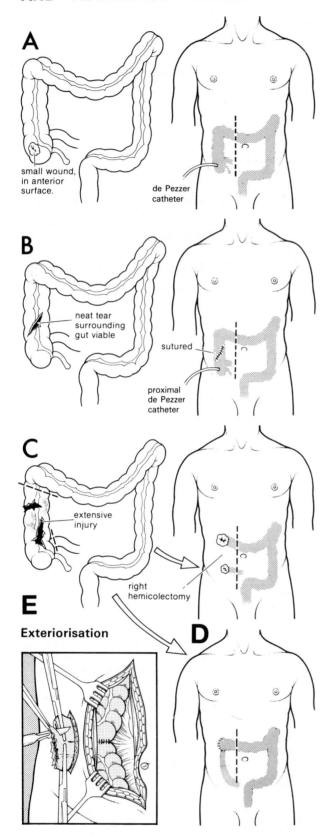

Fig. 66-19 WOUNDS OF THE CAECUM AND ASCENDING COLON.
A, shows the insertion of a de Pezzer catheter into a wound in the
caecum. B, shows its insertion into a wound of the ascending colon.
C, shows a right hemicolectomy, with an ileostomy and colostomy. D,
shows a right hemicolectomy done for the same injury as in C, but with
an end–to–side anastomosis. E, exteriorizing a wound of the ascending colon. *Modified, by the kind permission of Peter London.*

insert this into the hole. Apply a purse string of 2/0 catgut
round the catheter, and tie it, making sure that the bowel wall
inverts around it as in Fig. 66-18. Tie the purse string, and then
put another one round it (C, and D).

Now make a small hole in the patient's abdominal wall, just
big enough to take the catheter. Make it over the place where
his caecum will lie comfortably when his abdomen is closed.
Push long artery forceps through this hole, right up to their
handles, from outside inwards (D). They will make a useful
retractor.

Put 4 or 5 sutures in the peritoneum round the abdominal
hole, and in the peritoneum on his caecum round the
caecostomy. For the moment, leave these sutures loose.

Grasp the end of the de Pezzer catheter with the forceps,
and pull it through his abdominal wall. Now tighten the
sutures, so as to anchor the caecostomy to his abdominal
wall (E).

Spigot the caecostomy, close his abdominal wall, and leave
his skin for delayed primary suture (9.7).

POSTOPERATIVELY Join the de Pezzer catheter by a wide bore
connector to a large tube which drains into a bottle of
disinfectant beside the patient's bed. After 36 hours do a gentle washout through the tube. Repeat this frequently
thereafter.

As soon as he is well and has good bowel sounds, you can
spigot the tube, so that he can walk about. Leave the
caecostomy tube in place for 3 weeks.

REMOVING THE TUBE Premedicate him. Tell him you are
going to remove it on the count ". . .three". Place a swab round
its base where it enters his skin. Hold the end of tube firmly
in one hand and its base and his skin in the other. Then, count
"One, two, *three!*" and firmly pull out the tube. His caescostomy
will heal spontaneously.

66.13 Injuries of the right colon from the caecum to the hepatic flexure

The usual options are a right hemicolectomy or exteriorization.
A hemicolectomy is best. If you don't feel capable of doing an
anastomosis, you can bring the ends of the patient's gut out
as an ileostomy and a mucous colostomy.

INJURIES OF THE RIGHT COLON BEYOND THE
CAECUM

If the wound is in the anterior wall only, you may be able
to insert a large de Pezzer catheter, as for a caecostomy, as
in A, Fig. 66-19.

**If the wound is less than 2 cm, and its excised edges have
a good blood supply,** suture it in two layers and drain the
paracolic gutter. Do a proximal caecostomy with a de Pezzer
catheter (B).

If the wound cannot safely be sutured do a right
hemicolectomy (as described below). If you are skilled, do an
end to side anastomosis (D). If you are less skilled, bring the
ileum and the transverse colon out of the wound (C).

An easier but less satisfactory alternative is to mobilize the
peritoneum in the paracolic gutter, so as to bring the damaged

---

Fig. 66-20 RIGHT HEMICOLECTOMY. A, incising the peritoneum
on the right of the patient's ascending colon. B, using blunt dissection
to reflect his right colon medially. C, freeing his colon from his
duodenum. D, a fan shaped piece of the mesentery of the right colon
is being excised. E, the end of his transverse colon is being closed with
continuous catgut over a straight non–crushing clamp. F, a single layer
of mattress sutures is being placed in the end of his colon. G, his small
intestine, still held in its clamp, is being drawn upwards. H, a crushing
clamp is being placed on the anterior taenia. I, the serosal surfces of
the two pieces of gut are being joined. J, part of the anterior taenia
is being excised. K, the mucosa is being approximated. L, the anterior
wall of the anastomosis is being closed. M, some extra mattress sutures
are being inserted. N, the final result. This figure does not show the
final closure of the mesentery—don't forget to do this. *Partly after Ellis
with kind permission.*

RIGHT HEMICOLECTOMY

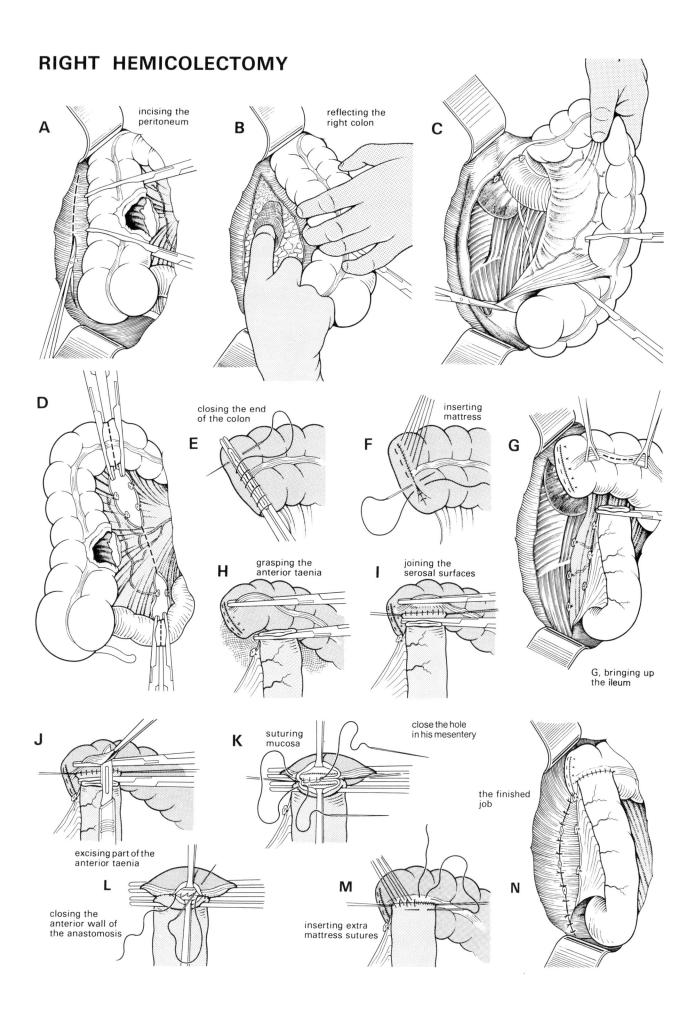

A incising the peritoneum

B reflecting the right colon

C

D

E closing the end of the colon

F inserting mattress

G G, bringing up the ileum

H grasping the anterior taenia

I joining the serosal surfaces

J

K suturing mucosa / close the hole in his mesentery

L excising part of the anterior taenia / closing the anterior wall of the anastomosis

M inserting extra mattress sutures

N the finished job

part of the colon out through an appropriate incision in the abdominal wall without tension or torsion. You can then close the abdominal wound, and resect the injured colon to leave a double barrelled colostomy (E).

HEMICOLECTOMY FOR AN INJURY OF THE RIGHT COLON

Wall off the patient's intestines with gauze or place them in a sterile plastic bag. Expose his caecum. Incise the peritoneum in his right paracolic gutter close to his colon, from the tip of his caecum upwards to his right hepatic flexure (A, in Fig. 66-20). There will be little bleeding.

Divide his hepatocolic ligament and tie the small blood vessels in it.

Using finger dissection reflect his right colon medially (B). Cover the raw surface that remains with moist packs.

CAUTION ! Don't injure: (1) His right ureter. (2) The second or third parts of his duodenum (C).

Clamp and divide the mesentery of his colon just distal to his hepatic flexure (D). Tie the branches of his ileocolic and right colic, and some of the terminal branches of his middle colic arteries. You are not operating for malignancy, so you can conveniently tie them fairly near the gut.

Dissect his greater omentum off the proximal part of his transverse colon.

Prepare his terminal ileum at its mesenteric border, and divide its mesentery to join the incision that you have just made in his mesocolon. Doubly tie any vessels you cut in his mesentery.

Place a pair of crushing clamps obliquely across his ileum, 1 cm from its mesenteric border.

Place a pair of crushing clamps across his colon, divide it between these clamps, and remove his right colon complete with its fan shaped piece of mesentery and the piece of his terminal ileum.

Cover the end of his ileum with a saline pack until you are ready to anastomose it.

Close the end of his colon with continuous catgut on a straight or curved needle by passing the sutures over the end of the crushing clamp (E). Remove the clamp and pull the sutures tight. Use 2/0 atraumatic silk or chromic catgut (if infection is present) to place a continuous line of Halstead mattress sutures 1 cm from the suture line, taking care not to include any fat (F). Invert the first line of sutures as you pull these mattress sutures up.

END–TO–SIDE ANASTOMOSIS Bring the patient's ileum, still held in its clamp, close to the anterior tenia of his colon (G).

If you have not previously excised his omentum, retract it upwards, and grasp the anterior taenia of his colon with Babcock forceps at the proposed site of the anastomosis.

Apply a small straight crushing clamp to the anterior tenia, so as to include a small bite of colon (H).

Arrange the clamps so that you can join the serosa of his colon and the ileum with mattress sutures of 2/0 silk (I). Leave the sutures at either end long to act as stay sutures. Cut into his colon by excising the protrusion from the crushing clamp on the anterior taenia (J).

Apply an enterostomy clamp behind each crushing clamp, remove the crushing clamps, and excise the crushed edges of both his ileum and his colon. If necessary, enlarge the opening in his colon.

Approximate the mucosal surfaces of both organs with continuous fine catgut, starting in the midline posteriorly and continuing round on either side (K). Continue the sutures round the angles and anteriorly as Connel inverted sutures (L). Complete the anastomosis with an anterior row of mattress sutures (M). Reinforce the angles with some additional mattress sutures.

Suture the edges of the mesentery of his ileum and colon, so that his intestine cannot later herniate through it.

CAUTION ! Test the patency of the stoma, it should be big enough to admit your index finger.

POSTOPERATIVE CARE Continue nasogastric suction and intravenous fluids for 3 to 5 days. Don't remove his naogastric tube until there is clear evidence that the stoma is patent, as shown by the absence of abdominal distension after the tube has been clamped for at least 12 hours.

WOUNDS OF THE TRANSVERSE, SIGMOID AND DESCENDING COLON

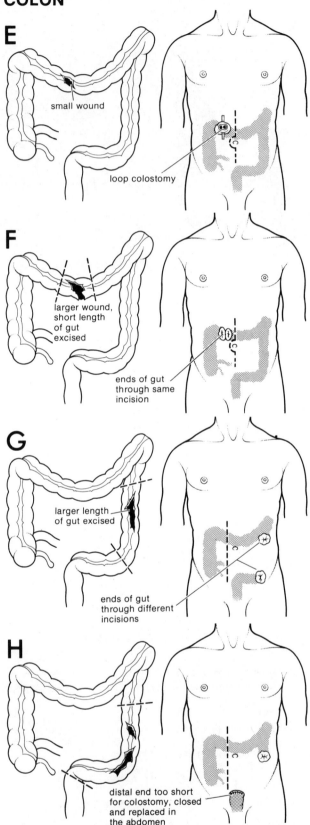

Fig. 66-21 WOUNDS OF THE TRANSVERSE, DESCENDING, AND SIGMOID COLON. E, a small wound, exteriorized on a loop colostomy. F, a small length of gut excised and a double colostomy made through the same wound. G, a longer length of gut excised in the descending colon and colostomies made through separate incisions. H, part of the colon resected and the rectum closed. *By kind permission of Peter London.*

66.14 Injuries from the hepatic flexure to the rectum

There are three possibilities: (1) If the wound involves part of the circumference of the gut, you can make a loop colostomy without dividing the gut, as in E, Fig. 66-21. Loop colostomies are easier in the transverse or sigmoid colon. But if you mobilise the colon properly you can use them anywhere at or beyond the hepatic flexure. The loop must lie easily on the abdominal wall without tension. If it is tight, it will gradually retract and cause great problems with abdominal wall abscesses. (2) If you have to resect a short (5 cm) length of gut you can bring the cut ends out through same incision (F). (3) If you have to resect a longer length of gut (more than about 5 cm), you cannot bring the two cut ends out of the same incision. So you will have to bring them out through separate incisions as faecal and mucous colostomies (G). If the lower end of the gut is too short to bring out to the surface, you will have to use Hartmann's procedure (H). To make a colostomy, goto Section 9.5.

INJURIES OF THE TRANSVERSE, DESCENDING, AND SIGMOID COLON

If the patient has a short, clean–cut stab wound, suture it, drain it, and watch him closely. A good procedure for a single small wound is to close it, and to do a loop colostomy, incorporating the suture line in the part which is exteriorized. *Don't open the colostomy.* If the suture line heals, replace his gut in his peritoneal cavity. If it leaks, no harm is done.

If the wound involves only part of the circumference of his gut, make a loop colostomy (E in Fig. 66-21).

If it involves the whole circumference of his gut, make a double colostomy (F). If the resected segment is short, bring the two ends out through the same incision as a double colostomy (F). If the resected segment is long, bring them out through separate incisions as faecal and mucous colostomies (G). These can if necessary be far apart, because the cut ends of the gut can easily be joined up subsequently. If the distal end is too short to bring out to abdominal wall, close it in two layers and drop it back into the pelvis (H). This is Hartman's procedure as described for sigmoid volvulus (10.10).

LOOP COLOSTOMY varies slightly according to the site. For details, see Section 9.5.

If the wound is in the patient's descending colon, divide the peritoneum of his lateral paracolic gutter, and mobilize bluntly behind his colon, which will come away up to the surface. This will also allow you to inspect its retroperitoneal surface.

If the wound is of moderate size, close it in layers transverse to the axis of his gut, and make a loop colostomy in his transverse colon proximally. Make a separate incision for the colostomy a reasonable distance away from his iliac spines.

If he has several wounds, bring out the most proximal one as a colostomy. Excise the more distal ones back to healthy, bleeding tissue. Either bring the distal end out as a mucous fistula, or do Hartman's procedure.

CAUTION ! (1) If his peritoneum has been contaminated with faeces, put a drain through a stab wound in his flank. (2) Do Lord's procedure (21.5).

TO CLOSE THE COLOSTOMY wait several weeks until he is well and cheerful. If his gut needs reanastomosis, refer him; if it merely needs closing, you may be able to do this as in Section 9.5.

66.15 Injuries of the rectum

A patient's rectum can be harmed by injuries which reach it from his abdomen or from his buttock. An abdominal wound of the rectum inevitably involves the peritoneum. A buttock wound may involve only his perirectal tissues, or it may enter his peritoneal cavity. His bladder, his urethra, his pelvis, his sacrum, and sometimes even the lower end of his subarachnoid space can be injured at the same time. The main danger is that

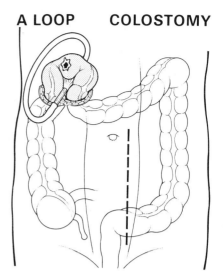

A LOOP COLOSTOMY

The blood supply of the colon

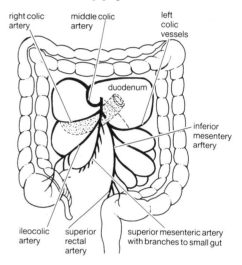

Fig. 66-22 MORE METHODS for injuries of the colon. A, a wound of the transverse colon has been exteriorized on a loop colostomy. B, the vascular supply of the colon.

faeces will leak into the tissue round his rectum and infect it, perhaps fatally.

You cannot bring wounds of a patient's rectum and rectosigmoid outside his abdominal wall as you can elsewhere in his colon. So aim to: (1) Divert faeces from his rectum by doing a diversionary colostomy above it. This is much safer than merely inserting a large rectal tube. (2) Empty his gut beyond the colostomy. (3) Drain the wound.

The main distinction is between wounds which involve his peritoneum, and those which do not.

Intraperitoneal wounds should be managed like wounds of the distal colon. Make a left iliac colostomy, close the rectal wound, and drain it.

Extraperitoneal wounds make an opening from a patient's rectum into the tissues round it below the reflection of the peritoneum. There are problems: (1) Diagnosis can be difficult, as in the patient JANE described below. (2) Other structures, especially the bladder and the pelvis, are often injured too. (3) The rectum is difficult to expose from below, so expose it from above, and make a drainage incision down from above, into the peritoneum.

JANE (5) fell from a tree on to a dead branch. Later, she complained of vague lower abdominal pain. There was a little blood in her rectum. She was examined under anaesthesia. A probe entered a wound in her rectal wall and tracked far upwards. Exploration showed that a twig had passed behind her peritoneum

189

lateral to her rectum, in front of her right common iliac vessels, avoiding her right ureter, and up alongside her inferior vena cava as high as her right kidney. Fortunately, no vital organs were damaged. A temporary defunctioning colostomy was done and she recovered.

JAKE (24), a performer in a disco bar, jumped in the air and fell on his microphone stand, injuring his perineum. Accompanied by much singing, he was brought in laughing by his friends. His fresh minor looking perineal wound was toileted and closed by immediate primary suture. Although he had no abdominal signs, the cautious house officer admitted him. The next morning his pulse rate had a risen (a very important sign). Later in the day he became very ill with a high fever and signs suggesting peritonitis in his lower abdomen. Laparotomy showed a 10 cm wound in his perineum. This led to an area of severe cellulitis, but had not injured any viscera. Large doses of broad spectrum antibiotics cured him. LESSONS: (1) Wounds in some parts of the body can be closed, if you see them early enough. In other areas, including the perineum, this is very dangerous. (2) Wounds may be deeper than they seem, and need radical toileting.

WHENEVER THE RECTUM IS INJURED DO A DEFUNCTIONING COLOSTOMY

INJURIES OF THE RECTUM

EXAMINATION If a patient might possibly have a rectal injury, study the wound track carefully. Put him into the lithotomy position and examine him with your finger and with a sigmoidoscope. If necessary, examine his rectum under anaesthesia. Is his anal sphincter torn? Does the injury involve the urethra or vagina? (68.3). Carefully examine the patient's abdomen for signs of peritonitis (6.2). If necessary, take an erect film and look for gas under his diaphragm (66-4).

PERIOPERATIVE ANTIBIOTICS In all but the most trivial rectal injuries, antibiotic protection is critical, particularly protection against anaerobes (2.7). The patient will need intravenous metronidazole 7.5 mg/kg 8 hourly, for 3 or 4 days before switching to the oral route. Combine this with chloramphenicol, gentamicin, or co-trimoxazole.

INTRAPERITONEAL INJURIES OF THE RECTUM

Make a lower midline incision. Control haemorrhage. This can be severe, and you may very occasionally even have to tie the patient's iliac arteries on both sides. If so, watch his ureters. Wash out his peritoneal cavity to get it absolutely clean (6.2). Squeeze out any faeces in his rectum into the normal bowel above the lesion, or wash them downwards. Excise the edges of the perforation.

If the patient's rectal wound is small, suture it, and insert a large rectal tube.

If his rectal wound is large, do a defunctioning colostomy (9.5). Make this as close to the injury as possible. The most convenient place is likely to be his sigmoid or transverse colon. The more worried you are about closure, the more important it is for the colostomy to be fully defunctioning. Insert a drain down to the site of the repair. If his injury is really severe, you may have to resect a length of rectum or rectosigmoid, do a terminal colostomy, and close the blind end of his rectum as for Hartman's procedure (10.10).

Do Lord's procedure (21.5).

EXPERITONEAL INJURIES OF THE RECTUM

Do a laparotomy (66.3). Excise the wound track from the patient's perineum. Clean out his perirectal space from above. Incise his pelvic peritoneum on each side of his abdominal rectum. If necessary, use blunt dissection with your fingers to peel his prostate and seminal vesicles off the front of his rectum. Remove all foreign bodies, pieces of clothing, etc. Make sure his wound is clean.

If possible try to stitch up: (1) his rectum using inverted sutures, (2) his anal sphincter.

Make a double defunctioning colostomy, preferably with his sigmoid colon. Wash out all faeces below the colostomy.

Incise the skin obliquely beside his coccyx. Using a pair of artery forceps, open up a track from his rectovesical pouch to your skin incision. Bring down a large corrugated rubber drain.

POSTOPERATIVE CARE (both kinds of injury) Wait several weeks before referring him for the closure of his colostomy (9.6).

DIFFICULTIES WITH RECTAL INJURIES

If a patient shows SIGNS OF PERITONITIS, do an immediate laparotomy. Put him into the Trendelenberg position, and examine his abdominal cavity through a low midline or paramedian incision. Examine his pelvic viscera.

If his BLADDER HAS RUPTURED INTRAPERITONEALLY, repair it (68.2).

If his URETHRA MIGHT HAVE BEEN INJURED, explore the wound to make sure. If it is normal leave it. If it has been injured, drain his bladder through a suprapubic catheter, and treat him as in Section 68.3.

If he presents late with a FISTULA draining in his buttock, do a proximal defunctioning colostomy in his left iliac fossa. Wait a month or two until his fistula has healed, then close the colostomy.

If digital examination of his rectum shows an injury which FEELS LIKE A TEAR, but he has no signs of peritonitis, assume that he has an extraperitoneal penetrating injury. Drain his pararectal tissues, and do a sigmoid colostomy. Don't try to suture his rectum.

If his ANAL SPHINCTER IS PARTLY TORN, but his anorectal ring feels intact, toilet and drain his wound.

If his ANAL SPHINCTER IS COMPLETELY TORN across (rare), don't try primary repair, unless the wound is clean cut.

DRAINING EXTRAPERITONEAL WOUNDS OF THE RECTUM

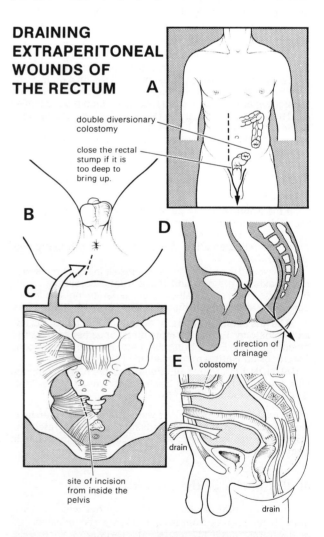

Fig. 66-23 DRAINING EXTRAPERITONEAL WOUNDS OF THE RECTUM. A, the rectum closed and a colostomy made. B, the external incision. C, the internal incision beside the rectum. D, the direction of drainage. E, a colostomy has been done and drains are in place.

After various authors.

Better, do a colostomy, toilet his peritoneal wound, and refer him for a definitive repair later.

66.16 Duodenal injuries

If a patient hits the steering wheel of his car, he can crush both his duodenum and his pancreas against his spine. The combination of a leaking duodenum and traumatic pancreatitis usually kills him. Diagnosis and treatment are difficult, and may be delayed for days because both organs lie at the back of his abdomen behind his peritoneum. These injuries are difficult even for the most skilled surgeon, and you will have to manage the patient as best you can. Fortunately, injuries of the duodenum are rare.

The patient's injured duodenum leaks into his peritoneal cavity or behind it and causes a deep seated pain in his epigastrium and back, which gets steadily worse. This is accompanied by severe vomiting, fever, toxaemia, and sometimes by shock. His epigastrium becomes tender, silent, and a little distended. When you open it, you find an oedematous red mass behind his stomach. The tear itself is difficult to find, and you may need to lift his duodenum and pancreas forwards from the right (Kocher's manoeuvre).

You should be able to suture small tears into the peritoneal cavity, and some of the tears behind it. If you cannot do this, the unsatisfactory alternatives are: (1) A duodeno–jejunostomy, which is difficult, (2) a gastroenterostomy which does not divert bile from the wound, or (3) a Foley catheter which does not provide enough drainage.

INJURIES OF THE DUODENUM

At laparotomy you find a large oedematous mass at the back of the patient's upper abdomen, displacing his hepatic flexure downwards to the left.

Find the triangle of peritoneal tissue which lies, with its apex pointing medially, between his colon and his duodenum. Explore any haematoma at the base of his mesocolon, or over the convexity of the second part of his duodenum.

Divide the bloodless fold of peritoneum above and lateral to the hepatic flexure of his colon. Draw this downwards and medially; if necessary, use a sponge stick.

You should now see his duodenum, except for its distal part underneath his mesenteric vessels.

If there is no injury on the front of his duodenum, move to the left side of the table. Incise the peritoneum lateral to the second part of his duodenum. Put your hand under it and under the head of his pancreas, and reflect them forwards. Look for staining with bile and blood, and dissect gently to reveal the tear. This is usually in its second or third parts.

Look carefully at the last part of the patient's duodenum, and at his duodeno–jejunal flexure. If necessary, reflect the peritoneum off it with blunt-tipped scissors.

BRUISING OF THE DUODENUM Don't try to suture a bruised duodenum. Instead, leave it and insert a drain.

A SMALL TEAR OF THE DUODENUM Suture this with nonabsorbable sutures as a single layer. If it is longitudinal, don't try to sew it up transversely. Stitch omentum over the tear and drain the area for several days.

A LARGE TEAR OF THE DUODENUM If the tear is too large or too ragged to suture, there are three possibilities:

If you are skilled, you can close the hole by bringing a loop of gut up onto it, so as to make a duodeno – jejunostomy.

If you are less skilled, repair the tear, and do a gastroenterostomy.

Alternatively, drain the patient's duodenum through a large bore Foley catheter, with two extra holes cut near its tip. Pass it down into the tear. Partly inflate the balloon, to keep it in place. Bring it out through a stab wound in his flank to provide dependent drainage. If possible, apply continuous suction. Drain the retroperitoneal area. Two weeks later deflate the balloon, and slowly withdraw it over several days. The fistula will usually dry up within a month.

If stenosis develops, the patient will need a feeding jejunostomy.

COMPLETE TRANSECTION AT THE DUODENO–JEJUNAL FLEXURE You may be able to do an end-to-end anastomosis. If the anastomosis breaks down, it will at least convert the leak into a fistula instead of a spreading peritonitis.

DRAINS The suture line may leak, so always insert a drain through a separate stab wound in the patient's right flank.

POSTOPERATIVE CARE For all lesions do a feeding jejunostomy (9.6a), except when you have already done a gastroenterostomy. You will have to feed the patient through his injured duodenum. The ileus that follows duodenal lesions can last for several weeks.

66.17 Pancreatic injuries

These injuries range from mild bruising to a pancreas which has been cut vertically in half. The patient may have few physical signs until a spreading retroperitoneal abscess develops.

If his pancreas is only bruised, you can drain it. This can be life–saving. A pancreatic fistula will probably form, but it can be treated after he has recovered from his acute injury. Pancreatectomy is the treatment of choice for major injuries. This is difficult, so close his abdomen and if possible refer him rapidly. The only exception is an injury to the tip of the tail of the pancreas.

THE PANCREAS

At laparotomy you find that the peritoneum over an injured patient's pancreas is discoloured and oedematous, sometimes with yellow opaque areas of fat necrosis.

Open his lesser sac by detaching his greater omentum from his transverse colon. Reflect his stomach upwards, and his transverse colon downwards, to expose his pancreas.

If his pancreas is only bruised, insert a drain and close his abdomen.

If there is a tear in the surface of his pancreas, suture it.

If the tail of his pancreas has been torn off, remove it, cut it across in a fish tail incision, find the end of the duct, and tie this with a nonabsorbable suture. Then join the two ends of the fish tail, using nonabsorbable sutures through its capsule. Drain the area.

If his pancreas is hopelessly torn, insert a drain and close his abdomen.

66.18 Injuries of the gall bladder

If only the fundus of the gall bladder is injured, do a cholecystostomy (13.3). With severe injuries the best treatment is usually cholecystectomy, which is difficult (13.6). You can do a cholecystostomy with a de Pezzer catheter in much the same way as a caecostomy.

CHOLECYSTOSTOMY Put a de Pezzer catheter into the patient's gall bladder as in Figs. 13-1 and 66-18. Anchor it to his abdominal wall in a similar way. If you find any stones in his gall bladder, remove as may as you can, before closing the purse string suture round the tube. A temporary biliary fistula will form, and then slowly heal.

66.19 Other difficulties with abdominal injuries

There are many of these. They include the patient who is brought in late, the patient whose injured abdomen or abdominal wall becomes infected, the development of a fistula, or the collapse of a lung.

DIFFICULTIES WITH AN ABDOMINAL INJURY

If a PATIENT IS BROUGHT IN LATE, more than 18 hours after an injury, manage him like this:

If he looks well, feels well, his temperature is normal, he has no signs of peritonitis or abscess formation, and if the site of his wound is only minimally tender, **a laparotomy may not be necessary.** None of his viscera may have been perforated, or the perforations may have sealed themselves off. Watch him, and if he deteriorates, operate.

If his condition is not good, but he looks as if he could withstand an operation, **operate.**

If he is in severe shock, **resuscitate him.** Give him intravenous fluids, and antibiotics. Pass a nasogastric tube. He will probably die anyway, but give him a chance. Operate, unless he clearly has only minutes to live. *If you refer him, resuscitate him first.*

If a patient's PULSE RATE RISES POSTOPERATIVELY, and his abdomen becomes increasingly tender and rigid, there is sepsis inside it. After an abdominal injury a patient is in danger from: (1) Generalized peritonitis (6.2). (2) Subphrenic (6.4) or other abdominal abscesses (6.3). (3) Retroperitoneal abscesses.

Treat peritonitis as in Section 6.2. Prevent it by: (1) closing lacerations in a patient's small gut carefully, (2) managing injuries to his large gut as in Section 66.11, (3) inserting drains appropriately, (4) cleaning out his injured peritoneum with saline before you close it, and (5) using perioperative antibiotics as in Section 2.7.

If a FISTULA forms, treat it as in Section 9.14. Sometimes you cannot avoid one, so prepare for one deliberately: (1) After a bladder injury do a suprapubic cystostomy (22.6 and 22.7). (2) After pancreatic or duodenal injuries, insert a drain. (3) When the large gut has been injured, do a colostomy (9.5).

If his ABDOMINAL WOUND BECOMES INFECTED and sloughs, lay it open, treat him with antibiotics, hypochlorite ('Eusol') dressings, and delayed skin grafting. This may happen when: (1) His unprepared colon or ileum has been opened. (2) There has been major trauma. (3) Much blood has been lost. (4) Perioperative antibiotics have not been given, or have not been properly timed. Delayed suture of the abdominal wall will make infection less likely.

If parts of a patient's LUNG COLLAPSE, or an entire lung collapses, treat him as in Sections 9.9 and 9.10. Prevent lung complications after any laparotomy by early breathing exercises. Occasionally, you may need to slap his chest, or bronchoscope him to remove mucus plugs. Very rarely, you may need to do a tracheotomy, or to ventilate him artificially. This is one of the complications of any operation under general anaesthesia. It is more common after an abdominal injury because: (1) His chest may have been injured at the same time. (2) Major abdominal wounds make breathing difficult.

67 Kidney injuries

67.1 The general method

A blow in a patient's loin can injure his kidneys. Mild kidney injuries are common. They cause a small break in the renal capsule, a small haematoma, and haematuria. More severe kidney injuries tear the renal capsule, pelvis, and calyces; they can tear away the poles of a patient's kidneys, and pulp them, or they can tear his kidneys from their pedicles. Fortunately, you can treat all but the severest kidney injuries conservatively.

After a closed injury the perirenal fascia usually keeps the escaping blood close to the injured kidney, unless the patient is a child. But after an open injury blood tracks in all directions and may enter the peritoneal cavity. If an extensive retroperitoneal haematoma forms, it may be accompanied by ileus.

Haematuria is the major sign; it is usually mild, and stops spontaneously. If a patient passes blood in his urine after an accident, but has no other signs, it is probably coming from his kidneys. If bleeding is more severe, blood may clot in a ureter and block it, so that the passage of blood stops. This may lead you to think that the patient is recovering, when really he is getting worse. Secondary haemorrhage and severe haematuria can occur up to three weeks later, so observe even minor kidney injuries carefully.

Kidney injuries do not usually cause much shock, so if a patient is severely shocked, suspect some other disaster also, such as a rupture of his spleen, or liver.

The loin over a patient's injured kidney is tender, and if he has a large haematoma round it, his loin may be flattened. You will not find a renal haematoma easy to feel in the early stages, because of the tenderness and guarding of the abdominal wall over it. Feel gently, or bleeding may start again.

THE GENERAL METHOD FOR A KIDNEY INJURY

This extends Section 51.3 on the care of a severely injured patient. If the patient also has a severe abdominal injury, this takes precedence over his injured kidney. Treat him conservatively and only operate on the indications listed in the next section (67.2).

THE CONSERVATIVE TREATMENT OF KIDNEY INJURIES

RESUSCITATION Transfuse the patient as necessary.

OBSERVATION Record his pulse every 15 minutes initially, and less often later. Examine his abdomen often for a gradually increasing loin mass.

X-RAYS An intravenous pyelogram is useful, so take one. The only contraindication to it is a low blood pressure which will allow insufficient excretion to give you a useful film. Do a pyelogram as soon as you can, without waiting for haematuria to stop, and before gas in the patient's gut has had time to obscure the films. Give him a double dose of contrast medium, but otherwise take the pyelogram exactly as usual, except that you should not compress his abdomen. Take a control film, followed by films at 5 minutes and 15 minutes; take another film at 30 minutes if you do not see the normal kidney well at 5 and 15 minutes.

Look for: (1) A functioning kidney on the other side, (2) delayed or absent function on the injured side, and (3) blood clots in the calyces. A normal pyelogram does not necessarily mean a normal kidney. You may also see fractures of the transverse processes of the lumbar vertebrae, which are often associated with kidney injuries, and obliteration of the psoas shadow.

URINE Save a sample of all the urine the patient passes, so that you can compare succeeding specimens. If his injured kidney is healing, his urine will change from red to brown. If it becomes red again, further bleeding has started.

FLUIDS AND GASTRIC ASPIRATION Adequate fluid and electrolytes will help him to pass clots without too much pain. Paralytic ileus is a risk in severe cases and may complicate the administration of fluid (10.14).

If there is no indication for an operation, and no distension which might indicate ileus, give him plenty of fluids by mouth.

If you have to operate, or there are signs of ileus, pass a nasogastric tube and aspirate it repeatedly, as long as there is any fluid to aspirate. Give him fluid intravenously.

Keep him quiet in bed for at least a week until all bleeding has stopped, and his pyelogram shows no gross abnormality. If necessary, sedate him thoroughly. Observe him for 3 weeks if necessary.

67.2 Operations for kidney injuries

Should you operate on a patient with an injured kidney? Probably not. If you transfuse him adequately, he will probably recover, even if he has severe haematuria, a large mass in his loin, and a falling blood pressure. This is fortunate because the kidneys

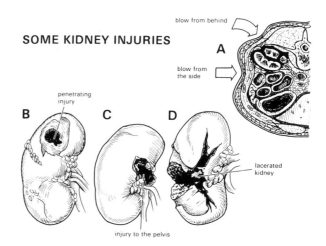

Fig. 67-1 INJURIES OF THE KIDNEYS. A, a blow from the side can drive the kidney against the transverse processes of the lumbar spine; a blow from behind can drive the twelfth rib into it. B, a penetrating injury. C, an injury of the renal pelvis. D, a severe laceration. *Adapted from an original painting by Frank H. Netter, M.D. from the CIBA Collection of Medical Illustrations, copyright by CIBA Pharmaceutical Company, Division of CIBA–GEIGY Corporation. With kind permission.*

are difficult to get at, and trying to approach them through a mass of blood clot is not easy, even for an expert. The indications for operating are: (1) Persistent haematuria causing a continuing fall in the patient's haemoglobin. (2) A haematoma of the kidney which continues to enlarge. (2) Some open injuries, such as stab or bullet wounds. If possible treat these by packing.

If you have to abandon conservative treatment, you can: (1) Drain a perirenal haematoma. (2) Pack a patient's bleeding kidney. (3) Suture a tear. It is also possible to remove his entire kidney or part of it. This is a heroic task for an experienced operator. For an inexperienced one it is almost impossible, so it is not described here.

Drainage is the simplest operation, and is all that is indicated when there is extensive bleeding and no major damage to the kidney. When a patient's condition is poor, and you do not feel capable of suturing or excising either all or part of his kidney, an easier alternative is to insert a pack, and remove it at 48 hours.

OPERATING ON AN INJURED KIDNEY

INDICATIONS FOR EXPLORING THE KIDNEY *Avoid exploring a patient's injured kidney if you can.* Try to refer those patients who need an operation. If you cannot refer a patient you may have to operate on the indications given above.

EXPOSING THE KIDNEY FROM THE LOIN

POSITION This is critical. Lie the patient on his normal side, with his back near the edge of the table. Flex his hip and his knee on the side next to the table. Extend his upper leg and place a soft pillow between his legs. If your table does not have a kidney bridge to extend his loin, place a large sandbag under his normal loin. If possible, support his upper arm. This will relieve the pressure on his chest, and help to hold him in place.

Find your landmarks by feeling his vertebral column, his iliac crest, and his twelfth rib.

CAUTION ! Don't mistake his twelfth rib for his eleventh or you will incise too high and open his pleura. Sometimes the twelfth rib is very short, so examine his ribs on the films from his pyelogram.

Start the incision just medial to the angle between his erector spinae muscle and his twelfth rib. Deepen it to show the muscles. The tissue planes will be more easy to identify if you infiltrate them with adrenaline and saline.

In the upper half of the incision, cut latissimus dorsi in the line of the incision.

In the lower half of the incision cut the patient's external oblique almost in the line of its fibres.

The next layer is the internal oblique. Cut this almost across the line of its fibres.

If you see his twelfth thoracic nerve, try not to cut it. Avoid clamping it with forceps when you clamp the artery that runs with it.

Place retractors under the edges of the incision, and you will see his transversalis muscle anteriorly, attached to the dorsolumbar fascia posteriorly.

Incise the dorsolumbar fascia first, and use a gauze swab to push the peritoneum lying under transversalis forwards and laterally.

Complete the division of the dorsolumbar fascia and transversalis muscle in the line of the incision.

Underneath you will find the patient's perirenal fascia and the fat round his kidney.

DECIDING WHAT TO DO NEXT Base your decisions on the following indications.

Drainage There is a mass of blood clot which may be infected over the kidney.

Packing (1) You are not sure if the patient has a normal kidney on the other side, or not. (2) He is in such poor condition that he will not stand a further operation. (3) You are inexperienced, and have little help and few facilities.

Suturing tears Linear tears which can be sutured.

DRAINING A PERIRENAL HAEMATOMA Avoid the patient's peritoneal cavity by approaching the mass well to the side. Incise its most fluctuant part. Scoop out the blood clot, then either pack the area or close it with a wide corrugated rubber drain.

PACKING A RUPTURED KIDNEY Clear the blood clot from the patient's perinephric space. Put one roll of gauze on the medial side of his kidney, and another on the lateral side. Fill the wound with a third roll of gauze. Tie them together so you can later pull them all out together.

Bring the skin edges together loosely, watch him carefully, and transfuse him as necessary.

If he has severe haematuria, or excessive oozing, reopen the wound immediately.

48 hours later, remove the packing in the theatre. His kidney will probably be dry and not bleeding. Insert a drain.

SUTURING A RUPTURED KIDNEY Pass catgut mattress sutures about 5 cm through the kidney tissue. Don't tie them too tightly or they will cut out, or strangulate the renal tissue. Tighten the knot steadily, and avoid a sudden jerk.

Put three further stitches through the kidney, one at the middle of the tear and one at either end. If you cannot control bleeding insert a pack. Alternatively, use haemostatic gauze.

Take a small corrugated drain down to the patient's renal pelvis, and leave it protruding from the wound.

68 The lower urinary and genital tract

68.1 The general method for an injury of the lower urinary tract

The two sexes injure their lower urinary tracts in different ways. A woman's urinary tract is vulnerable to obstetric disaster, but seldom to trauma, whereas a man may sustain any of the injuries in Fig. 68-1. He can occasionally rupture his bladder into his peritoneal cavity (A). Much more often, he ruptures it extraperitoneally (B). He can also rupture his posterior urethra (C), his membranous urethra (D), his bulbous urethra (E), or his penile urethra (F). His prostatic urethra is protected by his prostate and is seldom injured. Blows to his lower abdomen burst his bladder (A). Fractures of his pelvis cause injuries B, C, and D. Blows to his urethra cause injuries D, E, and F. He may have more than one injury, and combinations of injuries B, and C, are not uncommon. A penetrating wound can injure any part of his urinary tract.

Always explore, repair, and drain a ruptured bladder. Ruptures of the urethra, on the other hand, are often incomplete and may heal themselves if you treat them conservatively, by diverting a patient's urine with a suprapubic cystostomy for three weeks. This will allow him to recover from any other injuries he may have, and give you time to refer him for endoscopy and expert repair, should the rupture of his urethra unfortunately turn out to have been complete. If you cannot refer him, you may have to repair him yourself.

Diagnosis is seldom difficult. The important sign in all injuries of the lower urinary tract is that *the patient cannot pass urine after an injury.* If his bladder bursts into his peritoneal cavity (A), he has the signs of a slowly developing peritonitis. If it bursts extraperitoneally (B), his urine slowly extravasates, and may eventually become infected. With both of these injuries (A, and B) his bladder usually fails to distend, but occasionally it may do, if there is a flap–like injury to its wall. So failure to pass urine after an injury, combined with failure of the bladder to distend, is usually an indication of injuries A or B.

In all more distal injuries (C, D, E, and F) the patient's bladder, including its internal sphincter, is intact, so after a few hours it always distends with urine. The combination of retention of urine with a distended bladder is characteristic of all injuries below the bladder neck, and occasionally of those above it. Another critical sign of injury of the lower urinary tract is blood at the patient's external meatus (even a drop is significant) in all urethral injuries (occasionally in C, and almost always in D, E, and F). His penis, scrotum, and perineum may also be injured.

Injuries to a patient's urinary tract are less urgent than some other abdominal catastrophes. If he has a ruptured spleen or liver, he needs an urgent laparotomy, but you have a few hours (never more than 24) in which to explore his ruptured bladder. Most surgeons would agree that you should not try to pass a urethral catheter, because it may introduce infection, and it can be misleading.

**CAN THE PATIENT PASS URINE AFTER AN INJURY?
IS THERE BLOOD AT THE TIP OF HIS MEATUS?
IS HIS BLADDER DISTENDING?**

THE GENERAL METHOD FOR INJURIES OF THE LOWER URINARY TRACT

This extends Section 51.3 on the care of a severely injured patient. Suspect that a patient may have injured his lower urinary tract if: (1) he has some injury which makes this likely (especially a fractured pelvis), or (2) he cannot pass urine after an accident, or (3) there is blood at the tip of his urethra.

CAUTION ! Don't pass a diagnostic catheter up the patient's urethra because: (1) The information it will give you will be unreliable. (2) You may contaminate the haematoma round the injury. (3) You may damage the slender bridge of tissue that joins the two halves of his injured urethra.

IMMEDIATELY AFTER AN INJURY OF THE LOWER URINARY TRACT

How did the injury occur? This will tell you the kind of injury to suspect.

Has the patient passed urine since the accident? If he wants to pass urine, let him try, *gently without straining.* If he strains, urine will extravasate into his tissues.

If he has passed blood–free urine since the accident, his urinary tract has not been seriously injured. If he can pass no urine, or only a little blood stained urine, with frequency and dysuria, his urethra has been injured.

If his bladder is distended, you may have to needle it to reduce his distress.

Has he ever had even a little bleeding from the external orifice of his urethra? If necessary, milk his urethra to demonstrate blood at its tip. You will usually find this bleeding

INJURIES OF THE LOWER URINARY TRACT

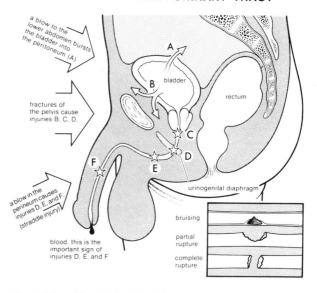

Fig. 68-1 INJURIES TO THE MALE LOWER URINARY TRACT. A, rupture of the bladder into the peritoneum. B, rupture outside the peritoneum. C, rupture of the posterior urethra. D, rupture of the membranous urethra. E, rupture of the bulbous urethra. F, rupture of the penile urethra.

if you look for it. It confirms a rupture (complete or partial) of some part of his urethra (injuries D, E, or F, and occasionally B, or C). He needs a suprapubic catheter.

The absence of bleeding is of no significance.

Is there a vague swelling in the patient's perineum, scrotum, or upper thigh? Early, this may be due to bruising, later, it may be caused by urine extravasating from injuries C, D, or E.

Is he tender above his pubis? The swelling may be more severe on one side than on the other. It indicates an injury, but not necessarily his urinary tract. The swelling may be due to bleeding, or to a mixture of blood and urine from injuries B, C, or D.

If he has a perineal haematoma, its size is no guide as to the probability of a urethral injury. Injuries E, and F, always cause a perineal haematoma; C, and D, may do.

Examine him rectally. Feel his prostate. This will not be easy if his pelvis is fractured. He may have so much tenderness and swelling that you cannot feel anything, except perhaps an indefinite doughy swelling (blood and urine) where his prostate should be. You may feel his prostate displaced upwards, floating freely, and running away from your examining finger as in Fig. 68-2. If so, he has ruptured his urethra in sites C, or D. The rupture is complete and he needs primary expert repair, or 'railroading', as in Section 68.5 as soon as his general condition permits. A dislocation of the prostate which you can be sure about on rectal examination is rare. This is such a difficult sign that some surgeons consider it valueless.

At the same time feel for a rectal injury. Can you feel a spicule of bone from a fractured pelvis penetrating his rectum? Is there blood on your glove? If so, goto Section 66.15 on rectal injuries.

If the patient's bladder is distended, aspirate it with a needle and look at his urine. If this is blood stained, either his bladder is bruised or ruptured, or the blood may have come from his kidney.

If you have to do a laparatomy for other trauma, you can examine his bladder with his other viscera.

INTRAPELVIC RUPTURE OF THE URETHRA

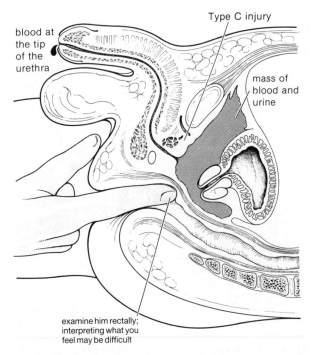

blood at the tip of the urethra

Type C injury

mass of blood and urine

examine him rectally; interpreting what you feel may be difficult

Fig. 68-2 RECTAL EXAMINATION FOR RUPTURE OF THE POSTERIOR URETHRA (injury C). This patient's urethra is completely ruptured. If you cannot refer him, 'railroad' him immediately. *With the kind permission of Hugh Dudley.*

X-RAYS If you suspect that a patient has ruptured his posterior urethra, X-ray his pelvis. A fracture is usually but not always present. The severity of his bony injuries is no indication of the probability of rupture.

An IVP is useful to establish a kidney injury, but is not useful for the bladder. You may need it for diagnosis.

SOME HOURS AFTER AN INJURY OF THE LOWER URINARY TRACT

Can you feel the dome of the patient's distended bladder distinct from the rest of the swelling? If his bladder is intact, it will now have had time to distend, and you may be able to feel it. In the presence of other signs, a distended bladder makes an injury to his urethra (C, D, E, or F) very likely, and a ruptured bladder (A or B) impossible.

CAUTION ! (1) A distended bladder is a useful but not invariable sign in distinguishing ruptures of the urethra inside the pelvis (C, or D) from intraperitoneal or extraperitoneal rupture of the bladder (A, or B). (2) A bladder can only distend if it has urine to distend with, so make sure you correct the patient's hypovolaemia and dehydration, so that he has some urine to secrete.

FURTHER MANAGEMENT OF AN INJURY OF THE LOWER URINARY TRACT

Read on for the management of rupture of the bladder (A, and B), and injuries to the urethra (C, D, E, and F). If you refer a patient with a suprapubic cystostomy, try to send someone with him to help him during the journey.

NEVER PASS A DIAGNOSTIC CATHETER IF THERE IS BLOOD AT THE EXTERNAL MEATUS

68.2 Rupture of the bladder

Intraperitoneal rupture A drunk patient with a distended bladder staggers in front of a motor vechicle. He receives a blow to his abdomen which bursts the dome or the posterior surface of his bladder, and floods his peritoneal cavity with urine (injury A, in Fig. 68-1). He feels sudden intense pain followed by shock and fainting. These immediate acute symptoms soon pass; there is no lower abdominal swelling, and his pain improves temporarily before signs of peritonitis follow after about 24 hours.

Extraperitoneal rupture Commonly, a patient is brought in with multiple injuries, one of which is a fracture of his pelvis which has ruptured his bladder outside his peritoneal cavity (injury B). Although he may want to pass urine, all he can produce is a drop of blood. The broken ends of his pubic bones have torn the anterior wall of his bladder close to its neck. Sometimes, his posterior urethra has ruptured also. Blood and urine fill his prevesical space and track between his peritoneum and his transversalis fascia. They infiltrate laterally towards his anterosuperior iliac spines, and down towards his prostate. If he is not treated, this mixture of blood and urine becomes pus, which may ultimately discharge through his sacrosciatic notches into his buttocks, through his obturator foramina into his thighs, or out through his inguinal canals. There is such devastating necrosis within his pelvis that he becomes severely toxaemic and may die.

In the first few hours after the accident, you may not be able to tell if a patient's fractured pelvis has ruptured his bladder, or has merely caused bleeding behind his pubic bones. But, even if his bladder has been ruptured, nothing much happens for the first 24 hours, so you have a day in which to observe him. *Don't delay more than 24 hours, and take great care not to infect the injured area by passing a diagnostic catheter meanwhile.*

You can usually tell quite easily if a patient's bladder has ruptured inside or outside his peritoneum from: (1) The history of the injury—a blow to his abdomen suggests rupture inside the peritoneum, whereas a fractured pelvis suggests rupture outside it. (2) The distribution of the tenderness—in extraperitoneal rupture this is narrowly localised suprapubically, in intraperitoneal rupture it is more diffuse over his lower abdomen and ends in obvious peritonitis.

If you are in doubt, there are two investigations that may confirm that his bladder has ruptured, and show you where it has ruptured, but they are usually not necessary: (1) You can do a retrograde cystogram. Unfortunately, this requires the use of a catheter, and with it the risk of infection. (2) You can do an intravenous pyelogram, which is safer but less reliable.

You will be wiser to wait a few hours to confirm the diagnosis, rather than to operate unnecessarily and find only a haematoma which bleeds profusely or even disastrously when you open it. If you have to do an immediate laparotomy for other reasons, say for a suspected rupture of the patient's spleen, you can easily examine his bladder at the same time.

If you diagnose any kind of rupture of the bladder, you will have to refer the patient urgently, or operate. A lower midline incision will bring you into his prevesical space outside his peritoneum just above his pubis. If this is full of urine and blood, his bladder has ruptured extraperitoneally. If it is normal, open his peritoneal cavity. If it contains blood and urine, his bladder has ruptured into it. The easiest way to find a tear is to open his bladder, put a finger into it, and feel for the tear. If an extraperitoneal rupture is large and easy to reach, it should not be too difficult to suture. But if the tear is difficult to get at, leave it, insert a suprapubic Foley catheter into his bladder and let it drain. An intraperitoneal rupture is usually larger, so always suture it and insert a suprapubic catheter drain.

Be sure to close a patient's bladder mucosa with catgut. If you use any other sutures, they may form a focus for the formation of stones. If his bladder has ruptured extraperitoneally, be sure to drain his prevesical space adequately.

RUPTURE OF THE BLADDER

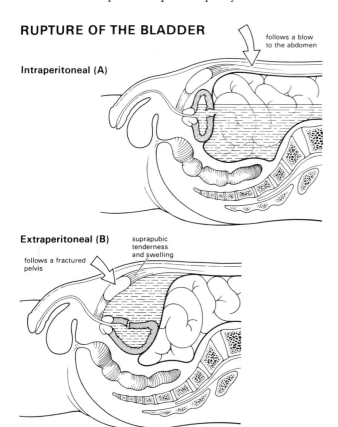

Fig. 68-3 INTRAPERITONEAL AND EXTRAPERITONEAL RUPTURE OF THE BLADDER If you diagnose any kind of rupture of the bladder, you will have to refer the patient urgently, or operate. *With the kind permission of Hugh Dudley.*

RUPTURE OF THE BLADDER

INDICATIONS Inability of the patient to pass urine within 24 hours of an injury, combined with: (1) The absence of a distended bladder (A, or B, in Fig. 68-1). (2) Increasing peritoneal irritation (A). (3) The appearance of a suprapubic swelling that might be extravasated blood and urine (B, or C). (4) Penetrating injuries that might have involved his bladder.

Make sure you have corrected the patient's hypovolaemia and dehydration, so that if his bladder is intact, it will contain some urine and be easier to find.

EQUIPMENT A general set. 2/0 plain catgut for the mucosa of the bladder, and 2/0 chromic catgut for its muscle wall.

ANTIBIOTICS Give the patient perioperative antibiotics (2.7).

OPERATION Take him to the theatre as carefully as you can, so as not to displace the broken fragments of his pelvis any further. Lie him supine with his legs slightly apart, so that you can, if necessary, pass a catheter. Drape him so as to expose his whole abdomen. Clean his urinary meatus, and its surroundings. If you are right handed, you may find it convenient to work from the left side of the table.

INCISION Make a midline incision from just below the patient's umbilicus to 1 cm above his pubic symphysis. Cut through the aponeurosis, and retract his rectus muscles. This will expose his prevesical space. Open it up with your fingers and inspect the front of his bladder. If you find urine, look where it is coming from.

CAUTION ! (1) Don't open his peritoneum yet. (2) If there is any danger that he may have other abdominal injuries, inspect the rest of his abdominal organs later in the operation.

If blood and urine flood up from his prevesical space, his bladder has ruptured extraperitoneally. Suck and mop the blood away. If bleeding is excessive, pack the space with gauze. Proceed as for extraperitoneal rupture, as described below.

If no blood and urine flood up from his prevesical space, find the upper surface of his bladder with its peritoneal reflexion, and use gauze dissection to displace this upwards. You will recognize that it is his bladder from the muscle fibres on its surface.

Incise his peritoneum by making a generous opening just above its attachment to his bladder. Enlarge the incision upwards as far as is necessary. Examine his abdominal organs and look for a retroperitoneal haematoma. If you find any other injuries, treat them first.

If his peritoneal cavity is normal, close it.

If his peritoneal cavity contains urine mixed with blood, his bladder has ruptured into it. Suck and mop away the blood and urine. The tear will probably be on its upper surface and you will find it easily. Proceed as for intraperitoneal rupture of the bladder, as described below.

If you are in doubt, open the patient's bladder as described below and inspect it from inside. Tears are more easily found from inside. Be prepared to find more than one tear.

EXTRAPERITONEAL RUPTURE OF THE BLADDER

The tear will probably be in the anterior wall of the patient's bladder, just above his prostate. It may be difficult to find when his bladder is empty and there is clot everywhere. Recognize his bladder by the muscle bundles in its walls, and the prominent veins on its surface.

If the tear is small, or difficult to find, don't suture it, or try to look for it in the blood and urine in front of his bladder. Instead, insert a suprapubic catheter, drain his retropubic space, and close his abdomen.

If the tear is large and easy to repair, suture it from inside. Open the bladder between stay sutures, as for a Freyer's prostatectomy (23.19). There will now be two (or more) holes in its wall—the original tear, and the incision you have just made. Put your finger into it, and feel the tear from inside.

CAUTION ! If the tear is near the ureters, pass a fine catheter up them to help to prevent you tying them off.

Go round to the left side of the table, if you are not already there. Suture the tear with a single layer of plain catgut stitches going deeply into the muscle.

Repair the patient's bladder in two layers, as for a prostatectomy (22.17), with an inner layer of continuous 3/0 plain catgut, and an outer layer of continuous chromic 2/0 catgut.

DRAINING THE BLADDER You will now need to drain the patient's bladder.

If there has been no blood at his external meatus, his urethra is probably unharmed. So drain his bladder through an indwelling 22 Ch Foley catheter passed up through his external meatus.

If there has been any blood at the patient's external meatus, his urethra has probably been injured. Avoid a urethral catheter. Instead, insert a 26 Ch Foley catheter through the cystotomy wound and sew his bladder wall round it with catgut (22.7).

Drain his prevesical space with a *large* (6 corrugations) rubber drain, or leave the wound partly open. Close the wound and anchor both his suprapubic catheter and his prevesical drain to his skin with stitches.

INTRAPERITONEAL RUPTURE OF THE BLADDER

Tilt the head of the table slightly downwards, and pack off the patient's intestines to make more room in his pelvis.

If there is an obvious tear in his bladder, feel and if possible look at the interior of his bladder through it. Alternatively, open his bladder through a separate incision anteriorly. Be sure to find and protect his ureters before you insert any sutures.

Control all bleeding inside the bladder, so as to reduce the risk of clot retention. Close the tear in his mucosa with continuous plain catgut, and its serosa with chromic catgut.

Remove the packs, level the table, mop up any free fluid in his peritoneal cavity, and close it. Drain his bladder with a urethral or suprapubic catheter, and drain his suprapubic space on the indications given above.

If there is frank peritonitis, insert a suprapubic peritoneal drain.

THE POSTOPERATIVE CARE OF A BLADDER INJURY

This is the same for both kinds of rupture. Connect the catheter to a closed drainage system, and check that it is draining. As soon as the patient has recovered from shock, raise him gradually into the sitting position.

If he has an extraperitoneal rupture, give him a broad spectrum antibiotic for 5 days in the hope of preventing the huge haematoma in his pelvis from becoming infected.

Prevesical drain **Remove this at 5 days.**

Indwelling urethral catheter. **Remove this at 7 to 14 days.** When it is removed he should be able to pass urine normally.

Suprapubic catheter (if you decide to insert one). **Keep this in** until after you have removed his urethral catheter. Remove this at 10 days. Try spigotting it first to see if he can pass urine.

DIFFICULTIES WITH BLADDER INJURIES

If there is SEVERE BLEEDING as you open the patient's prevesical space, fragments of his fractured pelvis have torn the vessels of his pelvic wall. The bleeding vessel may be impossible to find. When you remove the blood, most of the bleeding will probably stop. If it does not, pack his prevesical space and its lateral recesses, and leave the pack in for 15 minutes. Then, with an enlarged incision and a good light, have another look. You may find and be able to tie the bleeding vessel. If you don't find it, replace the pack, give him antibiotics, and remove it 24 hours later.

If he has an OPEN WOUND of his bladder, explore it, close the tear in its wall, do a suprapubic cystostomy, and drain his prevesical space. The tear may be posterior, in which case you may be forced to cut open the front of his bladder, in order to repair it from the inside.

If you have OPENED HIS BLADDER ACCIDENTALLY during the course of another operation, what you should do depends on when you recognize it.

If you recognise an accidentally opened bladder during the operation, **close it in two layers and insert a suprapubic or**

urethral catheter. Leave it to drain for about two weeks before removing it.

If you recognize it only some days later, **insert a catheter as** above, and also a peritoneal drain through a stab incision in one of his rectus muscles, being careful to avoid his inferior epigastric arteries. Don't put the suprapubic tube and the peritoneal drain too close together.

You are most likely to injure the bladder accidentally during Caesarean section (18.8), or when you repair a sliding hernia (14.2), or when you drain a patient's peritoneal cavity suprapubically for peritonitis. The main way of preventing injury is to catheterize a patient's bladder after you have anaesthetized him, before doing any of these procedures. If you decide to catheterize him first, leave the catheter in place to prevent his bladder filling up before you come to operate.

If he gets CLOT RETENTION, wash out his bladder thoroughly through his urethral or suprapubic catheter to remove all clot.

68.3 Rupture of the posterior urethra (injuries C, and D)

Suspect that a severely injured patient has ruptured his posterior urethra, if he has: (1) A fractured pelvis, particularly if he has a 'butterfly fracture' (D, Fig. 76-1), or a 'hinge fracture' (E, in this figure). (2) Bleeding from his external meatus. (3) A distended bladder. (4) A boggy swelling displacing or partly concealing his prostate.

If a patient's prostate is not widely displaced, and there is no boggy feeling when you examine him rectally (a difficult and unreliable sign), the rupture of his posterior urethra is probably incomplete. and will heal itself if you leave it for 3 weeks, and insert a suprapubic catheter to prevent his urine extravasating meanwhile. If a small bridge of urethral tissue survives, his urethra may reform with very little stricture—provided that the infection which may follow catheterization does not destroy it. The prevention of this infection one of the reasons why you should not try to catheterize him. The other reason is that you may make his injury worse. If his rupture heals during three weeks of waiting, it was incomplete. The best test of this is to see if he can pass urine normally when you clamp off the suprapubic tube. If he cannot, the chances are that the rupture was complete, so *try to refer him for expert repair at 3 weeks.* Don't leave him longer than this because increasing fibrosis will make repair more difficult. Repair at 3 weeks is seldom easy, but it is no more difficult than it would have been immediately after the accident.

If his prostate is widely displaced, and there is a boggy feeling when you examine him rectally, his urethra is probably completely ruptured. If you cannot refer him, you will have to try to 'railroad' him, as in the next section.

The great advantage of conservative treatment is that it will usually avoid railroading, which is difficult and bloody. Your first sight of the retropubic space of a patient with a fractured pelvis and a torn urethra will be daunting indeed.

POSTERIOR URETHRAL INJURIES

This follows from Sections 51.3, and 68.1, and is the same for injuries in sites C, and D, in Fig. 68-1.

IS IMMEDIATE REPAIR INDICATED?

If a patient's prostate is widely displaced immediately after the injury (rare), and there is a boggy feeling on rectal examination, he probably has a complete rupture. Insert a suprapubic catheter, and refer him immediately. Experts can do primary repair. If this is impractical, goto Section 68.4 and railroad him yourself immediately. If you are not sure his rupture is complete or not, because displacement on rectal examination is such a difficult sign, treat him conservatively, as described below.

If his prostate is not displaced, his urethra may not be completely ruptured, conservative treatment is indicated, and his prognosis is good.

CONSERVATIVE TREATMENT Put him to bed with a suprapubic catheter on continuous drainage. Use a fine plastic, suprapubic tube (23.6 and 23.7), not a suprapubic Foley catheter.

Insert the catheter by open exposure of his bladder (23.7). Do this at a laparotomy which will: (1) enable you to examine any other abdominal viscera which may also be injured, and (2) let you assess the extent of his prostatic dislocation. You don't want to bring him back to the theatre for another operation soon afterwards.

Pass a long 26 Ch suprapubic catheter (this is about the size of intravenous plastic tubing) with side holes, and anchor it with a stout stitch.

CAUTION ! Remember that exploring his bladder converts a closed fracture of his pelvis into an open one, so give him perioperative antibiotics (2.7).

TREAT HIS PELVIC FRACTURE If he has a hinge fracture, use a sling or traction as in Section 76.2. Ignore butterfly compression fractures.

THREE WEEKS AFTER A POSTERIOR URETHRAL INJURY

Clamp the patient's suprapubic tube, and see if he can pass urine.

If he can pass no urine, he probably has a complete rupture. Refer him for accurate open repair by an expert. If you cannot repair him, railroad him.

If he can pass urine, his outlook is good. When he has passed as much urine as he can through his urethra, empty his bladder thoroughly through his suprapubic tube. This is his residual urine. Measure it.

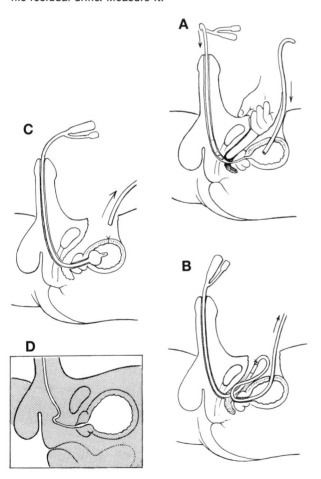

Fig. 68-4 RAILROADING WITH CATHETERS. A, feeling for the tip of the Foley catheter in the patient's retropubic space. B, the two catheters have been joined together. C, the Foley catheter has been pulled through into his bladder, which has been closed. D, a tortuous stricture is sure to form. You will have to use sounds to get the feel of it before it becomes tightly fibrotic. Record in the patient's notes how the stricture is best negotiated—it may not be sounded by you next time, and your successor will be grateful! *Kindly contributed by Peter Bewes.*

If his residual urine is less than 75 ml, his urethra is sufficiently healed for you to remove his suprapubic tube.

If his residual urine is more than 75 ml, leave the tube in for a few more days and try again.

If it remains more than 75 ml, and gets steadily worse, he has a complete rupture, and his prognosis is poor, especially if repair is delayed beyond 3 weeks. This situation is rare. Usually, he either recovers completely, or can pass no urine. If referral really is impossible, attempt railroading.

CAUTION ! Beware of: (1) The elderly man with an enlarged prostate. (2) The young boy who may have considerable difficulty starting micturition and whose rupture is likely to be just below his bladder neck.

If railroading fails or is impossible, he will be left with a permanent suprapubic catheter, unless he can be referred for urethral reconstruction.

68.4 'Railroading'

This is a method of passing a catheter through a patient's urethra when it is torn, and when the two ends of the urethra are widely separated. 'Railroading' is not easy, and should very rarely be necessary. If there is much fibrosis, you will have to use sounds, but you should start by using a catheter. Pass one catheter up his urethra from below, feel for it in his retropubic space and bring it out into the wound. Pass another catheter down through his bladder from above. Find it in his prevesical space and bring it too out into the wound. Push the end of the lower catheter into the cut end of the upper one, and stitch them if necessary. Then use the upper one to pull the lower one through into his bladder.

If you use sounds, pass one sound up his urethra from below, and another down through his bladder from above. You will feel them meeting in the blood clot where his posterior urethra should be. Use the upper sound to guide the lower one up through his prostatic urethra into his bladder. When the lower sound is in his bladder, fix a rubber tube to it and use this to pull a Foley catheter up into his bladder. There is a great danger that you will create false passages, so be careful!

RAILROADING

Refer the patient if you can.

INDICATIONS (1) A severely displaced prostate immediately after the injury. (2) Failure to pass urine after 3 weeks of conservative treatment with suprapubic catheter drainage. (3) Increasing residual urine after attempted conservative treatment.

INVESTIGATIONS If possible, do an ascending urethrogram, and a micturating cystourethrogram. Use the suprapubic tube to get the contrast medium into the patient's bladder. Fill his bladder as full as you can, and then get him to pass urine as a film is taken.

ANAESTHESIA Give him a general anaesthetic with a relaxant, and lie him supine. Have blood cross-matched.

USING CATHETERS FOR RAILROADING

Lubricate the patient's urethra and try to pass a 16 or 18 Ch soft rubber catheter. If this passes immediately after the injury, your diagnosis was at fault. Remove it at once but leave the suprapubic catheter in for the full 3 weeks.

If a Foley catheter fails to enter his bladder, make a lower midline incision to expose and open his bladder with a suprapubic cystotomy as in Section 68.2. Make a fairly large vertical incision in his bladder. An opening of a reasonable size will make the procedure much easier. The catheter will present in his pelvis through the torn lower end of his urethra. If necessary, use 'finger dissection' deep in his retropubic space. Finding it may not be easy, and there may be a lot of clot to be swept away. Pass another larger 24 Ch catheter down through his bladder, into his internal urinary meatus and then through into his retropubic space. Bring it out into the wound. Remove its tip and eyes and push the end of the Foley catheter into it. If necessary, suture them together. Try to make a smooth join that will cause the minimum of trauma. Then pull the Foley catheter into his bladder.

If (in late cases) the Foley catheter fails to pass into his retropubic space, because there is too much fibrosis, you will have to use sounds.

USING SOUNDS FOR RAILROADING

EQUIPMENT Two curved metal sounds, a piece of rubber or plastic tube that will fit tightly over one of them, as in A, Fig. 68-5, and will not come off when you draw it through the patient's uretha. A 20 Ch silicone latex Foley catheter.

SOUNDING If a rubber catheter does not pass, gently try to pass a curved Lister's sound. If this does not pass, find where it is held up; see under difficulties' below.

If all is well the sound should pass easily into the patient's retropubic space. Pass another sound down through his bladder. You should feel a metallic 'clink' as the sounds touch (B). If you don't, mobilize the apex of his prostate a bit more and try to feel the ends of the two sounds in the wound. Or, ask your assistant to put his finger in the rectum and feel the ends of the two sounds.

Keeping the two sounds in contact with one another, use the upper one to guide the lower one into the bladder (C). Fix the piece of tube to the tip of the lower sound (D), and use it to draw this tube down through his urethra.

Alternatively, pass your finger through his prostatic urethra, try to feel the sound and guide it into his bladder, as in H, Fig. 68-5.

Stitch the tip of a Foley catheter snugly to the tube and use this to pull the catheter up into the patient's bladder (E). If the tube and the catheter do not fit snugly, the join will further injure his urethra as it passes through.

WHEN THE FOLEY CATHETER IS IN PLACE stitch a stout monofilament suture to its tip, and bring this out through the patient's abdominal wall (F).

Blow up the balloon of the Foley catheter, and close the patient's bladder as usual (23.7). Keep the monofilament suture long, roll it round a swab and fix it to his abdominal wall. If the balloon bursts, you can use it to railroad another Foley catheter into place without doing a second laparotomy.

Send the patient back to the ward with the catheter on continuous drainage. If there was a tendency for the bladder to 'ride high' far from the pelvic diaphragm, tie the distal end of the catheter (perhaps its side tube) with a long string to a 20 ml specimen bottle full of water. Lead this over the end of his bed; it will exert just enough traction to keep his prostate in place (G).

CAUTION ! (1) Keep the balloon blown up. (2) Don't exert too much traction, or you will pull the balloon out of the patient's bladder into his retropubic space, or cause the base of his bladder to necrose. Most surgeons don't exert any traction if the bladder doesn't 'ride high'.

Keep up this gentle traction for 3 weeks. Then remove the catheter, and see if he can pass urine.

As soon as possible, bougie him with a large Lister bougie. Repeat it after 3 weeks, then 4, then 5 weeks until he is stable. He will certainly have a difficult stricture, so follow him up for life.

Alternatively insert a second Foley suprapubically, and drain his bladder through this. A Foley catheter which is exerting traction is not ideal for draining the bladder at the same time.

DIFFICULTIES WITH URETHRAL INJURIES

If the SOUND IS HELD UP IN THE PATIENT'S PERINEUM, cut down on its tip, as for external urethrotomy (23.9), and continue as for this operation.

If the SOUND IS HELD UP AT HIS PERINEAL MEMBRANE, remove it, and do a laparotomy as for Freyer's prostatectomy (23.17), but with a lower midline abdominal incision. Open his retropubic space right down to his perineal membrane. Use the index fingers of both your hands to open up this space. Then open up his bladder as for Freyer's prostatectomy. Find

RAILROADING

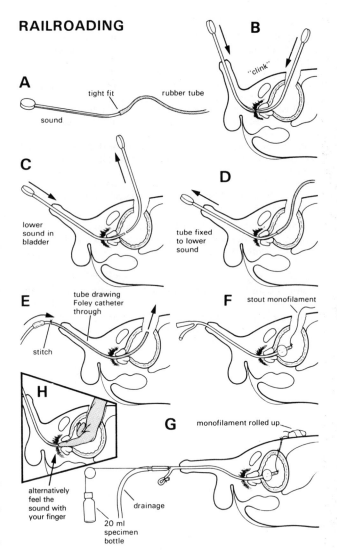

Fig. 68-5 RAILROADING WITH SOUNDS. A, shows how the rubber tube must fit tightly over the sound. B, the two sounds meeting in the patient's retropubic space. C, the lower sound has entered his bladder. D, the rubber tube has been fitted on to the lower sound and it is now being drawn through his urethra. E, the rubber tube has been stitched to the Foley catheter and is drawing it through. F, monofilament has been fixed to the Foley catheter, so that if it slips out, another one can be drawn through. G, traction is being exerted. H, an alternative, guiding a sound into the bladder with your little finger. *Kindly contributed by Peter Bewes.*

his internal meatus. You may be able to guide a Foley catheter past the obstruction into his bladder. If you fail, reintroduce the urethral sound, and pass another one down through his bladder and his internal urinary meatus as in B, Fig. 68-5.

68.5 Injuries of the penile urethra (injuries E, and F)

Rupture of a patient's anterior urethra resembles that of his posterior urethra (68.4) except that: (1) It is caused by a blow to his perineum rather than by a fractured pelvis. (2) He has a severe perineal haematoma. (3) He is more likely to bleed through his urethra, and when he does bleed, the bleeding will be more severe. (4) The diagnosis is easier, and he is less likely to die. Treatment with a trial of conservative treatment is similar. You will hardly ever have to operate on the injured area itself, because the injury is nearly always incomplete. But, if conservative treatment fails, and the rupture turns out to be complete, you can cut down on his anterior urethra, as if you were doing an external urethrotomy (23.9), which is less difficult. Scar tissue forms more readily in Africans, so strictures are a major problem in these patients.

INJURIES OF THE PENILE URETHRA

If the patient can pass urine, let him do so; his urethra is not seriously injured.

CONSERVATIVE TREATMENT OF INJURIES OF THE PENILE URETHRA **If he cannot pass urine,** take him to the theatre, do a formal cystostomy (23.7), insert a suprapubic catheter, and leave it in for 3 weeks. Use a fine plastic tube, not a Foley catheter. Provided that the haematoma in his scrotum or perineum is not so tense as to endanger the skin over it, leave it. Otherwise, open it, evacuate it, and tie any bleeding vessels.

If his wound is open, goto Section 68.9.

If at 3 weeks he cannot pass urine, he has a complete tear and you will have to refer him for repair, or repair him yourself by the method which follows.

REPAIRING THE PENILE URETHRA AFTER AN INJURY

ANAESTHESIA (1) Caudal epidural anaesthesia (A 7.3). (2) Subarachnoid anaesthesia (7.4). (3) General anaesthesia (A 11.3).

METHOD Put the patient into the lithotomy position. Pass a straight bougie. See how far it goes. Mark the obstruction site by your usual method (23.8).

Cut down on his bulbospongiosus at the site of the obstruction, as for an external urethrotomy (23.9).

If you cannot find the proximal end of his urethra, open his bladder, and pass a catheter down from above.

If his whole urethra is disrupted, mobilize his bulbospongiosus proximally and distally as necessary, so that it will stretch to meet without tension (it is a very elastic organ).

Repair his urethra and bulbospongiosus end to end with 3/0 plain catgut and leave a silastic Foley catheter in for 6 weeks on intermittent drainage.

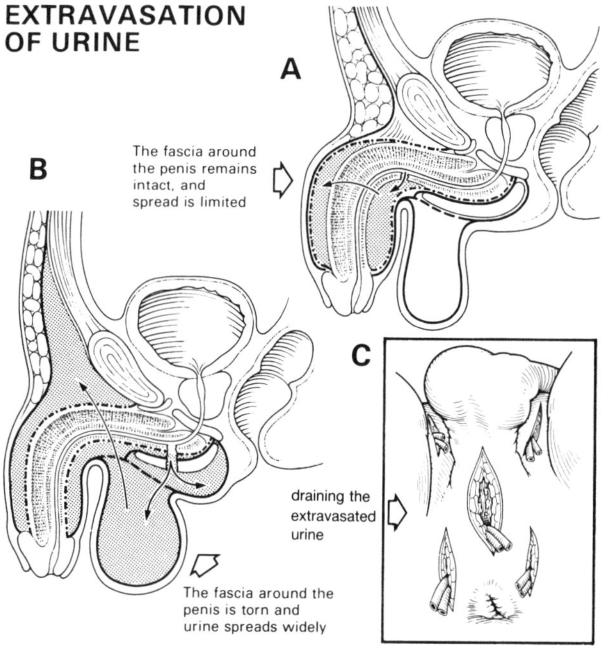

EXTRAVASATION OF URINE

Fig. 68-6 EXTRAVASATION OF URINE. Urine leaking from the bulbar urethra may at first be limited to the penis if the fascia around it (Buck's fascia) remains intact, as in A. If this fascia is breached, urine can spread much more widely, as in B. *Adapted with kind permission from an original painting by Frank H. Netter, M.D. from the CIBA COLLECTOION OF MEDICAL ILLUSTRATIONS, copyright by CIBA Pharmaceutical Company, Division of CIBA–GEIGY Corporation.*

At 6 weeks remove the catheter, and follow him up for a stricture. He will need bouginage for life.

If you don't have a silastic catheter, insert a suprapubic catheter, at the same time as the repair, and leave the repair without a splint. Use the next 3 weeks to get one of the bougies in Fig. 23-9 made. At the end of 3 weeks gently pass it under lignocaine anaesthesia. Measure his residual urine. When this is 75 ml or less, remove the suprapubic catheter.

`POSTOPERATIVE CARE All patients need repeated dilatation, starting at 6 weeks, and eventually every 3 months for life.

68.6 Extravasation of urine complicating urethral injuries

A patient's urine extravasates if he tries to pass it through a ruptured urethra. Try to prevent this happening by draining his bladder. In injuries B, C, and D, in Fig. 68-1, combine this with draining his prevesical space. Extravasation can also complicate a urethral stricture (23.10).

Extravasation can be superficial or deep. Superficial extravasation appears as a large, expanding, tender swelling of the patient's penis, or a swelling in his scrotum, perineum, or lower abdomen. Provided he has not been catheterized, the urine which has escaped is unlikely to be infected. If it is infected, severe necrotizing cellulitis will follow.

EXTRAVASATION OF URINE If a patient presents late with a large red oedematous swelling, insert a suprapubic catheter into his bladder (23.6), and let out the stinking fluid through multiple wide incisions in the swelling. Give him antibiotics (2.7) and wait. This is not the time to start repairing his urethra.

If you cannot refer him, you can try the residual urine regime (68.3) after a month or so of suprapubic drainage. If he has only a little residual urine, try bouginage. If that is satisfactory, remove his suprapubic catheter when his residual urine is less than 75 ml. If the overlying skin sloughs, graft his wound.

68.7 Strictures after urethral injuries

Unfortunately, a stricture usually follows an injury to any part of the urethra, *so any patient who has ever had a urethral injury* must be regularly reviewed (22.8). Monitor his stream with a bucket and tape measure as in Fig. 23-9, or with a stop watch. If there is any deterioration at all, pass bougies to calibrate the size of his stricture, and decide whether or not to start life long bouginage. He may have an 'S' bend deformity of his membraneous urethra, resulting from partial backwards displacement of his prostate. If you instrument him forcibly, you can easily make a false passage at the 'S' bend. If his stream is diminishing, bouginage for life is inevitable. The secret of success is *to diagnose an impending stricture early, and to start bouginage before he notices his stream is tailing off.* If he has an anterior stricture, he may be able to bougie himself with the homemade bougie in Fig. 23-9. Tell him to boil it and leave it in the water until the water becomes tepid. Warn him also that he will probably have urinary infections and should present early for treatment. The strictures that follow injuries will be easier to manage if you don't leave them too long before you start to bougie them.

A STRICTURE ALMOST ALWAYS FOLLOWS A URETHRAL INJURY

68.8 Injuries of the penis and scrotum

When the skin of a patient's penis is avulsed, its shaft is usually uninjured, and you can graft it quite easily. When there is a

201

defect in the skin of his scrotum, you can usually close the wound with the skin which remains. Don't try to graft the scrotum, because there is no way of applying pressure to the graft.

INJURIES OF THE PENIS AND SCROTUM

BRUISING is the result of injury to the patient's non–erect organ. Treat it as a urethral injury. Can he pass urine? If he can, his urethra is not seriously injured.

If he cannot pass urine, insert a suprapubic catheter, and treat him as a urethral injury.

If his penis starts to swell with blood or urine, treat him as for a fractured penis as described below.

OPEN WOUNDS Do a wound toilet, you will probably not need to excise any skin. The urethra may be very difficult to recognize in the bleeding tissue–don't injure it! If in doubt, assume that injured tissue will recover. Use delayed closure. If the penis needs bandaging, let this mimic the erect position. If the urethra is injured, insert a suprapubic catheter.

AVULSION (DEGLOVING) INJURIES If any flaps of skin remain on a patient's injured penis, even if they are completely detached, replace them immediately, because they will probably live.

If any part of the shaft of his penis is bare, cover it with split skin, allowing for contraction. Cover the graft with a firm, even dressing. Or, if the deep layer of his foreskin remains attached to the shaft proximal to the corona, you may be able to use both layers to make a high quality flap or graft.

Alternatively, bury the shaft of a patient's penis in his scrotum and release it later.

If any flaps of scrotal skin remain, remove them.

If the skin of his scrotum has been avulsed, but enough remains, try to make a bag for his testes. If necessary, undercut the skin of his thighs. Or, make incisions in his thighs to hold his testes and cords until you can refer him for a plastic repair.

FRACTURE OF THE PENIS is the result of the sudden posterior angulation of an erect penis. Open up the huge swelling with an incision over the most swollen part and evacuate the clot. Then suture the capsule of the ruptured corpora cavernosa.

If the patient's corpus spongiosum and urethra have been fractured, insert a suprapubic catheter for 3 weeks and proceed as for a urethral injury (68.5).

DIFFICULTIES WITH INJURIES OF THE PENIS AND SCROTUM

If a patient's TESTIS IS INJURED, toilet his wound, then clean and close his tunica albuginea. Drain his scrotum only and don't insert a drain under his tunica.

If his PENIS IS JAMMED in a circular object, the distal part becomes engorged and swollen. In early cases try sucking some of the blood from his corpora cavernosa with a needle and syringe, then compress the distal part with cold compresses for 15 minutes. In later cases you will have to open up the circular object, if necessary under general anaesthesia.

If the distal part of his penis becomes gangrenous, amputate it, and proceed as for carcinoma of the penis (Chapter 32).

INJURY OF THE TESTIS

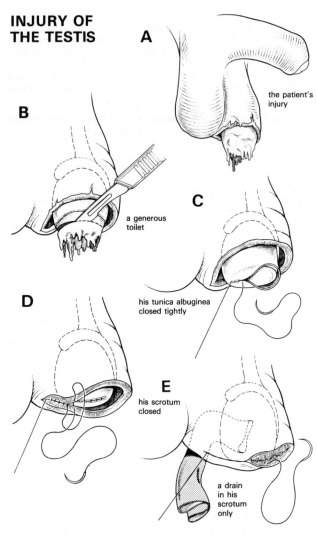

Fig. 68-7 AN INJURY OF THE TESTIS. A, the patient's injury. B, a generous toilet. C, his tunica being closed. D, his scrotum being closed. E, a drain in his scrotum. *From the Early Care of the Injured Patient. The Committee on Trauma of the American College of Surgeons. Edited by A.J. Walt. With kind permission.*

69 Broken bones

69.1 Examining an injured limb

The penalty of having a stiff skeleton is that it may break, especially the bones of the arms and legs. You can treat injuries to the soft tissues of the limbs in more or less the same way, wherever they occur, but each part of each limb bone is different—hence the space we devote to them. Treating them provides many opportunities for disaster, but none is more common or more serious than: (1) Primary closure of an open fracture (or a contaminated wound) (54.1). (2) Applying a cast over a recent injury without splitting it, especially in minor fractures with little initial swelling (70.4). More limbs are lost from these two causes than from anything else.

THE GENERAL METHOD FOR AN INJURED LIMB

HISTORY

Always take a careful history. Most fractures are the result of some characteristic injury, so enquire carefully about the force which caused an injured limb. For example:

If a patient landed on his heels from a height, he may have fractured his calcaneus, and also perhaps his spine.

THE NEUTRAL POSITION

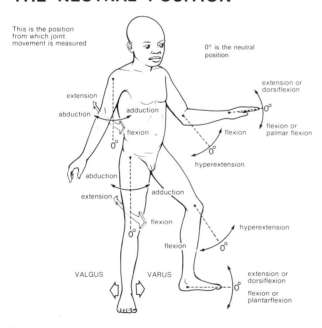

Fig. 69-1 THE NEUTRAL POSITIONS from which flexion and extension, and adduction and abduction can be measured. The positions of rest, and function (for ankylosis) are both quite different and are shown in Fig. 7-16. The position of safety for the hand is shown in Fig. 75-8. Note that in a valgus deformity the distal part of the limb deviates away from the midline and in a varus one it deviates towards it. *Kindly contributed by John Stewart.*

If he fell on his outstretched hand, he may have any of the injuries to his upper limb listed in Section 74.1.

If a very small force was able to break his bone, it may have been weakened by some other disease so that the fracture is pathological.

If he is a child, he may have fallen because he is feeling ill.

CAUTION ! Osteomyelitis and septic arthritis are the most important differential diagnoses. If you take a careful history you will not miss them.

EXAMINING AN INJURED LIMB

Many methods of examination are the same for an injured patient as for an orthopaedic one, so modify those in the list below appropriately.

The important signs of a fracture are: (1) tenderness and abnormal mobility at the fracture site, and (2) an abnormal X-ray. Sometimes you may be able to feel crepitus—the grating feeling as bone ends move over one another. It is acutely painful so don't examine for it unless it is necessary. If you expect to feel it and don't feel it, there may be soft tissue between the fragments.

LOOK Remove the patient's clothes and look for abnormal attitudes, contour, and shortening. If displacement is gross, one glance will tell you he has a fracture or a dislocation—deformity, shortening, rotation, or overlap will be obvious. You can diagnose most dislocations merely by looking at them.

Are both limbs the same? Compare one side carefully with the other. One joint may look larger than the other, either because it is swollen, or because the muscles round it are wasted. If necessary, measure shortening with a tape measure (77-3).

FEEL Ask the patient to point to exactly where the pain is. Often, his whole joint is acutely tender; if it is not, feel carefully for the place of maximum tenderness, particularly if you suspect a fracture of his wrist or ankle. You will then know which bone to X-ray. Tenderness to gentle pressure is a more useful sign than tenderness to deep pressure.

If a bone is tender, assume it is broken (or he has osteomyelitis) until an X-ray shows it is normal, or until you are quite sure he has not got osteomyelitis—see Section 7.3. If a ligament is acutely tender, it may be ruptured.

Feel the patient's bones carefully, for example, are the three bony points of his elbow (72-2) in their normal places?

If you suspect infection, test for warmth. Test for this first, because your other examinations may increase it. (1) Use the back of your hand to compare the abnormal side with the normal one. Or, (2) move the palm of your hand down the patient's limb. It usually gets progressively colder, if it gets warmer anywhere, the warm part may be abnormally vascular, usually because of infection.

MOVE Ask the patient to move his injured limb, as much as he can himself. This is active movement.

If he can use his arm actively, or walk on his injured leg without a limp, he has no serious injury. Many important injuries are missed, or unnecessarily overtreated, because nobody asks a patient to do this.

If he cannot move his limb actively, gently move it passively for him in all directions, as far as you can without hurting him.

Record the movement that is possible from the neutral position for each joint as shown in Fig. 69-1.

Most surgeons evolve their own particular routines, which they vary as necessary. Later we describe a detailed routine for the knee. Work out your own for the other joints.

Finally record your findings, and don't forget to include the soft tissue injuries. A patient's X-ray films are not a sufficient record of his injury.

15 GOLDEN RULES FOR FRACTURES

(1) If a patient is severely injured, save his life first; treat any airway obstruction (52.1), haemorrhage, or shock (53.2) before you treat his fractures.

(2) Splint him where he lies when you first see him (51.2); this will minimize soft tissue damage and avoid converting a closed fracture into an open one.

(3) Look for signs of nerve (55.8) and vessel injury (55.3) and record your findings.

(4) Handle his injured part as little as you can.

(5) If he has an obvious fracture, make sure that this is his only injury—it may be the least of his injuries. Don't let him die from a tension pneumothorax (65.5) while you are treating a fracture of his forearm!

(6) Don't be deceived by the absence of deformity and disability; sometimes he can continue to use his fractured limb.

(7) Take X-rays in 2 planes and examine them yourself.

(8) Reduce the fracture as soon as you can, don't wait for the swelling to go down, except sometimes in the ankle (82.4).

(9) If he has continuous severe pain, suspect circulatory impairment and treat it immediately (70.4).

(10) When you split a cast, divide the plaster and the padding right down to his skin.

(11) If you put him into traction, be sure to check this frequently (70.9).

(12) All joints that are not immobilized by the fracture must be kept moving (69.10).

(13) Remember that open fractures are contaminated wounds, so toilet them and use delayed primary closure (69.7).

(14) Aim to restore function. If a patient's arm is injured, try to restore the proper use of his hand; shortening and some misalignment are often acceptable. If his leg is injured, try to restore painless stable weight bearing; prevent misalignment; maintaining length is desirable, but a little shortening is acceptable.

(15) Finally, remember to treat him as a whole person; don't only treat his injured limb.

69.2 X-rays for bony injuries

You are more likely to make a mistake because you don't examine a patient than because you don't x-ray him. Although all fractures should in theory be X-rayed, this may be unnecessary with some of them, and you may have no X-rays. If films are scarce, keep them for injuries which involve a patient's joints, especially his elbows, hips or ankles. Always X-ray him if his symptoms seem to be worse than your present diagnosis suggests. A fracture is a three dimensional lesion, so you will need X-rays in two planes at right angles in order to visualise it. For most fractures take an AP (anteroposterior) and a lateral view. Even if there is a radiologist's report, look at all films yourself, *and if you are in doubt, compare them with views of the other side, if possible on the same film. This is especially important in young children.*

Make sure the films include enough of the patient. For example, a film of his forearm may fail to show an injury of his wrist, so *in all long bone fractures, X-ray the joints above and below the fracture.* Don't overlook a proximal injury, for example a fracture of the neck of the femur. It is a major error to treat a distal injury, and to fail to diagnose a proximal one.

If you are not sure if he has a fracture or not, ask him to come for another X-ray in 7 to 10 days time. If he does have a fracture you will see it more easily then. If his films are normal a week after the injury, the problem is not in his bones.

X-rays will not show you the position of his bones at the time of the accident. For example, an injury may have severely displaced the bones of the knee and torn its ligaments, after which they may have returned to their normal position. So a normal X-ray does not exclude a ligamentous injury.

Don't take 'X-rays for X-rays sake'. Many fractures can be diagnosed without them. Colles, Pott, Smith, Bennett, Monteggia and Maisonneuve all described their fractures before X-rays were invented. If your X-ray machine does not work, or your stock of film is almost exhausted, here is some help.

IF YOU DON'T HAVE X-RAYS make your diagnosis of a fracture or a dislocation on: (1) the violence of the injury, (2) the classical deformities of particular injuries, (3) tenderness over a subcutaneous bone (if this is absent a fracture is unlikely), (4) loss of function (a patient who can walk and bear weight normally is unlikely to have a serious injury).

The injuries which least need an X-ray include: (1) extension fractures of the wrist, (2) clavicle fractures, (3) many tibial fractures (you can detect angulation and rotation clinically), (4) greenstick fractures of the forearm in children.

The injuries which most need an X-ray include: (1) doubtful hip injuries, which might be a slipped epiphysis, or fracture of the femoral neck, (2) possible penetrating wounds of the skull in children by hoes or garden forks, (3) ankle injuries, (4) elbow injuries, and (5) any long bone fracture where there might be a dislocation at the upper end, (6) severe foot injuries where the patient cannot walk.

COMPARE THE ABNORMAL SIDE WITH THE NORMAL ONE

69.3 Adequate function with minimum risk

There are two main methods of treating fractures, and two corresponding schools of fracture surgeons who emphasize one method of treatment rather than the other method: (1) Fixing fractures internally with metal screws, plates, and pins. (2) Treating them without operating, if an operation can be avoided. Some fractures, such as those of the clavicle, should never be treated by internal fixation. A few, such as those of the neck of the femur, can only be fixed internally. Many other fractures, such as those of the shaft of the femur, can be treated by either method.

Fixing fractures successfully by internal fixation needs: (1) Much training, experience, and skill, and is not to be learnt merely by reading a manual. (2) A complex and costly set of equipment. (3) Expensive screws and plates. (4) A theatre environment of the highest sterility. (5) Much time, which you probably will not have. If you attempt internal fixation without *all* these necessary conditions, too many of your patients will end up severely disabled by ununited or infected bones, which drip pus through multiple sinuses for many years.

Because internal fixation is such a disaster when it is badly done, we have collected together here a system of non–operative methods for most of the common fractures and for many of the rarer ones. You will find that these methods will give you a much lower rate of infection and non–union.

Of the fractures which have to be fixed internally, some of those of the olecranon and patella are not too difficult, so we have included methods of internal fixation for them. The only common fractures for which we have no adequate method are those of the neck of the femur. These have to be fixed internally, but they need more skill and equipment than you are likely to have.

This is not the place to discuss the merits of the two schools, except to say that in the industrial world fracture treatment is dominated by internal fixation, and particularly by the Arbeitgemeinshaft für Osteosynthesenfragen, the Association for Osteosynthesis, or AO for short.

High technology methods of internal fixation, such as those of AO, are attractive, and give superb results with some difficult fractures. For example, they enable a patient to fall from his horse, break his radius, and yet be at work again the next week. *But these good results can only be obtained by master surgeons, when the risks of operating, and particularly the risk of infection, have been reduced to the lowest possible degree.* This is essential, because infection is a ten times greater disaster in orthopaedics than it is in general surgery, where a wound infection is usually only a minor problem. If you have equipment for internal fixation, don't use it, except occasionally in its simplest forms, as described here. Unless you can meet AO criteria, your results will be disastrous. Refer the more difficult fractures, if you can—the place for AO is in a referral hospital.

The non—operative school is less preoccupied with mechanical elegance, less visible, less organized, and lacks an obvious label. The thinking behind its work is to follow the natural healing processes of the body, to use closed methods wherever possible, to encourage the patient to start using his limb as soon as he can, and to interfere surgically only if absolutely necessary, and then only in the simplest way possible. If it is not essential to restore the exact anatomy after a fracture, the non—operative school does not try to do so. It argues that the perfect immobilization which AO methods try so hard to achieve is seldom even desirable, and that in many fractures a little movement is a good thing in that it encourages callus formation and union, and prevents the absorption of bone. The members of this school point out that: (1) perfect radiological reduction does not always mean perfect function, and (2) function may be perfect, even though reduction is not. In the 1920s Böhler was the main exponent of these methods, and in the 1950s George Perkins. More recently these methods have been developed by Sarmiento. Because internal fixation is so dominant, no systematic collection of non—operative methods exists—hence the need for this one.

THE POSSESSION OF EQUIPMENT FOR INTERNAL FIXATION SHOULD NOT BE A LICENCE TO USE IT

With fractures of the shafts of long bones, non—operative methods give excellent results. With more difficult ones, particularly fractures into joints, your results, and those of most surgeons, are unlikely to be perfect. With difficult fractures try to:

(1) Get a patient's injured limb to unite in the position of function. If it becomes fixed in this position it will be more useful to him than a limb which is septic, or has failed to unite, because you operated when the risks were too high. The measure of adequate function in a limb is its usefulness in relation to the patient's life and work. Adequate function is a state of his mind as much as of his joints; so, if he has a difficult fracture, warn him that function is unlikely to be perfect. Discuss the problems with him and let him prepare for them.

(2) Avoid unnecessary complications, especially infection and injuries to important structures. The patient may be in bed a little longer than if a master surgeon had treated him by internal fixation, he may perhaps be a little stiffer, and he will have less beautiful X-rays. But you will only get good results if you follow all the details carefully. How you apply a cast, when you should remove

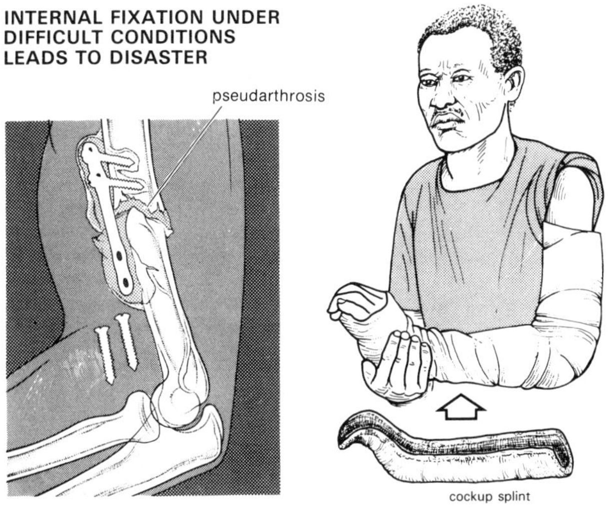

STAGES IN THE HEALING OF A LONG BONE

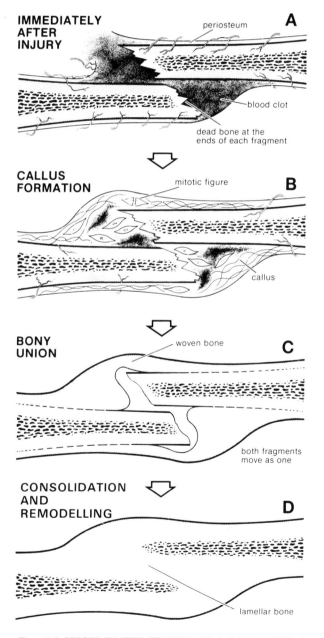

Fig. 69-3 STAGES IN THE HEALING OF A LONG BONE. A, immediately after the injury. B, callus formation. C, bony union. D, consolidation and remodelling. *Kindly contributed by Peter Bewes.*

Fig. 69-2 THE DISASTROUS RESULTS OF INTERNAL FIXATION UNDER DIFFICULT CONDITIONS. There were no indications for plating this patient's humerus; the plate is loose, and the screws have fallen out. He has a pseudarthrosis and a radial nerve palsy for which he is being treated in a plaster cockup splint. The method in Section 71.17 using active movements and a sling would almost certainly have resulted in union, besides being simpler and cheaper.

it, and exactly which exercises he should do are just as important as the mechanical niceties of internal fixation.

There are some important general principles: (1) The maintenance of alignment (2) The avoidance of rotation of the fragments. (3) The avoidance of distraction. (4) The encouragement of joint movement. (5) The careful application of casts and traction. In addition, each fracture has its own rules. Remember that the size of a fracture has little relation to its seriousness. For example, you can easily treat a fracture of the femur in a child, but a chip off the head of an adult's radius may have to be removed at an open operation.

THE DETAILS ARE CRITICAL

69.4 For the purposes of closed treatment there are three groups of fractures

They are: (1) Fractures of the shafts of long bones, including those of the mandible, the clavicle, and the ribs. (2) Fractures of the ends of long bones, often into joints, such as supracondylar fractures of the humerus, extension fractures of the wrist, and fractures of the tibial condyles. (3) Fractures with ischaemic or totally intracapsular fragments. Fortunately, there are only two fractures in this group—(a) intracapsular fractures of the neck of the femur, and (b) fractures of the neck of the scaphoid. These fractures can only be treated by replacing the fragments exactly and keeping them totally immobile, either in a cast (the scaphoid) or by internal fixation (the neck of the femur), until the ischaemic fragment has been vascularized from the more vascular one.

The first two groups of fractures need more discussion.

69.4a Fractures of the shafts of long bones

The shafts of long bones heal in four stages:

(1) Injury When a patient breaks one of his long bones, he injures the soft tissues round it, and tears the periosteum away from at least one of the fragments. This deprives the bone next to the fracture of its blood supply, and kills it.

(2) Callus formation During the next few weeks the periosteum and endosteum near the fracture produce soft vascular callus full of active spindle cells. Cancellous bone only forms a significant amount of callus when the two bony fragments are close together; cortical bone can form callus when they are not so close. Gentle movement stimulates callus formation in a fractured long bone; complete lack of movement depresses it. The non—operative school welcomes callus, and encourages gentle movements.

The newly formed callus forms a sheath round the broken bone, and is fixed to the fragments above and below the fracture, but not to the bone at the fracture site itself. The bone here is ischaemic and dead, and does not unite until it has been revascularized later.

After two weeks enough calcium has been deposited in the callus for you to see it on an X-ray. This calcified callus is slowly converted into loose open 'woven bone' which makes the bone ends 'sticky', and prevents them moving sideways on one another, although it still allows them to angulate.

(3) Clinical or bony union As time passes the woven bone round the patient's fracture becomes harder, and so firmly fixed to the fragments that they move as a single unit. This is clinical union and is a critical milestone in the healing of a broken long bone. It is the indication for a change in management, and is more important than the appearance of his X-ray. It usually occurs 4 to 8 weeks after the injury, but in the tibia it can take much longer.

EXAMINING FOR CLINICAL UNION

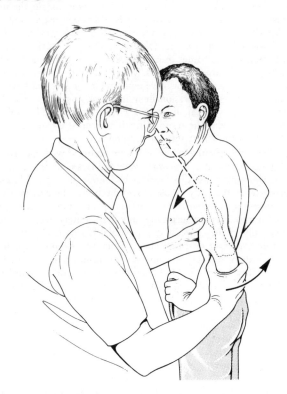

Fig. 69-4 EXAMINING FOR CLINICAL UNION. This is the indication for a change in management, and is more important than the appearance of the X-ray. It usually occurs 4 to 8 weeks after the injury, but in the tibia it can take much longer. *Kindly contributed by Peter Bewes.*

EXAMINING A LONG BONE FOR CLINICAL UNION

(1) Feel the fracture site for tenderness, looking at the patient's face as you do so. If it is not tender, his fracture has probably united.

(2) Feel the fracture site for warmth. If it feels warm, it has probably not united.

(3) Put one hand over the callus and grasp it firmly. Ask the patient to keep his limb muscles loose. With your other hand, move the lower end of his broken bone from side to side. If his fracture has united, the upper end of the bone should move in the opposite direction. Don't be too gentle, but don't move the bone so vigorously that you cause pain, or refracture it.

Pain, particularly pain at night, is a sign that a fracture has not united. Repeatedly examining a fracture in this way is useful, especially in the early days, because it promotes callus formation. If manipulation is painless and there is no movement, the fracture has united.

When a patient's fracture has united clinically, you can reduce splinting, *but you must continue to protect it from stress*, and especially from stresses that are likely to break it. For example, a patient must protect a fracture of the shaft of his humerus from the angulation stresses that dangling it out of a sling will cause while his elbow is still stiff (71.17).

(4) Consolidation and remodelling Bone continues to heal during this stage, which lasts several months. The broken fragments remain firmly held by callus, while the dead bone at the end of each fragment is slowly removed, and their ends joined by more callus and finally by solid bone. The more a patient uses his limb, the stronger this new bone becomes. Excess callus is slowly removed until his injured limb is as strong, or even stronger, than it was before. Consolidation takes as long again as clinical union, so if union took 8 weeks, consolidation will take 16 weeks. Don't allow him to do any violent sport until consolidation is complete.

69.4b How should you treat a broken long bone?

These guidelines follow from the above account of how long bones heal. They apply to fractures of the clavicle, the humerus, the ulna, and the shaft of the femur. The radius is for some reason an exception, perhaps because the healing processes described above are better adapted to angulation stresses than they are to those of rotation, and the radius is above all a bone that rotates. The tibia is also a bone which is best immobilized.

A little movement is a good thing in some long bone fractures because it promotes callus formation, especially in the early days, it increases the blood supply to a limb, and it improves muscle tone. Complete immobilization of a femur fracture is unnecessary, and by reducing callus formation, it delays union. So, allow the bone ends to move a little, and encourage the patient to keep exercising his muscles, even if they are inside a cast. Active movements in which he uses his own muscles, are better than passive ones.

A recent fracture is painful. This pain helps to limit excessive movement of the fragments. For the first three days after an injury pain prevents almost all movement. Thereafter a patient can move the fragments through a steadily increasing range of painless movement, but he must not move them so much that the flexible newly formed callus is broken. The limited range of movement increases the formation of callus and promotes union. So encourage him to use the joints on either side of his broken humerus or femur, within the range of painless movement. If he exceeds it, he may refracture his bone. Pain is subjective, so you will have to restrain some patients and encourage others. Exercise in the first few weeks after a fracture is the main factor in determining how much callus is formed, and it is callus which promotes union.

Cautious weight bearing speeds healing, so encourage a patient to walk on his broken leg—cautiously! He can only do this if you can prevent the fragments angulating. A plaster cast can prevent a patient's tibia doing this, but is much less satisfactory for his femur. So, if his tibia is broken, allow him to walk on it early, but if his femur is broken, keep him in bed on traction until it has united. His fracture will be so painful that he will seldom be able to bear weight until it is useful and safe for him to do so.

'Active movements' and 'weight bearing' are not the same. It is never too soon to start active movements, whereas bearing weight too soon may be disastrous. For example, if a patient tries to bear weight on a fractured femur too early, the fragments will gradually angulate, and may perhaps refracture.

**GENTLE MOVEMENT INCREASES CALLUS
EXERCISE IS NECESSARY, EVEN INSIDE A CAST
AIM FOR ACTIVE PAIN–FREE MOVEMENTS**

69.4c Fractures of the ends of long bones

If a fracture enters a joint, you will not be able or equipped to reduce the fragments precisely at an open operation, or to fix them internally. If you cannot refer a patient to have this done, the alternative is active movement, as early as pain will allow. This smooths the opposing joint surfaces, and lets them mould to one another as union proceeds.

It is often said that unless the fragments of all broken joint surfaces are replaced exactly, osteoarthritis always follows. Although this is true for the ankle, it is less true for such fractures as: (1) comminuted supracondylar fractures of the humerus in adults, (2) comminuted extension fractures of the wrist in elderly patients, (3) plateau fractures of the upper tibia, and (4) comminuted fractures of the calcaneus with injury to the sub-talar joint. With these fractures surprisingly good results follow from accepting the poor position of the fragments, and allowing early active movements to smooth out the irregular joint surfaces as union proceeds. These good results are in striking contrast to the poor results that average surgeons get when they try elaborate methods of internal fixation. Experts with the AO method may get excellent results with these fractures, but many of their followers do not.

69.5 Varieties of bony injury

When you see a fracture, think of it in terms of the variables in Fig. 69-5. Is it closed, or is there a tear in the skin over it, so that it is open (compound)? Spiral fractures have pointed tips, heal rapidly, and are caused by forces acting along the length of a limb, which remains fairly stable. Transverse and oblique

PATTERNS OF LONG BONE FRACTURE

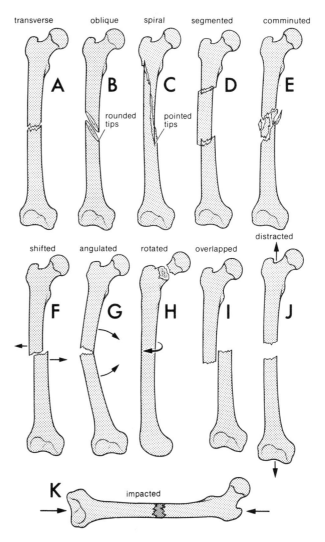

Fig. 69-5 PATTERNS OF LONG BONE FRACTURE. **Many fractures show several of these features at the same time. For example, a fracture can be transverse, shifted, and angulated.** *Kindly contributed by Peter Bewes*

fractures take longer to heal than spiral ones, and are caused by forces acting across a limb, which becomes unstable. Oblique fractures have rounded tips, heal particularly slowly, and have all the disadvantages of a transverse fracture, with the added one that you cannot easily get the fragments to hitch (73-13). Angulation can be anterior or posterior, the lower fragment can be in varus (directed towards the midline) or in valgus (directed away from it). Overlap is not always as undesirable as you might think (78.1), but always avoid distraction because, if the ends of two fragments do not touch, they may never unite.

Occasionally, the fragments are impacted into one another in a suitable position, so that you can preserve the impaction, as in some fractures of the necks of the humerus or the femur. Unfortunately, the fragments are usually in an unsatisfactory position, so that an important first step in reducing most fractures is to disimpact the fragments by pulling them apart.

JOINT INJURIES

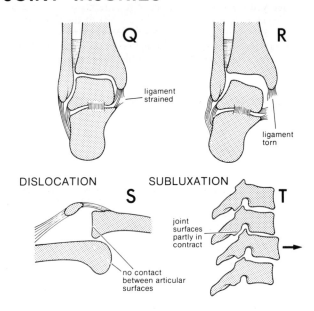

Fig. 69-6 SOME JOINT INJURIES. In a dislocation the joint surfaces are widely displaced, but in a subluxation they are still partly touching one another. *Kindly contributed by Peter Bewes.*

A ligament can be *sprained* and only partly torn, or it can be completely *ruptured*. In a *dislocation* the joint surfaces are widely displaced, but in a *subluxation* they are still partly touching one another. Both subluxations and dislocations are often combined with fractures.

Fractures and dislocations differ greatly in the urgency with which you must treat them. *Reduce all dislocations and fracture dislocations immediately,* because the longer you leave them, the tighter the ligaments will become, and the more difficult or impossible your task. If a dislocation is likely to be difficult to reduce, use a relaxant. With most fractures you have more time, and the best time to reduce a fracture is either immediately after the injury, before the tissues have started to swell, or up to a week later (not more), after the swelling has gone. If you are referring a fracture for internal fixation, the sooner the patient reaches the referral hospital the better. He should at least be there within two weeks.

Which fractures are common? Some fractures and dislocations are much more common than others, but the rarer ones are no less important to the patients who have them, and are not necessarily any more difficult to treat. The common ones are extension fractures of the wrist, clavicle fractures, supracondylar fractures of the humerus in children, fractures of both

BONY INJURIES IN CHILDREN

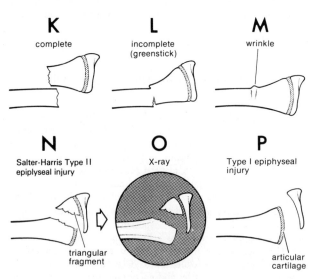

Fig. 69-7 BONY INJURIES IN CHILDREN. A child's bones are different from those of an adult; instead of breaking, they often bend like a stick. *Kindly contributed by Peter Bewes.*

forearm bones in children, fractures of the shaft of the humerus in adults, fractures of the tibia and fibula either alone or combined, fractures of the shaft of the femur, fractures of the radius and ulna, and fractures of the metatarsals and metacarpals. Most other fractures are rare.

DISTRACTION IS DANGEROUS
REDUCE DISLOCATIONS EARLY

69.6 Fractures in children

A child's bones differ from those of an adult. Instead of fracturing completely, they often bend like a stick (incomplete or greenstick fractures), or there may only be a small swelling of the cortex (wrinkle fractures). Fractures in children always unite if you treat them properly; they need immobilizing for a shorter time, and you can almost always manage them by closed methods. Skin traction is much more satisfactory in children than it is in adults, and, because a child's joints do not become stiff permanently, he seldom needs physiotherapy.

Although some severe malpositions slowly disappear as a child grows, other apparently mild ones become steadily worse. So you must know which positions you can accept, and which you cannot. Here are some general principles.

(1) Try to get the fragments into line. They need not necessarily be end to end.

(2) Try to stop them rotating, because growth will not correct a rotation deformity.

(3) Be cautious about how much angulation you accept. This depends on: (a) The age of the child, and particularly on whether his epiphyses have united or not. In Caucasians they typically unite at 14 in a girl and 16 in a boy, but in an African they may remain open almost to the age of 20. (b) The distance of the fracture from the end of a long bone. The younger the child, and the nearer his fracture to the end of his bone, the greater the angulation you can accept. Uncorrected angulated fractures near the middle of a long bone cause severe deformity, especially in the forearm, and also in the femur and tibia. But angulation near the end of a bone in the plane of a hinge joint, such as

208

the elbow, fingers, or knee, causes very little disability. Angulation in other directions is likely to be permanent.

(4) Overlap and moderate shortening are unimportant. In fractures of the femur and humerus in younger children, *they are even desirable,* because these bones readily regrow to their normal length. So you can leave a fractured long bone to unite with its fragments side to side up to the age of 10 in girls, and 12 in boys. The fragments unite rapidly, and the bone soon moulds.

69.6a Epiphyseal injuries in children

Among the endpages of this book you will see charts showing the epiphyses, and stating both the time they appear and when they unite. These charts are for Caucasians—African epiphyses unite later.

Some epiphyses are much more often injured than others. Epiphyses are of two kinds: (1) pressure epiphyses at the ends of long bones near joints, and (2) traction apophyses, to which muscles are attached. The cartilage joining epiphyses and apophyses to the shaft of a bone is weak, and is often the site of displacement. Except for an important injury to the medial epicondyle of the humerus, injuries to other apophyses are only a minor nuisance and are not discussed further here. Injuries to pressure epiphyses are much more important.

Suspect an epiphyseal injury whenever any patient under 20 has signs of an injury near the end of a long bone, even if it seems only to be a sprain. He may have displaced an epiphysis at the moment of injury after which it returned to its usual place, so a normal X-ray does not exclude a displaced epiphysis.

Fortunately, most epiphyseal injuries cause no growth disturbance. But if an epiphyseal plate is injured on one side only, or if it is one of a parallel pair, such as the radius and ulna, progressive angular deformity occurs slowly over several years, and can only be corrected by osteotomy. Salter and Harris have described the following five types of epiphyseal injury each of which needs managing differently, and has a different prognosis.

Type I The epiphysis slips completely off the end of the shaft, without a fracture. These injuries are common at birth and in early childhood. Reduction is usually not difficult, and the prognosis is good, except at the upper end of the femur (77.10).

Type II The line of separation runs through part of the epiphyseal plate and then out through the shaft, where it produces a characteristic triangular fragment (N, Fig. 69-7). This is a common epiphyseal injury, particularly at the distal end of the radius.

Type III The fracture extends from the joint surface into the epiphyseal line and then along it to the periphery. These are rare injuries, usually at the ends of the tibia. Accurate reduction is essential to restore a smooth joint surface and align the epiphyseal plates. An open operation may be necessary.

Type IV The epiphysis and part of the shaft split, particularly at the lateral condyle of the humerus (72.13). Perfect reduction is essential, and open reduction is often necessary.

Type V This is another rare injury, usually of the ankle or knee, with a poor prognosis. The epiphyseal plate is crushed and at least part of it subsequently closes early. The first x-ray may look almost normal, and you may think the child has only a sprain. Suspect an injury of this kind if he has a history of a crush injury, and don't let him bear weight for at least three weeks.

EPIPHYSEAL INJURIES IN CHILDREN

X-RAY **Take two views of the child's injured limb at right angles; if you find them difficult to interpret, compare them with exactly the same views of the other side.** *Failure to do this is responsible for most of the errors in treating children's fractures.* **Diagnosing an epiphyseal separation is difficult before the centres of ossification have appeared. Suspect epiphyseal separation if there is displacement of the shaft and soft tissue swelling.**

EPIPHYSEAL INJURIES

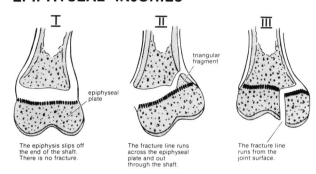

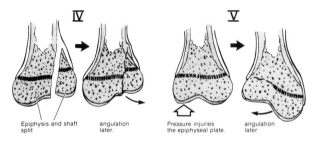

Fig. 69-8 EPIPHYSEAL INJURIES. Suspect an epiphyseal injury whenever any patient under 20 has signs of an injury near the end of a long bone, even if it seems only to be a sprain. *After Salter with kind permission.*

REDUCTION An epiphyseal plate is easily damaged, so reduce the displacement gently. If a Type I or II injury is more than 10 days old, leave it. The epiphysis will probably have stuck in its displaced position, so that you will have to use excessive force to replace it.

CAUTION ! Reduce these injuries immediately, especially in the lower limbs. Any delay will make reduction more difficult.

IMMOBILIZATION Injuries of the first three types need about half the time required for a shaft fracture at the same age. Immobilize Type IV injuries for the same time as for a shaft fracture.

FOLLOW UP See the child regularly. Compare X-rays of his injured and his normal sides. If there has been little growth see him every 6 months.

THE PROGNOSIS is good for injuries of the first two types and poor in the other three, particularly the fourth.

The younger the child the more growth he has ahead of him, and the worse the deformity that may follow a given injury. An injury in the last year of growth is likely to cause little disability.

REDUCE EPIPHYSEAL INJURIES IMMEDIATELY

69.7 Open fractures

A fracture is 'open' when a break in the skin over it brings it into communication with the organisms of the outside world. The break in the skin can be the result of either a wound from outside, or a bony fragment piercing the skin from inside, in which case the tissues are less likely to be contaminated.

Traumatic osteomyelitis as the result of infection is always a possibility in an open fracture, but it is much less likely to occur if you do a careful wound toilet, and close the wound by delayed suture. So toilet *all* open fractures carefully and close them by delayed suture (54.4), *even if the skin wound is a small one, and occurs from within outwards*. This is especially important if the patient presents late. If you fail to do this and the wound becomes infected, traumatic osteomyelitis will probably follow. *Failing to do an adequate toilet, and closing the wound by immediate primary suture are very common errors.*

Although some open fractures can be fixed internally, don't try it. The wound is already contaminated, and the plates and screws will probably become infected. An occasional Kirschner wire is the maximum amount of internal fixation that is wise.

If you apply the above principles rigidly, infection is unlikely, and antibiotics will make little difference (54.1). So give them only if an infection occurs which needs treating.

Gustillo, Ramon, and Anderson J.T. 'Prevention of infection in the treatment of 1025 open fractures of the long bones. Journal of Bone and Joint Surgery. 1976;58A:454

TWO OPEN FRACTURES OF THE FEMUR

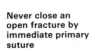
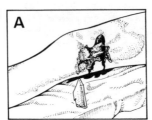

Never close an open fracture by immediate primary suture

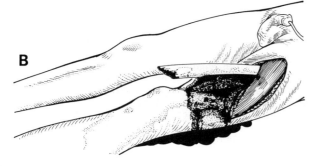

Fig. 69-9 TWO OPEN FRACTURES OF THE FEMUR. A, shows a small loose fragment of bone, and B, an extreme case in which the whole femur has been stripped bare of muscle. The important measures here are a thorough wound toilet and delayed primary suture, followed by traction. *Kindly contributed by John Lowrie.*

OPEN FRACTURES

This extends Section 51.3 on caring for a severely injured patient and Section 54.1 on caring for wounds. Open fractures of particular bones such as the tibia (81.12), the radius and ulna (73.6), and the femur (78.6), are discussed elsewhere.

All open fractures need *urgent* treatment, so don't leave them until the following day. Take the patient to the theatre and give him a general anaesthetic. Toilet his wound to remove all foreign material (54.1). Syringe out the whole of the inside of his wound with saline under pressure every 10 minutes all through the operation. Remove all dead tissue until you reach a healthy bleeding surface. *Then LEAVE THE WOUND OPEN!* But make sure you cover any arteries and nerves.

CAUTION ! (1) Don't close the wound by primary suture. (2) If the skin edges gape, don't try to bring them even partly together with stitches. (3) When you finally close the wound some days later, don't close it under tension.

If bone fragments have no attachments, remove them. But if they have any attached periosteum, leave them; they may live. If you remove them unnecessarily, you will leave a gap which can only be replaced by grafting.

Try to bring the fragments together end to end. If possible, keep them in place with traction rather than in a cast. If this

is difficult, at least try to maintain the alignment of the limb by applying traction. If convenient, you can combine traction with plaster slabs or a plaster gutter.

If you are going to apply a cast, don't do so until all risk of infection is past. If necessary, graft the patient's skin wound, and apply a cast on the same day.

Raise the patient's injured limb.

DIFFICULTIES WITH OPEN FRACTURES

If the SKIN IS BRUISED over the fracture, watch it carefully. It may break down so that a fracture which was closed initially becomes open.

If FRACTURE BLISTERS develop, they do not make the fracture into an open one. Prick them with a sterile needle, and cover them with vaseline gauze.

If a PIECE OF BONE IS MISSING, bringing the fragments into contact with one another is more important than maintaining length.

CLOSE *ALL* OPEN FRACTURES BY DELAYED PRIMARY SUTURE
TRAUMATIC OSTEOMYELITIS *IS* PREVENTABLE

69.8 Open joint wounds

Immediate primary suture is usually advised for joint wounds, but in knee wounds in particular, it can be disastrous. Although it is unwise to leave a joint widely open, it is equally unwise to close it tightly. An effective compromise is to do a thorough wound toilet, as for any other wound, and to close it immediately, leaving a corner of the joint open to improve drainage and the chance of healing. Some joints will be destroyed and need an arthrodesis, but this will happen anyway. Don't let the presence of an opening into a joint influence your decision as to whether to close the rest of a wound immediately, or by delayed primary suture.

Antibiotics have the same rather uncertain role that they do in other contaminated wounds (54.1).

OPEN JOINT WOUNDS

Excise the edges of all layers of the patient's wound, remove dirt and wash out the joint cavity forcibly with saline from a syringe.

If necessary, open his wound wider by the standard incision for the joint (7.17), and feel around inside it. You may feel a piece of the patient's trousers inside his knee!

Even if his injury is a recent one, don't sew up the joint capsule completely. Instead, leave the joint and the wound at least partly open, so that pus can discharge. Don't insert a rubber drain.

If the bones in a joint wound are dislocated and the wound is open, reduce it urgently. *Every hour's delay makes the loss of the joint more certain.* Leave the skin wound partly open and pack it with gauze.

If a patient's wound is already badly infected, it may be helpful to leave a plastic tube with side holes cut in it to irrigate it.

Don't try to immobilize a wounded joint, or it may never move again. Instead, encourage early gentle movements. Make these more and more vigorous as the joint heals. Close the wound as soon as the danger of infection has passed, usually after about 3 days. The superficial tissues may need a skin graft.

If the knee is involved, apply skin or skeletal traction (78.4) to take tension away from it. CAUTION ! Don't forget tetanus toxoid.

69.9 Pathological fractures

Two kinds of fracture can occur without major trauma: (1) Fractures in which normal bone is subjected to unaccustomed, frequently repeated normal movements, as in fatigue fractures of the tibia (81.8), and march fractures of the metatarsals (83.11). (2) Fractures in which the bone is abnormal. Under the age of 20 the common causes are a chondroma (in a finger or toe) or a bone cyst at the end of a long bone, and osteomyelitis (7.2). Over the age of 40 the common causes are a secondary carcinoma (in the spine, pelvis, humerus, or femur), or osteoporosis (in the spine or femoral neck).

PATHOLOGICAL FRACTURES

X-RAYS Benign lesions typically have a smooth margin, and malignant ones a ragged gnawed appearance.

BIOPSY If you decide to biopsy the lesion, take tissue from the border of the lesion and try to get normal and abnormal bone in the same specimen.

TREATMENT Most pathological fractures unite, many of them at the normal speed, so that you can treat most of them in the same way as fractures through normal bone. Even fractures through secondary metastases may unite.

If a fracture takes place through a bone cyst, it may unite. If it does not, refer the patient.

If a fracture takes place through a sarcoma, this may be an indication for amputation.

69.10 Active movements means active movements!

All fractures need some exercises from the first week onwards, if not before. Fractures must thus be firmly associated with exercises in the minds of everyone—including the patient. The decision to treat fractures by non–operative methods is thus not a decision to do nothing! Enthusiasm for exercises is a critical part of this method. Exercises are usually necessary for the injured joint itself, and are always important for the normal joints on either side of it. If these joints are not used, even for a few days, they soon become stiff. Encouraging, cajoling, and even bribing and bullying all have their place.

DEMONSTRATE THE EXERCISES YOURSELF

Who is to encourage the patient to move his joints? Few district hospitals have a physiotherapist, and even the elements of physiotherapy are not yet part of any nursing curriculum. So the responsibility is yours, as you go round the ward, to make sure that the patients do their exercises. Your staff must see the patients doing their exercises, and really care that they are done. Exercises are no less important with out–patients. Teach the exercises using examples of each kind of injury, and let your staff see you demonstrating them. Merely telling your nurses and medical assistants to get the patients exercising is not enough. Show them just how much trouble you are prepared to go to yourself.

Here are some exercises which all ward staff should know and teach patients. Carefully supervised walking is an important leg exercise and is discussed in Section 8.1. Active movements may be painful, especially to begin with, so ease the patient's pain with plenty of aspirin and persist in your persuasion.

ACTIVE MOVEMENTS ARE SAFER THAN PASSIVE ONES

SOME EXERCISES

You will need some exercises when a patient is in bed, and others later when he is able to walk.

JAW EXERCISES

Chewing Ask the patient to chew gum or sugar cane.

CLAVICLE EXERCISES

Shoulder bracing Encourage the patient to keep bracing his shoulders backwards; this will help to draw the fragments of his fractured clavicle out to length. Make sure he keeps his shoulder, elbow, and hand moving.

BACK EXERCISES

Arching exercises Ask the patient to lie on his back and arch it so as to make a tunnel that you can put your hand through. This is a good exercise for a stable fracture of his thoracic or lumbar spine.

Extension from the prone position Ask him to lie on his front. With someone holding his legs, ask him to arch his back so as to raise his shoulders from the bed without using his arms. This is a useful extension exercise later in spinal injuries.

SHOULDER EXERCISES

Arm dangling is useful for all arm fractures, especially those of the humerus when the patient's arm is in a sling. Ask him to stoop forwards and let his injured shoulder swing loosely in all directions. Let it swing under the influence of gravity, like a pendulum, as in Fig. 69-11. Don't let him tighten his shoulder with his arm to his side, because this may angulate a broken humerus. More shoulder exercises are shown in Fig. 71-7.

ELBOW EXERCISES

Flexion and extension Ask the patient to repeat flexion and extension movements gently many times within the limits of pain. Forceful exercises are particularly undesirable in elbow injuries (72.10).

PENDULUM EXERCISES

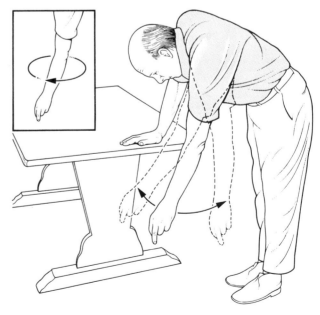

Fig. 69-11 PENDULUM EXERCISES FOR THE SHOULDER are useful for all arm fractures, especially those of the humerus when the patient's arm is in a sling. *Kindly contributed by John Stewart. This drawing is a good likeness of him.*

FOREARM EXERCISES

Pronation and supination Ask the patient to do this repeatedly with his elbow at 90°. This is the movement of turning the knob of a door.

WRIST EXERCISES

Flexion and extension Ask him to flex and extend his wrist as freely as he can.

FINGER EXERCISES

Squeezing a ball Ask the patient to keep squeezing a rubber ball, or a ball of cotton wool, inside a tight gauze bag.

HIP EXERCISES

Abduction Ask him to lie on his side and abduct his hip against gravity.

Flexion When he is lying on his back in bed, ask him to raise his leg from his hip with his knee straight.

KNEE EXERCISES

Quadriceps exercises While the patient is lying on his back, ask him to keep his leg straight and lift his knee off the bed. When he can do these exercises satisfactorily, let him do them with sand bags of increasing weight on his ankle.

Knee swinging If his knee is stiff, ask him to let it hang over the side of his bed, and swing until it is at least 90°. As the range of movement in his knee improves, he can get the last few degrees of flexion by grasping his lower leg in his arms and flexing his knee.

Cycling is superb knee exercise.

Knee bending with his foot raised on a step is useful in patellar fractures and is shown in Fig. 79-7.

ANKLE EXERCISES

Cycling is also one of the best ankle exercises. Make sure the patient flexes and extends his ankle as he rides.

ALL PATIENTS WITH FRACTURES NEED SOME EXERCISES, AND THEY MUST BE SUPERVISED BY SOMEONE WHO CARES

---

70 Plaster and traction

70.1 Plaster, and the equipment for it

Plaster of Paris is ideal for treating some fractures. But you must apply it skilfully, and only on the proper indications. If you apply a plaster cast carelessly, it can cripple a patient forever, and you may even have to amputate his limb. Use a plaster cast: (1) to immobilize bony fragments in the right position, (2) to protect his limb while his bones unite, (3) to make him comfortable. But casts have serious disadvantages. They can obstruct his circulation, they can cause pressure sores (70.3), they are heavy and inconvenient, they stiffen joints, and if you leave them on too long, the bones inside them become weak and osteoporotic.

Use standard casts, such as the long leg and short leg walking casts (81.3). The indications for each of them and the details as to how you should apply them are critical. These critical details include the position of the patient's limb, how far up and down it the cast should go, where you should put the padding, and the rule that a patient must exercise his muscles inside his cast. So follow the details we give exactly, and see that your assistants do so too. There are other ways of doing things, but you will not know which they are, and we do not have the space to describe them. Vary the methods we describe only if you have good reasons for doing so. For example, never apply any cast at the extreme range of movement of a joint. Pressure on the joint surface will make its cartilage necrose and cause osteoarthritis later.

EXERCISE THE MUSCLES INSIDE A CAST

• *PLASTER BANDAGES, normal, slow setting, best quality, 10 cm, 15 cm, and 20 cm wide.* Good quality plaster bandages make the strongest casts and poor ones are a mistake. If you use them, you will need twice as many, and the cast will be twice as heavy. If necessary, you can make plaster bandages locally from powdered plaster of Paris and rolls of gauze bandage. Plaster bandages are cheaper if you buy them as a long roll which you can cut off in the lengths you require.

• *CREPE BANDAGES* Many hospitals do not have these, so we have indicated alternatives when possible. You can use a plaster bandage instead of a crêpe one to hold plaster slabs, but this is far from satisfactory.

• *STOCKINETTE, woven tubular, orthopaedic, various widths, three rolls of each width.* Use this in suitable widths for the finger, the arm, the leg, and in small quantities for the trunk. If you thread it on to the limb before applying plaster, it will stop the plaster sticking to the hairs on the patient's skin, and will make casts and slabs more comfortable. It is not a substitute for adequate padding. If you don't have it, use ordinary cotton bandages, or a single layer of expanded cotton wool. Cotton bandages will also make a stronger cast.

• *PADDING, cotton wool, orthopaedic, ten rolls only.* If you do not have this, cut a roll of ordinary cotton wool into smaller rolls 10 or 15 cm wide. Unroll them, leave in the sun, and let them expand. Then split them into four or five layers of the thicknesses you want, and roll them up again, ready for use. Each of your new rolls of expanded cotton wool will be the same size as the original one, but it will contain more air and collapse down more easily when you roll it on to a limb and cover it with plaster.

• *STIRRUPS, locally made.* These support a patient's leg when he wears a walking cast. The cross pieces at the top are thin so that they bend easily to fit the shape of his leg and spread its weight through the cast.

• *PLASTER SHEARS, Lorenz, 380 mm, nickel plated, one only.* These large shears will open the strongest casts, but are unnecessary if you have an electric cast cutter.

• *PLASTER SHEARS, Guy, with shaped bows and flattened probe end, 250 mm, nickel plated, one only.* These shears are

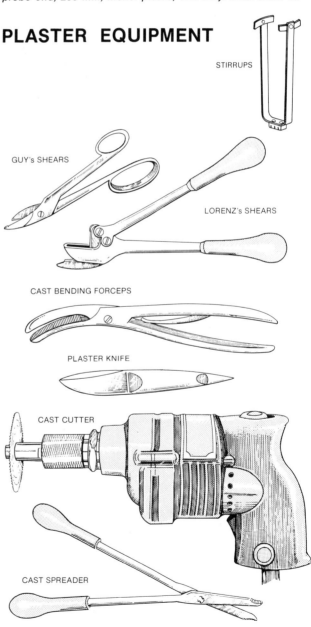

PLASTER EQUIPMENT

STIRRUPS

GUY's SHEARS

LORENZ's SHEARS

CAST BENDING FORCEPS

PLASTER KNIFE

CAST CUTTER

CAST SPREADER

Fig. 70-1 PLASTER EQUIPMENT. Use this equipment to make standard casts, such as the long leg and short leg walking casts. The indications for each of them and the details as to how you should apply them are critical.

smaller and easier to use for removing small casts than the Lorenz shears. If you don't have them, use ordinary pliers.

• *PLASTER KNIFE, Esmarch, solid forged, two only.* Use this for splitting circular casts after they have hardened; sharpen it on a stone. If necessary, you can use almost any knife.

• *PLASTER SAW, Bergman's, hand, one only.* If you don't have electricity, you will need this.

• *PLASTER CAST SAW, electric, oscillating, with four extra blades, 44 mm and 64 mm, state voltage, one outfit only.* These will be useful if you have electricity; unfortunately most plaster saws have a short life.

• *PLASTER CAST SPREADER, one only.* When a cast has been split, this will spread it, so that you can remove it from the limb.

• *PLASTER CAST BENDING FORCEPS, Böhler, one only.* These are large pliers for bending the edges of a cast and opening it.

• *PENCILS, INDELIBLE, for writing on a cast, six only.* When you apply a cast write on it the date you applied it and the date you expect to remove it, together with a sketch of the fracture inside, as in Fig. 70-6. If the plaster is still wet, you can use a ball pen, but an ordinary pencil is unsatisfactory. An indelible pencil containing a water soluble blue dye is ideal.

70.2 Slabs or a circular cast?

You can apply plaster, either as a slab covering part of the circumference of a limb, or as a circular cast all round it.

You can put a slab on one side of a limb, or on both sides, and hold it in place with a crêpe bandage. The advantage of slabs is that they allow a limb to swell without obstructing its circulation (70.4). As the swelling subsides, the elasticity of the crêpe bandage will hold the slabs against the limb without letting them become loose. If you don't have a crêpe bandage, you can use a few turns of plaster bandage, but remember: (1) to split it as you would a circular cast (70.3), and (2) to renew it as it becomes loose. Slabs are useful for the initial treatment of a severe fracture and are safer than circular casts.

But slabs don't immobilize some fractures securely enough. Slabs are weak, and easily break at the elbow or the knee. So for many fractures you have to use a circular cast which will hold the fragments in place more securely, and be stronger. But if you apply a circular cast unwisely, it will obstruct the circulation in a limb, and as the swelling subsides, it will become loose.

ALWAYS PAD THESE PARTS OF A LIMB

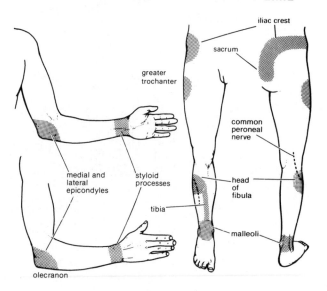

Fig. 70-2. ALWAYS PAD THESE PARTS OF A LIMB, or a cast will be uncomfortable and pressure sores may form. Protection of the common peroneal nerve as it winds round the neck of the fibula is especially important

So with a circular cast you have two choices, either: (1) wait for most of the swelling to go, before you apply it, or (2) renew it as the tissues shrink.

70.3 Splitting and spreading a cast

Always pad the prominent bony parts of a patient's limb, shown in Fig. 70-2, or the cast will cause pressure sores. You can choose whether or not you will put a layer of cotton wool or orthopaedic felt over the rest of his injured limb. Padding a cast completely: (1) makes it less likely to obstruct his circulation, (2) compensates to some extent for shrinkage of his limb because the padding expands a little as his limb shrinks, (3) makes the cast less likely to cause pressure sores, (4) makes it easier to remove, and (5) makes it easier to wedge. The only disadvantage of a padded cast is that it does not hold the bony fragments quite as still as an unpadded one. Be safe and pad all casts. The only exception is a cast for the scaphoid (Fig. 74-10).

If you have decided to apply a circular cast, the next question is whether or not you should split it, so that it can open as the tissues under it swell. If you put a circular cast on a freshly reduced fracture without splitting it immediately, *the cast may restrict the swelling of the tissues, increase the pressure in the limb, obstruct its circulation, and cause either ischaemic gangrene needing amputation, or the compartment syndrome followed by Volkmann's ischaemic contracture (70.4).* This can happen even if ischaemia lasts less than an hour, and is a particular danger with fractures of the forearm and lower leg. It is not a danger in casts for the scaphoid or Bennett's fracture, so there is no need to split these casts. *An unsplit circular cast is especially dangerous if a patient already has signs of circulatory impairment (70.4).* A hundred unsplit long leg casts may give no trouble, but the hundred–and–first may obstruct a patient's venous return, cause gangrene, and require that his leg be amputated. When you make rounds the following morning, it may be too late! Gangrene or Volkmann's contracture may have started at midnight!

Splitting a cast with a scalpel will not destroy its capacity to hold the bony fragments, and is easy if you do it while a cast is still soft. *Spreading* a split cast with a blunt object such as a screwdriver, so that its edges open, is a separate procedure. It is only necessary on the rare occasions when the circulation to a limb is impaired.

ALWAYS SPLIT THE FIRST CAST ON FRACTURES OF THE FOREARM AND LOWER LEG

70.4 Catastrophes with casts

Two disasters can befall the circulation of an injured limb. An unwisely applied cast can cause both of them: (1) If its circulation is completely obstructed, the limb becomes gangrenous, so that all its tissues die, including the skin. (2) If pressure builds up in a tight space, such as a fascial space, the *compartment syndrome* may develop, followed by *Volkmann's ischaemic contracture.*

The compartment syndrome is caused by the partially ischaemic muscle swelling, squeezing out its own blood supply, becoming hard and partly necrotic, and then slowly fibrosing over several months. As it does so, it strangles the vessels and nerves of the limb. The patient's skin remains intact, and although its nutrition may be impaired later, it does not become gangrenous. Volkmann's ischaemic contracture is the final result. This is usually an anaesthetic, crippled, clawed, forearm. But it can also be an ankle in extreme equinus, with flexion of its midtarsal joint and dorsiflexion of its MP joints and toes. Volkmann's contracture is one of the ultimate orthopaedic

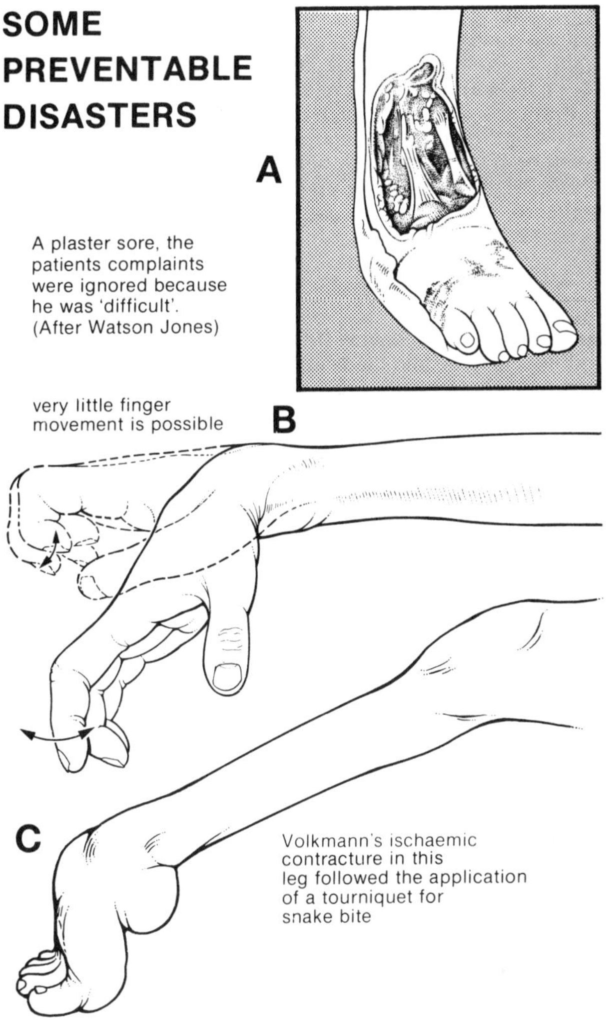

SOME PREVENTABLE DISASTERS

A

A plaster sore, the patients complaints were ignored because he was 'difficult'. (After Watson Jones)

very little finger movement is possible

B

C

Volkmann's ischaemic contracture in this leg followed the application of a tourniquet for snake bite

Fig. 70-3 SOME PREVENTABLE DISASTERS. A, a pressure sore. B, Volkmann's ischaemic contracture of the hand. C, Volkmann's ischaemic contracture of the leg.

disasters, because it cripples for life, it cannot be adequately treated, and *it is almost always preventable!*

In its less extreme forms Volkmann's ischaemic contracture is more common than most people think. It may only show itself later as a stiff foot, or a very stiff hand that gradually begins to develop severe contractures during the months that follow the injury.

A patient's forearm muscles are most commonly involved by Volkmann's ischaemic contracture, and occasionally the muscles of his lower leg, but never by the muscles of his upper arm, or his thigh, which are less firmly enclosed in fascia. Usually, the tight fascia of his forearm or leg is enough to restrain the swollen tissues and start the syndrome, but a tight bandage (including an Esmarch bandage), or a tourniquet, or gallows (78.2) or extension traction (78.3), or an unsplit cast can all precipitate it. Although a layer of cotton wool between a patient's skin and the cast reduces the risk, any cast all round a limb is a potential source of disaster. Most cases occur in the forearm of children following forearm fractures or supracondylar fractures (72.8). Some follow fractures of the tibia (81.14), and a few follow injuries to the thenar muscles, or dislocations of the elbow (72.4) or knee (79.8). Occasionally in adults, and very rarely in children, there is soft tissue injury only with no fracture.

Correct management will usually prevent ischaemia, but always be watchful for the early signs (55.3); these are *pain, paraesthesiae, pallor, and paralysis*. The presence of a peripheral pulse does not exclude the compartment syndrome. The critical symp-

toms are the patient's inability to use the muscles of his limb, and pain. The ordinary pain of an immobilized fracture is moderate and improves. Ischaemic pain is more severe and gets worse during the first few hours after an injury. Pain after 48 hours is more likely to be caused by infection.

A well applied circular cast should reduce the pain of a fracture. If a patient, especially a child, complains of pain, take his complaints seriously, it is probably due to: (1) pressure on a bony point which may only subside as his skin erodes away, or (2) ischaemic pain which you must relieve. Pain is *not* an indication for aspirin or pethidine, it is an indication to find out why there is pain, and to split, window or renew the cast. So, never apply a circular cast to a patient who is unconscious from other injuries, and so unable to complain of pain. He may develop the compartment syndrome only too easily.

SHANTI (8 years) had an undisplaced fracture of the distal end of her radius. There was almost no swelling. A circular cast was applied. She returned the next day crying in pain. She was given aspirin and sent home. Three days later she returned with a gangrenous hand and sloughing forearm muscles. Her forearm was amputated. LESSONS (1) An undisplaced forearm fracture does not require a circular cast; all she needed was a slab and a crêpe bandage. (2) Never treat a painful cast with analgesics only. (3) If you apply a circular cast, ALWAYS split it. (4) Pain, numbness, and paralysis are signs of impending Volkmann's ischaemic contracture.

ABDULLAH (8 years) had a supracondylar fracture. It was successfully reduced within an hour and a skin tight cast was applied. He returned the following day saying that his fingers hurt, but was sent home without removal of the cast. Five days later he returned again. This time all his fingers and thumb were black and gangrenous, and had to be amputated. LESSONS (1) A cast is not the treatment for this fracture. (2) Don't apply a skin tight cast immediately after an injury, before the limb has had time to swell—wait at least 12 hours. (3) Take any complaint of pain seriously and split or remove the cast immediately.

VOLKMANN'S CONTRACTURE—A PREVENTABLE CATASTROPHE Use procedures, particularly slabs and a crêpe bandage or a split cast, which will make the syndrome less likely.

Identify the patients at particular risk and examine them frequently. Record your findings carefully, and note at what time you made them.

Watch for pain, paraesthesiae, pallor, and finally paralysis, and teach your staff to do the same.

Check the sensation of the nerves in the involved area using two point discrimination, or a pin. In injuries of the forearm, *test for pain on passive extension of the fingers.* Test the strength of all involved muscles. Feel the compartment for tenderness and tenseness.

CAUTION ! Remember that a normal pulse does not exclude the compartment syndrome.

TAKE THE COMPLAINT OF PAIN UNDER A CAST SERIOUSLY

70.5 Make your own plaster bandages

This is almost a lost art, but if you can make plaster bandages yourself they will be a tenth the price of those you buy. The difficulty is that the powdered plaster tends to fall through the bandage. The trick is to make the bandage *just* damp before you cover it with plaster. This will help the plaster to stick to the gauze, without destroying its capacity to set later when it is thoroughly wetted in the normal way. 'Home made' bandages are not so convenient, and take longer to set, but the economy may be worth it.

MAKING PLASTER BANDAGES

MATERIALS Medicinal plaster of Paris (dried calcium sulphate BPC) is best, but you can use builder's plaster of Paris. Buy it by the kilo and keep it dry. Ordinary wide gauze bandages.

METHOD Take a gauze bandage, wet it, and squeeze it as dry as you can. It will now be only just damp and will hold the dry plaster in the next stage.

Rolls. Open the roll of damp bandage, lay a length of it flat, and sprinkle it lightly with powdered plaster. Sprinkle it from your hand, or with a sprinkler. Roll it up as you cover it.

Slabs. Double the bandage backwards and forwards as you cover it.

Dip the prepared rolls or slabs in water and use them just as you would commercially made ones.

Use them that day or store them in an airtight tin. Don't try to make slabs with preloaded bandages.

70.6 Plastercraft

Using plaster skilfully is a craft worth learning. A poorly applied malleolar cast, for example, can make it impossible to reduce an ankle fracture. A really critical cast can mean so much to a patient that you should try to apply it yourself. Less critical casts can be applied by an assistant, but only provided you train him carefully and continually supervise him. Ways of making each particular cast are described later, so here are some of the points of technique which apply to all of them.

WETTING A BANDAGE

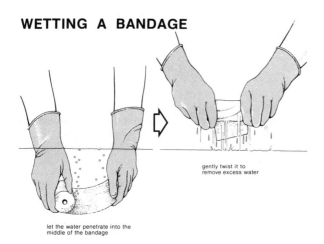

let the water penetrate into the middle of the bandage

gently twist it to remove excess water

Fig. 70-4 WETTING A PLASTER BANDAGE. Hold the bandage in your right hand. Unwind it half a turn, hold it with your left hand, and put both hands in water. Leave the bandage under the water for about 5 seconds until the bubbles have stopped. Hold it gently, so that water enters all its layers. Then, holding one end of the bandage in each hand, take it out of the water, and twist it gently. This will remove excess water, and yet keep the powdered plaster in the bandage. Don't wring it out, or squeeze it, because this will leave it too dry to make a good cast.

BASIC PLASTERCRAFT

For all slabs and casts, get everything ready before you wet the plaster bandages. So put stockinette on the limb, or cut and roll a layer of cotton wool directly on to the skin. Fold and trim the slab, and have your assistant ready.

Use 15 or 20 cm bandages wherever possible. Cold water is usually best, but hot water makes them set faster, so adjust the temperature to your needs.

SLABS

Take a dry bandage of suitable width, and use its loose end to measure the required length of the slab. Lay this length of bandage on a table and then double more bandage backwards and forwards over it until you have enough layers to make a slab of the right thickness. Usually, 5 to 10 layers are enough. If necessary, fold the bandage double.

Hold the dry slab in both hands, and dip it in water. Wait

for the bubbles to stop, remove it, gently squeeze it, and quickly smooth it out on a flat surface. This will remove the bubbles from between the layers of bandage, and prevent them separating later to weaken the cast.

Apply the wet plaster slab to a single layer of cotton wool, or to a tube of stockinette. Hold the patient's limb in the correct position and smooth out the slab.

CAUTION ! Don't let a plaster slab cover more than two thirds of the circumference of a limb, or it will become so nearly a circular cast that it may obstruct his circulation.

CIRCULAR CASTS

Pad the patient's bony points with particular care in *all* casts, as in Fig. 70-2, especially if he is thin. Be sure to pad well around his knee and his heel. Then pad the rest of his limb.

If you are fortunate enough to have tubular stockinette, thread this over his limb, leaving it long enough to extend several centimetres above and below the cast. If necessary, cut a hole for his thumb. If you have no stockinette, wind ordinary cotton bandages on to his limb.

Use special orthopaedic padding, or ordinary cotton wool expanded as in Section 70.1. Roll this smoothly over his whole limb, evenly with no folds or lumps, and without obscuring the shape of the limb. Don't pull it tight or it will tear. You may need 2 or 3 layers to build up a thickness of about 1 cm. Put extra padding over bony prominences. Apply it from well above to well below where the cast will end.

CAUTION ! (1) Don't apply so much padding that the patient's limb is able to move about freely inside the cast, as if it were inside a boot. (2) If there is a wound on his limb, put the padding on loosely, it may become wet with blood, contract, and impede the circulation.

Roll on the wet plaster bandage without lifting it off his limb, pressing each fold firmly with the base of your thumb, so that most of the tension is transmitted to the middle of the bandage, and not to its edges, where it might cause a sharp ridge. The tension you need will vary with the thickness and elasticity of the padding.

CAUTION ! (1) The correct tension is important or the cast will be loose. (2) The inside of the finished cast must be smooth, because ridges may cause sores. (3) Never pull a plaster bandage tight.

Apply each turn slowly, settle it carefully in position, and join it to the turn below by smoothing it with your hands to remove bubbles. Let it follow the way it wants to go. Leave about 3 cm between turns. Apply it as a spiral without reverses, and when you have to change its direction, make a quick tuck, and smooth it out. Don't twist the whole bandage, or attempt 'figures–of–eight', or apply two turns in exactly the same place, except at the ends.

While you are applying one roll of plaster, ask your assistant to wet the next one. Bandage from one end to the other, and back again, making the cast slightly thicker at its ends, where it will be most likely to fray. Don't build up its thickness over the fracture site, where extra thickness will be useless.

Trim its edges while they are still wet, not after they have dried. Bind the ends of the stockinette over into the cast with the last few turns of bandage. This will make it smooth and strong.

CAUTION ! (1) Don't press on a cast with your fingers or thumb while it is hardening, or they will leave a swelling inside it which will cause a pressure sore. (2) For the same reason don't let a cast, especially a cast over the heel, rest on a hard surface while it sets.

A large cast may not be completely dry for 72 hours, and will not be fully strong until then.

Alternatively, start by placing a slab of 4 thicknesses of bandage each side of the limb to strengthen it. Or, incorporate such a slab between layers of bandage.

If you want to strengthen a cast, let the cast dry thoroughly over the next day or two, then add more plaster. Wet plaster bandages stick to dry plaster better than they do to damp plaster.

SPLITTING A CAST

The cast *must* be padded, or you will cut the patient as you try to split it!

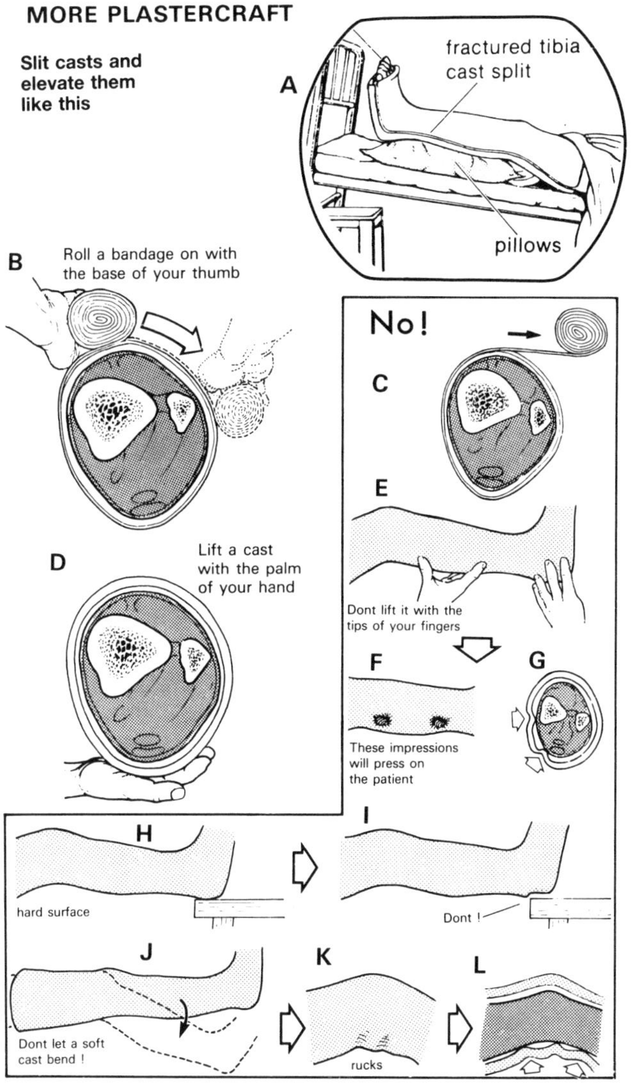

MORE PLASTERCRAFT

Slit casts and elevate them like this

A

fractured tibia
cast split

pillows

B Roll a bandage on with the base of your thumb

No!

C

D Lift a cast with the palm of your hand

E

Dont lift it with the tips of your fingers

F

These impressions will press on the patient

G

H

hard surface

I

Dont !

J

Dont let a soft cast bend !

K

rucks

L

Fig. 70-5 MORE PLASTERCRAFT. A, shows a cast which has been properly split. B, you are rolling a wet plaster bandage round a patient's cast with the base of your thumb—not taking it off his limb or pulling it too tight (C). D, lift a wet cast with the flat of your hand, not with the tips of your fingers (E). Fingers will leave depressions in the cast (F) which will press into the patient (G). H, don't rest a wet cast, especially its heel, on a hard surface, or a depression will form which will press into the patient (I). J, don't let a wet cast bend, or it will form folds (K) which will also press into him (L). *Mostly after Techniques Elementaires Pour Medecins Isoles. Les Agrégés du Pharo. Editions Maloines, with kind permission.*

INDICATIONS (1) All casts put on under emergency conditions. (2) A cast on a patient who is going on a journey. (3) Casts over any recent injury, whether swollen or not. The patient's limb may not be swollen now, but it may soon start to swell. (4) All first casts on tibia fractures. (5) You will be wise if you split all first circular casts, especially if nursing care is not good.

CAUTION ! Failure to split a cast is a common cause of disaster.

SPLITTING A CAST There are several ways to split a cast, but the secret is *to split it while it is still soft 3 or 4 minutes after you have applied it.*

(1) If the cast is still fairly soft, use a disposable scalpel blade to make a single cut through the plaster down to the padding. If it is already hard, use a sharp plaster knife, a solid bladed scalpel, or a pen knife. This will be hard work. When the cast is hard, widen the split a little with a screwdriver or a plaster spreader.

(2) Cutting a hardened cast will be easier if you start the cut with a knife, then wet it with an eye dropper, either with water, or with dilute acetic acid (vinegar). Let the plaster under part of the slit soften while you work on another part. Then return to the first part. This is particularly useful for removing casts from small children.

(3) Lay a rubber strip (such as a piece of car inner tube) on the skin where you intend to cut before you apply the cast. Then cut through it down to the strip.

(4) Lay a piece of greasy rubber tube about the thickness of your finger on the skin where you are going to split the cast. Pull the tube out before you split it. The cast will be thinner where the tube was and will split more easily.

SITES FOR SPLITTING OR REMOVAL Avoid the bony points, so cut an arm cast down the midline of its anterior surface. If there are anterior and posterior slabs, avoid them and slit the cast down its ulnar side. Split a leg cast down its lateral surface, cutting between the lateral malleolus and the heel.

BIVALVING A CAST Cut the cast right down to the skin, on both sides of the limb.

CARING FOR A CAST If the patient has to walk home in the rain, let his cast dry and then give it a coat of oil paint.

Lice and other insects may multiply under a cast, and cause such intolerable itching that they drive him to remove it piece by piece. If necessary, dust some insecticide powder down the ends of his cast.

Casts often become loose in time, so see him regularly, and repair and replace his cast as necessary.

AN EXPLANATION TO THE PATIENT FOR ALL CASTS

Explain why you are applying the cast, and when you expect to remove it.

Tell the patient not to use his limb or bear weight on his leg for 48 hours while his cast dries out. Warn him to raise it to prevent swelling, to keep it dry, and to return immediately if he has *pain, numbness, stiffness, or if his fingers or toes become cold, blue, or swollen.* He must also return if his cast becomes loose. Explain that he must exercise his muscles inside the cast,

A FRACTURE PASSPORT

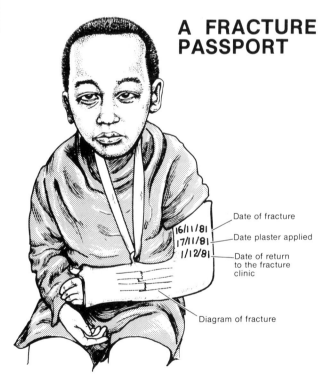

16/11/81 — Date of fracture
17/11/81 — Date plaster applied
1/12/81 — Date of return to the fracture clinic

Diagram of fracture

Fig. 70-6 A FRACTURE PASSPORT is a useful reminder to the patient, and yourself, especially if his notes are lost. Record both the date of his fracture, the date the cast is applied, and the date it is to be removed. Draw a sketch of the fracture. The best way to write on a damp cast is to use a blue indelible pencil. *Kindly contributed by Ruediger Finger*

and the joints which are not immobilized, especially his fingers and toes. He must understand these instructions, so if you cannot speak his language, find someone who does. If he can read, hand him a sheet telling him what to do.

CAUTION !If he comes back complaining of the above symptoms, take his complaint seriously.

REMOVING A CAST can be more painful than applying it, so look at the patient's face to see if you are hurting him. Let him see what you are doing, and let him help, where he can.

Snip the stockinette at the end of the cast and insert the blade of the shears between the stockinette and the cast. Keep the blade parallel to his skin, and avoid bony prominences. Alternatively, and especially in small children, soak the cast off in water. A mother can do this when her child's fracture has healed, or if he has a club foot.

CAUTION ! Use an electric plaster cutter only if: (1) You are sure there is padding under the whole length of the cut. (2) The patient is conscious. Use an up and down movement, and don't try to slide the blade of the cutter along his limb.

DIFFFICULTIES WITH CASTS

If your PLASTER BANDAGES ARE UNSATISFACTORY, use them with hotter water, make the cast thicker, and collect any loose powder that falls off, moisten it with a little water, make it into a paste, and rub it on to the outside of the cast. Use it on the less critical fractures, and keep your best plaster for malleolar fractures, and difficult forearm fractures.

If PLASTER BANDAGES ARE SCARCE, you may be able to economize in their use by making casts lighter, and strengthening them with strips of wood, bamboo, or tin. There are alternative methods for some fractures which do not require plaster, as described below.

Cut the bamboo into strips 300×10×3 mm. Wind a thin initial layer of plaster bandage round the limb. Then apply the bamboo strips all round, especially across the joints. Finally, apply a second thin layer of plaster to complete the cast.

If a CAST BECOMES LOOSE and plaster is scarce, cut a longitudinal strip out of it and then bind it together.

If you have NO PLASTER, you may be able to use strips of bamboo. Many traditional bone setters used strips of bamboo very effectively. Tie these over a well wrapped or padded limb, and hold them in place with string, or adhesive strapping, as in the next section. The traditional method of applying wet goatskin is dangerous, because it contracts as it drys and can cause Volkmann's contracture.

Fractures of the tibia have been treated by wrapping layers of cardboard round a leg.

If you suspect even the possibility of ISCHAEMIA, immediately split the patient's cast from end to end. If this does not cure his symptoms, remove it and examine it for signs of the compartment syndrome which may need incision (70.4). Loss of reduction is better than Volkmann's ischaemic contracture, or gangrene.

If a patient has a PRESSURE SORE on his heel, fish mouth his cast, and then repair it, as in A, Fig. 70-7. If he is in bed, with his cast removed, put a big sausage shaped dressing round his ankle, so that it raises the sore from his bed.

NEVER SEND A PATIENT IN A CAST HOME WITHOUT EXPLAINING THE COMPLICATIONS

70.7 Windowing casts and wedging them

Windows If a patient has an open fracture, a soft tissue injury, or osteomyelitis, you may occasionally need to make a window in his cast, so that his lesions can be dressed. Fortunately, most wounds and sinuses don't need a dressing, because plaster readily absorbs pus and blood. Avoid a window when you can because: (1) if a patient walks about, his tissues may swell and herniate through it, so that his wound will not heal, and (2) windows

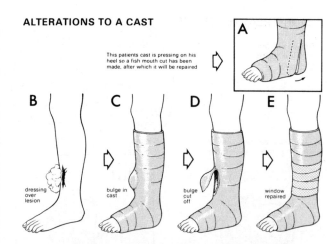

Fig. 70-7 ALTERATIONS TO A CAST. A, if a cast is pressing on a patient's heel, you can open it with a saw, and then repair the cut with plaster bandages. **B,** to **E,** the easiest way to make a window is to put some dressings over the lesion, make the cast, saw off the bulge, and then repair the cast. *Kindly contributed by John Stewart.*

which are not closed and strengthened can weaken a cast so much that it bends with each step he takes.

Wedges If a patient's fractured forearm or lower leg is angulated inside a cast, you can straighten it in two ways, provided the fragments have not yet united: (1) You can open or close a wedge in the cast. This is not as easy as it looks because you may make a wrinkle inside the cast which will cause a pressure sore. *So wedging needs care and skill!* (2) You can wait until his fracture is healed enough not to displace, but is still soft enough to be bent. This is 3 to 6 weeks after the injury in an adult, and sooner in a child. You can then remove the old cast, straighten the patient's limb under anaesthesia, and apply a new cast. If you don't have X-rays, always use this method. *Changing a cast is safer than wedging it,* but if you are very short of plaster you may have to wedge it.

Opening a wedge is easier; it lengthens a cast slightly, and if the fragments are overlapped, it helps to distract them. Closing a wedge by cutting a piece out of a cast and then closing up the gap is more difficult, and is less often necessary. It closes up the fragments a little, so it is useful if they are distracted.

AVOID WINDOWS IF YOU CAN DON'T LET WEDGES CAUSE PRESSURE SORES

WINDOWING A CAST

Make the windows as small as is conveniently possible, as in Fig. 70-7. Put a firm ball of cotton wool over the lesion where you want a window, and make the cast over it. While the cast is still soft, hold a knife parallel to the patient's skin, and cut off the swelling over the wool, so as to make the window. Or, cut a square hole in a dry cast with a plaster saw.

Prevent the tissues of the lesion herniating through the window by raising the limb and by applying a firm pressure dressing through the window. This acts like a piston in a cylinder and helps to prevent herniation. Dress the wound and plaster over the window to strengthen the cast.

WEDGING A CAST

Study the X-rays and plan the geometry of what you intend to do carefully. Draw a line round the cast where you want to cut.

OPENING A WEDGE is better than trying to close one, because you are less likely to make a wrinkle inside a cast that will cause a pressure sore. Do this as in Fig. 70-8.

OPENING A WEDGE

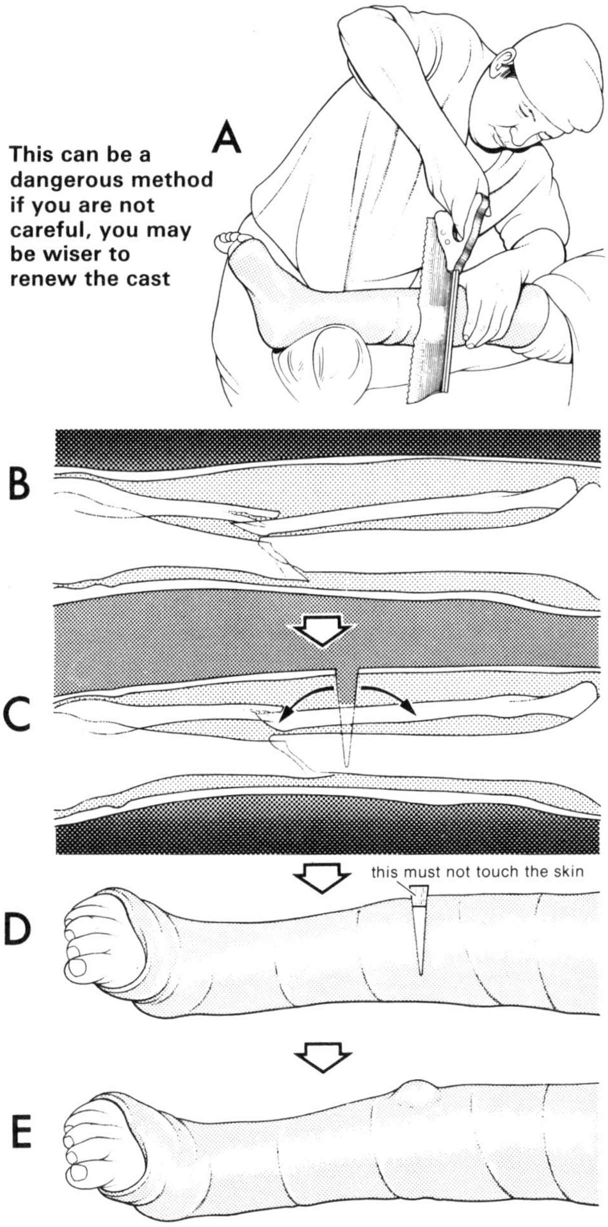

A

This can be a dangerous method if you are not careful, you may be wiser to renew the cast

B

C

D

this must not touch the skin

E

Fig. 70-8 OPENING A WEDGE. Obtain some small blocks of wood to hold the wedge open. Cut through the whole circumference of the cast except for 2 or 3 cm on its convex side, so as to leave a hinge on which it can bend (A, and B). Make the cut about 2 cm proximal to the fracture (C), so that if there is a wrinkle inside the cast, it will not be directly over the fracture, where it may erode the skin. Use a saw or plaster knife. Cut down to the padding, and not into the limb! Carefully bend the cast the way you want it. If necessary hold it open with a block of wood (D), but make sure that the block is clear of the skin. Then repair the cast with a few turns of plaster bandage (E). X-ray the limb to check alignment. *Kindly contributed by Peter Bewes.*

CLOSING A WEDGE On the side of the cast which is to be made concave, mark out a wedge about 1 to 3 cm across at its widest part. Cut out the wedge, and gently bend the cast so as to close the wedge. Repair the cast with some turns of plaster bandage. X-ray the limb to check alignment.

If more than one wedge is needed in different planes, replace the cast.

CAUTION ! Wedge a limb, especially an arm, with care—it can precipitate Volkmann's ischaemic contracture. Watch the circulation in the limb carefully afterwards.

THE GEOMETRY OF WEDGING

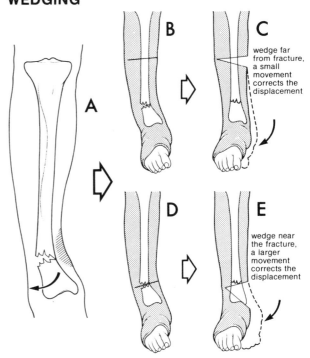

wedge far from fracture, a small movement corrects the displacement

wedge near the fracture, a larger movement corrects the displacement

Fig. 70-9 THE GEOMETRY OF WEDGING. A, the angulation that requires correction. B, if the wedge is far from the fracture a small movement will correct the displacement. B, if the wedge is near or over the fracture, a larger movement is necessary. *Kindly contributed by Peter Bewes.*

70.8 Chinese wooden splints

You can use splints made of strips of wood padded with paper and cloth for fractures of the humerus, radius, and ulna, and for extension fractures of the wrist. There is no evidence that they are better that plaster casts, but if you don't have plaster, you may find them useful. Wooden splints are light, tenacious, elastic, radiotranslucent, permeable to the natural moisture of the skin, and can be moulded to the shape of the limb.

CHINESE WOODEN SPLINTS

INDICATIONS Some fractures of the upper limb.

CONTRAINDICATIONS (1) Open fractures. (2) Severe bruising. (3) Severe soft tissue swelling. (4) Signs of peripheral circulatory insufficiency. (5) Nerve injuries.

MATERIALS (1) Make thick cloth bandages 1.5 to 2 cm wide from two layers of calico or four layers of bandage sewn together. (2) Make paper or cotton wool pads. These must be absorbent and soft and elastic enough to mould easily to the shape of the limb. (3) Thin pliable strips of wood or bamboo.

METHOD Bandage the patient's limb. Place four or five layers of pads outside the bandages and fix them there with strips of adhesive tape. Outside these place the wooden splints. Bind them in place with about four strips of cloth.

Take a check X-ray. Raise the limb and monitor its circulation carefully. If the fracture displaces or the paper pads shift, adjust them immediately.

DON'T FORGET THE PATIENT AFTER YOU HAVE APPLIED THE CAST

CHINESE WOODEN SPLINTS

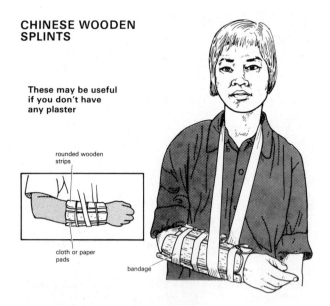

These may be useful if you don't have any plaster

rounded wooden strips

cloth or paper pads

bandage

Fig. 70-10 CHINESE WOODEN SPLINTS. You can use splints made of strips of wood padded with paper and cloth for fractures of the humerus, radius, and ulna, and for extension fractures of the wrist. *Kindly contributed by Cai Ru Bin.*

70.9 Traction

To exert traction is to pull. You can use traction: (1) to pull fractured bones into place to begin with, or (2) to keep them moderately immobile until they have united, or, (3) to do both these things, one followed by the other. To apply traction successfully you will have to find some way to grasp a patient's limb safely, for several weeks if necessary. There are two ways you can do this: (1) You can stick adhesive strapping to his skin (skin traction). (2) You can pass a Steinmann pin, a Denham pin, or Kirchner wire through his bone (bone traction). Cord has then to be attached to the strapping, pin, or wire, passed over a pulley, and fixed to a weight. The weight may pull the patient out of his bed, so you usually need to exert countertraction by raising the foot of his bed. One of the main purposes of traction is to allow a patient to exercise his muscles and move his joints, so make sure he does this. Traction takes time to apply and manage, but it can easily be managed by assistants—if you teach them!

Traction is mostly useful in the leg. In the arm it is uncomfortable, inconvenient, difficult to maintain, and frustrating for the patient. For all these reasons arm traction is only useful in rather exceptional circumstances. Elaborate kinds of traction, such as that of Hamilton and Russell for the leg, require equipment you are unlikely to have, so we have only described the simpler kinds here.

PATIENTS IN TRACTION MUST EXERCISE

TRACTION METHODS SUMMARIZED

ARM TRACTION METHODS

FOREARM TRACTION Adhesive strapping is applied to a child's forearm when his elbow is so swollen from a supracondylar fracture that it cannot be reduced immediately (72.6, Fig. 72-11). Uncommon.

CAUTION! Don't let the strapping interfere with the circulation in his hand.

SKIN TRACTION FOR A FRACTURED HUMERUS is only necessary when a patient is confined to bed (Fig. 71-16). Rare.

OLECRANON TRACTION A Kirschner wire or a small Steinmann pin is passed through the olecranon for some lower humerus fractures (Fig. 72-14). This is the preferred method of treating comminuted supracondylar fractures in adults. Uncommon.

METACARPAL TRACTION A Kirschner wire through the first two metacarpals is used for for some forearm fractures, especially if the circulation of the forearm is impaired so that you cannot apply skin traction (Fig. 70-13). Rare.

LEG TRACTION METHODS

'90 – 90 TRACTION' is useful when the proximal fragment of a fractured femur is sharply flexed. A Steinmann pin is put through the supracondylar region of a patient's femur, or his upper tibia, and his hip and knee are flexed to 90° (77.12). Uncommon.

GALLOWS TRACTION The legs of a small child with a fractured femur are suspended from a bar with adhesive strapping (78.2). Very common.

EXTENSION TRACTION Adhesive strapping is used to treat fractures of the femur in an older child or teenager with his knee extended. Also useful for some fractures of the neck of the femur (78.3). Very common.

PERKINS TRACTION An upper tibial pin is used to treat most fractures of the femur in an adult. The patient's knee is flexed and he exercises it (78.4). Very common.

BOHLER–BRAUN TRACTION using a special Böhler–Braun frame is useful for some supracondylar fractures of the femur (79.13). It can also be used for other fractures, expecially those of the tibia (79.3), but we describe better methods. Uncommon.

DISTAL TIBIAL TRACTION A pin through the distal tibia is used to treat some fractures of the proximal tibia (80.5). Fairly common.

CALCANEAL TRACTION A pin through the calcaneus is used to treat some tibial fractures (81.12, Fig. 81-10). Fairly common.

The purpose of traction is to reduce overlap and bring the displaced bone ends together—not to pull them so far apart (distract them) that they cannot unite! So: (1) Check the length of a patient's injured limb by measuring it, or with X-rays, and

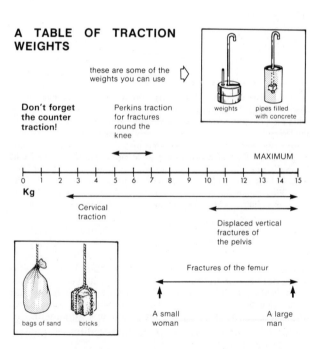

A TABLE OF TRACTION WEIGHTS

these are some of the weights you can use

Don't forget the counter traction!

Perkins traction for fractures round the knee

weights   pipes filled with concrete

MAXIMUM

0 1 2 3 4 5 6 7 8 9 10 11 12 13 14 15
Kg

Cervical traction

Displaced vertical fractures of the pelvis

Fractures of the femur

A small woman

A large man

bags of sand   bricks

Fig. 70-11. A SCALE OF TRACTION WEIGHTS showing the range of weights needed for various fractures. Adjust them: (1) to the patients's build, and (2) during the course of treatment.

adjust the traction accordingly. (2) Vary the traction you apply to the needs of the patient—small patients need less weight than large ones. Don't apply too much traction, and be prepared to adjust it. To begin with you need to apply more traction than is necessary later, when the soft tissues have stretched. For example, for femoral fractures you may need to apply 15 kg to start with, and then reduce it kilo by kilo on the following days.

Ideally, traction should be checked with X-rays, but unfortunately the BRS X-ray machine (1.13) is not portable, and you will probably not have a machine which you can take to the wards. The solution is to have a few beds with large castors which you can wheel to the X-ray department without taking down the traction.

Applying traction to a cast is dangerous because the skin through which pressure is applied is likely to necrose. The only safe way to apply traction to a cast is to pass a pin through the patient's bone and to incorporate this in the cast. Never apply traction to a plaster boot without a proximal tibial pin in place, because it too easily causes pressure sores on the dorsum of the foot.

ADJUST THE TRACTION CAREFULLY

EQUIPMENT FOR BONE TRACTION

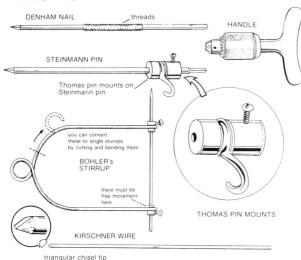

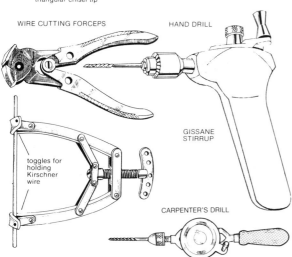

Fig. 70-12 EQUIPMENT FOR BONE TRACTION. Both the handle and the hand drill are cannulated so that a Kirschner wire can pass right through them and be held close to the skin. If you don't have any other kind of drill, use an ordinary carpenter's drill.

• *STRAPPING, traction, adhesive, 50 mm×10 mm, six rolls only.* This is elastic across its width, but not along its length. If you don't have it, use ordinary zinc oxide strapping. 'Elastoplast', which is elastic in both directions is useless.

• *PIN, Denham, (Denham threaded Steinmann pin), stainless steel, 4 mm, tapered, self tapping, with long coarse screw thread, triangular shank, packet of 5, two packs only.* This is the ordinary Denham pin, but made with a triangular shank. If possible, buy the kind with a long length of thread which will grip both cortices of the tibia.

• *PIN, Steinmann, triangular shank, stainless steel, trocar pointed at one end, (a) 2×180 mm, (b) 3×180 mm, (c) 4×180 mm, six only of each size.* The small size is for the olecranon and the larger ones are for the tibia.

• *HANDLE, with Jacobs chuck, 4 mm capacity, and key attached by chain, fully cannulated, stainless steel, one only.* This is an ordinary drill chuck in a handle. This chuck has three jaws, and although it is intended for Kirschner wire and for pins and nails with triangular shanks, you can use it with square shanks. It will not grip the round section of a pin.

• *STIRRUPS, Böhler, for Steinmann pins, with rotating swivel fixation pieces, (a) 102×89 mm, three only. (b) 165×144 mm, three only. (c) 241×152 mm, five only.* These stirrups can be used for Steinmann or Denham pins. The small ones are for the calcaneus and the olecranon and the large ones are for the tibia. If you don't have these stirrups, take a wire coat hanger and bend it to shape, or tie the cords over corks as in E, Fig. 70-14.

• *PIN MOUNTS, Thomas, stainless steel with rotating collar for Perkins traction, four pairs only.* These are much the best mounts for Perkins traction. If you don't have them, you can make them by cutting a Böhler stirrup and bending the wire. The hooks must rotate freely round the collars.

• *STIRRUPS, for wire traction, adjustable, tensioning, Gissane, 216 mm, with two cord hooks, two only.* These are for exerting tension on Kirschner wire. They are more expensive than the standard Kirschner wire stirrups, but there are no loose parts to get lost. Use these stirrups for exerting traction on the olecranon in fractures of the humerus, on the metacarpals in fractures of the radius, and on the metatarsals in some fractures of the foot.

• *WIRE, Kirschner, plain unthreaded, stainless steel, drill pointed at one end, packet of 5, (a) 0.75×254 mm, four packets only. (b) 1 mm×254 mm, four packets only. (c) 1.5 mm×254 mm, four packets only.* These are the standard Kirschner wires. Unfortunately, Kirschner wire is seldom available in district hospitals at the present time. It is one of the purposes of this system of surgery to promote its use.

• *INTRODUCER, for Kirschner wire, Pulvertaft's, one only.* This will make introducing Kirschner wire much easier.

• *CUTTERS, Kirschner wire, one only.* If you don't have these, sterilize a pair of ordinary pliers, but take care to oil them carefully afterwards.

• *HAND DRILL, for Kirschner wires and drills, 4 mm capacity cannulated throughout, one only.* The chuck of this drill has a hole through it so that long Kirschner wires can be passed down it and supported close to the skin. If you don't have one of these drills, use a small ordinary carpenter's hand drill and the bits for it and keep them oiled after use. Unfortunately, a carpenter's drill is not cannulated, so you can use it only with drill bits, not with Kirschner wire. The main use of a drill is to exclude osteomyelitis (7.3). If you don't have any kind of drill, you may be able to hammer in a Steinmann pin through cancellous, but not through cortical, bone.

• *DRILL BITS, twist, bone, 4 mm, six only.* Use these to: (1) Drill a hole for a Steinmann pin. (2) Explore for pus in patients with osteomyelitis. Don't drill so vigorously that the bit becomes too hot, because the heated bone around the bit may die and form a ring sequestrum.

• *FORCEPS, wire cutting, compound lever action with pliers jaws, 170 mm.* These can cut and bend Kirschner wire up to 1.6 mm diameter.

• *CORD, braided, for traction, local purchase.* If you don't have this use a length of bandage.

• *PULLEYS, orthopaedic, assorted, ten only.* If you don't have pulleys for Perkins traction, wrap a strip of old X-ray film loosely round the bar of the bed so it can rotate. Hold it there with adhesive strapping and let the traction cord run over it.

• *BARS, for overhead traction.* These are needed for '90–90' traction (Fig. 77-11), for some pelvic fractures (Fig. 76-2), and for humerus fractures in unconscious or supine patients (Fig. 71-16). Make them from welded tubing.

• *WEIGHTS, for traction, local manufacture.* Use bags of sand, or bricks suspended in stockinette, as in Fig. 70-11; each brick weighs about 3 kg. Or, use lengths of pipe filled with concrete into which a hook has been placed before the concrete sets. For example, 45 cm of 7.5 cm pipe filled with concrete weighs about 7 kg.

70.10 Skin traction

The great advantage of skin traction is that there is no need to pass any instrument through the tissues. But: (1) You cannot apply more than 5 kg, and even then not for long, so it is not suitable for Perkins traction. (2) Joints which are crossed by the strapping cannot flex and exercise. (3) The patient's skin may become sensitive to the strapping. (4) Skin traction is poorly tolerated in old patients and easily causes blisters. (5) If it is not carefully managed, the strapping slips off completely. (6) It is very uncomfortable in hot climates. (7) It can occasionally cause ischaemia followed by Volkmann's contracture (78.2).

Nevertheless, skin traction is particularly useful for treating: (1) elbow fractures in adults and children, (2) fractured femurs in children, (3) fractured femurs in adults where pin traction cannot be used or has caused complications.

SKIN TRACTION

If possible, use special traction strapping. If you use ordinary zinc oxide strapping, help it to stick by applying compound tincture of benzoin (compound tincture of benzoin BPC) to a patient's skin. This is an alcoholic varnish which becomes sticky as it dries. Let it get sticky and then apply the strapping to it.

If necessary, shave the patient's skin. Apply strapping to *both* sides of his limb, up to but not above the fracture line, or it will fail to exert any traction. Finally, wind a crêpe bandage spirally over it. *Never wind circular turns of adhesive strapping round a limb, because the strapping can become too tight.*

Either fix a piece of wood in a loop of strapping, as in Fig. 78-3, making it slightly wider than the patient's ankle so that the strapping does not compress his malleoli. Or, fold each end of the strapping, and tie a cord to it.

CAUTION ! (1) When you apply skin traction to an adult's leg, especially a thin, bony, old one, take great care that the strapping does not press on his common peroneal nerve, as it winds round the neck of his fibula. This could paralyse it and cause foot drop. (2) Don't let the strapping extend above the fracture line onto the proximal fragment, or it will be useless. (3) Don't let it interfere with his circulation.

If you don't have any crêpe bandage, take some 2 cm zinc oxide tape and wind it in two long right and left spirals round the limb. The spirals should cross each other twice as in Fig. 78-1. This will be safer than applying circular strapping.

DON'T APPLY STRAPPING PROXIMAL TO THE FRACTURE LINE

70.11 Skeletal traction

Steinmann pins are stainless steel rods 2 to 4 mm in diameter. A Denham pin is similar, except that it has a few large threads on it, which you can screw into the cortex of the bone to stop it slipping from side to side. Denham pins are better than Steinmann pins for Perkins traction (78.4) and for calcaneal traction (81.12). But Steinmann pins have other uses, so you will need both. Insert them with the chuck shown in Fig. 70-12. If you don't have a chuck, you can, if necessary, hammer in a Steinmann pin, if you follow the instructions below, but you cannot

SITES FOR SKELETAL TRACTION

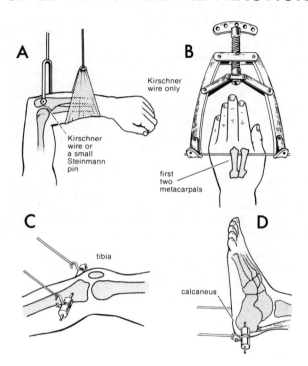

Fig. 70-13 SITES FOR SKELETAL TRACTION. Pins can spread or introduce infection, so put them through healthy tissue some distance from a fracture, and not through the fracture site itself where injured tissue is easily infected. *After de Palma with kind permission.*

hammer in a Denham pin, because of its threads. If you wish, you can drill a hole for a pin before you insert it. One difficulty is finding the hole after you have drilled it.

These pins are stiff, so you can apply traction to them without tensioning them. You can use: (1) A Böhler's stirrup (Fig. 70-12) and a single traction cord and weight. (2) Two Thomas pin mounts (swivels) with two traction cords and two weights. (3) If you don't have either of these, you can put corks on the ends of the pin and tie the cords to them. If you tie the traction cords directly to the ends of a pin, they usually slip off and cause agony as they do so. Join the cords together and run them through a pulley attached to a single weight, so as to equalize the pull on either end of the pin as in B, Fig. 70-14.

Pins can spread or introduce infection, so: (1) Put them through healthy tissues some distance from a fracture, and not through a fracture site where the injured tissue is easily infected. You can use them to treat open infected fractures, but the further they are from the site of the infection the better. (2) Keep them still. The pin must stay motionless in the bone, and rotate freely in the stirrup or pin mount. This is why a Denham pin which is firmly screwed into the bone is better than a Steinmann pin. If your pin mounts have set screws, don't tighten them. (3) Never put a pin through a joint capsule. The most serious complication of skeletal traction is infection of the knee joint, or osteomyelitis, particularly in the calcaneus (7.13). If sequestrectomy does not cure this, it may be necessary to remove the whole calcaneus.

A LOOSE PIN PROMOTES INFECTION

STEINMANN'S AND DENHAM'S PINS

EQUIPMENT A sterile sharp pin. A blunt one promotes infection, so sharpen a pin each time, if necessary on a grindstone.

TIBIAL TRACTION RIGHT AND WRONG

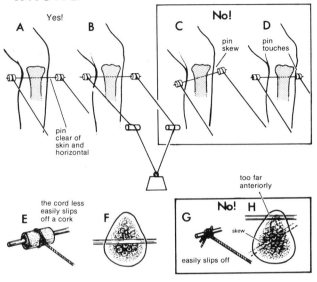

Fig. 70-14 TIBIAL TRACTION RIGHT AND WRONG. A, and B, at all sites the pin must be at 90° to the axis of the limb and in a horizonal plane. There must be the same length of pin each side of the limb. If the pin is very skew, one of the cords will slide along it and press into the skin (C, and D). E, if you don't have a Thomas swivel, tie the cord to a cork, not to the pin directly (G). Don't put the pin in too far anteriorly or put it in skew (H). *Kindly contributed by John Stewart.*

A scalpel and local anaesthetic. Some surgeons sterilize the chuck, others use an unsterile chuck and a no–touch technique.

INSERTING THE PIN In most district hospitals this is best done in the theatre. If nursing and ward equipment are very good, you can do it in the ward under local anaesthesia.

If you are going to hammer a pin in, do it through the cancellous bone near the end of a long bone, and not through the thick cortical bone of the shaft, because this may split. Take the patient to the theatre, find two assistants, and give him a general anaesthetic.

If you are using local anaesthesia, sedate him, and apply iodine to the skin where the pin will go in and come out. Inject local anaesthetic into the skin, subcutaneous tissue, and periosteum of both sides, making sure it goes under the periosteum.

Make a small nick in the skin with the point of a sharp scalpel. Put the pin in the chuck, and push it through the skin into the bone, twisting it slightly from side to side as you do so. Ask one assistant to hold the patient's leg. Take great care to get the direction of the pin right. Ask your other assistant to check its direction by observing its alignment from the foot of the table. Putting it in is hard work!

As the pin comes out of the bone on the other side of the limb, its point will raise the skin, so nick this with a scalpel, and push the pin through it.

When the threads of a Denham pin reach the bone, screw them in about six turns, so that some of them enter its cortex. The threads should lie in the cortex, not in the medulla.

Finally, secure the pin in a Böhler's stirrup or, preferably, with Thomas pin mounts. If the sharp point might injure the patient's other leg, put a cork or a cap on it.

PARTICULAR SITES FOR PIN FIXATION

THE UPPER FEMUR is occasionally used for the central dislocation of the head of a patient's femur (77.4). Insert the pin vertically through his greater trochanter.

THE LOWER FEMUR is one of the less satisfactory sites. Insert the pin at the level of the flare of the condyles, opposite the upper pole of the patella, slightly anterior to the midline of the leg.

THE UPPER TIBIA is much the most important site, and is used for most fractures of the femur, and many fractures around the knee. If you insert the pin from the lateral side, you are less likely to injure the patient's common peroneal nerve. There are two alternative sites.

If you are using a chuck, put a 4 mm pin through firm cortical bone 3 cm distal to the patient's tibial tuberosity. Go from the lateral to the medial side. Feel the neck of his fibula where his common peroneal nerve will be winding round it, and insert the pin anterior to that point.

If you have no chuck and you have to hammer a pin in, do so from the lateral to the medial side 1 cm distal to the tibial tuberosity through the junction of cortical and cancellous bone, that is, through the flare of the condyles. The pin will be less firmly held here but the bone is less likely to shatter.

CAUTION ! In either site, don't insert the pin too far anteriorly, because there will not be enough bone to hold it.

If his tibia is osteoporotic, apply a short leg cast around it and incorporate the pin in this.

LOWER TIBIA For some fractures of the upper tibia (80.5). Insert the pin from the lateral side 4 to 6 cm above the patient's medial malleolus immediately in front of his fibula. This makes sure it is well clear of his ankle joint, and avoids injuring his superficial peroneal nerve. Align it carefully so that it is at right angles to the long axis of his limb and is in the coronal plane.

CALCANEUS For some fractures of the tibia (Fig. 81-10). Insert a 4 mm pin from the lateral side medially through the posterior part of the patient's calcaneus, as in Figs. 70-13 and 70-16. Put the pin in, or just behind, a vertical line joining the tip of his lateral malleolus to the lower border of his heel. If you drive it in at right angles to the axis of his limb, it will emerge well clear of his posterior tibial vessels.

CAUTION ! (1) If you put the pin in too far posteriorly, you will dorsiflex the patient's foot. (2) If you leave it in more than 15 days you will increase the risk of osteomyelitis.

OLECRANON For some fractures of the radius and ulna. Use a thin 2 mm Steinmann pin, and insert it from the medial side laterally, avoiding the patient's ulnar nerve. A Kirschner wire is better, if you have the equipment to apply it.

DRESSINGS Keep the pin track clean. Apply dressings to the entry and exit wounds of the pin and inspect them regularly.

CAUTION ! If there are any signs of infection round a pin at any site, remove it immediately. If you cannot put it back through uninfected skin elsewhere in the bone, change to skin traction.

REMOVING A PIN Use an antiseptic such as iodine to clean the projecting point of the pin that will be drawn through the tissues. Pull it out with the chuck. Don't remove it by hitting the point of the pin with a hammer. Unscrew a Denham pin, and don't merely pull it.

IF A PIN TRACK BECOMES INFECTED, REMOVE THE PIN

70.12 Skeletal traction with Kirschner wires

These are thin flexible stainless steel wires 0.75 to 1 mm in diameter. Use them for applying traction: (1) Through the heads of the metacarpals in open forearm fractures. (2) Through the olecranon in comminuted fractures of the lower humerus, or when the patient must lie supine. Kirschner wires are thin and flexible, so you must drill them in, and you can only apply traction to them with an expensive tensioner, such as the Gissane stirrup which will hold them taut. Unlike a Steinmann or Denham pin, where movement takes place between the pin and the pin mount, movement with Kirschner wire traction takes

SETTING UP CALCANEAL TRACTION

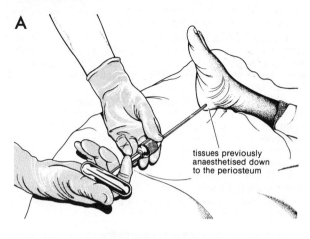

A

tissues previously anaesthetised down to the periosteum

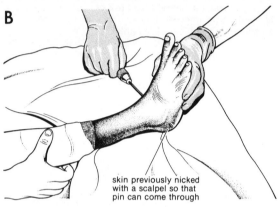

B

skin previously nicked with a scalpel so that pin can come through

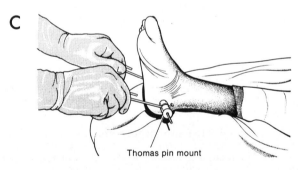

C

Thomas pin mount

Fig. 70-16 INSERTING A STEINMANN PIN THROUGH THE CALCANEUS. If you put the pin in too far posteriorly, you will dorsiflex his foot. If you leave it in for more than 15 days you will increase the risk of osteomyelitis. *Kindly contributed by Peter Bewes.*

place between the wire and the tissues. This limits the amount of exercise that is practical. Kirschner wires can only be used if they are straight, and because they always bend in use, you cannot use the bent parts again, although you may be able to cut off the straight parts which remain and reuse them.

KIRSCHNER WIRE TRACTION

Sharpen the wire on a stone to a chisel or a triangular point as in Fig. 70-12. Cut it to length with a pair of pliers.

Drill it in with a hand drill (Fig. 70-12). Use the chuck to hold the wire near the end. In the softer bones of children, you may be able to put it in with pliers.

OLECRANON For some comminuted supracondylar fractures when the patient must lie supine. Insert the wire from the medial to the lateral side, taking care to avoid his ulnar nerve.

METACARPALS For open or comminuted fractures of the radius and ulna. Insert the wire through the second and third metacarpal from the medial to the lateral side, avoiding the fourth and fifth metacarpals which are more mobile and lie anteriorly. Metacarpal bone is hard, and drilling may be difficult. Don't go too far anteriorly, or you may injure the patient's digital vessels and nerves. Some surgeons claim that metacarpal traction is seldom necessary and prefer skin traction on all the four fingers, while watching the circulation of the fingers with care!

CALCANEUS Kirschner wire traction is an alternative to a Steinmann pin for fractures of the tibia.

DRESSINGS These are the same as for Steinmann pins.

DISTRACTION IS ONE OF THE GREAT ENEMIES OF UNION

70.13 Kirschner wire for bone fixation

Kirschner wire fixation is useful for some severe hand injuries and in some fractures of the olecranon. If you put a short piece of Kirschner wire through two pieces of bone it will keep them aligned, but it is less successful in preventing them coming apart. The easiest way to prevent this happening is to bind the fragments in place with soft stainless steel wire. This is most effectively done by drilling a hole, through the bone, passing the wire through the hole and then looping it in a figure of eight around the bent ends of the pieces of Kirschner wire as in Fig. 72-26. This is Kirschner wire hemicirclage, and is an AO method; it is the most practical way of fixing those fractures of the olecranon (72.18) which must be fixed internally.

INTERNAL FIXATION WITH KIRSCHNER WIRE

INSERTION If you are going to fix a fragment with Kirschner wire alone, use two wires in slightly different planes, avoiding the plane at right angles to the fracture plane.

Use wire cutting forceps to bend over the outer 3 mm of the wires. These bent ends will be easier to find and remove later if necessary; they will not pierce the skin, and they can be used to anchor soft wire for hemicirclage.

Drill the bone and thread soft stainless steel wire thorugh it, as in Figs. 72-26, 79-8, and 75-9a.

CAUTION ! Don't leave Kirschner wire sticking out of the skin, because this increases the chances of infection.

REMOVAL If the wire is causing no trouble, leave it. If the ends of the wire are painful under the skin, or if there is infection, or a sinus, remove it. Feel for the end of the wire under the skin and take it out under local anaesthesia. Make a nick in the skin and remove it with bull nosed pliers filed to a sharp point, or with any convenient instrument. If you cannot find the end of the wire, you may have to give the patient a general anaesthetic and remove it after first applying a tourniquet.

71 The shoulder and upper arm

71.1 Introduction

Most shoulder injuries are caused by a patient falling on the point of his shoulder, or on his outstretched hand. If he does this, he can dislocate the joints at either end of his clavicle, or break it anywhere. He can injure his brachial plexus. He can also break his scapula, dislocate his shoulder, or break the neck of his humerus. Occasionally, he breaks the neck of his humerus and dislocates its head.

We have already discussed the general principles of examining an injured limb (69.1), so here are some more detailed methods, which will be particularly useful, if you don't have X-rays. Do them gently, because they can be painful, particularly examining for crepitus.

EXAMINING THE SHOULDER AND UPPER ARM

THE CLAVICLE EXAMINATION

Look carefully at either end of the patient's clavicle. Are they same on both sides? (abnormal prominence suggests a dislocation).

Stand behind him, feel the entire subcutaneous surface of his clavicle, and the joints at either end. Where exactly is it swollen and tender? (fractures).

Is there any abnormal movement between his clavicle and his acromion? (acromio–clavicular dislocation). If so, can you reduce the dislocation by raising his humerus with your hand under his elbow, and depressing his clavicle?

THE SCAPULA EXAMINATION

Palpate the spine of the patient's scapula and his acromion. Tenderness and swelling probably indicate a fracture.

Flex his arm to 90° and rest it on your forearm. Gently move his whole arm up and down. Provided his clavicle is intact, abnormal mobility or crepitus in his shoulder suggests that he has fractured the neck of his scapula.

THE SHOULDER JOINT EXAMINATION

INSPECTION Is the outline of the patient's shoulder flattened, and the normal roundness of his deltoid muscle lost as in Fig. 71-4? (dislocation, or a circumflex nerve injury causing wasting of his deltoid).

Is his anterior axillary fold lowered, his deltopectoral groove swollen, or his elbow displaced away from his body? Does the axis of his humerus point towards the middle of his clavicle as in Fig. 71-4? (these are all signs of an anterior dislocation of the shoulder).

Is his shoulder grossly swollen? (the neck of his humerus is probably fractured, perhaps with dislocation of its head. In a fracture dislocation swelling of the shoulder joint hides the flattening caused by the dislocation, so this injury is often missed).

PALPATION Can you feel the head of the patient's humerus dislocated into an abnormal position? Feel high up into his axilla. You may be able to feel a thickened capsule, or an effusion.

Are the tip of his acromion, the tip of his coracoid, and the greater tuberosity of his humerus in their normal places?

MOVEMENTS OF THE SHOULDER Stand behind him. Put one hand round in front of him and hold the outer end of his clavicle firmly. With your other hand hold the tip of his scapula still. With his scapula held, you can now be sure that any movements he makes are those of his shoulder, not those of his scapula moving over his chest. If pain begins as soon as he starts to move his arm in any direction, there is something seriously wrong with his shoulder.

Abduction How far can the patient abduct his shoulder? He should be able to abduct it to 90° before his scapula starts to move. If his scapula starts to move earlier, abduction of his shoulder is limited.

Adduction With his forearm flexed, and his scapula held, can he bring his elbow across to the midline in front?

Rotation Can he externally rotate his flexed forearm, so that it reaches the coronal plane? Can he rotate it internally enough to scratch the small of his back?

If any of the above active movements are limited, repeat them passively. Finally, ask him to lift his arm from his side, at first to 90° and then above his head. If he can do this, he has no serious shoulder injury.

OTHER SIGNS IN THE SHOULDER Stand behind the patient and rest your hands on the point of each of his shoulders. Try to insert the tips of your fingers under the edge of each acromion, between it and the head of his humerus. You may be able to feel that the head of his humerus is dislocated on the injured side.

Put one hand on his shoulder, and grasp his elbow with your other one. Bring your hands together so as to compress his humerus. If this is painful it may be fractured.

Grasp the top of his shoulder, so that your thumb lies over the head of his humerus, and your fingers over the spine of his scapula. Flex his forearm and use it to rotate his humerus. If you cannot feel the head moving under your thumb, or if there is crepitus, the neck of his humerus has fractured. If the fracture is impacted, this sign is absent. If, at the same time, the head is displaced, he has a fracture dislocation.

The shoulder joint is hidden under muscles, so you cannot see if it is swollen, but you can see swelling of the subacromial bursa, especially if you look from behind and above, and compare both sides.

UPPER ARM EXAMINATION

Palpate the lower half of the patient's humerus for the signs of a fracture. This is more difficult in its upper half, which is hidden by muscles.

Support his forearm and gently abduct his arm. Pain, tenderness, angulation, or crepitus, indicate a fracture of the shaft.

On both sides, measure the distance from the tip of his acromion to his lateral epicondyle. Shortening indicates a fracture. This test is particularly useful if you suspect it is impacted.

NERVES AND VESSELS In any injury of a patient's shoulder and upper arm, test his median, ulnar, radial and, axillary nerves (Fig. 55-6). If his clavicle is injured, check his subclavian vessels and listen to the breath sounds in his lungs.

X-RAYS Ask for the following views.

Clavicle An X-ray is usually unnecessary for the clavicle.

SUPPORTING AN INJURED ARM

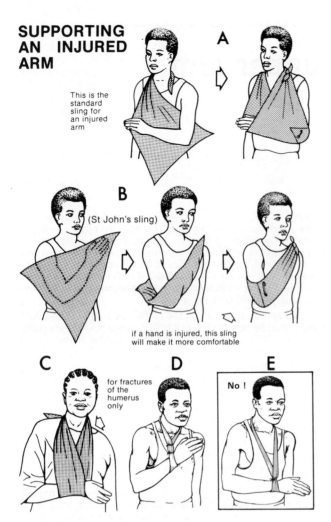

This is the standard sling for an injured arm

A

B (St John's sling)

if a hand is injured, this sling will make it more comfortable

C for fractures of the humerus only

D

E No !

Fig. 71-1 SLINGS FOR AN INJURED ARM. Most injured arms are best in sling A. If a hand is injured, the St John sling B, will raise it. Fractures of the humerus need sling C, in which the patient's elbow hangs free. Supracondylar fractures need the collar–and–cuff D. The narrow bandage sling E, is commonly used but is much less satisfactory.

Acromio–clavicular joint Ask for an AP view of the injured shoulder. Dislocation may be difficult to see, so if you suspect it, ask for a distraction view in which the patient holds a weight.

Shoulder Ask for an AP and a lateral view. If you suspect a posterior dislocation ask for an axillary view. This is difficult, because he may be holding his arm to his side, so you may have to take it yourself.

Shaft of humerus Ask for an AP and a lateral view.

71.2 Casts, slings, and exercises for injuries of the upper limb

Later chapters start with a description of the appropriate casts. These are seldom needed for injuries of the elbow and almost never for injuries of the shoulder and upper arm. The slings in Fig. 71-1 are important for ambulant patients with injured arms. An injured or infected arm which hangs down is painful—a sling makes it much more comfortable and alows it to be exercised when necessary. Many hospitals supply plaster casts and sell or hire out crutches. They should do the same for slings. A loop of bandage (E, in Fig. 71-1) is not good enough. *An important principle in all shoulder injuries is for the patient to start exercising his elbow and fingers as soon as he can.* Even in a sling he can do some of the exercises in Fig. 71-7.

ACTIVE MOVEMENTS FOR INJURIES OF THE SHOULDER GIRDLE

INDICATIONS (1) All fractures of the clavicle. (2) Most dislocations of the sterno–clavicular and acromio–clavicular joints.

METHOD A sling will relieve the patient's pain. Make it with a triangular bandage, and rest his arm in it for 2 or 3 weeks, or until the fracture site is no longer tender. Start elbow and finger exercises immediately. Begin shoulder exercises in 2 or 3 days. If his clavicle is fractured, bracing his shoulders back will help him to hold it to length. Encourage him to move his arm as soon as he can.

Don't leave a sling on too long. Remove it at a set time, some patients develop a 'sling neurosis' and are unwilling to part with it.

ELBOW AND FINGER EXERCISES MUST START IMMEDIATELY

71.3 Injuries of the brachial plexus

If an injured patient has a totally paralysed insensitive arm, he has a brachial plexus injury in which he has injured all three cords of his brachial plexus. He can also injure them separately. These injuries can be the result of falling from a tree, or from a motor cycle, as in Fig. 51-6. If a patient is lucky, he merely stretches his nerve roots, if he is unlucky he pulls them away from his cord. In both types of injury he loses the power and feeling in his arm, but in a stretch injury, he can usually still move his rhomboid muscles, because the nerve which supplies them leaves the brachial plexus close to the cord. In an avulsion injury, this nerve is torn from his cord with the rest of his brachial plexus, so that his rhomboid muscles no longer function on the injured side.

BRACHIAL PLEXUS INJURY Ask the patient to pull his shoulder blades together. If he can do this, the function of his rhomboids is intact.

If his rhomboids are intact, support his arm in a sling, protect it from injuries, such as cuts, bruises, and burns, until its sensation returns. Make sure that one of his relatives exercises his shoulder, elbow, and hand for 6 months or longer, because his arm may continue to recover for at least a year.

If his rhomboids are paralysed, he has probably torn the roots of his brachial plexus away from his cord, so that his injury is permanent. If he shows no signs of recovery at 6 months, consider amputating his upper arm through skin which has sensation.

FRACTURE OF THE CLAVICLE

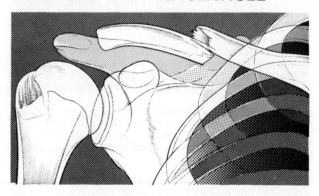

Fig. 71-2 FRACTURE OF THE MIDDLE THIRD OF THE CLAVICLE If an adult breaks the middle third of his clavicle, his sternomastoid muscle pulls the medial fragment up, while the weight of his arm pulls the lateral one down.

71.4 Fractures of the clavicle

The clavicle often breaks, especially in a child. He crys when he moves his arm, but there may be little to suggest that he has broken his clavicle. Feel carefully, and you will find an area of tenderness but no swelling. The fracture may be greenstick and difficult to see on an X-ray. Sometimes there is a swelling without any history of injury.

If an adult breaks the middle third of his clavicle, his sternomastoid muscle pulls the medial fragment up, while the weight of his arm pulls the lateral one down. Often there is a third middle fragment. If the fracture is lateral to his coraco–clavicular ligament, the medial end of his clavicle is little displaced, because these ligaments hold it. If it breaks medially to the ligaments, its outer end may appear to be displaced backwards and upwards, so that it forms a lump under his skin. Without an X-ray these fractures are difficult to distinguish from subluxation of the acromio–clavicular joint.

Treat all fractures of the clavicle with a sling and active movements, as in Section 71.2.

The clavicle almost always unites with no loss of function, and although the patient has a lump, this will disappear in a child and usually does so in an adult. If it is unslightly, it can be removed.

71.5 Dislocations of the sterno–clavicular joint

The clavicle can dislocate anteriorly or posteriorly.

An anterior dislocation makes a patient's sterno–clavicular joint swollen and tender. This distinguishes it from a fracture of the medial end of his clavicle, where tenderness is immediately lateral to the joint. Reduction is usually unnecessary, so encourage him to use his arm (71.1). It will be weak for some months, but movement will in time become full and painless.

A posterior dislocation is rare and is usually combined with a chest injury, in which several of the patient's ribs may be broken at the same time. The dislocated end of his clavicle obstructs his superior mediastinum and causes severe pain, a tight feeling in his throat, difficult swallowing, and fullness of the veins of his neck.

Try closed reduction first. Place a sandbag between his scapulae, and press his shoulders back. If this fails, refer him.

71.6 Dislocation of the acromio–clavicular joint

There are two varieties of this injury, depending on whether the ligaments joining the patient's clavicle to his scapula are partly or completely torn.

If only the ligaments between a patient's clavicle and his acromion are torn, those joining his clavicle to his coracoid can prevent severe displacement. His clavicle is stable and you cannot move it backwards or forwards. If you want to see whether the gap between his acromion and his clavicle is greater than normal, compare it with an X-ray of the other side.

If all the ligaments joining his clavicle to his scapula are torn, the weight of his arm pulls his shoulder downwards, while his sternomastoid muscle pulls his clavicle upwards, as in A, Fig. 71-3. The joint is so wildly unstable that the lateral end of his clavicle rides free, high above his acromion, and you can easily move it backwards and forwards. X-ray him standing, and holding a 2 kg weight to distract his acromio–clavicular joint, because the dislocation may reduce itself spontaneously when he is lying down.

Treat a mild dislocation with a sling and active movements (71.2) until pain subsides. If a patient has a major dislocation, stick pads to his acromion and his elbow, and reduce his dislocation by binding them together with adhesive strapping; then put his arm in a sling, as in B, Fig. 71-3. Don't refer these injuries for surgical repair.

71.7 Fractures of the scapula

The scapula can break in several ways. Direct blows occasionally break it into several pieces. Its coracoid process can fracture, either with no displacement, or with downward displacement. Its neck can fracture, so that its glenoid articulation breaks off and is displaced. This is the most common scapula injury, and provided it does not involve the joint surface, it needs only symptomatic treatment. The acromion may fracture with only a crack, or with severe communition and displacement.

These fractures cause much pain and bleeding and are difficult to diagnose without sophisticated X-rays. A patient's clavicle, his ribs, or his spine may be broken at the same time.

The scapula is splinted on both sides by muscle, so treatment is easy. Give him a sling and encourage him to move his shoulder, elbow, and fingers actively and early.

71.8 Anterior dislocation of the shoulder

Dislocation is the most common shoulder injury. It is usually anterior and only occasionally posterior. In an anterior dislocation the head of a patient's humerus passes forwards and

DISLOCATION OF THE ACROMIOCLAVICULAR JOINT

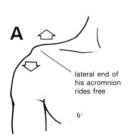
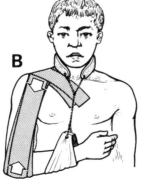

A

lateral end of his acromnion rides free

B

Fig. 71-3 DISLOCATION OF THE ACROMIO–CLAVICULAR JOINT. A, shows the characteristic deformity of the shoulder. B, shows the method of strapping it.

ANTERIOR DISLOCATION OF THE SHOULDER

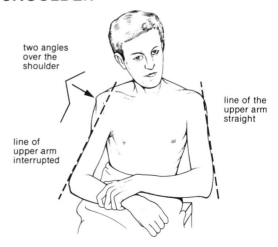

two angles over the shoulder

line of upper arm interrupted

line of the upper arm straight

Fig. 71-4 AN ANTERIOR DISLOCATION OF THE SHOULDER. Note the characteristic profile of the patient's shoulder.

ANTERIOR DISLOCATION OF THE SHOULDER

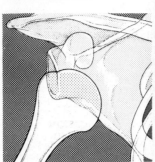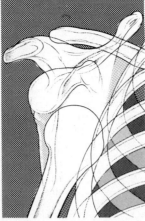

Fig. 71-5 THE X-RAY APPEARANCES of an anterior dislocation of the shoulder. Always take an AP and an oblique view before you try to reduce what might seem to be an ordinary dislocation. If you take an oblique view routinely, you will not miss a rare posterior dislocation. A quarter of all acute dislocations are associated with a fracture, most commonly a fracture of the greater tuberosity.

downwards to lie in front of his scapula. In the common subcoracoid variety, the normal outline of his shoulder is broken by the two sharp angles shown in Fig. 71-4. He is in great pain.

This dislocation is often missed because nobody examines the patient for loss of movement, which is the critical sign. Typically, he holds his elbow fixed away from his side, and he cannot make it touch his chest. His injured arm looks longer than his normal one, his shoulder joint is fixed, his elbow is flexed, and his forearm is internally rotated. Although you can make his scapula move over his chest, you cannot make his humerus move on his scapula. If his shoulder is not too swollen, you may be able to feel the displaced head of his humerus below his coracoid process.

The main differential diagnoses of an anterior dislocation are: (1) a fracture of the neck of the humerus, and (2) a fracture dislocation. Both are much less common than a simple dislocation. The treatment for these injuries differs. If you treat either of the latter two injuries as if it were a simple dislocation, the results can be disastrous, so always take an AP and an oblique view before you try to reduce what might seem to be an ordinary dislocation. If you take an oblique view routinely, you will not miss a rare posterior dislocation (71.9). An oblique view is more difficult to take than a true lateral view but is easier to interpret.

Three signs will help you in the differential diagnosis: (1) Can you make the patient's elbow touch his side? (2) Will his humerus move on his scapula? If one or both these signs are present, he may have fractured the neck of his humerus, or he may have a fracture dislocation. (3) Much swelling also makes a simple dislocation unlikely.

We have not described Kocher's method for reducing a dislocated shoulder. If you use it and are inexperienced, you may fracture the neck of a patient's humerus.

LACK OF SHOULDER MOVEMENT AND AN ABNORMAL CONTOUR ARE THE CRITICAL SIGNS OF A DISLOCATED SHOULDER

ANTERIOR SHOULDER DISLOCATION

Reduce the patient's dislocation immediately. If his injury is recent, reduction is usually easy.

INDICATIONS Anterior dislocations less than 3 weeks old. If the dislocation is older than this, see below.

TWO METHODS FOR A DISLOCATED SHOULDER

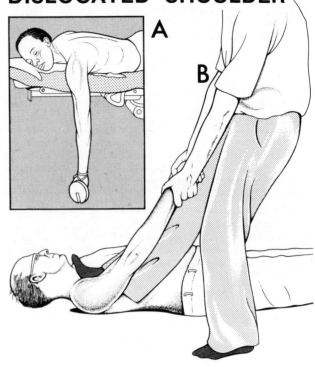

Fig. 71-6 TWO METHODS FOR REDUCING A DISLOCATED SHOULDER. A, the arm swinging method, and B, the Hippocratic method. The editor is on the floor; the sock belongs to Peter Bewes! *A, kindly contributed by Gerald Hankins.*

Have you X-rayed him to make sure your diagnosis is correct? Check his axillary nerve (Fig. 55-6), and his radial pulse.

ANAESTHESIA If the patient's injury is recent, he may not need an anaesthetic. Good relaxation is required if it is more than a few hours old, or if he is very muscular. (1) General anaesthesia with a muscle relaxant. (2) Ketamine and diazepam (A 8.2). (3) Intravenous pethidine with diazepam (A 8.8).

THE ARM SWINGING METHOD FOR A RECENT ANTERIOR DISLOCATION

Try this first, especially if the patient's dislocation is very recent, using pethidine, preferably with diazepam.

Lie him on a table, face downwards, with his arm over its edge.

Ask him to relax his arm as much as he can. If the table is high enough, tie a 2 kg weight to his wrist. Dead weight traction of this kind is often more successful than manual traction, because it is easier for him to relax. Leave him alone for a while. When you return you may find the dislocation reduced.

If it is not reduced, bend his elbow and move his arm in all directions. At the same time pull on his arm. His shoulder will usually go back into its socket with a sudden spontaneous click.

THE HIPPOCRATIC METHOD FOR A RECENT ANTERIOR DISLOCATION

METHOD Lie the patient on the floor. If he has dislocated his right shoulder, remove your shoe and put your right foot in his axilla, lean backwards, and pull on his abducted arm. If you are agile, you can also use this method while he is on a table, by raising your foot and placing it in his axilla.

Pull gently and steadily for 5 minutes.

CAUTION ! Don't exert excessive force. You may injure his brachial plexus.

SHOULDER EXERCISES

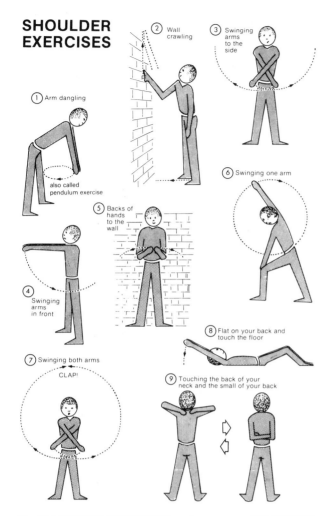

① Arm dangling

also called pendulum exercise

② Wall crawling

③ Swinging arms to the side

④ Swinging arms in front

⑤ Backs of hands to the wall

⑥ Swinging one arm

⑦ Swinging both arms CLAP!

⑧ Flat on your back and touch the floor

⑨ Touching the back of your neck and the small of your back

Fig. 71-7 SHOULDER EXERCISES are in two groups. EARLY EXER-CISES should be done smoothly and rhythmically with gradually increasing amplitude. Here are the instructions to a patient. (1) Stoop forwards and circle your arm ('arm dangling'). (2) Put your arm against a wall. With your arm straight, move steadily closer to it ('wall crawl-ing'). (3) Stand astride with your arms crossed and swing them sideways and upwards. (4) Stand astride and swing your arms forwards and upwards. (5) Lean against a wall with your arms bent, turn your arms to touch the backs of your hands against the wall. LATE EXERCISES should be done more vigorously. (6) Put one leg in front of the other, put your hand on your knee, and swing your arm. (7) Stand astride with your arms crossed, swing your arms sideways and upwards, and clap them above your head. (8) Lie on your back with your arm stret-ched and press downwards to touch the floor. (9) Stand astride; alter-nately touch the back of your neck and fold your hands behind your back. *Kindly contributed by Michael Wood.*

If this does not reduce the dislocation, ask an assistant to exert traction as above. While he does so, press the head of the patient's humerus backwards with both your thumbs in the direction of its socket. Or, grasp his arm with both hands and pull laterally.

If you fail and are not using general anaesthesia, try again using it and a relaxant.

POSTOPERATIVE CARE (both methods) As soon as the patient is awake ask him to abduct his arm gently. Check that you have not injured his axillary or musculocutaneous nerves during reduction. Examine him to make sure that you have reduced his dislocation, and check with an X-ray.

Put his arm in a sling for 3 weeks, and start pendulum exer-cises in the sling immediately. Then start most of the other early exercises in Fig. 71-7. Avoid abduction and external rota-tion exercises, because they are dangerous and may redislocate his shoulder.

DIFFICULTIES WITH DISLOCATED SHOULDERS

If you suspect that a patient has a dislocation but you have NO X-RAYS, anaesthetize him and move his shoulder gently. A dislocation may reduce spontaneously, and you are unlikely to harm him.

If PART OF HIS GREATER TUBEROSITY HAS BROKEN OFF, it will probably return to its bed as you reduce his disloca-tion. If it does so, well and good. But if it fails to do so, and prevents him abducting his arm, try the methods in Section 71.10. *A quarter of all acute dislocations are associated with a fracture, most commonly a fracture of the greater tuberosity.* You can easily see this in routine X-ray views of a patient's shoulder. The external rotator muscles of his shoulder pull a piece of bone away from the head of his humerus as his shoulder dislocates.

If you FAIL TO REDUCE HIS DISLOCATION under diazepam or ketamine, try general anaesthesia with a relax-ant. This usually succeeds. If it fails don't try again using more force. Instead, refer him for open reduction.

If his DISLOCATION RECURS after 6 weeks, it will probably continue to do so, so refer him for an operative repair. A dislocated shoulder is usually stable after you have reduced it. But, if it dislocated after only a very minor injury, it pro-bably did so because the labrum separated from the glenoid ring. Adult cartilage does not usually unite with bone, so his shoulder may continue to dislocate with increasing ease. Finally, it may dislocate even when he sneezes or turns over in bed.

If the HEAD OF HIS HUMERUS DROPS OUT OF HIS GLENOID because his axillary nerve has been paralysed, sup-port his arm in a sling for several months until his nerve recovers. Tighten the sling regularly so as to keep the con-tour of his shoulder normal, and show his spouse how to do the same. This is not the same condition as recurrent disloca-tion of the shoulder. Suspect it when a patient is anaesthesic over his deltoid, and is totally unable to abduct his arm.

If his SHOULDER REMAINS STIFF after a dislocation, explain that movements will eventually return. Active exer-cises are safer and more effective than passive ones. Avoid excessive force, because this will only make the stiffness worse. His shoulder is more likely to become stiff if he fails to move it early.

If a patient's BRACHIAL PLEXUS IS INJURED, it will pro-bably recover in a year. Meanwhile, put his shoulder through a safe range of movements to prevent contractures. Some nerve injury is common after a dislocation, and may involve any of the three cords of his brachial plexus. His axillary and musculocutaneous nerves are commonly involved. Sometimes his whole brachial plexus is torn from his spinal cord, paralysis is permanent, and his useless aneasthetic arm has to be amputated (71.3).

If his AXILLA RAPIDLY SWELLS after a shoulder injury, his axillary artery has been torn. This is a very rare disaster in an old patient with hard arteries, and may follow a frac-ture dislocation. It is more likely to occur if you are trying to reduce a fracture dislocation, particularly an old one, or if you use greater force than the original injury. The patient's torn artery bleeds and forms a large arterial haematoma (55.5) round his shoulder. Suspect this disaster if a rapidly increas-ing swelling in a patient's axilla follows a shoulder injury. If you don't diagnose a torn axillary artery, and it is not repaired (55.6), he may bleed to death. Tying it is a desperate opera-tion, but you will not have time to refer him. Firm axillary pressure may stop the bleeding, so try it. If this fails, you may have to clamp or tie his subclavian artery (3.4).

If the CIRCULATION IN HIS ARM IS POOR before his dislocation is reduced, reduce it gently. If this does not restore his circulation, his axillary vessels should be explored and his axillary artery repaired, if necessary. So, refer this rare com-plication quickly.

If a patient with a DISLOCATED SHOULDER PRESENTS LATE (more than 3 weeks after the dislocation), refer him. A difficult open operation may be justified, especially if pressure on the structures in his axilla causes symptoms, but the results may be poor. If you cannot refer him, movement bet-ween his scapula and his chest may give him a useful range of painless movement. Ask him to do active exercises, so that he can preserve as much movement as possible in his other joints.

Reduction becomes increasingly difficult and dangerous as time passes. Initially, every hour is important, and after 6 weeks reduction may be impossible. Using force may break the neck of a patient's humerus, or tear his axillary vessels or nerves.

A PATIENT WHO CANNOT MOVE HIS SHOULDER AFTER AN INJURY HAS A DISLOCATION UNTIL PROVED OTHERWISE
REDUCE ALL DISLOCATIONS *IMMEDIATELY*

POSTERIOR DISLOCATION

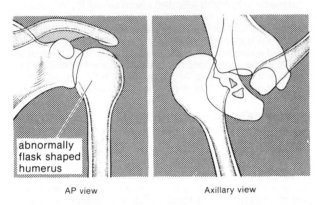

abnormally flask shaped humerus

AP view   Axillary view

Fig. 71-8 POSTERIOR DISLOCATIONS OF THE SHOULDER are often missed because the AP view looks almost normal. The closeness of the head to the film does however make it look abnormally small. The head also looks flask shaped. You will not miss a posterior dislocation if you always take an oblique or a lateral view whenever you X-ray an injured shoulder. An axillary view (if you can move the patient's arm far enough from his side to get the tube into his axilla) shows the dislocation best.

71.9 Posterior dislocation of the shoulder (rare)

If a patient has pain, swelling, and reduced movement after a shoulder injury, together with an apparently normal AP X-ray, suspect that he has a posterior dislocation. Typically, he cannot move his arm, which is locked in adduction and internal rotation. The outline of his shoulder is abnormal, but not as abnormal as in an anterior dislocation. His coracoid process is prominent, and in late cases he has a characteristic dimple on the front of his shoulder. *Looked at from above, his shoulder bulges posteriorly. Also, you may be able to feel the head of his humerus posteriorly under the spine of his scapula.* His shoulder movements are poor and his humerus feels as if it is fixed to his scapula. You will probably be able to reduce his dislocation without too much difficulty.

POSTERIOR DISLOCATION OF THE SHOULDER

Give the patient a general anaesthetic. Try to put his shoulder through a normal range of movements, while pulling upwards on his humerus, with his arm above his head, and his elbow flexed to relax his biceps tendon. The dislocation will usually reduce promptly.

If this fails, try the alternative method in Fig. 71-9. If this also fails, refer him.

If reduction is successful, put his arm in a sling for 3 weeks and encourage him to move it as soon as he can.

AN ALTERNATIVE METHOD FOR A POSTERIOR DISLOCATION

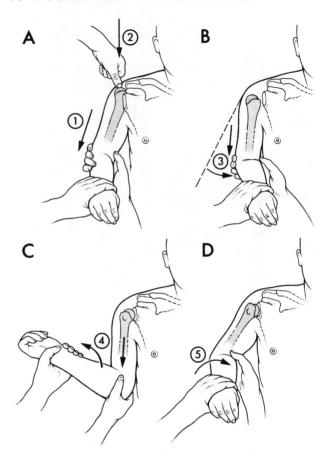

Fig. 71-9 AN ALTERNATIVE METHOD FOR REDUCING A POSTERIOR DISLOCATION. Flex the patient's elbow, and exert traction in the long axis of his arm (1). Ask an assistant to press downwards on the head of his humerus with his thumb (2). Adduct his arm while still maintaining traction (3). When the head reaches the glenoid cavity, rotate his arm externally (4), then gently rotate it internally (5). His axillary nerve may be injured, so support his arm in a sling to prevent his humerus dropping out of his glenoid. *After de Palma, with kind permission.*

DIFFICULTIES WITH A POSTERIOR DISLOCATION OF THE SHOULDER

If the patient's DISLOCATION IS OLD, reduction may be possible, so refer him. If this is impractical, ignore the dislocation, and concentrate on active movements and exercises. Occasionally, an arthrodesis is necessary for severe and persistent pain. Posterior dislocations are often overlooked in early stages, so they are often diagnosed too late.

POSTERIOR DISLOCATIONS OF THE SHOULDER ARE OFTEN MISSED

71.10 Fracture of the greater tuberosity

The greater tuberosity of a patient's humerus can be fractured by a direct blow, or it can be torn off when he dislocates it. Treatment depends on how far displaced the fragment is.

FRACTURE OF THE GREATER TUBEROSITY

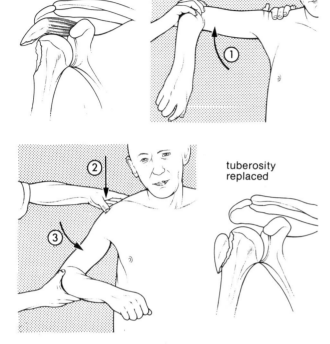

tuberosity detached

tuberosity replaced

Fig. 71-10 FRACTURE OF THE GREATER TUBEROSITY. Infiltrate the fracture site with local anaesthetic. Abduct the patient's arm (1), and press firmly on the fragment with your thumb (2), continue to press on the fragment while you lower his arm (3), so that it stays in place while you do so. *After de Palma, with kind permission.*

FRACTURES OF THE GREATER TUBEROSITY

MINIMAL DISPLACEMENT Begin active shoulder, elbow, and finger movements immediately. If necessary give the patient a sling for a few days.

MORE THAN MINIMAL DISPLACEMENT Try the following methods in this order, until you find one which works.

First try abducting the patient's arm. This will cause the fragment to press against the under-side of his acromion and may push it into place. If this fails try the method in Fig. 71-10.

If reduction is successful, put his arm in a sling and encourage active movements.

If reduction fails, repeat it again 2 weeks later, when the fragment will have become 'sticky'. If this too fails, and abduction is severely limited, refer him for operative treatment. Meanwhile encourage active movements, as above.

71.11 Fractures of the neck of the humerus

The surgical neck of the humerus is the region between the tuberosities, and the insertions of the pectoralis and teres major. When it breaks the soft tissues hold the fragments together very satisfactorily, and provided there is some contact between them, they always unite. There is such a wide range of movement in the shoulder joint that the exact position of the fragments is unimportant. Even if the joint surfaces do not fit together perfectly, good function is still possible, *but only if the patient starts to move his shoulder early.* Most of these fractures need not be reduced. The only ones which you should reduce are those in which there is no contact between the broken surface of the

FRACTURE OF THE NECK OF THE HUMERUS

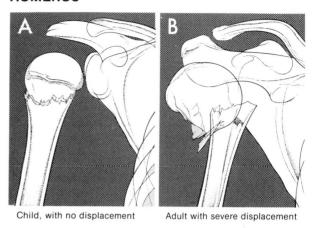

Child, with no displacement   Adult with severe displacement

Fig. 71-11 FRACTURES OF THE NECK OF THE HUMERUS. A, is an incomplete fracture in a child. B, shows considerable displacement of the shaft. There is such a wide range of movement in the shoulder joint that the exact position of the fragments is unimportant.

neck and the shaft. Fractures of the surgical neck are common in children, and are not common again until middle age.

71.12 Fractures of the neck of the humerus in adults

The patient, who is typically an older woman, falls on her outstretched arm and injures her shoulder. Her osteoporotic humerus breaks across its neck. Sometimes, its head is comminuted. In spite of her pain, she may be able to use her swollen, tender shoulder, so the diagnosis is often missed. Soon, she has severe bruising extending to her elbow. If the head of her humerus is impacted on the shaft, the fracture is more likely to heal with reasonable function. These fractures are less common in young adults, but when they do occur, they usually heal well.

FRACTURES OF THE NECK OF HUMERUS IN AN ADULT

Check the patient's axillary nerve (55.8) and his radial pulse.

REDUCING A FRACTURE OF THE NECK OF THE HUMERUS

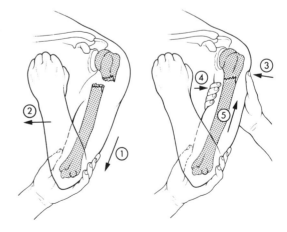

Fig. 71-12 REDUCING A FRACTURE OF THE NECK OF THE HUMERUS with wide separation or severe angulation. *After de Palma, with kind permission*

X-RAYS Take two X-rays at right angles. The fragments may be widely separated, but overlie one another in a single view.

Is the fracture impacted? If you can move the patient's arm through a reasonable range without causing severe pain, it is impacted.

IMPACTED FRACTURES OF THE HUMERAL NECK IN AN ADULT

Begin active and assisted shoulder movements immediately. Between these exercises, put the patient's arm in a sling for 4 to 6 weeks. Make sure that it supports his elbow, and so prevents disimpaction. He must not lift heavy objects for 3 months.

UNIMPACTED FRACTURES OF THE HUMERAL NECK IN AN ADULT

Treatment depends on how widely separated the fragments are.

THERE IS NO SEPARATION AND ONLY MILD ANGULATION (1) The broken surfaces of the fragments are in contact. And, (2) angulation between the head and the neck is less than 90°.

Shoulder exercises are too painful to begin immediately. So put the patient's arm in a sling and give him an analgesic. If pain is unbearable, bandage it to his chest. Begin elbow, wrist, and finger movements. Wait for 3 weeks before starting active shoulder exercises.

THERE IS WIDE SEPARATION OR SEVERE ANGULATION (1) There is no contact between the broken surfaces of the fragments. Or, (2) there is angular deformity of more than 90°.

Get good muscle relaxation with a general anaesthetic. Flex the patient's elbow and pull on the humerus as in Fig. 71-12 (1).

While still pulling, adduct his elbow across his chest and flex it in the frontal plane of his body. (2) The combination of these movements will restore the length of his humerus.

Place your other hand in his axilla. Press on the head with your thumb (3), and pull the shaft outwards (4). After the fragments are aligned, release traction gradually, so that the fragments engage (5).

If the fracture is stable after reduction, put his arm in a collar and cuff. Keep it to his side for 3 weeks, then gradually begin progressive movements as pain lessens, starting with pendulum exercises and continuing with wall crawling exercises (Fig. 71-7).

If the fracture is unstable after reduction, put him in forearm traction as in Fig. 72-11 for 2 weeks, then give him a sling and arm dangling excercises.

IF THERE IS SO MUCH SEPARATION THAT THE SHAFT OF THE PATIENT'S HUMERUS IS IN HIS AXILLA, laceration of his axillary artery is the danger, so check his pulse at his wrist before you try to reduce his fracture.

If his pulse is obliterated, bind his arm to his side and refer him. If you cannot refer him, take him to the theatre, and be prepared to tie his subclavian artery above his clavicle (3.4). As you do the reduction, you may pull a spicule of bone out of his axillary artery and cause massive bleeding.

CONSCIENTIOUS EXERCISES WILL OFTEN RESTORE MOVEMENTS TO A STIFF SHOULDER

71.14 Fractures of the neck of the humerus in children

Some children with a fracture of the neck of the humerus are in great pain and are quite unable to move their arms; others have little pain and a surprising range of shoulder movement. If a child is in pain, don't try to examine his shoulder—X-ray it. Take two views to determine the position of the fragments.

In young children the fracture is transverse and is about 2 cm below the epiphyseal line. When the fracture is complete,

the shaft rides up in front of the upper fragment, and overlaps it. In an older child the fracture line passes through the epiphyseal line, so that the epiphysis separates. Sometimes, the fragments bow outwards, but do not separate, or they may separate so that the end of the shaft lies under the skin.

FRACTURES OF THE NECK OF THE HUMERUS IN CHILDREN
Check the child's radial pulse and his axillary nerve (55.8). Treat incomplete and complete fractures in the same way.

If the fragments are not widely separated, put his arm in a sling and encourage him to move it.

If the fragments are widely separated, try to get them to hitch, as described above for widely separated unimpacted fractures in adults (71.12).

If you fail to get the fragments to hitch, put him in traction for 2 weeks, as in Fig. 72-11.

DIFFICULTIES WITH FRACTURES OF THE NECK OF THE HUMERUS IN CHILDREN

If the SHARP END OF THE DISTAL FRAGMENT HAS POKED THROUGH THE CHILD'S SHOULDER MUSCLES, and you can feel it under his skin, anaesthetize him and manipulate the broken end of his humerus back through his muscles. Use a combination of pulling and twisting movements, and get it to hitch with the proximal fragment. Sometimes the distal fragment goes right through the skin.

If you CANNOT MAINTAIN REDUCTION with his arm in a sling, apply skin traction, using overhead suspension (Fig. 72-11), a pulley, and enough weight to keep his arm raised—2 kg will probably be about right. Don't tie his arm to a pole, because if he sits up, reduction is lost. Continue traction for 2 weeks until the fragments are sticky. Then put his arm in a sling and start pendulum exercises (Fig. 7-7).

REDUCING A FRACTURE DISLOCATION

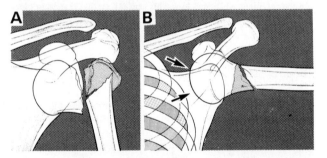

Fig. 71-13 REDUCING A FRACTURE DISLOCATION OF THE NECK OF THE HUMERUS. A, before reduction. B, during reduction. The arrows show where to push with your thumbs to return the head of the patient's humerus back into his glenoid.

71.15 Dislocation of the shoulder with fracture of the neck of the humerus

This is a serious injury, usually of older people. The neck of the patient's humerus breaks, either at the time of the accident, or while a simple dislocation is being reduced with excessive force. The head of his humerus lies in front of his glenoid, or it may be displaced into his axilla. His axillary vessels and his brachial plexus are sometimes injured at the same time.

FRACTURE DISLOCATION OF THE HEAD OF THE HUMERUS

If possible refer the patient, particularly if he is a child, because the results of operating are better in children.

If this is not possible, give the patient a general anaesthetic and proceed as follows. Good relaxation is essential.

REDUCTION Try the following methods in turn, until you find one which works.

(1) Try the arm swinging method for a dislocated shoulder (71.8). Combine this with gently trying to push the head back into place with your thumbs.

(2) Try the Hippocratic method with a foot in the patient's axilla (71.8).

(3) Ask an assistant to pull the patient's arm into abduction, as in Fig. 71-13. As he does so, use both your thumbs to press the head of his humerus towards its socket.

If possible, X-ray his shoulder to check reduction while he is still anaesthetized.

If you can reduce the head, treat him as if he had an uncomplicated fracture of the neck of his humerus (71.12).

If you cannot reduce the head the first time, try only once more. If you fail again, and cannot refer him, accept the position and start 'pendulum' exercises immediately (Fig. 69-11). Later, attempt wall 'crawling exercises' (Fig. 71-7). Function will not be perfect, and he will not be able to raise his arm above his head, but he will be able to use it at waist level without pain.

71.16 Displacement of the upper humeral epiphysis

In children between 5 and 15 years the head of the humerus sometimes becomes detached from the shaft, and may take a piece of the shaft with it. The head of the humerus is very mobile, so reduction can be difficult. Perfect reduction is not necessary because the head readily remodels. Anaesthetize the child, reduce the displacement by abducting his arm. Maintain traction in bed for 2 weeks as in Fig. 72-11. Then protect it in a sling for another week.

IF AN ADULT INJURES HIS SHOULDER, EXERCISE HIS ELBOW AND FINGERS FROM THE BEGINNING

FRACTURES OF THE HUMERUS

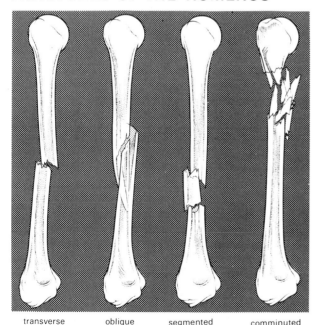

transverse   oblique   segmented   comminuted

Fig. 71-14 FRACTURES OF THE SHAFT OF THE HUMERUS. Put the patient's arm into a narrow sling, so that half the weight of his forearm acts on the lower fragment to reduce the overlap and the angulation. All these fractures can be treated in the same way.

71.17 Fractures of the shaft of the humerus

Babies A baby's humerus is often fractured during a difficult delivery, or in a non–accidental injury. It heals rapidly with massive callus formation and needs no treatment. Bind his arm loosely to his chest wall for a week to prevent further injury. At the end of a year there will be no trace of the fracture.

Adults Fractures of the shaft of the humerus are not common again until adult life. They are of many kinds, but you can treat them all in the same way. If you do this properly, they cause no problems. Union is the first priority, then elbow movement. Moderate angulation is no disability.

Put the patient's arm in a narrow sling, as in C, and E, Fig. 71-15, so that half the weight of his forearm acts on the lower fragment to reduce overlap and angulation. Put his arm across his chest to correct rotation. The muscles attached to his humerus will hold the fragments in place. Overlap and shortening are unimportant. In young children they are even desirable. There are no indications for internal fixation unless the patient also has other injuries, or must be back at work quickly.

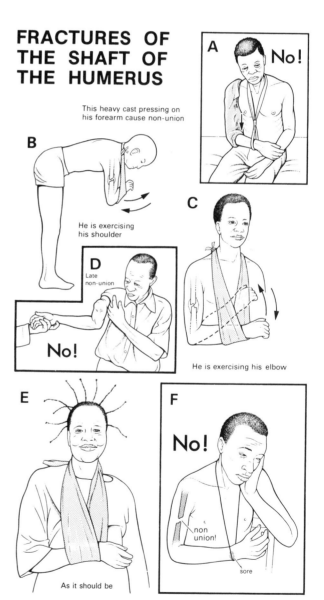

Fig. 71-15 TREATING A FRACTURE OF THE SHAFT OF THE HUMERUS. A, how it should not be done. This heavy cast will press on the patient's forearm and distract the bone ends. **B,** a properly treated patient exercising his shoulder. **C,** the same patient exercising his elbow. **D,** non–union after a fracture 30 years before. This patient had surprisingly little disability. **E,** success. **F,** failure. *Kindly contributed by Peter Bewes.*

Some surgeons (including ourselves) treat these fractures without a splint, and argue that a little movement is a good thing in fractures of the shaft of the humerus because it promotes union; others splint them to reduce pain, and protect the patient's arm in case he should fall. The ideal splint is a stiff, light cuff with 'Velcro' fastenings, which will allow active shoulder and elbow movement. Failing this, you can apply a *light* U–slab, or you can use strips of bamboo as described below. If you use a plaster splint, it must be a *light* one, or its weight will distract the fragments and cause non–union. The traditional splint in Fig. 56-1 is admirable.

FRACTURES OF THE SHAFT OF THE HUMERUS

INDICATIONS If the patient is ambulant, use this method for all fractures of the mid–shaft of the humerus, whether they are spiral, oblique, transverse, or comminuted.

CONTRAINDICATIONS If the patient is unable to sit or stand because of other injuries, treat him in traction as described later.

X-RAYS are not essential, unless there are signs which suggest that the patient's shoulder may be dislocated also, or unless the fracture is so low in the shaft as to be supracondylar (72.11).

TREATMENT FOR FRACTURES OF THE SHAFT OF THE HUMERUS

Before starting, check the patient's peripheral pulses, and test the function of his radial nerve *and record it (Fig. 75-3)*. Can he dorsiflex his wrist or extend his fingers? If his radial nerve is injured and fails to recover, he will not be able to blame your treatment.

If the fracture is grossly angulated, reduce it under anaesthesia. Manipulate him carefully. His radial nerve is close to the fracture site. You can use local anaesthesia of the fracture haematoma, provided you do it in a sterile manner (A 5.6). Alternatively, wait for the bone ends to become sticky in about 10 to 20 days and then manipulate them.

Make the patient a sling 10 cm wide which supports only the distal part of his forearm. It must not include his elbow, which must be at 90°. Make it by folding a triangular bandage several times, as in Fig. 71-15.

CAUTION ! The width of the sling is critical. Use a narrow wrist sling which supports only the distal half of the patient's forearm. Don't use: (1) an elbow sling which raises and supports his elbow, or (2) a collar and cuff, or (3) a bootlace or piece of bandage. If his elbow is supported in a full sling, the weight of his forearm cannot reduce the overlap. A collar and cuff will draw the lower fragment forwards and angulate the fracture. A bootlace or a single turn of bandage will be acutely uncomfortable.

If you decide to splint the patient's arm: (1) Ideally use a plastic splint with 'Velcro' fastenings. Or, (2) pad his arm well with cotton wool, place some strips of bamboo (ideally sewn between two pieces of cloth) along it, and cover these with a crêpe bandage. Or, (3) apply a *light* U–slab.

CAUTION ! If you decide to put a U–slab on his arm (and you will usually be wise not to), it *must* be as thin and light as possible. Apply it during the first few days only. It is unnecessary later, and may distract fragments undesirably.

Tell the patient that he may hear and feel crepitus for the first week or two, but that this is a good sign. He may think he needs a splint. Reassure him that he does not.

If he is to avoid a stiff shoulder, he MUST exercise it. If he has a transverse fracture, the only safe exercises are the rhythmical pendulum exercises shown in A, Fig. 71-7 and B, Fig. 71-15. Show him how to bend forwards, and to move his arm in all directions from his shoulder.

Tell him to use his hand *actively,* and to flex and extend the muscles of his elbow a little inside the sling, as in C, Fig. 71-15. He must not take off his sling until there is clinical union, or the bone may angulate at the fracture site, and break again. Passive movements are unnecessary and potentially

dangerous. Supervise these exercises carefully, or the fracture may not unite. If he is 100% on your side and smiling (patient E), you have won. If he looks like patient F, expect failure.

CAUTION ! (1) Exercises must start within a day or two of the injury, or the fracture will be slow to unite. (2) If he has a transverse fracture, warn him that he must not abduct his arm at the shoulder or let his forearm hang by his side until his fracture is solidly united. He should wait for you to tell him that it is safe for him to do this. Extending his arm when his elbow is stiff will cause forward bowing and may fracture the callus, or cause delayed union or malunion.

If you wish to correct the position, do it at about 15 days when the bone ends are sticky. This is seldom necessary, because almost any position is acceptable.

Good callus usually forms in 4 weeks. Wait for signs of consolidation (Fig. 69-4). These are: (1) No tenderness over the fracture site. (2) Attempts to angulate the bone at the fracture site fail, and do not cause pain.

When, and only when, there are definite signs of clinical union, cautiously remove the sling for longer periods each day, until the patient has good elbow movements.

Consolidation usually takes 2 months in spiral fractures and 3 months in transverse ones; it normally takes twice as long as clinical union. So, if consolidation takes 6 weeks, the patient should continue to wear his sling for 12 weeks. If there is any danger of his humerus refracturing, as in a crowded bus, he must wear his sling, but he can take it off at other times.

CAUTION ! (1) A hanging cast, as in A, Fig. 71-15 is the most common cause of non–union. (2) Forced movements of his elbow may refracture his humerus. So, be careful!

DIFFICULTIES WITH FRACTURES OF THE SHAFT OF THE HUMERUS

If the patient's ARM IS PULSELESS AND COLD, reduce it and apply gentle traction. If this does not restore his circulation immediate exploration of his artery is indicated (55.3). Meanwhile keep his arm cold. If its circulation is not restored, his arm may need amputating.

If his SHOULDER OR ELBOW IS STIFF, he may complain about it long after his arm has healed. But, provided it has not been injured, his shoulder should not become stiff, if he does his dangling exercises properly. A stiff shoulder is a serious disability.

Loss of movement is less serious in the elbow, because people commonly use only a limited range of elbow movements.

If UNION IS DELAYED, or fails, assist it by encouraging him to contract his arm muscles vigorously, so that he can hear the bone ends grating! Unless there is vigorous muscular action, little callus will be formed, and union will be poor. Be patient if it is slow. Keep his arm in a sling and make him use the flexors and extensors of his elbow. These cross the fracture site and their action will encourage union.

Delayed union or non–union can be the result of: (1) Removing the sling too early, so causing posterior angulation of the fracture. (2) Using a sling which supports the elbow. (3) Other injures which confine the patient to bed, (4) Applying a heavy cast which distracts the fragments. (The more plaster you apply to these fractures, the less likely they are to unite.) (5) Unskilled internal fixation, as in Fig. 69-2. (6) Traction. (7) Soft tissue between the bone ends.

When non–union has occurred, if the patient is painfree, encourage him to accept the disability, as in D, Fig. 71-15 and continue his daily activities. If he cannot accept his pain and disability, consider referring him for internal fixation and a bone graft. This may fail, even in the best hands.

If he CANNOT DORSIFLEX HIS WRIST after a fracture of his humerus, he has injured his radial nerve. He can do this in various ways: (1) It can be bruised or stretched at the time of the injury and slowly recover. (2) It can be torn at the time of the injury and not recover. Or, (3) a radial nerve paralysis can develop during treatment, as the result of fibrosis and constriction of the radial nerve tunnel. Whatever the cause, he will probably recover. Refer him for exploration of his radial nerve if: (1) it shows no signs of recovery in 6 months, or (2) the paralysis develops some weeks after the injury.

Meanwhile, use a cock–up splint to support his wrist in dorsiflexion and prevent a contracture, as in Fig. 69-2. Sometimes passive exercises are enough. Ask him to extend his fingers several times a day with his other hand.

If he has FRACTURED THE SHAFT OF HIS HUMERUS AND DISLOCATED ITS HEAD, the dislocation will be almost impossible to reduce, because traction on his arm will not move the head of his humerus. So refer him rapidly for open reduction and internal fixation.

If he has fractured the shaft of his humerus and has OTHER INJURIES WHICH PREVENT HIM SITTING OR STANDING, you can treat his fracture in a sling as usual, if he can sit. If his other injuries prevent this, you will have to use traction instead.

Either apply skin traction, as in Fig. 71-16, or drill a Kirschner wire through the thick part of his olecranon, and hold it in a Gissane stirrup, as in Fig. 70-13. Pass a cord from the stirrup over the foot of his bed. Use skin traction to suspend his forearm with his elbow flexed at 90° and his humerus slightly abducted.

CAUTION ! Start with 2 kg in an adult, and check reduction with X-rays once or twice during the first week. Adjust the weight so as not to distract the fragments. As soon as he can sit up, change to the sling method of treatment.

Alternatively, **make a light plaster gaiter (Fig. 81-6)** round the shaft of his humerus, and encourage early active movements.

DON'T LET THE PATIENT TAKE HIS ARM OUT OF HIS SLING TOO SOON!
HEAVY CASTS ENCOURAGE NON–UNION

71.18 Fractures of the humerus, radius, and ulna

If a patient has broken his humerus, his radius, and his ulna, concentrate on his radius and ulna; his humerus will probably heal itself. Management depends on the type of humerus fracture he has.

MULTIPLE ARM FRACTURES

If a patient's humerus fracture is spiral, distraction is less of a problem and it will probably unite, so reduce his forearm fracture and apply a *thin* long arm cast with his elbow at 90° and his forearm in mid–pronation, so that if rotation is reduced subsequently, his hand will be in the best position. Support the cast in a sling so that its weight does not distract his humerus fracture.

If his humerus fracture is transverse, a long arm cast will probably cause serious distraction. So refer him for open reduction and internal fixation.

TRACTION FOR FRACTURES OF THE SHAFT OF THE HUMERUS

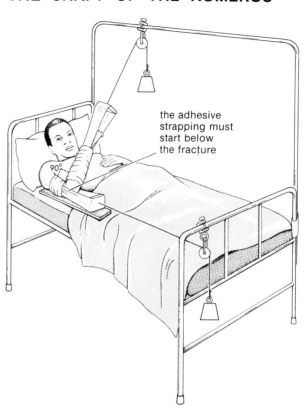

the adhesive strapping must start below the fracture

Fig. 71-16 TRACTION FOR FRACTURES OF THE SHAFT OF THE HUMERUS when a patient is confined to bed. Use skin traction to suspend his forearm with his elbow flexed to 90° and his humerus slightly abducted. *Kindly contributed by John Stewart.*

If referral is impossible, there are four things you can do: (1) You can risk applying a forearm cast, and support it well in the hope that it will not distract his humerus. (2) You can put a thin (not more than 4 mm) Steinmann pin through his olecranon (Fig. 70-13), and a Kirschner wire through his metacarpals (70.11). When you have done this, you can suspend his arm vertically with his forearm horizontal, supported by a stirrup. (3) You can apply traction, as in Fig. 71-16, but using metacarpal traction instead of skin traction. (4) You can splint his forearm fracture in a light cast in a position of function. Splint his humerus fracture with a light slab on its lateral side, held in place with a crêpe bandage. Finally, support his arm in a sling as in A, Fig. 71-1.

72 The elbow

72.1 Introduction

Injuries of the elbow fall into two groups—those of children and those of adults. A child seldom suffers from any of the adult fractures and vice versa. But dislocations can occur at any age. The penalty for mismanaging any of these injuries is likely to be a stiff painful elbow always.

The ligamentous injuries of the elbow include: (1) epicondylitis (tennis elbow) in adults, in which the attachment of the extensor muscles to the lateral condyle is strained, and (2) pulled elbow in children in which the head of the radius jams inside the annular ligament. In pulled elbow there is usually a history of a specific injury, but not in epicondylitis.

The signs in the list which follows should enable you to diagnose most injured elbows, even if you do not have X-rays. They are especially useful in children whose X-rays are difficult to interpret. You cannot remember all these signs, so consult the following section with the patient in front of you.

EXAMINING THE ELBOW

First, check the patient's median, ulnar, and radial nerves and his radial pulse, and record your findings (Fig. 75-3).

If his elbow is normal he can: (1) flex it by putting his hand on his shoulder, (2) extend it by holding his arm out straight, and (3) pronate and supinate it 90° in either direction, as in Fig. 69-1. Limitation of any movement suggests disease.

Is the contour of the posterior of his arm abnormal? If so, he may have a supracondylar fracture or a dislocation. If very little movement is possible, he has a dislocation, or supracondylar fracture, or a T–shaped fracture. If his elbow is fixed in 45° of flexion with almost no movement, he almost certainly has a dislocation.

Does the head of his radius move normally? Bend his elbow to 90°. If he can rotate his forearm, the head and neck of his radius are probably normal. Place your middle finger on his lateral epicondyle, and your index beside it over the head of his radius. Pronate and supinate his arm. If the head of his radius is intact, you can feel it moving under your index finger.

Can you feel the 3 bony points, as in A, in Fig. 72-2 Are they in their normal position in relation to the lower end of his humerus? If his elbow is severely swollen, you will not be able to feel them.

If the 3 bony points are displaced in relation to one another, he may have a dislocation. If his olecranon is displaced, has it moved medially or laterally in relation to an imaginary line down the back of his arm? You will need to know this when you come to reduce a supracondylar fracture or a dislocation.

If his 3 bony points are in their correct relation to one another, but are displaced in relation to the lower end of his humerus, as in D, Fig. 72-2, he may have a supracondylar fracture. *This is a critically important sign in very young children before much ossification has taken place in the lower end of the humerus so making the X-rays difficult to interpret.*

Where is the greatest tenderness? Just above the patient's elbow? (supracondylar fracture). On the medial side of his elbow? (fracture of the medial epicondyle). Over his lateral condyle and the outer part of his antecubital fossa? (fracture of the lateral condyle, or epicondylitis). Over the head of his radius? (fractured head of radius). If the tenderness is over his olecranon, can you feel a gap in it, or move it in relation to the shaft of his ulna? These are signs that it may be fractured.

Can you move the end of his humerus or its condyles on the shaft? Use your finger and thumb to feel the bony ridges running up from his medial and lateral epicondyles. Steady his arm with your other hand. Then very gently try to move the lower end of his humerus sideways, and backwards and forwards on the shaft. If it moves, he has a supracondylar fracture. This is painful, so only do it if it is absolutely necessary.

If his elbow is obviously broadened, can you move one condyle in relation to the other, perhaps with crepitus? (T–shaped fracture).

Can he extend his elbow as in Fig. 72-23? If he can, his extensor mechanism is intact.

Is there an effusion? You can rarely diagnose an effusion because of swelling of the soft tissues. Look at his elbow from the back. Are the normal hollows on either side of his olecranon obliterated or bulging? If they are, he has an effusion. You may be able to observe fluctuation between these swellings, or between them and the fullness on the anterior surface of his elbow. When compared with the other side, does his ulnar nerve feel abnormally superficial in its groove behind the medial epicondyle, or even displaced from it by the effusion?

SUMMARY OF THE MAJOR FEATURES IN ELBOW INJURIES

Dislocated elbow Any age. Contour abnormal. Severe swelling. Elbow fixed at 45°. The 3 bony points are not in their

THE AGE INCIDENCE OF INJURIES ROUND THE ELBOW

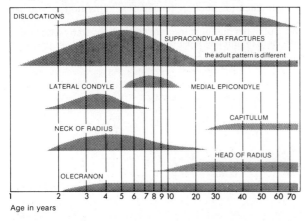

Fig. 72-1 INJURIES AROUND THE ELBOW have a characteristic age incidence. You will see dislocations at all ages. Supracondylar fractures are the most common elbow injuries with a modal age of about 7. They are much less common in adults, and when they do occur are more often T–shaped or comminuted. The medial epicondyle is injured in teenagers, and the lateral condyle in young children. Fracture of the capitulum is a rare adult injury. The neck of the radius fractures in children, and its head in adults.

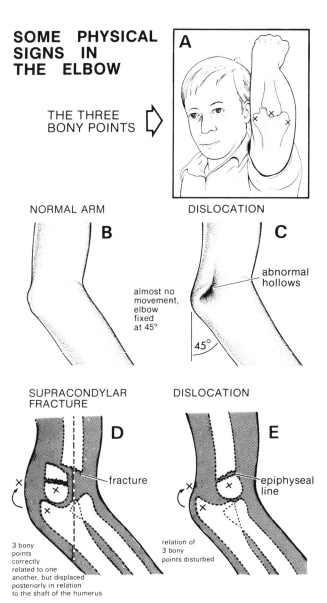

THE THREE
BONY POINTS ⇨

A

NORMAL ARM

B

DISLOCATION

C

abnormal
hollows

almost no
movement,
elbow
fixed
at 45°

45°

SUPRACONDYLAR
FRACTURE

D

fracture

3 bony
points
correctly
related to one
another, but displaced
posteriorly in relation
to the shaft of the humerus

DISLOCATION

E

epiphyseal
line

relation of
3 bony
points disturbed

Fig. 72-2 SOME PHYSICAL SIGNS IN THE ELBOW. A, the 3 bony points on the back of the elbow. B, and C, the contour of a normal arm and a dislocation compared. D, in a supracondylar fracture the 3 bony points are correctly related to one another, but are posteriorly displaced in relation to the shaft of the humerus. E, in a dislocation their normal relationship to one another is disturbed. *Kindly contributed by John Stewart.*

normal relation to one another. Olecranon displaced posterior to the epicondyles. Lower end of humerus not abnormally mobile, no crepitus. Distance between lateral epicondyle and radial styloid abnormal.

Supracondylar fracture Common in children. Contour abnormal. Severe swelling. Some movement possible. Olecranon not displaced above the epicondyles. The 3 bony points are in their correct places in relation to one another, but they lie posteriorly to the shaft of the humerus. Abnormal mobility of the lower humeral fragment with crepitus. Distance between lateral epicondyle and radial styloid normal.

T-shaped fracture Adults. Severe swelling. Contour abnormal. Condyles move in relation to one another. Some movements of the elbow still possible. Crepitus. Swelling obscures the 3 bony points.

Fractured medial epicondyle Older children and youths. Contour normal. Medial epicondyle tender and swollen. Some flexion and extension possible. Rotation normal.

Fractured lateral condyle Children. Contour normal. Lateral condyle tender and swollen.

Fractured capitulum Rare. Adults. Very little flexion or extension. Some rotation possible. The 3 bony points are normal. Tenderness difficult to localize.

Fractured neck of radius Common. Children under 4 years. Contour normal. Flexion and extension less painful than rotation. No rotation. The head of the radius may be tender.

Pulled elbow Young child. Contour normal. The child refuses to use his arm. No rotation.

Fractured head of radius Adults. Contour normal. Moderate swelling. Some flexion and extension possible but no rotation. The 3 bony points are normal. Head of the radius tender.

Fractured olecranon All ages. Contour normal. Moderate swelling. The olecranon is tender, and a gap may be palpable. There are two varieties of fracture depending on whether active extension is possible or not (72.18).

THE ELBOW OF
A CHILD OF 10.

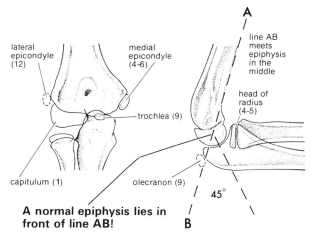

lateral
epicondyle
(12)

medial
epicondyle
(4-6)

trochlea (9)

capitulum (1)

olecranon (9)

A

line AB
meets
epiphysis
in the
middle

head of
radius
(4-5)

45°

B

A normal epiphysis lies in front of line AB!

Fig. 72-3 AN X-RAY OF THE ELBOW OF A CHILD OF 10 YEARS. Six centres of ossification can be seen in an AP view, but they are not always present at the same time. A large centre for the capitulum appears in the first year. A smaller one for the medial part of the trochlea appears at about 9 years. A centre for the medial epicondyle appears about the fifth year. It is entirely outside the capsule and unites with the shaft at 20. The lateral epicondyle starts to ossify at about 12. The centres for the capitulum, the trochlea, and the lateral condyle join one another and the shaft at puberty. A centre for the head of the radius appears in the fourth or fifth year, and unites with the shaft at puberty. There is also a centre of ossification for the olecranon, and another centre for the trochlea (not shown). These appear at about 9 years and unite at puberty.

In a lateral view, the shaft of the humerus and its lower epiphysis overlap one another and obscure most of the epiphyseal space, which is wider behind than it is in front. A normal epiphysis lies in front of the lower end of the shaft, so that a line AB drawn down the anterior border of the shaft, meets the epiphysis at its middle. A supracondylar fracture disturbs these relationships. *After Perkins with kind permission.*

72.2 X-rays of the elbow

Always X-ray an injured elbow. Ask for an AP and a lateral view. Minor fractures such as small chips off the capitulum are difficult to diagnose without an X-ray. In a severe elbow injury the medial epicondyle is easily detached, so it is the first thing to look for. The films of a child's injured elbow are not easy to interpret, so *X-ray his other elbow in the same position, and compare the two.* Also consult the diagrams inside the back cover, but remember that these apply to Caucasians, and that African epiphyses unite later. If you are still in doubt, X-ray the patient again in a week. The fracture, if there is one, will then be easier to see. Note that: (1) in children a mildly oblique X-ray can both resemble and disguise a dislocation, and (2) that the head of the radius and the medial and lateral epicondyles can be displaced before their centres of ossification appear. This makes diagnosis difficult.

If a child's injured elbow looks normal on X-ray, the three bony points are in their normal places, and diagnosis is difficult, consider pulled elbow (72.16). Some of these injuries are mild subluxations. Try gently manipulating the elbow under anaesthesia. You may feel a sudden click after which it moves normally.

IS THE MEDIAL EPICONDYLE OF AN INJURED ELBOW IN ITS NORMAL PLACE?

ASPIRATING THE ELBOW

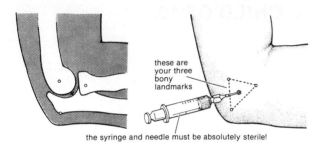

the syringe and needle must be absolutely sterile!

Fig. 72-4 ASPIRATING AN ELBOW JOINT. Use an absolutely sterile needle and feel for the bony landmarks.

72.3 Elevating and aspirating the elbow

An injured elbow rapidly swells, and makes reduction of a fracture difficult. As with the knee, aspirating the blood from a tensely distended elbow joint relieves pain, and allows the patient to move his elbow much earlier. Some surgeons consider this an an important part of the active movements treatment of comminuted supracondylar fractures in adults (72.11), and especially of fractures of the head of the radius (72.15). Other surgeons never aspirate an injured elbow.

If an elbow is dislocated reduce it immediately. If it is fractured and too swollen to reduce immediately, put the patient's arm up in forearm traction as in Fig. 72-11.

ASPIRATING THE ELBOW Clean the patient's skin carefully, paint it with iodine, and taking the most careful aseptic

DISLOCATION OF THE ELBOW

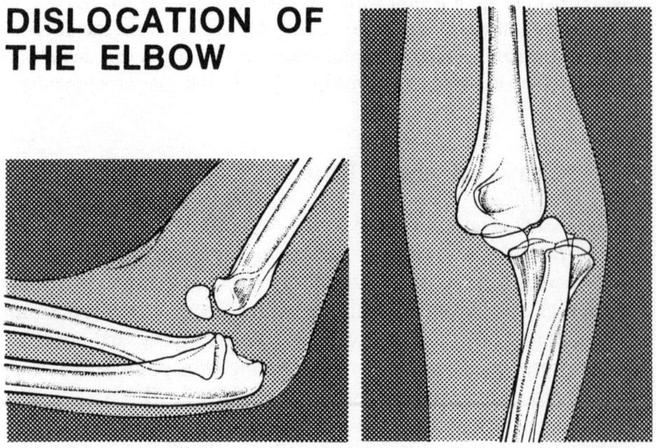

Fig. 72-5 AN X-RAY OF A DISLOCATED ELBOW. The sooner you reduce a dislocated elbow the easier this will be, and the fewer the complications.

precautions, aspirate at the summit of the swelling between the 3 bony points on the outer side of the elbow, as in Fig. 72-4.

CAUTION ! Don't put anything into the joint except the tip of a sterile aspirating needle.

72. 4 Dislocation of the elbow

A patient of any age can dislocate his elbow if he falls on his outstretched hand. In this common injury a force travels up his forearm and pushes his radius and ulna posteriorly, or his humerus posteriorly and laterally. He cannot move his elbow, and holds it at about 45°. The posterior outline of his arm, instead of being normally rounded, or showing a slight prominence over his olecranon, bends abruptly backwards as in C, Fig. 72-2. The three bony points of the elbow are not in their normal places. There may be other injuries also: (1) A child may fracture his medial epicondyle which may become trapped inside his dislocated elbow. (2) His lateral condyle may also fracture.

A patient may also have severe soft tissue injuries, and occasionally the circulation of his forearm is obstructed, with the danger of Volkmann's ischaemic contracture (70.4).

REDUCE A DISLOCATED ELBOW IMMEDIATELY

REDUCING A DISLOCATED ELBOW

The sooner you do this, the easier it will be, and the fewer the complications. If it is very recent, the alternative method described below may work.

Check the patient's radial pulse, and his median, ulnar, and radial nerves (Fig. 75-3).

ANAESTHESIA Good relaxation is essential in adults, but is less necessary in children. (1) General anaesthesia. (2) Give a child ketamine (A 8.2) or a general anaesthetic. (3) Axillary (A 6.18) or brachial plexus blocks are satisfactory if you do them well.

REDUCTION Lie the patient on his back with his upper arm vertical, and his forearm flexed across his chest, as in A, Fig. 72-6.

Find an assistant and ask him to exert traction on the patient's hand from the other side of the table (1), and at the same time, to flex the elbow gradually (2). While he does this, grasp the patient's elbow in both hands, with your fingers round the front of his humerus, and your thumbs behind his olecranon, then push it forwards (3).

The patient's olecranon should lie in the centre of his arm midway between his two epicondyles as in A, Fig. 72-2. If it is shifted sideways, first move it into the midline with your thumbs as you reduce it, then push it forwards over the lower end of the humerus. The dislocation will reduce with a scrunch.

When you think that you have succeeded, move the patient's elbow through its normal range. Unless you can get full flexion, you have not reduced it. If it feels stable, treat it as described below.

ALTERNATIVE METHOD If the dislocation is very recent, method B, in Fig. 72-6 may work without an anaesthetic.

Sit the patient sideways on a chair. Put a pillow over the top of the chair's back, and let his forearm hang over it.

Ask an assistant to exert traction on the patient's wrist, while at the same time you press on the back of his olecranon. Using the same movements described above, you may be able to coax his olecranon back into place.

Alternatively, and with experience, you may be able to caress his elbow and then suddeny flick it into place before he knows what has happened, and without using an anaesthetic.

X-RAYS Check: (1) that reduction is satisfactory, and (2) that there is no bony fragment trapped in the joint. If there is, it will have to be removed by opening the joint. If you are not able to do this, refer the patient.

CAUTION ! If you neglect to X-ray a patient after trying to reduce his dislocated elbow, you may fail to diagnose that reduction is incomplete, until after the swelling has gone. Reduction will then be possible only at open operation.

POSTOPERATIVE CARE FOR A DISLOCATED ELBOW

As soon as a patient recovers from the anaesthetic, re-examine his radial pulse, and his median, ulnar, and radial nerves to make sure that you have not injured them during reduction.

If reduction is stable, rest his arm in a sling for 3 weeks in the hope of avoiding post traumatic ossification. While it is in the sling he should move it as much as possible. Start shoulder, finger, and wrist exercises within the sling immediately. Don't let him take the sling off for 3 weeks. If there are no complications, his elbow will recover slowly, but he may always have some limitation of full extension.

CAUTION ! Never perform passive stretching exercises. These encourage post traumatic ossification.

If reduction is unstable, flex his elbow as far as it will go in a collar and cuff sling, or with a posterior slab, for 3 weeks. Then start active movements.

If reduction is very unstable in all directions: (1) there is a fracture, or (2) his medial epicondyle is trapped inside his elbow (see below), or (3) his ligaments are torn. Apply a temporary plaster backslab and refer him.

DIFFICULTIES WITH A DISLOCATED ELBOW

If the patient's dislocation occurred MORE THAN TWO WEEKS AGO, every day's delay will have made the prognosis worse. If the dislocation occurred less than 6 weeks ago, try to reduce it by manipulation. If it is already 2 weeks old, this will be difficult. If you fail, refer him for open reduction. An arthrodesis or elbow excision may be necessary.

REDUCING A DISLOCATED ELBOW

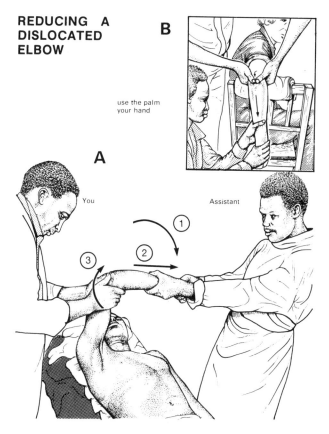

Fig. 72-6 TWO WAYS OF REDUCING A DISLOCATED ELBOW. If a dislocation is very recent, method B may work without an anaesthetic. Sit the patient sideways on a chair. Put a pillow over the top of the chair's back, and let his forearm hang over it. *Kindly contributed by John Stewart.*

If his dislocated elbow has been INCOMPLETELY REDUCED: (1) A child's medial epicondyle may have broken off and be inside the joint. If you are in doubt, X-ray his other elbow, and look for a small centre of ossification in an abnormal position. (2) There may still be a sideways displacement after the backward displacement has been corrected. If so, try to reduce the dislocation again. If you fail, refer him without delay because there is probably soft tissue between the joint surfaces.

If the patient's elbow REDISLOCATES EASILY and is very unstable, make sure there are no fractures. Apply a collar and cuff to maintain the stable position for 2 weeks. If it still redislocates, refer him.

If his MEDIAL EPICONDYLE IS TRAPPED inside his elbow, he is likely to present as failure to reduce a dislocation and a very unstable elbow. A trapped medial epicondyle is easy to find because the flexor muscles are attached to it. If it really is in his elbow joint and his elbow is unstable in all directions, apply a temporary posterior slab, and refer him.

If he has OTHER FRACTURES, he may have a flake off his capitulum, or a fracture of his coronoid, or a fracture of the head of his radius. First reduce the dislocation, and then treat the fracture as if the dislocation had never existed. If it is a major flake, refer him immediately to have it removed.

If a NERVE HAS BEEN INJURED, particularly his ulnar nerve, it may need to be explored by an expert if it does not recover spontaneously in a month. Any of the nerves crossing the elbow may be injured, especially the ulnar.

If 2 or 3 weeks after an injury the MOVEMENT OF A PATIENT'S ELBOW BECOME LESS, a firm mass forms near the joint, and his soft tissue starts to calcify, he is suffering from POST TRAUMATIC OSSIFICATION (myositis ossificans). When an elbow dislocates the periosteum is torn off the back of the humerus and brachialis is torn from the front. These injured tissues may calcify and ossify, particularly in children. The same complication can follow a supracondylar fracture, and is made worse by: (1) repeated manipulations in an attempt to reduce the injury, and (2) forceful movements subsequently.

Watch the patient carefully for the first few weeks after reduction. If at any time movement of his elbow becomes less, stop him moving it for a few days. Continue to immobilize it, until unrestricted use of it no longer dminishes its range. Allow him full activity, *but avoid forced movements and exercises.* The only safe movements are those that are possible using the injured

SUPRACONDYLAR FRACTURES

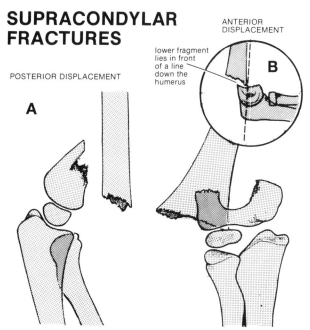

Fig. 72-7 SUPRACONDYLAR FRACTURES. A, posterior displacement is much more common. B, in an anterior displacement a line down the front of the humerus passes behind the distal fragment.

239

elbow's own muscles, without the help of his normal hand. X-ray his elbow and look for soft tissue calcification, usually anteriorly in brachialis. See also Section 72.10.

Don't try to remove any bony lumps or refer him for their removal *until at least a year after the injury.* Sometimes, in spite of the best care, a patient's elbow becomes stiff permanently. If this starts to happen, keep it in its most useful position, according to his needs. This is usually flexed to about 90°, with his forearm in mid–pronation (Fig. 73-1).

AVOID FORCED ELBOW MOVEMENTS

72.6 Posteriorly displaced supracondylar fractures in children

This a particularly important children's fracture—the wrong treatment can easily make it worse. Supracondylar fractures are common between the ages of 3 and 11, and are rare after the age of 20.

A child falls on his outstretched arm, and breaks the lower end of the shaft of his humerus just above the epiphyseal line in one of four ways: (1) In a third of cases there is no displacement, or the fracture is incomplete, so that the child needs no treatment except for a collar and cuff. (2) In the remaining two thirds of cases the distal fragment is displaced posteriorly. The child is tender just above his elbow, which swells rapidly and obscures the bones round the fracture. (3) Occasionally, the lower fragment is displaced anteriorly (72.7). (4) Occasionally, separation takes place at the epiphyseal line and displaces the epiphysis. Treat these epiphyseal displacements exactly as if they were supracondylar fractures. Reduce them immediately. Like all epiphyseal injuries, they unite rapidly.

There is one rare immediate danger and two common later ones.

The rare immediate danger, both with this fracture and with posterior dislocations of the elbow, is that they can impair the blood supply to a child's lower arm, and so cause the compartment syndrome followed by ischaemic fibrosis of his forearm muscles (Volkmann's ischaemic contracture), or gangrene requiring amputation (70.4). Contracture from a supracondylar fracture is much rarer than contracture as the result of failing to split a circular cast on a fracture of the forearm.

The force causing the injury pushes the distal fragment posteriorly and proximally, and the proximal fragment anteriorly and distally. The sharp proximal fragment pierces the periosteum, and comes to lie under brachialis. If the force continues the proximal fragment goes straight through brachialis into the child's antecubital fossa, and may even penetrate his skin. As it moves forwards it may tear his brachial artery, or make the artery go into spasm, or it may injure his median or occasionally his radial nerve. The artery and the nerve may also come to lie between the proximal and distal fragments, and so prevent reduction. Worse, the antecubital fossa fills with blood. This: (1) obstructs the collateral vessels which might otherwise bypass the injured artery, and (2) impairs the venous return from his arm. The ischaemic forearm muscles swell and the compartment syndrome develops (73.7). Bending such an acutely swollen elbow is like trying to bend a balloon.

The most common later disability is a very stiff, or fixed elbow. This is caused by the post traumatic ossification that may follow repeated manipulation. *So try to reduce the fracture with the minimum of manipulation.* One attempt at manipulation followed by one more is the most you should try. Your first attempt is the most likely to succeed, and later ones will become more and more difficult.

The other common late disability is a deformed elbow. Some displacements remodel and others do not.

The displacements which remodel are: (1) Moderate angulation

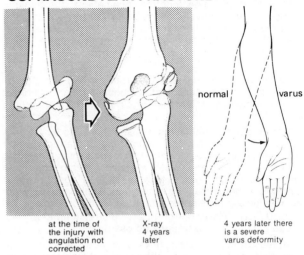

at the time of the injury with angulation not corrected

X-ray 4 years later

4 years later there is a severe varus deformity

Fig. 72-8 UNCORRECTED ANGULATION IN A SUPRACONDYLAR FRACTURE. Varus angulation is common and results in a loss of carrying angle in mild cases, or in an ugly varus deformity in more severe ones, like this child. It does not affect flexion and extension, so that disability is mild, but it does not look good. *After Perkins with kind permission.*

of the lower fragment in the plane of the elbow. (2) Posterior displacement of the lower fragment; growth of the epiphysis corrects this.

The displacements which do not remodel are: (1) Severe angulation of the lower fragment in the plane of the elbow. If you leave this unreduced, or reduce it badly, the child will be left with permanent hyperextension and severe loss of flexion. (2) Valgus or varus angulation. This does does not remodel, however mild it is or however young the child. Varus angulation is common and is usually accompanied by internal rotation and medial displacement. The result is a loss of the normal carrying angle in mild cases, or an ugly varus deformity in more severe ones, like the child in Fig. 72-8. This is common, and although it does not affect flexion or extension, so that disability is mild, it does not look good, and makes it difficult for the patient to carry a basket.

The principles of reduction are: (1) To exert traction on the child's elbow, and while doing this to correct the sideways displacement of the distal fragment. Then, (2) to flex his arm while still exerting traction, so as to use his triceps tendon to hold the lower fragment in place. A common error is to try to correct sideways displacement *after you have flexed his arm.*

Never treat these fractures with a circular cast. The risk of Volkmann's ischaemic contracture is great. If you do apply plaster, it *must* be a backslab.

NEVER PUT A CIRCULAR CAST ON A SUPRACONDYLAR FRACTURE

A CHILD'S SUPRACONDYLAR FRACTURE POSTERIORLY DISPLACED

The following description assumes that the child's fracture is on the right side, and follows Fig. 72-9.

If possible, reduce the fracture immediately. If there are signs of ischaemia this is urgent.

If immediate reduction is impossible because his arm is swollen like a balloon, apply forearm traction as in Fig. 72-11, and reduce the fracture as soon as the swelling has sub-

REDUCING A SUPRACONDYLAR FRACTURE

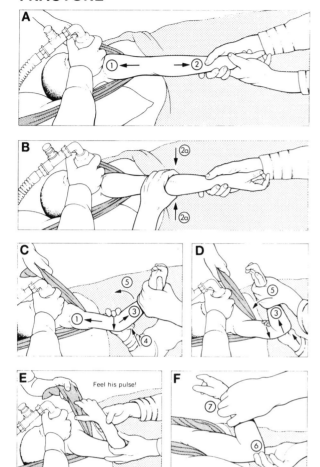

Fig. 72-9 REDUCING A SUPRACONDYLAR FRACTURE. The principles of reduction are to exert traction on a child's elbow and while doing so to correct the sideways displacement of the distal fragment. Then, flex his arm while still exerting traction, so as to use his biceps tendon to hold the lower fragment in place. *Kindly contributed by Peter Bewes.*

sided sufficiently for you to feel the fragments. If the skin of his forearm is blistered, so that you cannot apply traction to it, elevate it in a stockinette sleeve or towel pinned together and suspended from a drip stand, as in Fig. 75-1. Reduction is possible up to a week later, but not more.

If the fracture is more than a week old, it will be difficult to manipulate, so leave it. Six months later, if there is a severe deformity, refer him for a corrective osteotomy.

Check his median, ulna, and radial nerves (Fig. 75-3).

ANAESTHETIC: **(1)** Intravenous ketamine (A 8.3). **(2)** General anaesthesia.

REDUCTION OF A SUPRACONDYLAR FRACTURE

Flex the child's normal elbow, feel its bony anatomy carefully, and compare it with his injured elbow. Feeling the bony parts

of the injured elbow may be impossible if it is very swollen. Note especially the position of his olecranon in relation to the axis of his humerus. This is a useful guide to satisfactory reduction.

Feel how much external rotation of his flexed elbow is possible on the normal side. Later, when you come to reduce a medially displaced fragment, you will need to rotate his injured forearm externally to the limit of what is possible on the normal side, and a bit more. This external rotation may be critical. Sideways displacement either corrects itself, or is easily corrected.

What happens to his pulse if you flex and exert gentle traction on his arm? If his pulse disappears when you do this and only reappears when his arm is nearly straight, it may merely be due to the swelling round his elbow, or he may have a brachial artery lesion.

DIAGRAM A, REDUCING A SUPRACONDYLAR FRACTURE

Steady the child's shoulder. Ask your assistant to hold it by passing a towel round it (1).

Pull to disimpact the fracture and correct angulation Extend the child's elbow gently. Grip his wrist and distal forearm. Pull hard in a longitudinal direction *for at least 1 minute by the clock* (2). You will feel the fragments disimpact and release the soft tissues trapped between them. Check that you have disimpacted them by feeling that the lower fragment is free.

DIAGRAM B, REDUCING A SUPRACONDYLAR FRACTURE

Correcting medial and lateral displacement. The distal fragment is usually displaced medially. Traction usually corrects this. If it does not, now is the time to try to correct it. Feel the distal fragment, although the child's elbow may be so swollen that this is impossible. If necessary, move the distal fragment towards the midline of his arm (2a).

DIAGRAM C, REDUCING A SUPRACONDYLAR FRACTURE

Correct the posterior displacement. While still exerting longitudinal traction with your right hand (3), press the olecranon with your thumb (4).

Begin flexing (5) with your thumb pressing on his olecranon. Do this while your assistant maintains traction in the child's axilla. Keep pressing his olecranon with your left thumb as you do so. Externally rotate his forearm a little more than was possible on the normal side. This will help to restore the normal carrying angle.

Continue flexing. As the child's arm reaches 90°, pull posteriorly on his humerus, and anteriorly on his forearm.

CAUTION ! Use only moderate tension as his arm reaches 90°. If you pull too hard at this stage, it is possible to pull the distal fragment in front of the end of the humerus. Fortunately this is rare.

DIAGRAM D, REDUCING A SUPRACONDYLAR FRACTURE

Complete flexing. Beyond 90° further flexion does not improve reduction, but it does stabilize reduction by wrapping the child's triceps tendon round the distal fragment and fixing it. This also impacts the fragments. Lateral displacement of the distal fragment cannot now be corrected.

The position of the point of the olecranon is the best guide to satisfactory reduction. It should be in line with the axis of the humerus or perhaps little anterior to it (6). You should also be able to feel both epicondyles forming, with the tip of the olecranon, the 3 bony points of the elbow in A, Fig. 72-2.

DIAGRAMS E, F, and G, REDUCING A SUPRACONDYLAR FRACTURE

Check the child's pulse (7). This may be difficult because of oedema. If his pulse disappears when you flex his arm, extend it until his pulse reappears.

If he has a good radial pulse, put his arm in a collar and cuff in as much flexion as his pulse will allow. His hand should be able to reach his mouth. If you cannot feel his pulse, extend his elbow until you can free it. Make a cuff out of two lengths of stockinette filled with cotton wool (8).

If you cannot get his arm beyond 70° without his pulse disappearing put him in forearm traction (Fig. 72-11), as described below.

If you are not sure if you can feel his pulse or not, don't worry for the moment. But immediately he wakes from the anaesthetic, ask him if he can flex his fingers. If he cannot do this, proceed as in Section 72.8.

CAUTION ! (1) Make the knot of the collar and cuff so secure that neither the child, nor his parents, nor his grandparents can remove it. A good way to secure it is to cover it with plaster. Provided there are no complications, it will need to stay on for 3 weeks. In whatever way the child twists and turns, he must not be able to extend his elbow more than 90° or reduction will be lost. (2) Don't fit a plaster backslab, it is unnecessary and make it difficult to flex his elbow sufficiently.

As soon as he awakes, make sure he can flex and extend his fingers. Check the function of his median and ulnar nerves. They may be injured, but they usually recover eventually.

CHECKING REDUCTION

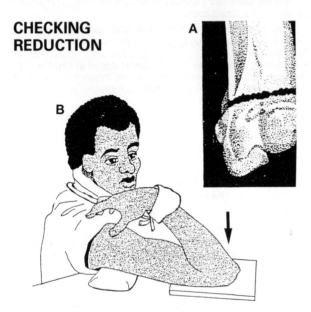

Fig. 72-10 CHECKING THE REDUCTION OF A SUPRACONDYLAR FRACTURE. A, the post reduction X-ray; This is schematic only and is from an older patient. B, positioning the arm and the film to take the X-ray. Don't let the X-ray assistant remove the child's collar and cuff to X-ray his arm. Take a lateral X-ray, and an AP view through the point of his elbow as shown: (1) There should be no angulation of the lower fragment in the AP view, (2) There should be no significant forward bowing in the lateral view. (3) The fragments must be in contact. If these criteria are met, reduction is satisfactory. Sideways and posterior displacement are not important.

CHECK REDUCTION The post reduction X-rays are of less help than they might be in seeing if angulation has been successfully reduced or not, because: (1) the child's arm must be kept flexed after reduction, and (2) the centres of ossification in the lower fragment may still be small. However, do your best by the the X-ray criteria in Fig. 72-10. If they are not met, have *one further attempt at reduction,* not more, or you will damage the child's elbow, and increase the chances of post–traumatic ossification.

PREVENT ISCHAEMIC PARALYSIS Don't send the child home because he may return with an irreversible Volkmann's contracture! Admit him to the ward and monitor the circulation in his hand carefully for 36 hours. Watch him for early signs of ischaemia. Check his pulse, and then press on his nail beds and see how quickly his capillaries refill. *The first signs of ischaemic paralysis are: (1) pain on passive extension of his fingers, (2) paraesthesiae, (3) pallor, and (4) paralysis as shown by the inability to use his fingers.*

Make sure the ward staff know why they are monitoring the child's circulation and what signs they should watch for. If

they don't know this, they may be quite content to feel the pulse in his normal arm!

CAUTION ! Don't give him morphine or any analgesic until you are sure that ischaemia is no longer a danger.

POSTOPERATIVE CARE AFTER REDUCING A SUPRACONDYLAR FRACTURE

If you have to reduce the flexion of a child's elbow, because of his impaired circulation, flex it again as his swollen elbow recovers. Then, X-ray him again.

Keep his collar and cuff on for 3 weeks. Don't let him take it off during this period. Make sure his parents understand this.

At 3 weeks his fracture will have united, so remove his collar and cuff, and replace it by a sling for 3 more weeks.

If, when you remove his collar and cuff, he ceases to be able to touch his mouth, replace it, and gradually tighten it until he can.

His elbow will be stiff for a long time. Encourage him to use it, but let movement return on its own, using its own active movements. Even when movement is slow to return, you can assure his mother that it will be better at the end of a year.

CAUTION ! (1) Forceful passive movements will make the stiffness worse. (2) Don't try to straighten his elbow by making him carry weights.

DON'T SEND HIM HOME FOR 36 HOURS AFTER REDUCTION

72.7 Supracondylar fracture of the humerus in children with anterior displacement of the distal fragment

Anterior displacement of the distal fragment of a supracondylar fracture is rare, and the signs are milder than with posterior displacement. Make the diagnosis from the lateral X-ray, as shown in B, Fig. 72-7. This may be difficult to interpret because the lower end of the diaphysis overlaps the epiphysis, especially in a young child, so that the epiphysis may appear to be displaced when it is not. The best test is to look at a lateral X-ray and to see where a line drawn down the front of the humerus cuts the curved lower border of the epiphysis, this is the line A–B in Fig. 72-3. It should bisect it as in Fig. 72-3. The epiphysis should not lie in front of this line.

A CHILD'S SUPRACONDYLAR FRACTURE ANTERIORLY DISPLACED

Anaesthetize the child as for forward displacement (72.6). Extend his forearm. Ask an assistant to exert steady traction in the line of his arm with his forearm supinated.

While your assistant is doing this, steady the lower end of his humerus with one hand, and correct the sideways displacement of the lower fragment with your other hand.

Either, put his arm up in traction as in Fig. 72-11, or apply a 10 cm plaster slab along the back of his arm and forearm with his elbow extended. Keep it in place with a crêpe bandage.

Confirm reduction with an X-ray. Remove the slab in 3 weeks in a child and put his arm in a sling.

Alternatively, flex his elbow to 90°, and push his forearm posteriorly on his upper arm so as to convert the anterior displacement to a posterior one. Then, treat it as you would a posterior displacement (72.6).

72.8 Ischaemia following a supracondylar fracture

This is a child who cannot move his fingers after the reduction of a supracondylar fracture. His arm shows some or all of these

FOREARM TRACTION

Extension traction

A

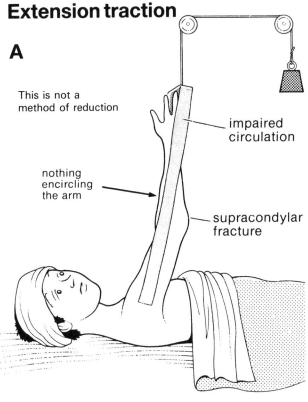

This is not a
method of reduction

nothing
encircling
the arm

impaired
circulation

supracondylar
fracture

B Dunlop traction

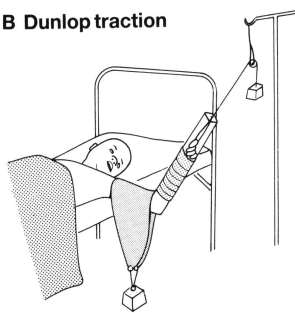

Fig. 72-11 FOREARM TRACTION is useful first treatment for ischaemia following a supracondylar fracture. Only if this fails to restore a child's circulation need you explore his arm. A, traction in extension. B, Dunlop traction. B, is more widely recognized, A is easier and adequate. *After Mercer Rang with kind permission.*

signs: (1) He has severe, deep, poorly localized, pain in the flexor muscles of his forearm. Pain when you extend his fingers passively is a serious late sign. So is flexion of his fingers. Occasionally, the syndrome is subacute and painless. (2) Paraesthesiae develop. First he feels 'pins and needles', then his arm becomes numb with anaesthesia of glove distribution. (3) The skin of his arm (if his is conscious) becomes white or blue (if he is Caucasian). There is no circulation in his nail beds. (4) His arm is weak, and he

cannot use his fingers. (5) Palpable induration of his forearm muscles is a diagnostic sign, but it occurs late. (6) His radial pulse may be weak or absent. An absent pulse is an unreliable sign, because the pulse is sometimes present even when there is severe ischaemia. Teach your staff the importance of the four 'Ps'—pain, paraesthesia, pallor (if they are caring for Caucasians) and paralysis, in that order.

Be vigilant, quick, and decisive. Recognize these signs early. If they are getting worse decompression is urgent. This is a very rare acute emergency, and there is no time to refer him. It is one of the few occasions where doing something is always better than doing nothing. *If you are lucky, extending his forearm in traction, as in Fig. 72-11, will be enough to restore his circulation.* If this fails, you will have to explore his antecubital fossa, and decompress the muscles of his arm. The penalty for not doing this will be Volkmann's ischaemic contracture (70.4).

EARLY SIGNS OF IMPENDING ISCHAEMIC CONTRACTURE
Temporarily ignore the child's fracture. Take off all bandages. If a plaster cast has been applied, remove it.

FOREARM TRACTION Apply longitudinal traction to the skin of the child's forearm. Use adhesive strapping and pass the cord over a pulley, so that if he moves about, traction will still be maintained. Suspend his arm as in Fig. 72-11.

Slope his bed slightly to stop him falling out, by putting a pillow under one side of the mattress.

Monitor the circulation in his arm.

If the pain goes, his circulation improves, and he is able to move his fingers, continue traction. When most of the swelling has gone, usually in about a week, reduce the fracture as described above, and put his arm in a collar and cuff. You should now have no trouble with his pulse. Usually, by this time the fracture is so firmly fixed that you will have to accept the malposition.

CAUTION ! If pain, paraesthesiae, pallor, and paralysis persist, for more than an hour, make preparations to take him to the theatre, explore his antecubital fossa and, if necessary, the volar aspect of his forearm, as described below. Don't be put off by a full stomach (16.1).

72.9 Forearm traction fails to restore the pulse of a child with a supracondylar fracture

This is the child whose supracondylar fracture is complicated by ischaemia of his forearm. He is unlucky in that signs of ischaemia persist, even with his arm extended in forearm traction and any tight cast or bandage removed. Take him to the theatre. There are two things you can do: (1) You can release the tension in his antecubital fossa and relieve the pressure on his vessels. (2) You can decompress his forearm muscles to relieve the compartment syndrome (73.7). Opinions vary as to which of these is the most important. Releasing the tension in his antecubital fossa is easier and may be all that is necessary. Don't delay; a wait of 3 or 4 hours may make all the difference between a normal and a totally useless arm. If you act promptly his prognosis is likely to be good. Don't try to inspect or repair his brachial artery—this is a highly skilled task, it is rarely necessary, and, because the collateral circulation round the elbow is so good, a blocked brachial artery does not necessarily cause Volkmann's ischaemic contracture.

WATCH FOR PAIN, PARAESTHESIA, PALLOR, AND PARALYSIS

OPERATING FOR ISCHAEMIA

Don't explore the child's antecubital fossa until you have tried to reduce the fracture, because this may itself be enough to improve the circulation his arm.

Make the lazy 'S' incision as in A, Fig. 72-12, beginning above the flexor crease on the inner border of his biceps tendon.

Pull back the flaps, incise his tight deep fascia and his bicipital aponeurosis (B). Pale or blue–black muscle will bulge from the wound. There may be a tight haematoma. Remove it. This may be enough to relieve the obstruction and restore his circulation.

CAUTION! Don't meddle with his brachial artery, or try to resect the spastic section.

EXPLORING THE ANTECUBITAL FOSSA

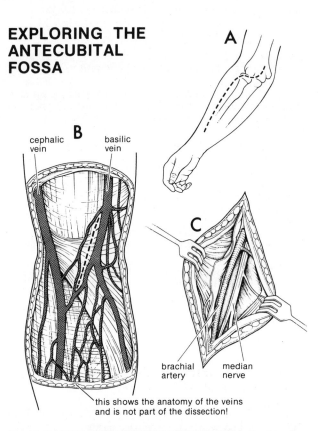

cephalic vein

basilic vein

brachial artery

median nerve

this shows the anatomy of the veins and is not part of the dissection!

Fig. 72-12 EXPLORING THE ANTECUBITAL FOSSA. Don't explore the child's antecubital fossa until you have tried to reduce the fracture, because this may itself be enough to improve the circulation his arm. *After Campbell permission requested.*

DECOMPRESSING A CHILD'S FOREARM MUSCLES **If the above methods fail, and his forearm is swollen, carry the incision down through it, as in Fig. 73-11. Slit his deep fascia in the length of the incision. Pale oedematous muscles will burst through the slit fascia. Decompress the superficial and deep volar compartments of his arm, as in Section 73.7.**

POSTOPERATIVE CARE **Leave the flaps open, and dress the child's wound. Don't sew it up. If the fracture is not reasonably reduced, apply forearm traction. If it is reduced, apply a collar and cuff.**

Skin graft the wound after 4 days. If a contracture develops, see Section 72.10.

TREAT THE EARLIEST SIGNS OF ISCHAEMIC PARALYSIS IMMEDIATELY

72.10 Other difficulties with supracondylar fractures in children

These include nerve injuries, post–traumatic ossification, a persistent varus deformity, and severe malunion. Most of these complications are difficult to treat. The principle is to prevent them by the methods described above if you possibly can.

OTHER DIFFICULTIES WITH A SUPRACONDYLAR FRACTURE

If a child has NERVE INJURIES after a supracondylar fracture, they will probably recover. They are more common than injuries to the brachial artery, but are less serious. Nerve injuries alone are not an indication for an immediate operation. If there is no recovery in a month, refer the child to have his elbow explored.

If the child's ELBOW WILL NOT MOVE after a supracondylar fracture, he is suffering from POST TRAUMATIC OSSIFICATION. After 3 weeks, when the collar and cuff are removed, his elbow will not move, or perhaps there is some movement which gradually becomes less. The front of his elbow is tender, there is muscle spasm and the tendon of his biceps stands out as a taut band. X-rays may show a vague shadow like callus in front of the joint, or it may be so dense that it looks like bone. Sometimes a stiff painful elbow with new bone around it is his presenting symptom.

Encourage his parents to put his injured elbow through several 15 minute periods of *gentle* active movements each day, both flexion and rotation. His parents must be patient, persistent and gentle. *Forced movements and even too vigorous passive movements will make his elbow worse.* Make this clear to them. If the movements of a child's arm are diminishing, put his arm in a collar and cuff until muscle spasm has disappeared, which may take months. If he cannot flex his elbow enough to get his hand to his mouth, put it in a loose collar and cuff and gradually tighten it until he can. After prolonged rest the spasm disappears and movement returns, but there is usually some permanent loss of movement. Unfortunately, post–traumatic ossification is common, and is a major disability, especially when pronation is lost. Osteotomy followed by an arthrodesis in the position of function (about 90°, see Fig. 7-16) may be necessary.

If SEVERE VARUS DEFORMITY PERSISTS, refer the child for corrective osteotomy not earlier than a year after the injury.

If the fracture was never properly reduced, and he now has MALUNION with only 30° of movement or less, management depends on where the movement is. If it is around the position of function (90°) an osteotomy is unlikely to improve him.

A COMMINUTED SUPRACONDYLAR FRACTURE IN AN ADULT

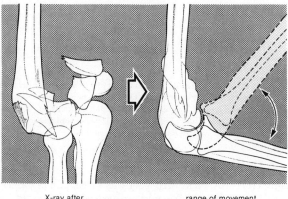

X-ray after the injury

range of movement a year later

Fig. 72-13 A COMMINUTED SUPRACONDYLAR FRACTURE treated by active movements showing the range of movement possible 18 months later. Note that the range of active movement is around the position of function (about 90°). This patient is right handed, so this enables his right hand to reach his mouth. *Kindly contributed by Peter Bewes.*

But if it is around full extension, an osteotomy may bring it into a more useful range.

NEVER MOVE AN ELBOW CONTRACTURE FORCEFULLY

72.11 Supracondylar fractures of the humerus in adults

Supracondylar fractures in adults differ from those in children, and are caused in a different way: (1) An old person falls and strikes his elbow on the ground. The force of the blow drives his ulna up against his humerus and either breaks off its lower end, as in a child, or, more often, splits it into two or more pieces which may separate widely and displace backwards or forwards. Or, (2) the patient rests his arm on the window of his car, and has it crushed by a passing vehicle (sidewipe fracture). In either case he cannot move his swollen and deformed elbow. Swelling obscures the bony landmarks and if you examine it carefully, you may be able to feel crepitus.

These fractures are usually T–shaped or comminuted. Rarely, they are transverse as in children; if so, you can manage them in the same way. If the fracture is T–shaped or comminuted, you cannot reduce the fragments by closed manipulation, and they are difficult to fix at open operation. Even when the fragments are fixed internally, the late results are often disappointing, so it is fortunate that the results of early active movement are usually better as shown in Fig. 72-13, and that patients have much less osteoarthritis than you might expect. *But the results will only be better, if the patient really does start moving his elbow early.* The function he will ultimately get depends on the relationship of his two condyles. If they are widely apart and shifted on one another, movement will be poor. If they are parallel and not shifted, movement will be better. Displacement of the fragments at the transverse fracture is less important. You can combine active movements with traction, as in Fig. 72-14.

SUPRACONDYLAR FRACTURES OF THE HUMERUS IN ADULTS

INDICATIONS FOR REFERRAL (1) If the lower end of the patient's humerus is in one or two fragments only, and you can refer him to a superb technician, he may benefit from internal fixation, especially if he is young. (2) Injuries to his median or ulnar nerves.

TRANSVERSE SUPRACONDYLAR FRACTURES
If the lower fragment is in one piece, treat it as for a child's supracondylar fracture (72.6).

T–SHAPED, Y–SHAPED, OR COMMINUTED SUPRACONDYLAR FRACTURES

EARLY ACTIVE MOVEMENTS If necessary, anaesthetize the patient and try to get the fragments into a better position. Try to start active movements as soon as possible. If his arm is very swollen keep it raised for a few days. Put his arm in a collar and cuff for not more than a week. During this time take it out several times a day and encourage him to move it.

CAUTION ! (1) Flexion and extension are subsequently likely to be limited, so make sure they are in the most useful range, as in Fig. 72-13. (2) For the same reason his forearm should be in mid–pronation.

Start pendulum exercises for his shoulder (Fig 71-7), and exercises for his wrist and fingers immediately after the injury.

After a week, provided he continues to be able to put his hand to his mouth, put his arm in a sling. Keep him in the sling for 5 weeks. Encourage him to use his hand and move his elbow as much as he can. Tell him that he will not regain any movement in his elbow unless he tries very hard to use it.

OLECRANON TRACTION If the patient's olecranon is intact, pass a Kirschner wire through it (70.10), and tension the wire with a Gissane stirrup (1), or, less satisfactorily, use a thin (less than 4 mm) Steinmann pin. The danger with a pin is that it is more likely to get in the way of his ulnar nerve. If the fragments are displaced, ask an assistant to exert traction on the stirrup while you press the fragments back into place (2).

Apply enough traction to keep his upper arm under tension (3) but not enough to lift his shoulder off the mattress. You may need to apply 2 to 5 kg.

Apply a sling (4) to keep his elbow at 90° and his wrist half–way between pronation and supinaton, with his hand over his opposite shoulder.

Apply 0.5 to 1 kg of backward traction on his upper arm (5). This is not essential.

Feel the bony prominences on the back of his elbow (6) and adjust the direction of traction so that the position of the prominences matches that on the normal side, and corrects any sideways shift. You may have to tie the traction cord to one of the outer holes in the stirrup (7).

CAUTION ! Check his radial pulse often. Don't apply too much traction, or you may obstruct the circulation to his arm, injure his nerves, or distract the fragments and so prevent union.

OLECRANON TRACTION

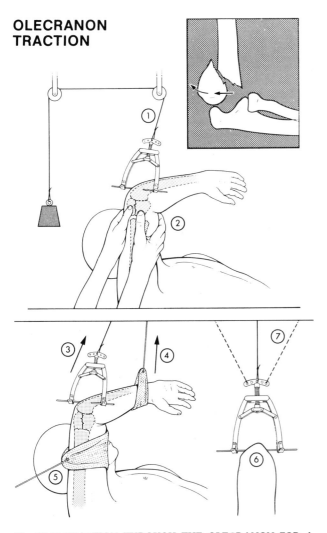

Fig. 72-14 TRACTION THROUGH THE OLECRANON FOR A T–SHAPED SUPRACONDYLAR FRACTURE. If a patient's olecranon is intact, pass a Kirschner wire through it (70.10), and tension the wire with a Gissane stirrup (1), or, less satisfactorily, use a thin (less than 4 mm) Steinmann pin. *After de Palma with kind permission.*

X-ray him. Slight backward displacement is acceptable, but there should be no angulation or lateral displacement.

While he is in traction, encourage him to move his elbow as much as he can. Let him take hold of the traction cord and assist his elbow movements himself.

Remove the traction at 2 to 3 weeks, put his arm in a sling with his elbow at 90° and his forearm in 45° of pronation. Start carefully graded active movements without using force. Recovery will take several months.

DIFFICULTIES WITH SUPRACONDYLAR FRACTURES IN ADULTS

If a patient's HUMERUS IS BADLY COMMINUTED AND OPEN, AND HIS RADIUS AND ULNA ARE INJURED TOO, this is likely to be the result of a car accident in which he had his elbow over the edge of the window. Toilet his wound. If his elbow is dislocated, reduce it. Suspend his arm in the position of function, and get it moving. Dress it, but do not close it by primary suture. Look at it in 4 or 5 days, and either close it or graft it. (1) Hang it up with metacarpal Kirschner wire (70.12), or (2) use skin traction on his fingers *while watching their circulation carefully.* Hang his hand up in the same position as for forearm traction.

INJURIES OF THE DISTAL HUMERAL EPIPHYSES

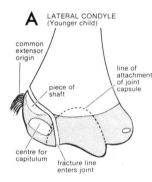
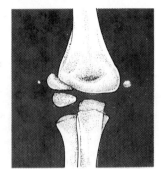
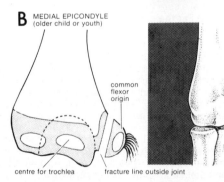

Fig. 72-15 INJURIES OF THE DISTAL HUMERAL EPIPHYSES. The medial epicondyle and lateral condyle differ considerably. A, The lateral condyle is a pressure epiphysis to which the common extensor origin is attached. It is fractured in young children. The fracture line enters the joint displacing the centre for the capitulum and sometimes part of the shaft. The displaced fragment must be accurately replaced. B, the medial epicondyle is a traction epiphysis outside the elbow joint to which the common flexor origin is attached. It is displaced in teenagers, and unless it happens to go inside the elbow joint it need not be removed or reattached.

72.12 Fracture of the medial epicondyle of the humerus

Between the ages of 5 and 20 the centre of ossification of the medial epicondyle is a separate piece of bone. The flexor muscles of the forearm are attached to it, and if these are pulled on hard enough by a fall on an outstretched hand, they can pull it away

from a patient's humerus. His detached medial epicondyle may remain outside his elbow joint or go inside the joint and lock it. Closed methods may succeed in removing it, but if they fail, an open operation is necessary. Removing the detached medial epicondyle would not be a difficult operation, if his ulnar nerve were not so close. Sometimes, his elbow is dislocated also (72.4).

After a fall an older child or youth complains of a painful elbow. The contour of his arm is normal, but his medial epicondyle is tender and swollen. Rotation is normal and some flexion and extension is usually possible. Compare the X-rays of both his elbows.

FRACTURES OF THE MEDIAL EPICONDYLE

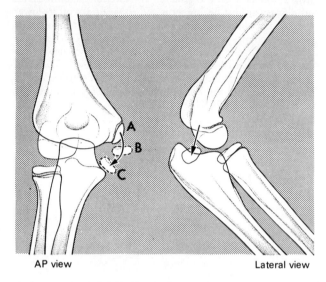

AP view   Lateral view

Fig. 72-16 FRACTURE OF THE MEDIAL EPICONDYLE. If the child is over 5, the age at which the centre of ossification appears, you will be able to see if it is in its normal position A or not. If it is displaced, it may not prevent his elbow moving (B), or it may be inside his elbow and locking it (C). *From Perkins with kind permission.*

FRACTURE OF THE MEDIAL EPICONDYLE

IF THE PATIENT CAN MOVE HIS ELBOW ADEQUATELY, put his arm in a collar and cuff for a week. Then give him a sling and encourage active movements. Full movements may not return for a year.

IF HE CANNOT MOVE HIS ELBOW ADEQUATELY, anaesthetize him. Extend his wrist to tension his flexor mucles. Flex, abduct, and supinate his elbow, then suddenly extend it. The fragment may reduce with a sudden clunk. X-ray his elbow, and repeat the manoeuvre twice if necessary.

If you can move his elbow through its full range of movement and it is stable, apply a collar and cuff as above.

If you cannot move his elbow through most of its full range, refer him for open reduction.

OPERATION If you cannot refer him, and are familiar with the procedures, consider operating. This is not an operation for the beginner, because the child's ulnar nerve will not be in its normal position and may be kinked into the joint with his medial epicondyle. Make all incisions in the line of the nerve, not across it.

Make a 5 cm longitudinal incision 1 cm anterior to his medial epicondyle. Find his ulnar nerve and take care not to injure it. You will see the fibres of the common flexor origin emerging from the joint cavity. Pull on these fibres with a hook or forceps, and pull the epicondyle out of the joint.

Find the rough place on the medial side of his elbow from which the epicondyle broke off. Either suture it in place by

FRACTURE OF THE LATERAL CONDYLE

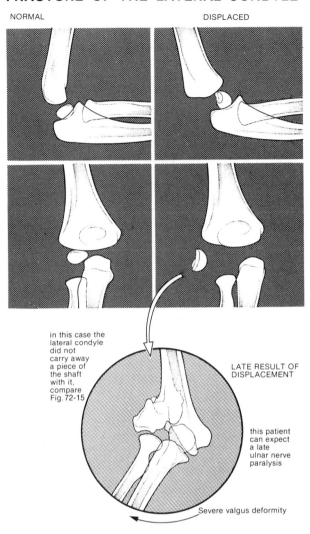

NORMAL   DISPLACED

in this case the lateral condyle did not carry away a piece of the shaft with it, compare Fig. 72-15

LATE RESULT OF DISPLACEMENT

this patient can expect a late ulnar nerve paralysis

Severe valgus deformity

Fig. 72-17 FRACTURE OF THE LATERAL CONDYLE is a serious Salter Harris Type IV epiphyseal injury; it occurs at a younger age than injuries of the medial condyle, and the fragment is larger. *Kindly contributed by John Stewart.*

drilling a small hole in it and in the neighbouring bone, or, anchor it in place with two short pieces of Kirschner wire with their ends bent over subcutaneously. Remove them 4 to 6 weeks later. If fixing the epicondyle is difficult, *and the fragment is small,* excise it. His flexor muscles will quickly find new attachments.

DIFFICULTIES WITH FRACTURES OF THE MEDIAL EPICONDYLE

If the patient's ULNAR NERVE IS INJURED, paralysis may be due to stretching and only be temporary. If recovery is delayed more than 6 weeks, refer him for transfer of the nerve to the front of his elbow.

If the FRAGMENT HAS BEEN LEFT INSIDE THE JOINT, and you discover it some time later, refer the child. If you cannot refer him, warn him that full movement may not return.

72.13 Fracture of the lateral condyle of the humerus (children)

A young child aged 4 to 15 falls on his outstretched hand. His wrist extensors, which are attached to his lateral condyle, pull it away from his humerus. His elbow is swollen and will not move. You can rotate his forearm, showing that his radius is

intact. The posteromedial side of his arm is not tender, showing that he has probably not got a supracondylar fracture. Sometimes his elbow is dislocated also.

This is a serious Type IV epiphyseal injury (69.6). It occurs at a younger age than an injury to the medial epicondyle, and the displaced fragment is larger. The fracture line runs from the middle of the articular surface of the child's elbow upwards and laterally, isolating part of his trochlea, the whole of his capitulum, and often a small part of the shaft of his humerus, as in Fig. 72-15. Sometimes, there is only a little lateral shift which need not be reduced. More often, the lower fragment turns over completely inside the joint. If it is not reduced, it unites to the shaft with fibrous tissue, and growth in the lateral half of his epiphysis stops. The result is a severe valgus deformity of his elbow which increases until growth ceases. Distortion of the path of his ulnar nerve round his severely deformed elbow causes a late ulnar paralysis with wasting of the small muscles of his hand.

The X-rays of his elbow are difficult to interpret, because a large part of the fragment is cartilage and casts no shadow. An AP view shows that the epiphysis of his capitulum is missing; instead, there is an abnormal mass of bone on the outer side of his elbow. In a lateral view this may be hidden behind his humerus, but it is usually displaced anteriorly. If he is under 12, you will not see the centre of ossification for his displaced lateral epicondyle, because it will not yet have appeared. If in doubt compare the X-ray of the injured side with that of the normal one. *Don't mistake this injury for a supracondylar fracture!*

FRACTURE OF THE LATERAL CONDYLE OF THE HUMERUS

IF THERE IS NO DISPLACEMENT, relieve the child's pain, if necessary, by aspirating his elbow joint (Fig. 72-4) using careful sterile precautions. Apply a backslab from his axilla to his kunckles with his elbow in 60° of flexion and his wrist dorsiflexed. Mould the backslab closely round his elbow, and hold it in a sling.

At 4 weeks replace the slab by a sling.

IF THERE IS DISPLACEMENT, suspend his arm in extension traction, as in Fig. 72-11, until the swelling is less. Find two assistants. Anaesthetize the patient.

Ask one assistant to apply traction to the child's partly flexed forearm. Ask the other assistant to apply counter traction to his upper arm. Ask them to slightly adduct his arm at the same time, so as to widen the space on the lateral aspect of his elbow joint.

THE LATERAL CONDYLE

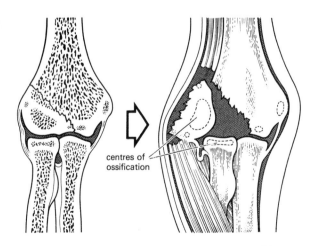

centres of ossification

Fig. 72-17a FRACTURE OF THE LATERAL CONDYLE. If this injury is not treated correctly, it will be followed by a severe valgus deformity which increases until growth ceases. *After Watson Jones with kind permission.*

While they are applying traction and adduction, try to manipulate the fragment back into place in contact with his humerus.

If closed reduction is successful, immobilize his elbow in a plaster backslab as above. Mould the backslab round the lateral side of his elbow to keep the fragment in place.

If closed reduction fails, do all you possibly can to refer the child for open reduction immediately. This involves fixing the lateral fragment with two fine Kirschner wires. The penalty for not doing so is likely to be a fixed elbow always. If the fragment is not replaced, warn his parents that a progressive valgus deformity and ulnar paralysis may occur, and that he must return early, so that an ulnar nerve transposition can be done.

DIFFICULTIES WITH FRACTURES OF THE LATERAL CONDYLE

If 10 to 30 years later the patient complains of NUMBNESS AND TINGLING in the distribution of his ulnar nerve, followed by wasting of the small muscles of his hand, he has an ulnar nerve paralysis. Warn his parents that this may follow the progressive valgus deformity of his elbow many years later, because he may not connect it with his injury. His ulnar nerve should be moved anteriorly in his elbow *before* the small muscles of his hand start to waste.

FRACTURE OF THE CAPITULUM

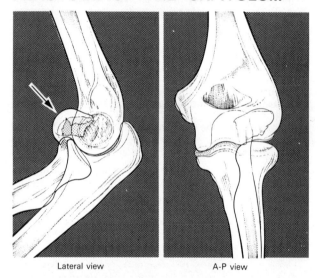

Lateral view   A-P view

Fig. 72-18 FRACTURE OF THE CAPITULUM is a rare adult injury. The arrow shows a large piece of the capitulum displaced anteriorly.

72.14 Fracture of the capitulum (adults)

In this rare fracture a piece of the patient's capitulum breaks off, tilts, and moves anteriorly. Unless it is reduced, he will have very little use in his elbow. The fragment varies in size from a small piece of cartilage, to the whole of the front of the patient's capitulum and part of his trochlea. The head of his radius may be fractured at the same time.

The patient holds his slightly swollen elbow at 90°, the contour of his arm is normal, and tenderness is difficult to locate. Rotation is fair, but very little flexion is possible. Small fragments consisting only of cartilage are difficult to see on the X-ray, so diagnose them from the history of locking and the signs of a loose body in the joint.

FRACTURE OF THE CAPITULUM

If the fragment is small, refer the patient for open removal.

If the fragment is large, try to reduce it.

Ask an assistant to exert traction on the patient's extended forearm. While he does this, press the fragment down firmly with your thumbs. Then when the fragment is in place, flex the patient's elbow to more than 90°.

If closed reduction is successful, apply a collar and cuff for a few weeks and start shoulder and finger exercises immediately.

If X-rays show that reduction has failed, refer him for external fixation of the fragment.

FRACTURES OF THE HEAD AND NECK OF THE RADIUS

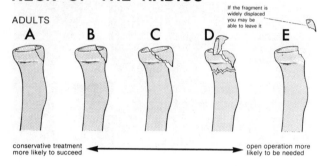

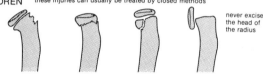

Fig. 72-19 FRACTURES OF THE HEAD AND NECK OF THE RADIUS are common injuries and can usually be treated conservatively. The patient's elbow and his X-ray may look so normal that the fracture is easily missed. *Kindly contributed by Peter Bewes.*

72.15 Fractures of the head of the radius (adults)

In this common injury a force travelling up the patient's arm drives the head of his radius against his capitulum. What happens depends on his age: (1) In a child the neck of the radius bends so that its head is displaced anteriorly and laterally, but the head itself almost never fractures. (2) In an adult the head may crack, a piece may chip off, it may break into many pieces, or the whole head may displace elsewhere in the joint. Treatment must be prompt and adequate.

Typically, the contour of the patient's arm is normal, and not greatly swollen. He is able to flex and extend his elbow a little, but he cannot rotate his wrist. The head of his radius is tender. His elbow and his X-ray may look so normal that the fracture is easily missed. If you think that he might have fractured the head of his radius, but his X-ray looks normal, treat him conservatively and X-ray him again in a week; the fracture will then be more obvious.

In the instructions below we advise you treat a patient conservatively if you possibly can. Although the operation itself is not difficult, you can easily cut the deep branch of his radial nerve (posterior interosseous nerve); so refer him if possible.

ROLF (37 years) fell on the ice, and broke the head of his radius, sustaining Fracture B, in Fig. 72-19. Instead of treating him with active movements, an 'expert' orthopaedic surgeon immobilized his arm, quite unnecessarily, in a cast for several weeks. When this was removed his arm was stiff for several more weeks. LESSONS there are many fractures for which a cast is NOT indicated!

DON'T OPERATE WITHOUT A TOURNIQUET

FRACTURES OF THE HEAD OF THE RADIUS

CONSERVATIVE TREATMENT

INDICATIONS Start by treating all fractures of the head of the radius this way.

METHOD Make sure that the patient's elbow is not also dislocated. If it is, reduce it first.

Aspirate the blood in his elbow joint (Fig. 72-4), inject 2 ml of local anaesthetic solution. You will now be able to flex, extend, and supinate his elbow. Start active movements (69.10) and encourage easy movements, *especially rotation*. Don't apply plaster. Observe him carefully.

If he improves, over the next few days, good. If not, refer him for operation as early as possible. By the time 5 days have elapsed you should know if conservative treatment is going to succeed or not. It is more likely to succeed in fractures A, and B, in Fig. 72-19 than it is in C, and D. Most skilled surgeons would operate immediately on C, or D, without attempting conservative treatment; you would probably be wise to try conservative treatment first. If the fragment in fracture E, is not much displaced, it may have to be removed at open operation. But if it is widely displaced, it may be not be restricting elbow movement, so conservative treatment may succeed.

If the patient improves under conservative treatment, so much the better, but warn him that full recovery will be slow.

OPEN OPERATION ON THE HEAD OF THE RADIUS

If possible refer the patient. This is not an operation for the beginner, or one to do if you have not seen it done. If you decide to operate, the sooner you do so the better. Try to operate within 5 days before dense scar tissue forms.

INDICATIONS Failure of conservative treatment. There is no need to remove a loose fragment (E) unless it is interfering with the movement of the elbow joint. *Don't remove the head of the radius in a child,* because this will interfere with the growth of the bone, and cause a severe valgus deformity.

TOURNIQUET Exsanguinate the patient's arm with an Esmarch bandage, and place a tourniquet (3.8) round his upper arm. Operating without a tourniquet will place the deep branch of his radial nerve in greater danger.

POSITION Lie him on his back and bring his arm over the front of his chest, so that the posterior surface of his elbow is uppermost. Leave his hand free so that you can rotate his wrist, and so turn the head of the radius. If necessary, attach a weight to his wrist, or tie it.

INCISION Make a 5 cm incision (A, in Fig. 72-20) over the posterolateral surface of the patient's elbow, extending downwards from his lateral epicondyle to his ulna over the interval between his extensor carpi ulnaris and his anconeus muscles.

Deepen the incision through the fascia between anconeus and extensor carpi ulnaris (B), to expose the joint capsule. If there is much bruising, and you cannot define these muscles, incise them between his lateral epicondyle and his olecranon.

CAUTION ! The deep branch of the radial nerve (posterior interosseus nerve) arises from the radial nerve 2 or 3 cm below the elbow. It winds round the lateral side of the neck of the radius, 1 cm below its head, between the two planes of the fibres of supinator. Don't dissect deeply in front of the radius, or distal to the annular ligament posteriorly. Unfortunately, its course may vary considerably.

Make a longitudinal incision in the capsule (C) to expose the head of the patient's radius and his capitulum (D). Syringe away the blood clot from the joint.

Find his annular ligament and divide the periosteum immediately proximal to it. Don't strip any of the periosteum from the bone.

Cut away the head of his radius with nibblers immediately proximal to the annular ligament (E). Don't cut this ligament.

Remove all loose pieces of bone (F). Reassemble the head

EXCISING THE HEAD OF THE RADIUS

CAUTION ! Keep his arm in full pronation

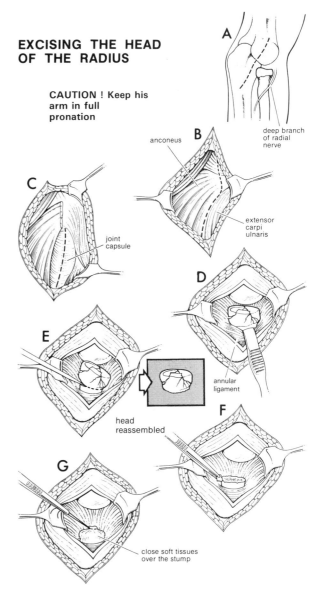

Fig. 72-20 EXCISING THE HEAD OF THE RADIUS. If possible refer the patient. This is not an operation for the beginner, or one to do if you have not seen it done before. If you decide to operate, the sooner you do so the better. Try to operate within 5 days before dense scar tissue forms. *After de Palma with kind permission.*

of his radius to make sure that no pieces are still missing inside the joint.

If possible, close the soft tissues over the broken neck of his radius with a purse string suture (G). This is not easy, and is not essential.

If his elbow has been dislocated, redislocate it to remove any loose fragments of the radial head that may be lying in other parts of the joint. Fragments are sometimes driven through the capsule and lie outside it. Inspect his capitulum for injury.

Rinse the wound forcibly with Ringer's lactate, or saline, and if possible insert a suction drain. Close the capsule and the muscle with one layer of interrupted sutures. Release the tourniquet and control bleeding.

POSTOPERATIVE CARE Flex the patient's elbow to 90°. Apply a pressure dressing to the wound and give him a collar and cuff.

Next day, encourage him to start exercising his fingers and shoulders. After a week encourage him to move his elbow. Avoid vigorous exercise or forced passive movement.

If he is in much pain or spasm, immobilize his elbow again for a few weeks, and then try again to mobilize it.

If a patient **PRESENTS LATE** with a fracture like that in **D, Fig. 72-19,** refer him. There is however little to be done.

If he has a **STIFF ELBOW,** watch the progress of his movements carefully. An injured elbow takes a long time to recover. The tissues round it sometimes ossify. If movements become fewer, stop them completely for a few days, then start them again cautiously. Don't push exercises if recovery is slow, because it increases the risk of post–traumatic ossification. X-ray his elbow and look for this.

MAKE SURE YOU REMOVE ALL THE FRAGMENTS

PULLED ELBOW

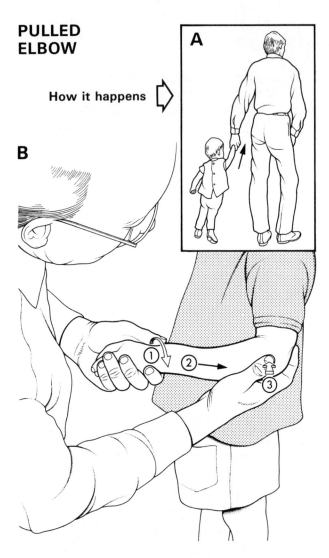

How it happens ⇨

Fig. 72-21 PULLED ELBOW. A, shows the mechanism of pulled elbow, and B, the method of manipulating it.

72.16 Pulled elbow (young children)

This common injury is the result of lifting up a child by one arm, or swinging him around on it. Many minor and otherwise undiagnosed injuries are probably pulled elbows. The head of a child's radius has no well defined neck, so that if it is pulled distally, it can be gripped by the annular ligament.

A child with a pulled elbow holds his hand in neutral, he refuses to use his arm, and he cannot rotate his wrist. Sometimes, the head of his radius is tender. His X-rays are normal. The differential diagnosis of a fracture of the neck of his radius.

Treatment is usually easy. Hold his hand in one of your hands as if you were shaking hands, and cup his elbow in the palm of your other hand. Suddenly supinate his arm and at the same time quickly push his hand towards his elbow, while pushing on the head of his radius with your thumb. This will usually free the head of his radius from the annular ligament. Sometimes, even extending his elbow to take an X-ray does the same. He will cry loudly, but he will usually be able to move his arm. If this fails, do nothing. He will usually recover completely in a few weeks; if he does not, refer him.

72.17 Fracture of the neck of the radius (children)

A child falls on his outstretched hand and breaks the neck of his radius just distal to the epiphyseal plate, proximal to the attachment of his biceps. The head of his radius angulates anteriorly and laterally on its broken neck, and usually remains attached to the shaft. The same injury may fracture his medial epicondyle, strain or rupture the medial ligament of his elbow, or fracture the upper third of his ulna.

The contour of his elbow is normal, and flexion and extension are less painful than rotation.

This injury can occur before the centre of ossification appears in the head of his radius at the age of 10. If it does, the only X-ray sign of a complete displacement of the head of his radius is this: the proximal end of his radius is closer to the lower end of his humerus on the injured side than it is on the normal one. If so, refer him.

REDUCING A DISPLACEMENT OF THE NECK OF THE RADIUS

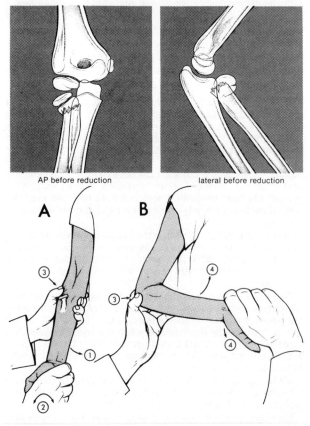

AP before reduction   lateral before reduction

Fig. 72-22 REDUCING A DISPLACEMENT OF THE NECK OF THE RADIUS. Treatment depends on the degree of angulation and on the child's age. Mild angulation needs no treatment, but moderate and severe angulation must be corrected. Closed reduction like this usually succeeds.

Treatment depends on the degree of angulation and on the child's age. Mild angulation needs no treatment. Moderate and severe angulation must be corrected, because the head may grow abnormally and ultimately dislocate, particularly after severe displacement in an older child. In very young children the head may grow almost normally, even after severe displacement. Never excise the head, because this is sure to cause a severe growth deformity.

FRACTURE OF THE NECK OF THE RADIUS

CHOICE OF PROCEDURE The following indications refer to angulation in the AP or the lateral view.

If the head is angulated less than 15°, put the child's arm in a sling for 10 days. Recovery will be complete.

If the angulation is more than 15°, try closed reduction, as described below. This may succeed even if the head is severely displaced.

If the child's elbow is also dislocated, reduce it and then treat the head of his radius.

If the head of the radius is completely separated (see above), refer him for open reduction.

CLOSED REDUCTION If the child's elbow is very swollen, suspend his arm in extension traction (Fig. 72-11), until the swelling his reduced.

Anaesthetize him, and ask an assistant to steady his upper arm. Extend his arm, grasp his wrist with one hand, and his elbow with the other, as in Fig. 72-22. Adduct his forearm at his elbow (1), so as to open the joint between his capitulum and the head of his radius a little.

Rotate his forearm (2) into the position in which the most prominent part of the displaced head lies laterally and superficially.

Put your thumb over the displaced head of his radius. While you adduct his forearm, press the head of his radius proximally and medially (3). Now flex his forearm and supinate it sharply (4).

If closed reduction fails to reduce the angulation to 15° or less, refer him for open reduction. If this is not possible, the head of his radius may remodel if he is young, so proceed with active movements only.

POST REDUCTION X-RAYS In the lateral view the forward angulation of the head should be corrected, and in the AP view the lateral angulation should also be corrected. In both views the surface of the head of the child's radius should be parallel to his capitulum.

POSTOPERATIVE CARE Bandage on a plaster backslab extending two thirds of the way around his arm. After 3 weeks replace it by a collar and cuff for another 3 weeks.

72.18 Fractures of the olecranon

A patient can fracture his olecranon in two ways: (1) He can receive a direct blow to the point of his elbow which fractures it *directly*. (2) He can fall on his outstretched hand at the same time as his triceps is contracting, and thus break his olecranon *indirectly*. In both cases his elbow is acutely tender and swollen. Sometimes the head of his radius is also injured.

Examine him. Can he extend his forearm against gravity, as in A, Fig. 72-23?

If he can extend his arm against gravity, the extensor mechanism of his elbow is intact, and active movements alone are enough, *whatever his X-ray may show.*

If he cannot extend his forearm against gravity, his extensor mechanism needs repair. Look at his lateral X-ray. If more than half his olecranon fossa is intact, excise the proximal fragments and suture his triceps to his ulna, as in Fig. 72-24. If less than half his olecranon fossa is intact, fix the two fragments of his olecranon by tension band wiring (Fig. 72-26). In this method two stiff Kirschner wires go obliquely through his olecranon

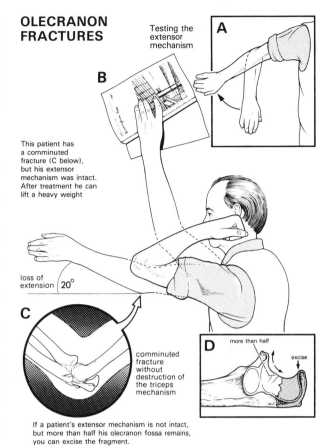

Fig. 72-23 CONSERVATIVE TREATMENT FOR AN OLECRANON FRACTURE. A, testing a patient's triceps mechanism by seeing if he can extend his elbow against gravity. B, early active movements with his arm in a sling gave this patient enough power to lift this heavy book, with only a little loss of extension. C, shows the extensive comminution of his olecranon. D, If a patient has lost his triceps mechanism and has more than half his olecranon fossa intact, excise the proximal fragment and sew his triceps tendon to his ulna. If less than half is intact use tension band wiring. *Kindly contributed by Peter Bewes and John Stewart.*

and are anchored in the cortical bone of the anterior surface of his ulna to give the fragment longitudinal stability. They are kept together by a band of flexible steel wire, wound in a figure of eight. If you don't have the equipment for tension band wiring, or if a patient's olecranon is in many fragments, you can excise the fragments and suture his triceps to his ulna.

If his elbow needs repair, but this is not possible, treat him with active movements, and warn him to expect some permanent loss of extension.

Olecranon injuries in children. A child may have several centres of ossification in his olecranon, so you may have difficulty deciding if he has a fracture or not. If in doubt, X-ray his other elbow. The epiphysis of the olecranon occasionally separates from the shaft of the ulna between the ages of 10 and 16. If it does, treat it in the same way as you would a fracture.

FRACTURES OF THE OLECRANON

ACTIVE MOVEMENTS TREATMENT

INDICATIONS (1) All patients in whom the triceps mechanism is intact, as described above, even if the fragments have separated slightly. (2) A patient who is too old to notice that active extension is lost, for example, he will never need to reach to lift a jam jar from a high shelf.

METHOD Put the patient's arm in a sling for a few days, and give him analgesics. Encourage him to use his arm, and to

EXCISING COMMINUTED FRAGMENTS OF THE OLECRANON

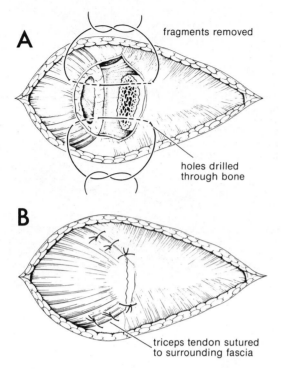

A fragments removed

holes drilled through bone

B

triceps tendon sutured to surrounding fascia

Fig. 72-24. EXCISING THE FRAGMENTS OF THE OLECRANON. This is only necessary if a patient has lost the use of the extensor mechanism of his elbow and if more than half his olecranon fossa is intact. *After Robb and Smith with kind permission.*

THE MECHANICS OF TENSION BAND WIRING

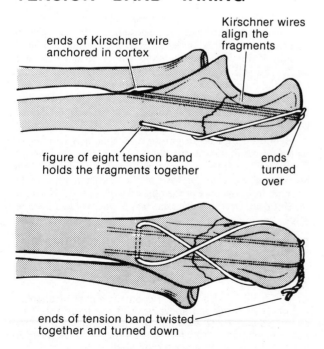

ends of Kirschner wire anchored in cortex

Kirschner wires align the fragments

figure of eight tension band holds the fragments together

ends turned over

ends of tension band twisted together and turned down

Fig. 72-25 THE MECHANICS OF TENSION BAND WIRING. The stiff Kirshner wires maintain alignment, while the figure of eight of soft wire holds the fragments together. *From the AO handbook.*

TENSION BAND WIRING

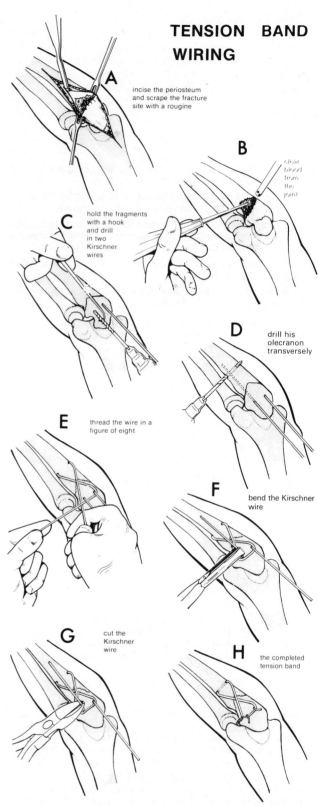

A incise the periosteum and scrape the fracture site with a rougine

B clear blood from the joint

C hold the fragments with a hook and drill in two Kirschner wires

D drill his olecranon transversely

E thread the wire in a figure of eight

F bend the Kirschner wire

G cut the Kirschner wire

H the completed tension band

Fig. 72-26 TENSION BAND WIRING. If less than half the patient's olecranon fossa is intact, fix the two fragments of his olecranon by tension band wiring like this. *From the AO handbook.*

take it out of the sling from time to time and let it dangle. Encourage him to return early to light work.

CAUTION! Don't splint his elbow, especially not in extension.

His elbow will heal rapidly. If there was less than 5 mm displacement, there will be bony union. Otherwise, there will

252

be a slightly unstable fibrous union with an excellent range of movement.

EXCISING FRAGMENT(S) IN OLECRANON FRACTURES

INDICATIONS (1) Loss of the extensor mechanism of a patient's elbow caused by a fracture involving half or less of his olecranon fossa. More than half of his olecranon fossa remains intact on the shaft. (2) Any fracture of his olecranon in which the extensor mechanism is lost and the equipment for tension band wiring is not available.

If possible, refer him. However, if you cannot refer him, proceed as follows.

INCISION Exsanguinate the patient's arm with an Esmarch bandage (3.8). Place a blood pressure cuff around his arm as high as possible. Lie him on his back and fold his arm over his chest so that his elbow lies uppermost.

Incise and expose his olecranon, as described below for tension band wiring. Remove the bone fragments, and cut them away from the tendon of his triceps. Drill two holes in the shaft of his ulna. If you don't have a drill, you can make holes at the edge of his ulna with a strong towel clip. Pass strong sutures through these holes, and then through his triceps tendon, as in A, Fig. 72-24.

CAUTION ! Watch his ulnar nerve. Find and gently retract it.

TENSION BAND WIRING FOR OLECRANON FRACTURES

INDICATIONS Loss of the extension mechanism of the elbow, due to a fracture involving more that half the patient's olecranon fossa, with a single proximal fragment suitable for wiring. If possible refer the patient. If you cannot refer him, proceed as follows.

EQUIPMENT Kirschner wire, 0.35 mm stainless steel wire, Faraboef's rougine, pliers, wire cutters, scoop, bone hooks or towel clips.

INCISION Make an 8 cm longitudinal incision just lateral to the point of the patient's elbow (A, in Fig. 72-26). Incise the periosteum and scrape it away from the fracture site with a rougine. Expose the smaller fragment. It may be in smaller pieces than the X-rays suggest. Open the joint and clear away any blood clot (B).

Hold the fragments together with a bone hook or towel clip so as to close up the joint line. Hold the hook so that it presses in the long axis of the ulna. Try to obtain hair–line reduction. The fracture line will be easier to see if you have previously stripped away the periosteum from around it. Drill in two Kirschner wires (C). Drill the olecranon transversely for the insertion of the tension band (D).

Thread the wire in a figure of eight through the hole in the ulna and round the Kirschner wires (E). Twist the ends of the wire loosely together. Bend the ends of a Kirschner wire upwards at 90° with pliers (F).

Cut the first Kirschner wire, leaving a few millimetres of its bent end projecting (G). Do the same thing for the other Kirschner wire. Turn the bent cut ends of both of them back against the bone. Twist the ends of the tension band together and cut them off (H).

POSTOPERATIVE CARE (both methods) Put the patient's arm in a collar and cuff and start active movements early.

CAUTION ! Don't let him try to extend his arm actively against resistance for at least a month.

DIFFICULTIES WITH OLECRANON FRACTURES

If the patient is a CHILD (rare), immobilize his elbow in extension for 5 weeks. Stiffness is unlikely to be a problem.

73 The forearm

73.1 Introduction

The results of treating fractures of the forearm are often so bad that the literature about them is only exceeded by that on the hip. Fractures of the forearm are mostly the result of a direct blow. When a patient's bones are broken, the muscles attached to the fragments pull them out of place, and make treatment particularly difficult.

(1) Either forearm bone can fracture alone. (2) Both bones can fracture simultaneously, usually in their middle thirds. When this happens in a child, the fracture is likely to be greenstick. (3) Either bone can fracture, and at the same time, the upper or the lower joint between them can dislocate. If the radius fractures, the lower radio–ulnar joint may subluxate (Galeazzi fracture). If the proximal third of the ulna fractures, the head of the radius may dislocate anteriorly (Monteggia fracture). These dislocations are often missed, *so always include a patient's wrist and his elbow on a forearm film,* particularly if the fragments are overlapped or angulated.

EXAMINING THE FOREARM Palpate the whole of the subcutaneous border of the patient's ulna, and the lower two thirds of his radius.

Squeeze his radius and ulna together in the lower part of his forearm. If this hurts him, he probably has a fracture.

Examine the head of his radius (72.1) (Monteggia fracture) and his inferior radio–ulnar joint (Galeazzi fracture) to make sure they are not dislocated.

Examine his elbow and his wrist.

X-RAYS should include the patient's wrist and a lateral view of his elbow. A line through the long axis of his radius should pass through his capitulum in both views, as in Fig. 73-4.

X-RAY THE PATIENT'S WRIST AND HIS ELBOW

Most fractures of the radius and all fractures of both bones are usually treated by open methods where skills and facilities are good. But if you are not a skilled surgeon, and your facilities are not perfect, closed methods are more likely to give your patients adequate function at minimum risk (69.3). Isolated fractures of the ulna are more easily treated than those of the radius, because the muscles attached to the ulna are much less likely to displace its fragments.

Closed methods of reduction use the long arm cast described below, modified by varying the position of the patient's wrist to suit the needs of particular fractures. If both his bones are broken you can gently squeeze the cast from front to back to correct the angulation of the fragments towards one another. A forearm cast is heavy, so hang it from his neck. If you don't, its weight may redisplace the fragments, or press on his radial nerve and paralyse it. Most casts for forearm fractures, especially those for fractures of both bones, must go above the elbow.

CASTS FOR THE ARM

A LONG ARM CAST The first cast on a forearm fracture should always be a long arm cast. Apply a single layer of cotton wool to the patient's arm, then put cotton pads over the bony points around his elbow, and in his antecubital fossa.

Apply the cast from just below his shoulder to his MP joints. Hold his elbow at 90°, and his thumb and fingers free. His thumb must be free enough to touch his little finger. If his thumb is held out in abduction, it will be so stiff when you remove the cast as to be temporarily useless.

Carry the cast to the base of his thumb and knuckles and to his distal palmar crease. If you carry it beyond this point, he will not be able to move his fingers.

Adjust the rotation of his forearm as is best for each particular fracture, as described later (73.5).

Take a narrow plaster bandage, mould a plaster eye over the centre of gravity of the cast, and tie it with a comfortable collar around his neck.

CAUTION ! If the fracture is recent, split the cast (70.4, 70.6).

Alternatively: (1) Instead of applying a circular cast, apply anterior and posterior slabs and bandage them in place. Or, (2) apply plaster to the patient's forearm first, and when this has set, complete the cast above his elbow.

A FOREARM CAST Use this to protect a patient's forearm bones from refracture for a few weeks after they have united, until they have consolidated.

73.2 Isolated fractures of the shaft of the ulna

A blow on the back of the patient's forearm breaks his ulna. The fracture is complete and transverse, with minimal displacement. There may be slight angulation and bowing, but there is no shift, no overlap, and no rotation. The subcutaneous border of his ulna is tender and swollen over the fracture. These fractures are common and easily treated, because the intact radius makes a good splint.

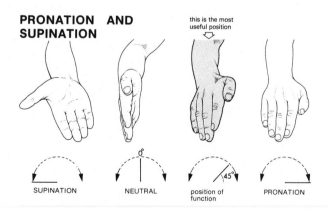

PRONATION AND SUPINATION

this is the most useful position

SUPINATION   NEUTRAL   position of function   PRONATION

Fig. 73-1 IF PRONATION AND SUPINATION ARE LIKELY TO BE LIMITED by the nature of the fracture, the patient's hand will be most useful to him if his forearm is in a position of mid–pronation. *Kindly contributed by John Stewart.*

A LONG ARM CAST

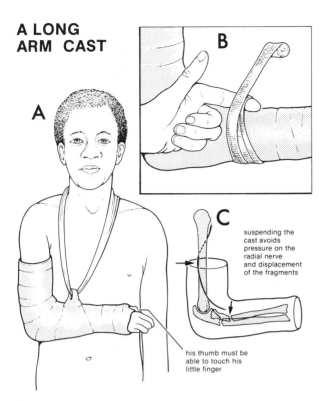

Fig. 73-2 A LONG ARM CAST. Suspending the cast avoids pressure on the patient's radial nerve. Make sure that his thumb is free and able to touch his little finger. *Kindly contributed by Peter Bewes.*

FRACTURES OF THE ULNA

Make sure that the head of the patient's radius is not dislocated by including his elbow in a lateral X-ray. If it is, he has a Monteggia fracture (73.3).

THE UPPER TWO THIRDS Treat him with active movements in a sling until he can use his arm without discomfort.

THE LOWER THIRD A small plaster slab may ease his discomfort.

Protect both types of fracture in a sling for 5 weeks, then test for union by squeezing his radius and ulna towards one another.

If there is no tenderness, he can use his arm for anything he likes, except heavy manual work.

If there is tenderness, the fragments have not yet united, so apply a skin tight cast from his elbow to his wrist, and continue active movements. Leave it on for five weeks, by which time it should have united.

ISOLATED FRACTURE OF THE SHAFT OF THE ULNA

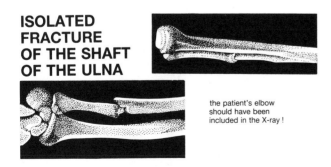

the patient's elbow should have been included in the X-ray !

Fig. 73-3 ISOLATED FRACTURES OF THE SHAFT OF THE ULNA. Make sure that the head of the patient's radius is not dislocated by including his elbow in a lateral X-ray. If it is dislocated, he has a Monteggia fracture. Unfortunately, this has not been done here!

73.3 Fractures of the proximal third of the ulna, with dislocation of the head of the radius (Monteggia's fracture)

In places where there is much personal violence, this is a common and nasty adult's fracture; elsewhere it is a rare children's fracture. An adult raises his arm to protect his head from a blow, and receives the full force of the blow on his forearm, breaking his ulna and dislocating the head of his radius. The important part of the injury is the dislocation of the head of his radius, not the fracture of his ulna, which is usually broken in its upper

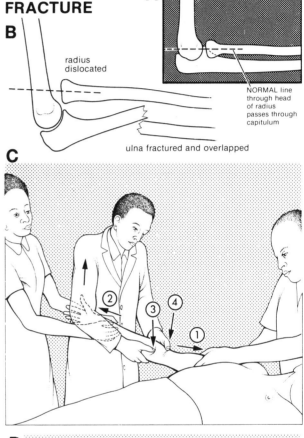

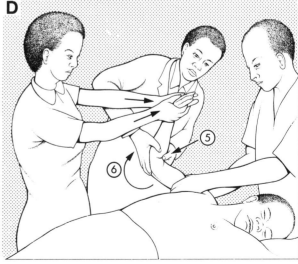

Fig. 73-4 MONTEGGIA'S FRACTURE. A, in a normal arm a line through the head of the radius passes through the capitulum. B, in Monteggia's fracture this line passes through the shaft of the humerus. C, and D, you will need two assistants to help you reduce the head of the radius. *After de Palma, with kind permission.*

third. Rarely, his ulna does not break, and dislocation of the head of his radius is his only injury. When his ulna does break, the fracture may be greenstick, and its fragments may only bow. Or, it may break completely and its fragments overlap, as in Fig. 73-4.

If you suspect that a patient has dislocated the head of his radius, take an AP *and a lateral view*, because you may see the dislocation in one view, but not in the other. A line through the centre of his radius should pass through his capitulum. If the fragments of his broken ulna overlap, either his radius must also be fractured, or its head must be dislocated.

Unless the dislocation of the head of a patient's radius is reduced, he will never be able to bend his elbow again. Closed reduction is usually possible in children, and sometimes in adults. Try to reduce this injury early, because the longer you delay the more difficult it will become.

MONTEGGIA'S FRACTURE

The method is the same, whether or not the patient has fractured his ulna.

Anaesthetize the patient and find two assistants. Extend his arm and supinate it. Ask one of your assistants to hold his upper arm (1, in Fig. 73-4) and your other assistant to exert traction on his wrist (2).

While your two assistants are maintaining traction, press the distal end of the proximal ulnar fragment posteriorly (3). Then try to press the head of the patient's radius posteriorly (4).

Next, while still pressing the head of his radius (5), flex his supinated forearm (6). The head of his radius should reduce with a 'clunk', and his ulna should finally straighten completely as it does so.

Apply anterior and posterior slabs directly to his skin from his axilla to the heads of his metacarpals, with his elbow flexed at about 80° and his forearm supinated. Bandage the slabs in place. They will help to keep the head of his radius in place.

Start finger and shoulder exercises immediately.

CAUTION ! The head of the radius is unstable after this injury and it can redisplace, so X-ray him at weekly intervals.

Hang the slabs from his neck for 3 weeks, remove them, change them for a collar and cuff, and add elbow movements to those he is already doing. Movements will take months to return—don't force them.

IF REDUCTION OF THE RADIAL HEAD FAILS OR THE PATIENT PRESENTS LATE, management depends on his age.

If he is an adult, refer him for immediate open reduction, as described below. If the head of his radius is not reduced, he will never be able to bend his elbow again.

If he is a child, and the injury is less than 3 months old, refer him. If the injury is more than 3 months old, leave him. Normal movements will usually return in spite of the unsightly hypermobility of his radial head.

IF REDUCTION OF THE ULNA FAILS so that it remains seriously angulated, refer him.

DIFFICULTIES WITH A MONTEGGIA FRACTURE

If the HEAD OF THE RADIUS WILL NOT REDUCE, it may have gone through a hole in the capsule, and so be irreducible by closed methods. Open reduction will be necessary, so refer the patient immediately. If the dislocation is an old one, reduction may be impossible by any method. If he is an adult, it may then be necessary to excise the head of his radius.

If a Monteggia FRACTURE IS OPEN, do a careful wound toilet. If there is an haemarthrosis, aspirate the patient's elbow (Fig. 72-4), and reduce the fragments into the best position you can. Provide skin cover by delayed primary closure or grafting, and then start early active movements.

73.4 Fractures of the shaft of the radius with dislocation of the lower radio–ulnar joint (Galeazzi's fracture)

These are rare, difficult fractures. In children the fracture of the radius is greenstick, and the only displacement is an anterior bow. Adults have a complete fracture of the radius in which the distal radial fragment tilts, shifts anteriorly, overlaps, and inclines towards the ulna. At the same time the distal end of the ulna dislocates from both the radius and the carpus, and displaces dorsally to make an ugly bulge on the back of the wrist.

Incomplete Galeazzi fractures (children) cause a child's lower forearm to bow forwards. He is tender over a greenstick fracture of his radius, usually in its distal third. The distal end of his ulna is also tender. Closed reduction is usually straightforward.

Complete Galeazzi fractures (adults) are often open, with the skin punctured on the front or back of the patient's forearm, and his radius sticking through it. There is usually no need to explore the wound because there is no dead tissue to remove. Instead, seal the puncture hole with a dressing, before you reduce the fracture.

GALEAZZI'S FRACTURE

INCOMPLETE GALEAZZI FRACTURES

If the fracture is in the distal third of the radius, even a 45° angulation in a small child does not matter, and soon corrects itself as he grows. The younger he is, and the closer the fracture to the epiphysis, the greater the angulation you can accept.

If the fracture is higher up in the middle third of the child's radius, moulding is less rapid and less complete, especially if he is older. So anaesthetize him, and bend his radius back

GALEAZZI's FRACTURE

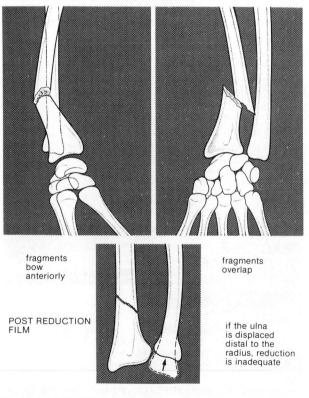

fragments bow anteriorly

POST REDUCTION FILM

fragments overlap

if the ulna is displaced distal to the radius, reduction is inadequate

Fig. 73-5 GALEAZZI FRACTURES are rare and difficult. In children the fracture of the radius is greenstick, and the only displacement is an anterior bow. Adults have a complete fracture.

into place. This reduces the fracture and the dislocation of his distal radio–ulnar joint. If the distal end of his ulna happens also to have been fractured, the overlap of the radius usually remains.

Apply a long arm cast with his elbow at 90°, his arm in mid–rotation, and his wrist slightly palmar flexed.

After 6 weeks, replace this cast by a shorter one extending from the upper part of his forearm to above his knuckles. This will hold his radius straight and prevent him dorsiflexing his wrist. Leave this short cast on for 6 weeks.

COMPLETE GALEAZZI FRACTURES

CLOSED REDUCTION Anaesthetize the patient, using a relaxant if possible. Then suspend his forearm over the side of the table from a drip pole as in Fig. 73-10.

Reduce the fracture until his forearm looks normal, apply a long arm cast, and mould it to give it a flat cross–section as in Fig. 73-9. Complete the cast, and include a ring in it.

X-ray him again, and consult Fig. 73-5. If his radial styloid is distal to his ulnar styloid, reduction is adequate. If his ulnar styloid is distal, reduction is not adequate.

If reduction is adequate, continue treatment as for a mid-shaft fracture of the radius and ulna (73.6).

If reduction is not adequate, his radius slips anteriorly into its displaced position, and his ulna slips distally to the head of his radius. If possible, refer him within the first week for open reduction of his radius. This will correct the position of his ulna at the same time.

DISASTER WITH A GALEAZZI FRACTURE

If the FRACTURE WAS MISSED, both bones will have united solidly, and the lower end of the patient's ulna will stick out as a lump on the back of his wrist, which will be stiff and painful. Refer him for the excision of the lower end of his ulna.

AN ISOLATED FRACTURE OF THE RADIUS

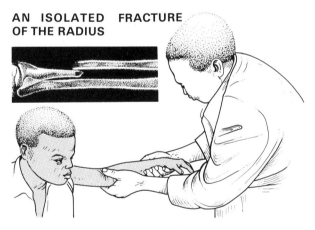

Fig. 73-6 ISOLATED FRACTURES OF THE SHAFT OF THE RADIUS. **Management depends on the degree of angulation. If angulation is minimal, bandage the child's arm. More than a minimal degree of angulation at the centre of the bone is not acceptable. If necessary, break the bone completely and realign the fragments.**

73.5 Isolated midshaft fractures of the shaft of the radius

The fact that a patient's radius rotates makes its fractures much more difficult to treat than those of his ulna. If there is no overlap, no reduction is necessary, and you can treat him with a plaster forearm splint. But if the fragments overlap, treatment is more difficult, because his intact ulna prevents you distracting and angulating his broken radius. Closed methods may work, but if they fail, this fracture needs open reduction and internal fixation. The radius usually breaks through its proximal third. If it breaks through the junction of its middle and distal thirds, closed methods are even less likely to succeed.

ROTATION OF FRAGMENTS OF THE RADIUS

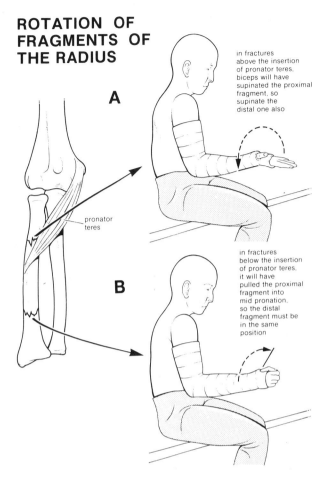

Fig. 73-7 ROTATION OF THE FRAGMENTS OF THE RADIUS. A, **in fractures above the insertion of pronator teres, biceps will have supinated the proximal fragment, so supinate the distal one also. B, in fractures below the insertion of pronator teres, this muscle will probably have pulled the proximal fragment into mid–pronation, so immobilize the distal fragment in this position also.** *Kindly contributed by John Stewart.*

A fracture allows the proximal fragment of the radius to rotate on the distal one. You cannot alter the position of the proximal fragment, so all you can do is to try to find out where it is, and line up the distal fragment with it, before you immobilize them both.

The supinating muscles, biceps, and supinator are attached to the proximal end of the radius, and the pronating muscles, pronator teres, and pronator quadratus are attached to its distal end. In fractures above the insertion of pronator teres (half–way down the radius) the supinators supinate the proximal fragment. In more distal fractures its position is more variable. There are several ways of finding out how far the proximal fragment has rotated.

(1) You can assume that, (a) in fractures of the proximal third of the radius (above the insertion of pronator teres), the proximal fragment will be in full supination, and (b) that in fractures of the distal two thirds below the insertion of this muscle, it will have pulled the proximal fragment into mid–pronation. This is a useful compromise because a forearm fixed in mid–pronation is only a minor disability, whereas one which becomes fixed in full supination will be a considerable handicap.

(2) The most accurate way is to take an AP X-ray of the upper end of the patient's injured radius, and use the position of his radial tuberosity as a guide to how far the proximal fragment has rotated. Either, (a) use Fig. 73-8 as a guide, or (b) better, if you have plenty of X-ray film and can spare it, take several X-rays of his normal radius, in various degrees of pronation and

supination, and find the position which best matches the fractured one. When you immobilize it, do so in this position.

Some surgeons routinely convert isolated greenstick fractures of the radius and greenstick fractures of both bones into complete ones. If this is done, they are said to be less likely to redisplace inside the cast after reduction.

IMMOBILIZE PROXIMAL THIRD FRACTURES IN SUPINATION
IMMOBILIZE MIDDLE AND DISTAL THIRD FRACTURES IN MID–PRONATION

HOW FAR HAS THE PROXIMAL FRAGMENT OF THE RADIUS ROTATED

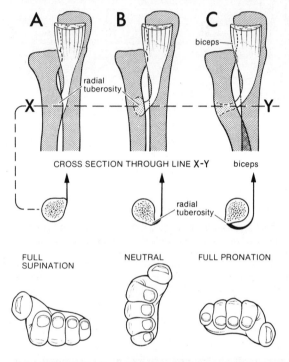

Fig. 73-8 HOW FAR HAS THE PROXIMAL FRAGMENT ROTATED? **Take an AP view of the elbow. Look for the position of the radial tuberosity. Match it with positions A, B, or C, and apply the cast with the patient's hand in the position shown.** *Kindly contributed by John Stewart.*

ISOLATED MIDSHAFT FRACTURES OF THE RADIUS

Examine the patient's lower radio–ulnar joint carefully to make sure it is not abnormally prominent and dislocated. If it is, he has a Galeazzi fracture.

ADULTS WITH AN ISOLATED MIDSHAFT FRACTURE OF THE RADIUS

If possible, refer the patient for internal fixation, particularly if: (1) the fracture is at the junction of the middle and distal thirds, or (2) you need to immobilize his forearm in either of these extreme positions, because subsequent rotation is more likely to be limited.

If you cannot refer him, proceed as follows.

WITHOUT OVERLAP No reduction is necessary, but the fragments need a splint to stop them rotating, so apply a long arm cast. Use the methods described above to decide the correct degree of pronation and supination in which to immobilise his arm. Flatten the cross section of his cast as

in Fig. 73-9. Don't pad it, except over the bony points at his elbow.

Start active finger movements immediately.

WITH OVERLAP Make one or even two attempts to reduce the fracture by the gentle 'squeezing grip', shown in Fig. 73-9. If you fail, refer him.

CAUTION ! Don't grip too hard, or you may impede the circulation in his arm.

CHILDREN WITH AN ISOLATED MIDSHAFT FRACTURE OF THE RADIUS

Management depends on the degree of angulation.

If angulation is minimal, bandage the child's arm.

If angulation is more than minimal, anaesthetize him, suspend his forearm, reduce the fracture, and apply a cast as above. To prevent the fracture slipping subsequently, slightly overcorrect the position.

CAUTION ! More than a minimal degree of angulation at the centre of the bone is not acceptable. If necessary, break the bone completely and realign the fragments.

Alternatively, apply the cast. While it is still wet and soft, quickly snap the greenstick fracture through completely. Hold the fragments reduced until the cast is hard.

THE POSITION OF FUNCTION IS THE POSITION OF MID–PRONATION

73.6 Midshaft fractures of the radius and ulna

These are common and difficult fractures: (1) The fragments are difficult to align, (2) they displace easily, and (3) cross–union may occur, and prevent the patient rotating his forearm. If he is under 18, open reduction and internal fixation are unnecessary, but in older patients this is one of the fractures which is generally treated by open methods—*if skills and operating conditions are good enough.* They seldom are in the district hospitals for which we write. So refer the patient immediately if you can; if necessary, internal fixation can be delayed 10 days. If you wait, make sure you correct overlap by applying traction meanwhile.

If you cannot refer the patient, treat him as we describe. Make quite sure that if rotation will later be limited, his forearm will at least be fixed in the most convenient position for him. This is in 45° of pronation, as in Fig. 73-1. For many patients a forearm fixed in this position is only a minor disability, because movements of the shoulder can compensate to some extent for pronation and supination of the forearm. Fixation in any other position is a completely unnecessary tragedy. Bowing may be ugly, but it is much less serious.

73.6a Greenstick midshaft fractures of the middle third of both forearm bones

These cause an obvious bowing of a child's forearm. Correct angulation carefully, because the fracture is in the centre of the bone and remodelling will not correct it later (69.6). Some surgeons deliberately break greenstick fractures through completely with the aim of reducing the risk of displacement recurring.

APPLY THE CAST IN MID–PRONATION

Anaesthesia is kind but not essential. Ketamine is satisfactory (A 8.2).

If the fracture is undisplaced, apply a plaster slab.

If the fracture is displaced, apply a circular cast from the child's knuckles to the middle of his upper arm with his forearm in mid–pronation. While the cast is still soft, straighten his forearm. Correct angulation carefully, especially in the lateral (coronal) plane, which moulds even less readily than angulation in the anteroposterior (sagittal) plane. CAUTION ! Split the cast. If you don't split it, he would be much safer with a plaster backslab. Some surgeons routinely treat displaced greenstick forearm fractures with slabs.

Start active movements of the child's shoulder and fingers as soon as possible.

X-ray him during the first 3 weeks, look for angulation, and if necessary, correct it under anaesthesia, as described below for angulation in complete fractures.

After 5 weeks, remove the long arm cast, and test for clinical union. If the fracture has united, replace it by a sling, and continue active movement. If it has not united, reapply the cast.

Alternatively, break his bones through with a sharp bending force, and slightly overcorrect the deformity. Suspend his forearm as for a complete fracture, apply a long arm cast, and be sure to split it!

DISTRACTING THE FOREARM BONES

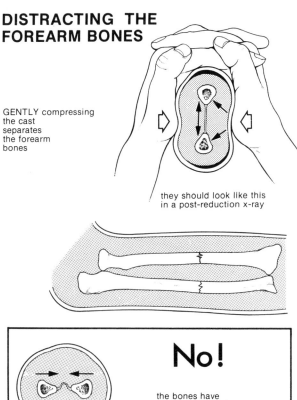

GENTLY compressing the cast separates the forearm bones

they should look like this in a post-reduction x-ray

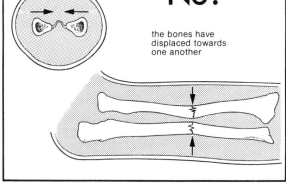

No!

the bones have displaced towards one another

Fig. 73-9 DISTRACTING THE FOREARM BONES. If you exert gentle pressure on a patient's forearm through a soft cast, this will separate his forearm bones and help to prevent cross–union. *Kindly contributed by Peter Bewes.*

73.6b Complete fractures of the middle third of both forearm bones

If both a patient's forearm bones are broken in the middle, his forearm is free to bend in the middle. You can easily correct this angulation; the difficult part is separating the fragments when they have inclined towards one another. In the following method the patient's arm is suspended vertically from a drip stand while a cast is applied. This: (1) prevents the fragments bending under the influence of gravity while the cast sets, (2) allows you to apply the cast in a single stage, and (3) lets you correct the inclination of the radius and ulna towards one another by *gently* squeezing the cast anteroposteriorly while it sets. This flattens its cross section, compresses the muscles of the patient's forearm, and so makes them push the two bones apart.

This is a potentially dangerous cast, so remember to split it as described below. If you split it correctly, you will not lose reduction. Never use an ordinary backslab, which is quite ineffective in complete fractures.

The details are critical. If you neglect them, your results will be bad. Try to enthuse the patient with the part he can play in getting his bones to unite by using his fingers early and actively. The muscles of his fingers arise from his broken bones, so active finger exercises will cause small movements of his muscles inside the cast, and promote union. Tell him to do up his own buttons, to feed himself, and to do anything he can with his hands.

GIVE THE CAST A FLATTENED CROSS SECTION

COMPLETE FRACTURES OF THE MIDDLE THIRD OF THE RADIUS AND ULNA

If you can refer the patient to an expert for open reduction, do so.

CAUTION ! If there is: (1) much swelling, or (2) weakness of finger movements, suspend the patient's arm from a drip stand using metacarpal traction (Fig. 70-13), or skin traction (70.10), until these signs have subsided. If he is unconscious, apply metacarpal traction until he recovers.

SETTING A MIDSHAFT FRACTURE OF THE RADIUS AND ULNA

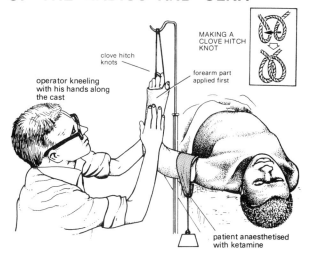

MAKING A CLOVE HITCH KNOT

clove hitch knots

forearm part applied first

operator kneeling with his hands along the cast

patient anaesthetised with ketamine

Fig. 73-10 SETTING A MIDSHAFT FRACTURE OF THE RADIUS AND ULNA. The forearm part of the cast is being applied while a sling and weight are applying traction to the upper arm. *Kindly contributed by John Stewart and Peter Bewes.*

Anaesthetize him. Ketamine is satisfactory (A 8.2). Find an assistant. If a spicule of bone has punctured his skin, wash and dress it before attempting reduction.

Find two assistants.

If the patient is already in metacarpal traction, leave it on until you have completed the cast.

If he is not in metacarpal traction, use a bandage and clove hitch knots to suspend his thumb and middle finger from a drip stand, so that you can later pass a plaster bandage across his palm.

Lie him horizontally close to the edge of the table. Adjust the height of the drip stand, so that his forearm is vertical, with his elbow flexed at 90° well clear of the table.

If any overlap remains, reduce it by applying a sling and a weight of 5 kg or more to his upper arm. Or, ask your assistant to press downwards on his arm, or to hold his elbow and pull it downwards.

Except in very fat, muscular, or swollen arms, you should be able to feel when the fragments are aligned. Traction usually reduces any overlap, but if it does not, proceed as follows.

If the patient is an adult, increase the deformity by angulating the fragments, getting them to hitch, and then straightening them, as in Fig. 73-13.

If he is a child, perfect end to end apposition is not necessary, and some overlap is acceptable.

CAUTION ! If you fail to correct the angular or rotational deformity in an adult or a child, loss of pronation and supination may follow.

APPLY A LONG ARM CAST When the arm looks and feels good, apply the cast. Apply the forearm part of the cast first, with the sling and weight still attached to the patient's upper arm to steady his elbow. First, apply a single layer of wool to his arm, then put cotton wool pads over the bony points round his elbow. These will make the cast more comfortable, and make rehabilitation easier.

Use cold water to make the plaster set slowly. First apply a cast from the patient's knuckles to his lower axilla. Apply it with his forearm in that position of rotation in which reduction is most easily obtained. Preferably apply it in mid–pronation, so that if rotation is limited later, it will be in the most useful range. Bring the cast as far as the IP joint of his thumb, and his midpalmar crease. This will help to prevent his thumb moving and dislodging the lower fragment of his radius. *The cast must allow free movements of his fingers, and of the distal phalanx of his thumb.*

As the cast sets, squeeze it *lightly* between your hands from front to back, to flatten it slightly and to separate his radius and ulna. Some surgeons mould anteroposterior grooves in the cast to separate the two bones.

Remove the sling and continue the cast to his axilla. Build a loop into the cast and support it in a sling. Later, support the cast with a sling through the loop.

CAUTION ! ALWAYS split the cast! Do this while it is still soft (70.6). Make a single cut along its ulna side, from the patient's hand to his axilla. If his arm is painful, or he is unable to move his fingers, spread the cast (70.6), and treat him as described below.

X-ray him immediately after reduction. If this is unsatisfactory, have one further attempt at reduction. If this fails, refer him for internal fixation.

If reduction is unsatisfactory, and you cannot refer him for internal fixation, accept the overlap and allow his forearm to heal in mid–pronation, which is the position of function. Provided his arm is in this position, he will probably have reasonable function, even if there is overlap.

POSTOPERATIVE CARE Watch the circulation in his fingers carefully. The compartment syndrome described below can occur.

CAUTION ! Can he move his fingers? Is passive extension painful?

Start shoulder and finger exercises immediately. Tell him to put his hand as far behind his head as he can. This will exercise his shoulder. Encourage him to use his hands.

X-ray him at 2 weeks, and again at 4 weeks, and make sure

that the rotation has remained in the position of function. If necessary, correct any angulation.

You can correct mild angulation by wedging (70.7), but a change of cast is safer. If you decide to wedge it, do this carefully, because it can precipitate Volkmann's ischaemic contracture. More severe angulation will need a new cast. After 4 weeks the bones will have united and it will be too late to do any correction.

If the patient is an adult, the cast must remain intact for 6 to 8 weeks. This is a long time, so it must be a good one. Examine for clinical union after 8 weeks. Gently spring his forearm bones. If these angulate or are tender, reapply the cast. Otherwise, put his arm in a sling, and encourage him to move his elbow and rotate his wrist.

If the cast needs to be changed for any reason, such as looseness, suspend his arm by his fingers to prevent the fracture angulating while you apply a new one.

If he is a child, keep his long arm cast on for 4 to 6 weeks, and then examine for union. He is very likely to refracture his arm, so apply a cast for another 6 weeks. This time, apply it to his forearm only. When you remove it, put his arm in a sling and encourage active movements.

DIFFICULTIES WITH MIDSHAFT FRACTURES OF THE FOREARM

If PAIN OR LOSS OF FINGER MOVEMENT DEVELOPS, split the cast if you have not already done so, spread it (70.6), and treat him as described in Section 73.7. The soft tissue swelling may be causing ischaemia which is much more serious than loss of position. You can correct this later by applying another cast.

If his FOREARM BONES WILL NOT UNITE, refer him. Reasons include: (1) sloppy plaster technique resulting in failure to immobilize his bones, (2) the failure to exercise his fingers, (3) not getting satisfactory reduction, soft tissue injury, or interposition and infection.

If his FRACTURED ULNA IS OPEN, there will probably be only a spike of bone projecting through his skin. Clean it and pull it back, or nibble it away. Toilet the wound, and suspend his forearm with Kirschner wire traction through his metacarpals (70.11) or skin traction on his fingers (70.10). Let his forearm hang vertically, so that the weight of his arm reduces the fracture. When the wound has begun to heal, treat him as for a closed fracture.

WATCH THE CIRCULATION IN HIS HAND CAREFULLY!
HE MUST KEEP MOVING HIS FINGERS!

73.7 The compartment syndrome in the forearm

If a patient with a forearm fracture suffers from the four Ps'—pain, paraesthesiae, pallor (if he is Caucasian), and paralysis, suspect that he has developed the compartment syndrome and may be in danger of its sequel, Volkmann's ischaemic contracture (70.4). This is more common with fractures of the forearm than it is with supracondylar fractures (72.8, 72.9).

The critical test is pain on passive extension of the patient's fingers. *A normal radial pulse does not rule out ischaemia.* If he cannot extend his fingers, there is compression in the anterior compartment of his forearm. If he cannot flex them, there is compression in the posterior compartment (rare). If, when you have removed the cast, the circulation and movement of his fingers does not rapidly return, decompress his forearm as described below. If possible, operate within a few hours of the onset of symptoms, but if he presents late, be prepared to operate even weeks later. If his muscles feel tense, swollen, and almost woody hard, decompression is urgent. Unfortunately, in splitting the cast you will lose reduction, so as soon as his circulation returns, apply skeletal traction. Later, reduce the fracture again, and reapply the cast.

Occasionally, a patient with a fractured forearm has signs of the compartment syndrome even before a cast is applied. It can also follow soft tissue injuries of his forearm, especially stab wounds, but sometimes even muscle contusion, as in the case below.

ASLAM (43 years) struck his forearm while waterskiing but did not fracture it. Eight hours later it became acutely painful and he could not extend his wrist or fingers. He consulted his neighbour, an orthopaedic surgeon, who decompressed his forearm within the hour, from wrist to elbow, as in Fig. 73-11, leaving his skin and fascia open. Dark swollen muscle bulged out of the wound. He was discharged the following morning, and his incision was closed 5 days later. He recovered completely. LESSONS (1) Remember the compartment syndrome. A happy outcome followed what might have been a major tragedy after a minor injury. (2) Be quick! Immediate decompression is imperative.

**INDURATION OF THE MUSCLES IS
PATHOGNOMONIC**

DECOMPRESSING THE
FOREARM

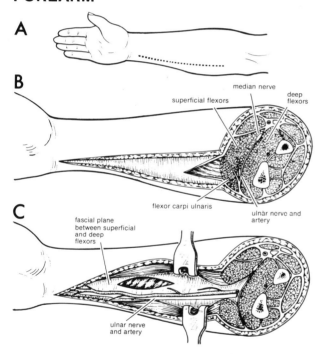

Fig. 73-11 DECOMPRESSION FOR THE COMPARTMENT SYNDROME showing a cross–section of the forearm with the positions of the ulnar nerve and artery. *After Matsen with kind permission.*

THE COMPARTMENT SYNDROME IN THE FOREARM

If a patient in a forearm cast complains of pain, believe him, and if he has a cast on, split it, spread it, and elevate his arm. If this does not rapidly relieve his symptoms, remove it. If the syndrome is advanced his arm will swell and become red. If his symptoms do not improve rapidly, proceed as follows.

Make an incision from his medial epicondyle to the ulnar end of the flexor crease on his wrist, as in A, Fig. 73-11. Incise the fascia over his flexor carpi ulnaris, and retract this muscle medially. Retract his superficial flexor muscles laterally, and incise the fascia over his deep flexors. Decompress each muscle by making a longitudinal incision through its sheath, carefully avoiding its nerve. The pale compressed muscle tissue will bulge up gratefully, as you release the pressure in its sheath. If you have acted in time, a conspicuous

hyperaemia will follow. If you are much too late, the deep flexor muscles will be yellow and necrotic.

CAUTION ! Don't cut his ulnar nerve or his ulnar artery. The nerve lies close to the artery underneath his flexor carpi ulnaris, and between it and his deep flexors.

Put Kirschner wires through his second, third, and fourth metacarpals (70.12), suspend his arm vertically, and leave the wound open and unsutured, under a vaseline gauze or a hypochlorite dressing.

Continue to apply traction. This usually reduces the fracture.

Leave the fascia open. If you can close the skin easily, do so. If you cannot close the skin easily, apply a gauze dressing and attempt secondary closure 5 days later. Apply a cast over the graft.

DIFFICULTIES WITH THE COMPARTMENT SYNDROME

If you have NO KIRSCHNER WIRE, decompress the patient's forearm, splint it with a plaster backslab, and refer him immediately.

If the SYNDROME IS ADVANCED when you decompress his forearm, maintain a high alkaline urine output, to assist the excretion of the myoglobin released from the necrotic muscle, and watch for renal failure (53.3).

If a CONTRACTURE DEVELOPS, apply splints to minimize the deformity as much as possible.

**DECOMPRESSING THE FOREARM IS AN ACUTE
EMERGENCY**

FRACTURE OF THE
LOWER QUARTER
OF THE RADIUS

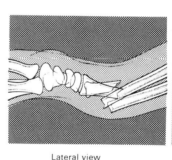

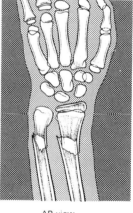

Lateral view   AP view

Fig. 73-12 FRACTURES OF THE LOWER QUARTER OF THE RADIUS AND ULNA usually occur in young children. There is posterior angulation and overlap, but very little angulation in the plane of the wrist. *Kindly contributed by John Stewart.*

73.8 Fractures of the lower quarter of the radius and ulna (usually young children)

In this common injury a young child breaks both his bones transversely about 4 cm above his wrist. The fracture is usually greenstick, and the lower fragments angulate radially and anteriorly. Sometimes his ulna remains intact, and the only X-ray sign is buckling of the cortex of his radius on one side (wrinkle fracture). If the fracture is complete, both lower fragments displace behind the shafts and produce a dinner fork deformity. The lower quarter of the forearm bones readily remodel, particularly in very young children, so that unless there is a significant degree of angulation, no reduction is necessary. Opinions vary as to whether you should reduce overlap or not. If necessary you can leave it. The younger the child, the more the displacement you can accept. See also Section 69.6 on the bony injuries of young children.

FRACTURES OF THE LOWER QUARTER OF THE RADIUS AND ULNA

ACCEPTABLE DISPLACEMENT This includes most greenstick fractures, especially those with any slight buckling of the cortex of the bone. (1) Angulation less than 30° in the plane of the wrist. (2) Lateral displacement without shortening. (3) Some surgeons also accept overlap.

Protect the child's arm with a slab and a crepe bandage, put it in a sling, and start active movements immediately.

UNACCEPTABLE DISPLACEMENT (1) More than 30° of angulation in the plane of the wrist. (2) Rotation. (3) Overlap is sometimes considered unacceptable.

In greenstick fractures anaesthesia is not essential. In complete fractures anaesthetize the child, preferably with ketamine.

CLOSED REDUCTION OF FRACTURES OF THE LOWER QUARTER OF THE RADIUS AND ULNA

If the lower fragment of the radius is angulated, straighten it. Disregard the ulna.

If you decide to reduce the overlap, increase the angulation as far as possible, press on the base of the distal fragments when they are fully angulated, get the ends to hitch, and then straighten and distract them as in Fig. 73-13. Apply a long arm cast in full pronation.

Consolidation takes 6 weeks. Keep the cast on for the full 6 weeks. The child may fall again and refracture his arm, so apply a forearm cast for another six weeks, *and split it!*.

IF CLOSED REDUCTION FAILS Attempts to correct overlap may fail because the pronator quadratus muscle comes between the bone ends. Management now depends on whether the child's epiphyseal growth lines have closed or not.

If the epiphyseal growth line at the lower end of the child's radius is open, it is not important if the fragments are end on or not, provided you get his radius reasonably straight. They will remodel themselves completely in 2 years, so some overlap is permissable. If you fail after two attempts, stop. Apply a long arm cast (73.1), and start exercises immediately.

If the epiphyseal growth line is closed, make a second attempt at closed reduction. If this fails, refer him.

Or, you can attempt open reduction if you are experienced. Do this as early as you can, but before 10 days.

OPEN REDUCTION Incise the back of the child's forearm longitudinally over the fracture, separate the muscles, open the periosteum longitudinally, and lever the displaced fragments into place with any convenient instrument, such as MacDonald's dissector. Close the wound in layers, and apply a backslab held in place with a crepe bandage. Take out the stitches a week later, and apply a long arm cast as for an extension fracture of the wrist (74.2), but extending above his elbow with his wrist in a neutral position.

Leave the long arm cast on for 6 weeks, and then apply a forearm cast for 4 more weeks.

73.9 Fracture separation of the distal radial epiphysis (10 to 15 years)

This is the most common epiphyseal injury. The fracture passes partly through the metaphysis of the child's radius, and partly through his epiphyseal line (Salter Harris Type II, Section 69.6). Its lower end usually displaces and tilts radially and posteriorly. There may also be a fracture of the styloid process of his ulna, or a separation of its epiphysis. Fortunately, if you reduce the epiphysis, subsequent disability is rare.

CHIBWE (7 years) had a minor fracture separation of his distal radial epiphysis. When he was first seen there was no displacement or swelling. A circular cast was applied and he was sent home. Next day he returned complaining of pain and stiff fingers. He was given aspirin and again sent home. Three days later he returned with a gangrenous hand and his forearm muscles sloughing under the cast. His forearm was amputated. LESSONS (1) Always split all circular casts on fresh fractures. (2) Where possible use slabs. (3) Take painful casts seriously. (4) 'Think Volkmann's'!

FRACTURE SEPARATION OF THE RADIAL EPIPHYSIS Give the child ketamine or a general anaesthetic.

If his radial epiphysis is displaced dorsally, press it firmly forwards into place. There is no need to exert traction, because his epiphysis is not impacted. It will hinge forwards on his intact dorsal periosteum, which will prevent over correction. Apply a well moulded cast extending above his elbow with his forearm pronated and his wrist ulnar deviated and slightly flexed. As always, split it (see the sad story above!). Leave it in place for 3 weeks.

His epiphysis may redisplace, so X-ray his wrist at short intervals. If it displaces, refer him for internal fixation.

The prognosis is good, even if there is slight residual angulation after reduction.

REDUCING OVERLAP

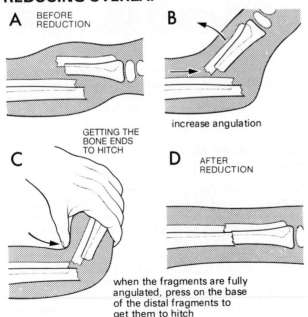

A BEFORE REDUCTION

B increase angulation

GETTING THE BONE ENDS TO HITCH

C when the fragments are fully angulated, press on the base of the distal fragments to get them to hitch

D AFTER REDUCTION

Fig. 73-13 REDUCING OVERLAP. Start by increasing the angulation, then get the ends of the bones to hitch (get their ends into contact). Finally, straighten them. *Kindly contributed by Peter Bewes*

DISPLACEMENT OF THE DISTAL RADIAL EPIPHYSIS

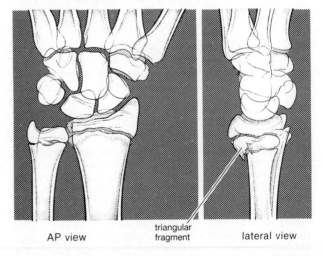

AP view

triangular fragment

lateral view

Fig. 73-14 FRACTURE SEPARATION OF THE DISTAL RADIAL EPIPHYSIS is the most common epiphyseal injury. A more typical appearance is that in N, and O, Fig. 69-7, which shows the fracture line passing partly through the metaphysis of the child's radius, and partly through his epiphyseal line (Salter Harris Type II).

74. The wrist

74.1 Introduction

One of the ways in which we use our hands is to protect our bodies from falling. Our outstretched hands are very good at doing this, but in doing so our wrists are particularly likely to get hurt in a variety of ways, which depend on how old we are. This chapter is entirely concerned with these injuries.

0–5 years A young child usually has a greenstick fracture of the lower third of his radius, and sometimes of his ulna also (73.6a). If his injury is severe, he may break both his forearm bones transversely just above his wrist (73.8).

5–10 years In an older child fractures of the lower quarter of the radius and ulna are more often complete (73.8), and the fragments may overlap.

10–15 years A child of this age typically has a fracture separation of his distal radial epiphysis (73.9).

Adults An adult is liable to two major groups of fractures at the lower ends of his forearm—those caused by hyperextension (common) of his wrist, and those caused by hyperflexion (unusual). These are most easily distinguished in a lateral X-ray.

(1) Hyperextension fractures comprise: (a) The common hyperextension (Colles) fracture in which the fracture line runs across the lower end of the radius parallel to the articular surface, with the distal fragment displaced posteriorly. (b) The much less common posterior marginal fracture in which the fracture line enters the joint. (c) Sometimes the distal fragment of the radius is comminuted.

(2) Hyperflexion fractures are rare. A lateral X-ray shows the fracture line running obliquely across the distal end of the radius. In (a) Smith's fracture, it does not enter the joint, but in (b) Barton's fracture, it does.

There is also *a group of minimal fractures,* including fractures of the radial styloid in which manipulation is rarely needed, and which you can immobilize as for a hyperextension fracture.

Falling on an outstretched hand occasionally causes *injuries of the carpal bones:* (1) The distal row of carpal bones can dislocate on the proximal row (intercarpal dislocation, 74.5), or (2) the lunate can dislocate. The wrist is seldom sprained, so that a 'sprain' is more likely to be a fracture of the scaphoid or of the triquetrum. Fractures of the triquetrum are difficult to see in an X-ray, so they are seldom diagnosed. Fortunately, they heal spontaneously.

Occasionally *the wrist can become dislocated on the forearm.* Reduce the dislocation immediately by exerting traction in the long axis of the forearm and hand.

EXAMINING THE WRIST

Observe the patient's wrist for swelling and deformity, and feel for warmth and tenderness.

Dorsiflexion Ask him to put the palms of his hands together, as in a position of prayer, and then to raise his elbows. This will let you compare the dorsiflexion in his wrists.

Palmar flexion Ask him to put the backs of his hands together and to depress his elbows. This will allow you to compare palmar flexion in his wrists.

Other movements Ask him to tuck his elbows into his sides. How far can he pronate and supinate them and deviate them in a radial or ulnar direction?

CAUTION! Have you examined his elbow? He may also have a fracture of the head of his radius.

SIGNS FOR PARTICULAR FRACTURES OF THE WRIST

Extension fractures (Colles fractures) Look at the back of the patient's wrist. Put the tip of one of your index fingers into the gap between his radial styloid and his wrist. Put the tip of your other index finger into the gap between his ulnar styloid and his wrist. This will show you the position of the two styloids clearly. The radial styloid is normally distal to the ulnar one. It is displaced proximally in an extension fracture. Its replacement is a useful sign of adequate reduction.

Examine both his wrists as if you were feeling his radial pulses. Has the normal concavity in front of his injured radius been filled out by a tender haematoma?

Is there a dinner fork deformity of his wrist? This is only present if backward displacement is gross, and is also seen in fractures of the lower quarter of the radius and ulna in children.

Flexion fractures (Smith's and Barton's fractures) Ask him to hold out his arm. Is his hand displaced anteriorly on his forearm, as in Fig. 74-7?

Fractures of the scaphoid (74.4) Three signs for this fracture are shown in Fig. 74-2.

(A) Hold the patient's hand with your left hand, and put the tip of your finger in the normal depression just distal to the end of his radius, between the two extensor tendons of his thumb (his 'anatomical snuffbox'). His scaphoid will be directly under it. *Deviate his hand towards his ulna,* and press. If he winces, he has probably fractured his scaphoid. The radial nerve passes over the snuffbox, and having this pressed can also be painful, so compare both sides carefully. Occasionally, there is mild swelling in the anatomical snuffbox.

(B) Does moving the patient's wrist cause him pain only at the extreme of its range?

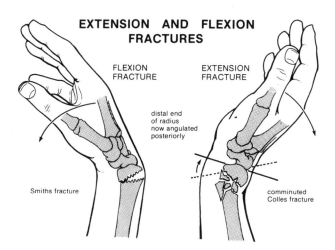

EXTENSION AND FLEXION FRACTURES

FLEXION FRACTURE

EXTENSION FRACTURE

distal end of radius now angulated posteriorly

Smiths fracture

comminuted Colles fracture

Fig. 74-1 FLEXION AND EXTENSION FRACTURES. In an extension fracture the normal volar angulation of the distal articular surface of the wrist shown in Fig. 74-3 is reduced or reversed. In this particular flexion fracture (Smith's) the fracture line does not enter the wrist joint.

THREE SIGNS FOR SCAPHOID FRACTURES

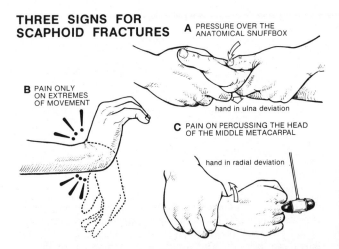

A PRESSURE OVER THE ANATOMICAL SNUFFBOX

hand in ulna deviation

B PAIN ONLY ON EXTREMES OF MOVEMENT

C PAIN ON PERCUSSING THE HEAD OF THE MIDDLE METACARPAL

hand in radial deviation

Fig. 74-2 THREE SIGNS OF A SCAPHOID FRACTURE. A, a patient's 'anatomical snuffbox' is the hollow between the tendons on the radial side of his wrist when his thumb is extended. Pressure here is painful if his scaphoid is fractured. B, pain only at the extremes of movement is typical of a scaphoid fracture. C, hit him with a patellar hammer over the head of his middle metacarpal and see if he feels pain.

(C) Ask him to clench his fist and deviate it radially. Percuss the head of his middle metacarpal. This is painful when his scaphoid is fractured. There may also be tenderness over the knuckles of his index and middle fingers, but none over those of his ring and little fingers.

Carpal dislocation Both carpal dislocations (intercarpal dislocation and dislocation of the lunate) produce a painful, swollen, immobile wrist. In addition, if a patient's lunate is dislocated, he may have any of these four special signs.

(1) Is there tenderness and an abnormally deep hollow on the back of his wrist just distal to his radius, in line with his first finger? Normally, the lunate occupies this hollow. If the lunate is dislocated this hollow is deep and abnormally tender.

(2) Ask him to clench both his fists. Compare their backs. If his middle metacarpal looks slightly shorter, his lunate may be dislocated (or his middle metacarpal may be fractured).

(3) Feel the volar aspect of his wrist, between his thenar and hypothenar eminences. If this is tender, and slightly full compared with the opposite side, his lunate may be dislocated. Percuss the fullness. This may produce paraesthesia in distribution of his median nerve.

(4) Examine his median nerve (75.3). A dislocated lunate may paralyse it, or produce numbness and tingling.

X-RAYS The routine views are an AP and a lateral. If you take a lateral view routinely you will not confuse flexion and extension fractures. If you suspect a fracture of the scaphoid, ask for oblique views. A lateral view is the easiest one in which to see displacements of the lunate, and the oblique view gives you another opportunity to see a fracture of the scaphoid. These three views can usually be taken on the same film.

CAUTION! If you suspect a scaphoid fracture, but the X-ray is negative, repeat it in 7 to 10 days.

COMPARE HIS INJURED WRIST WITH HIS NORMAL ONE

74.2 Extension (Colles) fractures

These are the most common human fractures. The patient falls on his outstretched hand, he hyperextends his wrist, he fractures the lower end of his radius, and he sometimes fractures the tip of his ulnar styloid in one of the following three ways.

A NORMAL LEFT WRIST

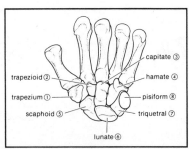

capitate ③
hamate ④
pisiform ⑧
triquetral ⑦
trapezioid ②
trapezium ①
scaphoid ⑤
lunate ⑥

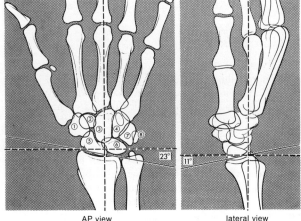

AP view   lateral view

Fig. 74-3 IN AN X-RAY OF THE NORMAL WRIST: (1) the lunate has a four-sided appearance, (2) the articular surface of the head of the radius is angled forwards about 11° and medially about 23°. The tip of the radial styloid should be about 2 mm distal to the tip of the ulnar styloid. These relationships are important in deciding if an extension fracture has been adequately reduced or not.

In all of them he complains of a swollen wrist, and of the signs described in Section 7.1.

(1) In the classical extension fracture he has a single transverse fracture about 2 cm from the lower end of his radius, which does not involve the surface of his wrist joint. The distal fragment is in one piece, shifted dorsally, tilted dorsally and radially, and impacted on the shaft. In the developing world these frac-

A COMMINUTED EXTENSION FRACTURE

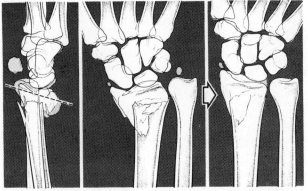

lateral view, the distal surface of the radius is angulated dorsally

AP view before reduction, the normal distal projection of the radius beyond the ulna has been lost

AP view after reduction, the distal projetion of the radius has been restored

Fig. 74-4 A COMMINUTED EXTENSION FRACTURE with considerable displacement. If the patient with this X-ray is old, treat him with active movements. If he is young, try to reduce it by one of the two methods described in the text.

tures are seen in adults of any age, and are not typically injuries of older women as they are elsewhere.

(2) In a T-shaped fracture the fracture line extends distally into the wrist joint, and divides the distal fragment into two.

(3) In a comminuted fracture the distal fragment is in many pieces.

X-rays are highly desirable, but not absolutely essential. You need them to make sure that the patient has not also got a fractured scaphoid, or some other injury of his carpus. If you are not sure what fracture he has, rely: (1) on the nature of the injury (flexion or extension) and remember that, (2) if there is any displacement, the distal fragment will be displaced backwards in an extension fracture, and forwards in a flexion one.

If a fracture is impacted in a reasonably good position with only moderate shift, and less than 15° of dorsal angulation, don't try to reduce it. Leaving it alone will let it heal faster, and will avoid the risk of anaesthesia. It will enable active movements to start earlier and thus reduce stiffness. Reducing a more severely displaced fracture is usually easy, but applying a cast in a way that will prevent the fragments slipping is not so easy, so follow the instructions carefully. Poor reduction is more often due to putting on the cast badly, than to manipulating the fracture incorrectly. Radial instead of ulnar deviation of the distal fragment is the common mistake. Prevent this by making sure the patient's hand is in moderate ulnar deviation when you apply the cast. Two methods of reduction are described; the disadvantage of the first one is that it takes a little longer.

FULL PRONATION WITH MODERATE FLEXION AND MODERATE ULNAR DEVIATION

EXTENSION (COLLES) FRACTURES OF THE WRIST

IF THE DISTAL FRAGMENT IS COMMINUTED OR T–SHAPED

If there is less than 15° of dorsal tilt and comminution is mild, apply a volar splint for protection and to relieve pain.

THE POSITION OF IMMOBILISATION FOR AN EXTENSION FRACTURE

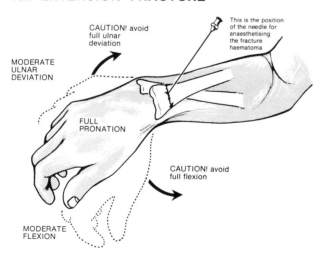

Fig. 74-5 THE WAY TO MAINTAIN REDUCTION IN AN EXTENSION FRACTURE is to apply the cast in full pronation, in moderate flexion and in moderate ulnar deviation. In this position the extensor tendons passing over the back of the distal fragment hold it reduced. Extreme flexion or extreme ulnar deviation will cause a stiff wrist. The needle shows the position for entering the haematoma for local anaesthesia.

Encourage the patient to start active movements of his fingers immediately.

If displacement or comminution is moderate or severe, management depends on his age. If he is young, attempt reduction as described below. If he is old, apply a backslab for a few days, and then encourage active movements as soon as pain allows.

If the distal fragments are in only two pieces and look as if they could be fixed internally, refer him if you can, especially if he is young.

If active immediate movements are indicated but pain is too great to allow them, apply an anterior plaster slab or a backslab for about 3 weeks, until the pain has lessened enough to allow the patient to begin using his wrist. If possible, hold the slab in place with crepe bandages. Remove the slab for periods of exercise and then reapply it. If you have no crepe bandages, use a plaster bandage, and split it (70.6).

IF THE DISTAL FRAGMENT OF THE RADIUS IS IN ONE PIECE

IF THERE IS MINOR DISPLACEMENT of the distal fragment, with less than 15° of dorsal tilt, don't reduce it. Apply a slab to the front of the patient's arm and wrist and start active movements, as above, as soon as the pain allows.

IF THERE IS MORE SEVERE DISPLACEMENT with more than 15° of dorsal angulation of the distal fragment, or the patient is in severe pain, or there are signs of pressure on his median nerve, reduce the fracture immediately, as follows.

ANAESTHESIA (BOTH METHODS) (1) Local anaesthesia of the fracture haematoma is very effective if the fracture is recent (A 5.6). Its disadvantages are that: (a) it converts a closed fracture into an open one, with the possible risk of infection, and (b) it does not relax the muscles. Using careful aseptic precaution, insert the needle on the back of the patient's forearm well above his wrist. Aim the needle obliquely, as in Fig. 74-5, so that it enters the fracture cavity; aspirate to make sure you are in the haematoma, then inject 10 ml, not more, of 2% lignocaine without adrenaline and wait 15 minutes. (2) Intravenous forearm block (A 6.19). (3) Supraclavicular block (A 6.17). (4) Axillary block (A 6.18).

FIRST METHOD FOR REDUCING AN EXTENSION FRACTURE OF THE WRIST

Lie the patient down. Suspend his arm from a drip stand, using clove hitches (Fig. 73-10) round his thumb, and index or middle finger. Put a strap round his upper arm, and apply 5 kg traction to it.

Wait 10 minutes while the traction corrects the impaction. At the end of this time the distal fragment will usually be free and you can move it into position with the minimum of effort.

Apply anterior and posterior plaster slabs. Suspension will have secured a suitable degree of moderate ulnar deviation, so you have only to make sure that you apply the plaster in moderate flexion and full pronation.

Don't let the anterior slab come further than the patient's distal palmar crease. Make sure the tip of his thumb can touch his index finger.

If possible, hold the slab in place with a crepe bandage. If you don't have a crepe bandage, pad his arm and hold the slabs in place with a plaster bandage. Split this while the cast is still damp.

If the fracture is unstable, continue the cast up his upper arm with the elbow at 90°. For stable or minimally displaced fractures, forearm slabs are enough,

SECOND METHOD FOR REDUCING AN EXTENSION FRACTURE OF THE WRIST

The following description assumes that the patient has a fracture of his right wrist.

Anaesthetize him and lie him down.

DISIMPACTION Ask an assistant to hold the patient's arm just above his elbow.

Hold his fingers in one of your hands and his thumb in the other.

REDUCING AN EXTENSION FRACTURE

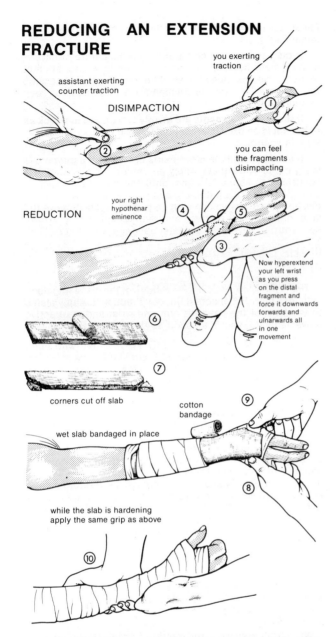

assistant exerting counter traction

you exerting traction

DISIMPACTION

you can feel the fragments disimpacting

your right hypothenar eminence

REDUCTION

Now hyperextend your left wrist as you press on the distal fragment and force it downwards forwards and ulnarwards all in one movement

corners cut off slab

cotton bandage

wet slab bandaged in place

while the slab is hardening apply the same grip as above

Fig. 74-6 REDUCING AN EXTENSION FRACTURE. This is the second of the two methods described in the text. Disimpact the fracture in steps 1 and 2. Reduce it in steps 3, 4, and 5. The critical movement is 5 in which the distal fragment is moved into a position of moderate flexion and moderate ulnar deviation, all in one movement. Hold the patient's fingers and thumb as in 8 and 9 while your assistant bandages on the slab.

Exert traction on his fingers and thumb (1) while your assistant pulls his elbow in the opposition direction (2). The younger he is the stronger the pull you need. Pull steadily for a minute timed by the clock. You will feel the fragments disimpact, and will sometimes hear them do so.

CORRECT THE DEFORMITY Abduct his forearm, stand with your back to him, and pronate his wrist.

Put your left thenar eminence (3) over the displaced distal fragment, with your fingers and thumb round the ulnar border of his wrist.

Put your right hand beneath his distal forearm with your right hypothenar eminence just proximal to the fracture line (4). Curl the fingers of your right hand round his lower forearm.

Using your right hypothenar eminence as a fulcrum, move the lower fragment into a position of moderate flexion and moderate ulnar deviation all in one movement (5).

If the ulnar styloid is fractured, disregard it.

IMMOBILIZE THE FRAGMENTS Apply a plaster backslab (6) with its corners cut (7) to allow movement of the patient's elbow, fingers, and thumb.

While your assistant bandages on the slab, hold the patient's fingers in one hand (8) and his thumb in the other (9). Lean backwards, exert gentle traction, and his wrist will fall into moderate ulnar deviation.

While the slab is still soft, move back to the inner side of the arm, and apply the same grip as you used to correct the deformity (10), but without applying any pressure. Allow the plaster to set while you maintain this grip.

CAUTION ! (1) Make sure his wrist is fully pronated, moderately flexed, and moderately ulnar deviated. (2) His MP joints must be free. If the slab extends too far distally it will splint them in extension, and give him a stiff useless hand.

CHECK X-RAYS The AP view should show that you have corrected the alignment.

The lateral view should show that the articular surface of the patient's radius is no longer facing dorsally. It should be facing 5 to 10° anteriorly, but a strictly vertical position is acceptable. If reduction is unsatisfactory, have one further attempt at manipulation. If you make further attempts in your efforts to get a good X-ray, the clinical result will only be worse.

POSTOPERATIVE CARE FOR AN EXTENSION FRACTURE (both methods)

Put the patient's arm in a triangular sling, with his elbow flexed at more than 90°. If his fingers become painful, tell him to return immediately, or to split the bandage with a pair of scissors. Encourage him to move his fingers, elbow, and shoulder actively, using the exercises in Fig. 71-7. Early shoulder movements are especially important because they will prevent the common complication of a stiff shoulder.

In a few days, or at the next fracture clinic, complete the cast around his forearm.

Where possible, X-ray him again 7 to 10 days later, so that if redisplacement has occurred, there will still be time to correct it. This is important in a younger patient, but if an older patient's fracture redisplaces, leave it, and encourage active movements.

A young adult Keep the cast on for 6 weeks.

An old adult Remove the cast after 3 weeks, and encourage him to move his wrist.

DIFFICULTIES WITH EXTENSION FRACTURES

If the patient's fracture has united, but his WRIST IS DEFORMED with an ugly radial deformity, pain, and limited rotation, you can refer him for excision of the head of his ulna, together with 2 cm of its adjacent shaft (Darrach's operation). This is a simple procedure with good results, so it is better than trying to remanipulate a badly reduced extension fracture with radial deviation. The pain over the head of his ulna will eventually improve, but it may last a year.

If he is SUDDENLY UNABLE TO EXTEND HIS THUMB some weeks or months after the accident, he has probably ruptured the tendon of his extensor pollicis longus. This sometimes happens suddenly long after the accident. Refer him to have it repaired.

74.3 Flexion fractures of the wrist (Smith's and Barton's fractures)

In these two fractures the patient falls on his flexed wrist to produce the characteristic deformity shown in Fig. 74-7, in which his hand is displaced anteriorly on his forearm. In a lateral X-ray, the fracture line runs obliquely across the distal end of his radius, instead of being parallel to its articular surface, as is usual in an extension fracture. Also, the distal end of the radius is displaced anteriorly in contrast to the posterior displacement of an extension fracture. In a Smith's fracture the fracture line does not extend into the joint, but in a Barton's fracture it does. In both the fragments are difficult to reduce and hold in place.

Although these two fractures should be easy to diagnose, they are so rare that they are often mistaken for extension fractures.

In Barton's fracture the fragments can seldom be held in a cast, so that open reduction and plating is usually necessary, but in Smith's fractures closed reduction may succeed. The fragment is displaced anteriorly, so that the patient's wrist must be held in *dorsiflexion, and his hand supinated* (the opposite to an extension fracture). If you treat either of these fractures badly, the loss of wrist movement will be severe.

A FLEXION FRACTURE (Barton's)

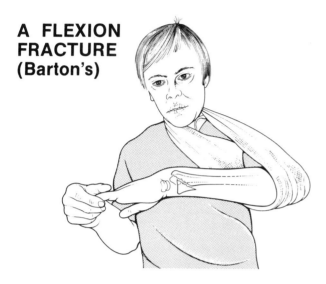

Fig. 74-7 A FLEXION FRACTURE OF THE WRIST. The fracture shown here is Barton's, in which the fracture line enters the wrist joint. *Kindly contributed by Peter Bewes.*

FLEXION FRACTURES OF THE WRIST

If the fracture involves the articular surface (Barton's fracture), refer the patient for internal fixation. If you cannot refer him, treat him as for a Smith's fracture described below.

SMITH'S FRACTURE Use local anaesthesia as for an extension fracture. Ask an assistant to apply traction in the axis of the patient's forearm.

While traction is being applied, supinate and dorsiflex his wrist fully. Apply a plaster slab to the front of his forearm, from just above his elbow to the proximal crease of his palm, and bind it on with a crepe bandage. Or failing this, pad his forearm and hold the slab on with a circular plaster bandage, split it, as for an extension fracture.

Take an X-ray to see if the fracture is reduced.

If the fracture is reduced, complete the cast on the third day; encourage him to use his hand, and keep his shoulder moving. Remove the cast after 6 weeks.

If the fracture is not reduced, have one more attempt at reduction. If this fails, refer him for internal fixation immediately.

DIFFICULTIES WITH EXTENSION FRACTURES

If the DISTAL FRAGMENT SLIPS, it will do so anteriorly and proximally, but this may not interfere with function. If the slipping is significant, refer the patient for the application of a plate.

74.4 Fractures of the scaphoid

These can occur at any age, even in children, but they are particularly common in young men. The patient falls on his hand and forcibly dorsiflexes the joint between the proximal and distal rows of his carpal bones. The scaphoid, which forms part of both rows, breaks across its distal pole, or its neck.

TWO FLEXION FRACTURES

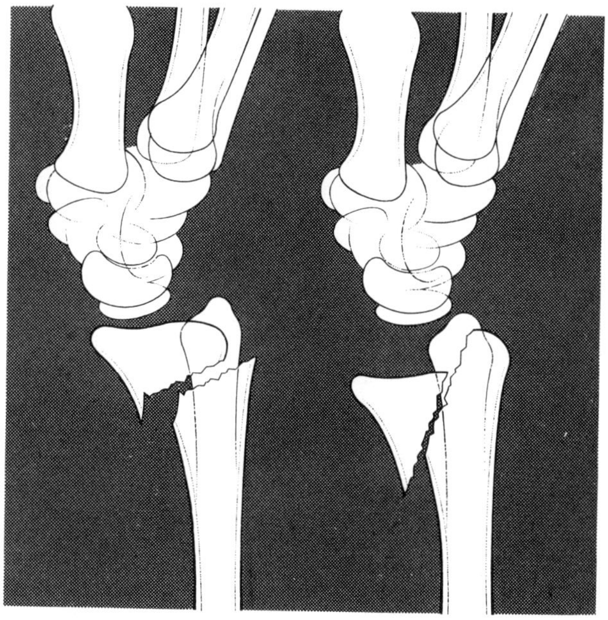

SMITHS   BARTONS

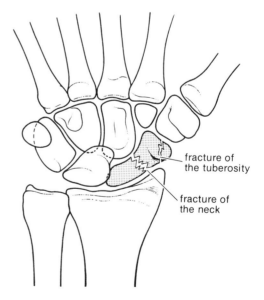

fracture line does not enter joint   fracture line enters joint

Fig. 74-8 TWO KINDS OF FLEXION FRACTURE. In Smith's fracture the fracture line does not enter the joint, but in Barton's it does. Barton's fracture should be referred for internal fixation. If this is impossible, you will have to treat it in the same way as Smith's.

Fracture of the distal pole (tuberosity) of the scaphoid is a minor injury, because the detached fragment has a good blood supply and unites readily. Treat this fracture by encouraging early active movements.

Fracture of the neck of the scaphoid is a more common and more serious injury, because non—union is frequent. The

FRACTURES OF THE SCAPHOID

fracture of the tuberosity

fracture of the neck

Fig. 74-9 FRACTURES OF THE SCAPHOID can occur at any age, even in children, but they are particularly common in young men. The patient falls on his hand and forcibly dorsiflexes the joint between the proximal and distal rows of his carpal bones. Fractures of the neck are much more important than those of the distal pole.

patient's wrist is normal, except for pain at the extremes of movement, and local tenderness in the anatomical snuffbox over his scaphoid. He may complain that his wrist continues to hurt after a 'sprain', but because the pain is so mild, he may continue to use his hand, with the result that this fracture is often missed. The signs in Section 74.1 should make you suspect the diagnosis, particularly pain on pressing the 'anatomical snuffbox'.

Take an AP, a lateral, and two oblique X-rays at 30° and 60°. The fracture line is a fine crack in the neck of the scaphoid *which you can easily miss.* Look for it on a dry film in a good light with a magnifying glass. If there is clinical evidence of a fractured scaphoid, but the X-ray is negative, apply a scaphoid cast and take another film after removing the cast 7 to 10 days later. The fracture line will then be much more obvious. If clinical signs are strongly suggestive, but the X-ray is still negative, assume that the patient has a scaphoid fracture, and treat it.

Neither fragment is significantly displaced, so they need not be reduced, but they do need to be splinted. If they are going to unite successfully: (1) splinting must be prolonged for 10 weeks, (2) the cast must be close fitting (there must be no movement at the mid–carpal joint), and (3) the cast must go above the elbow.

Non–union is the main difficulty with these fractures. This may be due to: (1) a poorly applied cast which allows movement at the mid–carpal joint, (2) interrupted splinting, (3) splinting for too short a time, or (4) aseptic necrosis of the proximal fragment, especially if it is small. All bandages and casts for the

A SCAPHOID CAST

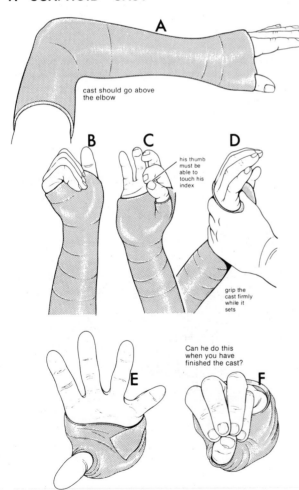

cast should go above the elbow

his thumb must be able to touch his index

grip the cast firmly while it sets

Can he do this when you have finished the cast?

Fig. 74-10 A SCAPHOID CAST. Note that it goes above the patient's elbow, that it ends just proximal to his distal palmar crease and the interphalangeal joint of his thumb, and that his thumb is able to touch his index finger. *Adapted from Perkins with kind permission.*

scaphoid, except the one we have described, are almost certainly useless, so whenever you apply a scaphoid cast, do so as in Fig. 74-10.

IF THE X-RAY OF A SPRAINED WRIST' IS NEGATIVE, BUT SYMPTOMS PERSIST, REPEAT IT 10 DAYS LATER

FRACTURE OF THE NECK OF THE SCAPHOID

In 15% of cases the patient has some other injury, so examine his wrist carefully. Anaesthesia is unnecessary.

APPLYING A SCAPHOID CAST Put a stockinette tube over the patient's lower arm and hand. Skilled surgeons usually apply an unpadded circular cast. If you are inexperienced, apply a thin layer of cotton wool.

Apply the cast from above the patient's elbow to just above his knuckles. Bring it just proximal to his distal palmar crease. Hold his elbow at 90°. Dorsiflex his wrist, and bring his thumb across his palm as if he were holding a glass. The plaster on his thumb should reach just short of its IP joint. Mould it firmly round his first metacarpal.

As soon as the cast is on, and before it has set, grasp his hand, so as to squeeze the cast from front to back, as in D, Fig. 74-10. Squeezing the cast like this will prevent his hand moving and straining the fracture line. If he can flex or extend his wrist even a little, the cast is useless. His wrist will not swell, so don't split the cast. Encourage him to use all the joints outside the cast. This will soon make it soft, so renew it as necessary.

THE POSTOPERATIVE CARE OF A SCAPHOID FRACTURE

At 6 weeks, renew the cast, but this time bring it below the patient's elbow. At 10 weeks, remove the cast and take another X-ray.

If his fracture has united, allow him to use his wrist progressively.

If his fracture has not united, proceed as follows.

(1) If wrist movements are very important to him, refer him. If you cannot refer him, apply another cast for 3 more weeks. Twelve weeks in a cast is the maximum time. If you leave it on longer than this, his wrist will become excessively stiff and osteoporotic.

(2) If wrist movements are less important to him, remove the cast, and allow a false joint to form. Often, there are no symptoms, even if the fragments fail to unite.

(3) If, later, he continues to have unacceptable disability, refer him for bone grafting, or removal of the avascular fragment.

DIFFICULTIES WITH A FRACTURED SCAPHOID

If the fracture has NOT UNITED and the PROXIMAL FRAGMENT LOOKS VERY DENSE on the X-ray, it has probably undergone avascular necrosis. It can be excised, but the operation is difficult. If you cannot refer him, encourage him to disregard his disability and use his hand as much as he can.

If you have NO PLASTER, aim for a pseudarthrosis and start active movements immediately.

REGARD A SPRAINED WRIST IS A FRACTURED SCAPHOID UNTIL PROVED OTHERWISE

74.5 Carpal dislocations

In these rare injuries, the patient falls on his hand and dorsiflexes his wrist violently, so that the second row of carpal bones dislocates on the first row. His lunate remains in its normal place in the proximal row, and in its normal place in relation to the

TWO CARPAL DISLOCATIONS

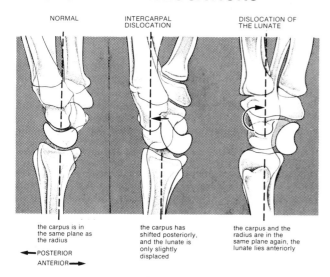

Fig. 74-11 TWO CARPAL DISLOCATIONS. A, a normal wrist. B, the carpus has been pushed backwards leaving the lunate in its normal position in relation to the radius (intercarpal dislocation). C, the carpus has sprung forwards and displaced the radius anteriorly.

radius. Sometimes the injury stays like this so that he has an *intercarpal dislocation*. But, if the distal row of carpal bones now springs forwards again, it may push his lunate forwards, out of its position in the proximal row, and away from its normal relation with the radius. He now has an *anterior dislocation of his lunate*. Rarely, the lunate dislocates posteriorly.

These dislocations are important, because you can usually reduce them. If you don't, severe disability follows, and the greater the delay, the worse it becomes. Exactly the same kind of injury fractures the scaphoid, so in injuries of the lunate, always look for a fractured scaphoid. Distinguishing between these two lunate injuries clinically can be difficult. The lateral X-ray is the critical one.

LOOK CAREFULLY AT THE LATERAL X-RAY

74.5a Intercarpal dislocation (perilunate dislocation)

This makes the patient's wrist swell. Neither he nor you can move his wrist, and its antero—posterior diameter is increased. His styloid processes are in their normal places. His radial pulse and the concavity of the lower end of his radius are normal, and you cannot localize tenderness anywhere.

The X-rays are difficult to interpret. Take a lateral view and compare it with one of his normal wrist. In an intercarpal dislocation the lunate is more or less in its normal place in relation to the radius, and is facing in its proper direction, but its distal cup—shaped articular surface is not in contact with the dome—shaped surface of the capitate. Instead, the patient's hand and his carpus lie in a plane posterior to his radius. This dislocation is less easy to see in an AP view. A useful sign is an increase in the normal space between the lunate and the scaphoid, as shown in B, Fig. 74-12.

The methods for reducing both these injuries are similar. The first step is to exert strong traction on the patient's hand. In an intercarpal dislocation, press over the back of his wrist and then flex it. In a dislocation of his lunate, press over the front of his wrist and then extend it.

INTERCARPAL DISLOCATION

Anaesthetize the patient. Bend his elbow to 90°, and secure his upper arm to the table with a bandage, as in C, Fig. 74-12. Supinate his forearm, and ask an assistant to pull strongly on his fingers for 10 minutes.

While your assistant is maintaining very strong traction, place both your thumbs against the *back* of the patient's wrist. Push forwards, and at the same time slowly flex his wrist (not illustrated).

Take an X-ray to make sure you have not dislocated his lunate by mistake. Look carefully to make sure that he has not also fractured his scaphoid. If reduction fails, refer him.

POSTOPERATIVE CARE If he has not fractured his scaphoid, apply a splint for 2 weeks to allow some healing, then encourage active movements immediately.

If he has fractured his scaphoid, apply a scaphoid cast, and split it. In a few days, when swelling has subsided, replace it with an unsplit cast.

DISASTER WITH AN INTERCARPAL DISLOCATION

If the DIAGNOSIS WAS MISSED, this may be because nobody listened to what the patient said. If he says "There is something wrong with my hand", believe him, even though his X-ray seems normal. If the dislocation was overlooked at

DISLOCATION OF THE LUNATE

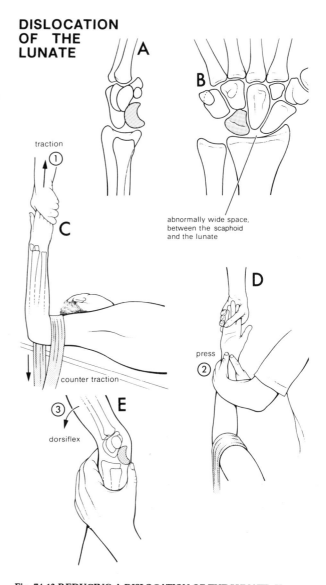

Fig. 74-12 REDUCING A DISLOCATION OF THE LUNATE. **You may find it easier to pull with the patient's arm horizontal and provide counter—traction by fixing his upper arm to the head of the table.** *After de Palma with kind permission.*

the time of the injury, refer him for open reduction. If this is not possible, his wrist movements will remain limited and painful.

74.5b Dislocation of the lunate

This is the second stage of an intercarpal dislocation. The displaced distal row of carpal bones springs back and rotates the lunate forwards. As it does so, the posterior radio–lunate ligament ruptures, but the anterior one remains intact. The displaced lunate presses on the patient's median nerve, and if it is not replaced, he may lose the function in it permanently.

The patient falls and injures his wrist, after which it is swollen and painful, and he can can only move it a little. His fingers remain partly flexed, and will not straighten. He may have any of the four signs in Section 74.1.

In a lateral X-ray, the proximal dome–shaped surface of the patient's lunate faces posteriorly, and is no longer in contact with his radius. Its distal cup–shaped surface faces anteriorly, and is no longer in contact with his capitate. His capitate and the carpus are in the same plane as his radius. Signs in the AP view are characteristic, but are often missed. The normal lunate appears to have four sides in an AP view, but when it is dislocated, it seems only to have three. *So look for a triangular lunate.* Look also for a widened space between the scaphoid and the lunate. Normally they touch. Dislocations of the lunate are so easily missed that the lunate is the first bone to look at in any X-ray of the wrist.

DISLOCATION OF THE LUNATE

Try to reduce a patient's lunate as soon as you can, before his median nerve is permanently injured. Every few hours make a difference. After 2 weeks, closed methods usually fail.

CLOSED REDUCTION Give the patient a general anaesthetic that will relax the muscles of his arm completely. Bend his elbow to 90° and fix his upper arm with a bandage to the table as in Fig. 74-12.

Supinate his forearm, and ask an assistant to pull strongly on the patient's fingers for *10 minutes* (1).

After 10 minutes of traction and while it is still being maintained, place both your thumbs against the *front* of the patient's wrist over his lunate, and press hard posteriorly (2) while dorsiflexing his wrist (3). Then flex his wrist while keeping up traction and pressure (not illustrated). If this fails, refer him for open reduction. If this is impossible, encourage early active movements. If he is lucky, he may have comparatively little disability.

POSTOPERATIVE CARE If his scaphoid has been fractured, apply a scaphoid cast. If it has not been fractured, encourage active movements from the start, and splint it only for the relief of pain. Irritation to his median nerve will improve quickly after you have replaced his lunate.

Alternatively, hang 5 kg of traction round the patient's upper arm, as for the first method for an extension fracture (74.2) of his wrist. Then try to manipulate his wrist.

IN AN X-RAY OF THE WRIST LOOK FIRST AT THE LUNATE

---

75 Hand injuries

75.1 The general method for hand injuries

Patients use their hands in very different ways. Some of them need nimble agile fingers, while others need a powerful grip. So one of your first priorities when you see an injured hand, is to find out what its owner does with it, and which functions you most need to preserve. Surgeons and labourers have quite different expectations of their hands, and yet provided their injuries are corectly treated, it is possible for each to hardly notice what might seem to be severe mutilation.

You can readily treat most of a patient's fractures and dislocations and injuries to his extensor tendons, but injuries to his flexor tendons will cause you and most experts much difficulty. Hand injuries are often worse than they look, and there are many opportunities for disaster: (1) You can easily miss cut nerves or tendons, so assume that all the structures under a wound have been injured, until you have proved they are normal. (2) If you neglect what is said later about splinting, movement, and amputation (75.22), a patient can easily end up with a stiff hand, or a stiff useless finger. The outcome of a hand injury mostly depends on how you care for it during the first few days. A patient is unlikely to return for such simple physiotherapy as you may have, so try to get his hand back into action as quickly as you can, even if this does mean radical surgery.

All the general principles of wound care (54.1) apply to an injured hand, with some extra ones. The principle that raw areas should be grafted as soon as is practicable is particularly important, because this minimizes infection and the fibrosis, and stiffness which follow.

Hand injuries are often multiple with several types of injury in the same hand, so be prepared to modify the methods for single injuries that we give here. Finally, operations on the hand are not easy, and only careful, dedicated, painstaking, and delicate work is good enough. Although a hand injury may look minor, it is never trivial—a fractured phalanx can disable a patient just as easily as a fractured femur.

• *FINGER SPLINTS, aluminium, padded, 50 lengths only.* These are strips of aluminium with foam rubber on one side. Cut them and bend them to suit a patient's needs, as in Fig. 75-9. If you cannot get them, you may be able to make them. Or, for most injuries, you can use a garter splint. There is no reason why aluminium finger splints should be any more expensive than plaster bandages; they should be in every medical store's list.

ASSUME THAT EVERYTHING UNDER A HAND WOUND HAS BEEN INJURED UNTIL YOU HAVE PROVED IT NORMAL

THE GENERAL METHOD FOR A HAND INJURY

IMMEDIATE TREATMENT FOR AN INJURED HAND

Bleeding is seldom severe. Plenty of gauze, a firm dressing, and raising the patient's injured hand, will usually stop it.

Keep the patient's hand raised at all times, before and after

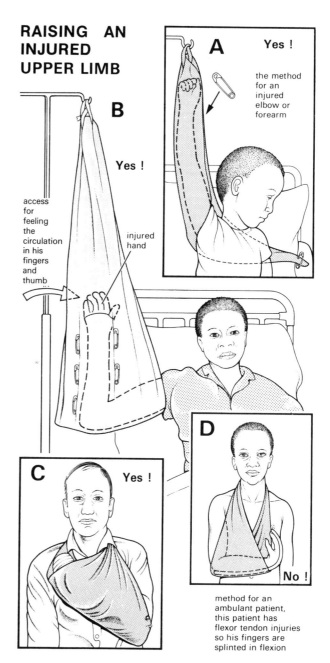

RAISING AN INJURED UPPER LIMB

Fig. 75-1 RAISING AN INJURED ARM AND HAND will reduce traumatic or infective oedema and minimize stiffness. A, if a patient's elbow (72.1) or forearm (73.1) is injured or infected, pin it in a towel, pass the end of it under him, and pin it to his bedclothes. B, if he is in bed with an injured hand, suspend it like this with his upper arm horizontal. C, if he is ambulant, raise his hand in a St John's sling, don't keep it horizontal as in D. Patient D's flexor tendons were cut, so his hand and wrist have been splinted in flexion. *Kindly contributed by Peter Bewes, Richard Batten, and John Stewart.*

271

HAND POSITIONS IN TENDON INJURIES

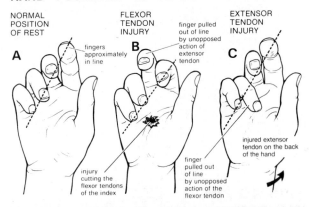

Fig. 75-2 HAND POSITIONS IN TENDON INJURIES. A, in a normal hand the fingers are approximately in line. B, in a flexor tendon injury the injured finger is extended. C, in an extensor tendon injury it is flexed. *Kindly contributed by Peter Bewes.*

the operation. Wrap it in a sterile towel, pin the towel together, and suspend it from a drip stand. Or, use stockinette traction, as for a malleolar fracture (Fig. 82-5). Cut a hole for his fingers to peep out. Keep it in this position while he is waiting for and recovering from his wound toilet. If his hand is severely crushed, suspend it for several days. This will relieve his pain, and minimize swelling and stiffness.

If he might have injured his flexor tendons, strap his hand and wrist in a flexed position (75.21). This will prevent him trying to flex his fingers and perhaps pulling his tendons out of their sheaths.

THE HISTORY IN A HAND INJURY

What caused the patient his injury? Clean knife injuries and those from a human bite, for example, require quite different treatment. What does the patient need his hand for? What is his job? Is he left handed or right handed?

What was the mechanism of the injury? Crushing, a force applied to a finger end on, hyperextension, or a sideways angulation all produce different injuries.

THE EXAMINATION IN A HAND INJURY

Follow the usual sequence of look, feel, move, and X-ray (69.1). You will need to answer five questions: (1) Is the viability of the hand or a finger in doubt? (2) Is the skeleton of the hand stable? (3) Is there actual or impending skin loss? (4) Have the nerves of the hand been injured? (5) Have its tendons been damaged?

IN WHAT POSITION IS THE PATIENT'S HAND? If his fingers are not in their normal position of rest, suspect a fracture or a dislocation, or a tendon injury in which the action of the unopposed normal tendon has pulled his injured finger into an abnormal position, as in Fig. 75-2.

Examine his skin, vessels, nerves, bones, joints, tendons, and muscles, and record your findings.

IS HIS CIRCULATION NORMAL? If you are worried about the circulation in an injured finger, check it for: (1) Pink finger nails which blanch on pressure, and then become pink again. (2) Sensation in the finger tip. (3) The patency of the patient's digital arteries. Raise his hand, compress the digital arteries at the base of his injured finger until it becomes pale. Still compressing them, lower his hand. Release one artery. If his finger becomes pink, that artery is patent. Repeat the process with the other artery (modified Allen's test).

ARE HIS NERVES INTACT? Test his median, ulnar, and radial nerves, as in Fig. 75-3. Test the sensory areas of his hand. In children this needs patience. If sensation is absent, it does not necessarily mean that it will be absent permanently, for a patient's injured hand may be oedematous, or heavily calloused, or he may be shocked. Absent movements are a more reliable sign of nerve injury.

TESTING THE NERVES OF THE HAND

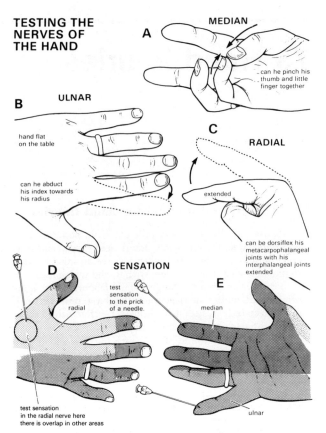

Fig. 75-3 TESTING THE NERVES OF A PATIENT'S HAND. A, his median nerve: can he pinch his thumb and little finger? B, his ulnar nerve: can he abduct his index towards his radius? C, his radial nerve: can he extend his fingers with his hand in the position shown? D, and E, test sensation with a pin.

Median nerve (1) Can he touch his little finger with his thumb? This tests the opponens muscle of his thumb. (2) Test sensation in the tip of his index with a needle.

Ulnar nerve (1) Lay the patient's hand palm downwards on a table. If he can abduct his index finger in the direction of his radius, towards his thumb, the deep branch of his ulnar nerve is intact. (2) Test the tip of his little finger with a pin.

Radial nerve A radial nerve lesion has to be high up in a patient's arm to affect the motor power in his hand. If only his sensation is affected, the injury is below his elbow joint. (1) Ask him to dorsiflex his wrist, extend both his IP joints, and flex his MP joints, as in C, Fig. 75-3. Can he now extend his MP joints? (2) Test the dorsum of the proximal phalanx of his thumb with a pin. There is extensive overlap in the area supplied by each nerve, so test the area outlined in a ring in Fig. 75-3, which is entirely supplied by the radial nerve.

ARE HIS TENDONS INTACT? You will need to test his superficial and deep flexor tendons, his wrist flexors, and his extensor tendons.

Profundus tendons Test each finger in turn. Hold its proximal IP joint extended, as in A, Fig. 75-4. If the patient can now flex his distal phalanx even 15°, the profundus tendon is intact. The profundus tendons are closely associated with the superficialis ones, so you have to immobilize them by flexing his other fingers.

Superficialis tendons Hold all his fingers, except the one you are interested in, fully extended, as in B, Fig. 75-4. If he can still flex the proximal IP joint of the finger in question, its superficialis tendon is intact. Holding his other fingers extended like this anchors his profundus tendons.

Wrist flexors Feel the tendons on the front of his wrist tightening as he flexes it against resistance, as in C, Fig. 75-4.

Extensor tendons Can he extend his fingers against resistance?

TESTING A JOINT FOR STABILITY—ARE THE COLLATERAL LIGAMENTS OF THE FINGERS AND THUMB INTACT? If you suspect that a patient has injured one of these: (1) look for swelling, and feel for tenderness over the injured joint, (2) hold the proximal bone of the joint you are testing steady, and move the distal one from side to side. Does it give? Do this with an IP joint extended, and a MP joint flexed. This is the position in which their ligaments are tight, see A, Fig. 75-8.

X-RAYS If you suspect fractures or foreign bodies, take AP and *lateral* X-rays. If you suspect an avulsion fracture at the base of a phalanx, make sure that the X-ray is centered on the right joint. X-ray all glass injuries.

Unlike the larger bones, the metacarpals and phalanges have an epiphysis at one end only. In the phalanges it is proximal and in the metacarpals it is distal, except for the first metacarpal in which the epiphysis is proximal. If you are in doubt, remember that something which is not tender is not a recent fracture.

CAUTION ! Don't confuse a fracture with: (1) A nutrient artery which passes obliquely through the cortex of a phalanx, usually at the junction of its middle and distal thirds. (2) The shadow of soft tissues. These may look like fracture lines but pass across a bone and are not confined to it. (3) Epiphyses.

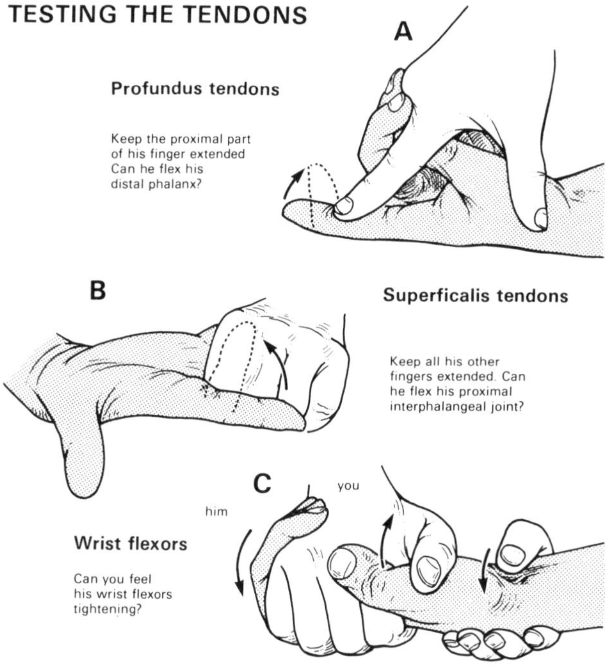

TESTING THE TENDONS

A

Profundus tendons

Keep the proximal part of his finger extended. Can he flex his distal phalanx?

B

Superficalis tendons

Keep all his other fingers extended. Can he flex his proximal interphalangeal joint?

C

you

him

Wrist flexors

Can you feel his wrist flexors tightening?

Fig. 75-4 TESTING A PATIENT'S FLEXOR TENDONS. A, test a deep flexor of a finger by keeping its proximal IP joint extended and asking him to flex its distal IP joint. B, test his superficialis tendons by keeping all his fingers, except the one you are interested in, extended. Then ask him to flex his proximal IP joint. C, feel his wrist flexor tendons tighten as he flexes his wrist against resistance.

THE TREATMENT FOR A SEVERE HAND INJURY

Admit all but the most minor injuries and operate on them in the main theatre.

ANAESTHESIA Find out and record which of the patient's nerves and tendons have been cut *before* you anaesthetize him. 'Peeking and poking' in his wound after you have anaesthetized him will tell you very little.

Anaesthesia must be adequate, so that you are not fighting with a moving hand. Relaxation is unnecessary. There are several possibilities. (1) Ketamine (A 8.2). (2) An axillary block is very satisfactory (A 6.8). (3) If you can find a suitable vein, you can use an intravenous forearm block (A 6.19). Often you cannot. If possible put the cuff on the patient's forearm, you will need less anaesthetic solution, and there will be less danger if the cuff fails. (4) Blocks of his median, ulnar, and

radial nerves (A 6.20). (5) Finger blocks are useful for the two distal segments only (A 6.21). If necessary, you can combine them with blocks of his median and ulnar nerves.

CAUTION ! Never use adrenaline in an intravenous forearm block, or in any block in the fingers or hand. The result will be gangrenous fingers.

EQUIPMENT Don't use the big instruments of a general set. Use fine forceps and needle holders. Cut the patient's bones with a bone nibbler, a Gigli saw, or a fine finger saw. Remove as little bone as you can. Don't use a big amputation saw, or you will damage his soft tissues unnecessarily.

TRACTION is of little value. It may be briefly necessary to reduce dislocations, or multiple displaced metacarpal fractures. Apply adhesive strapping along the sides of the patient's fingers and watch the circulation in them carefully. Don't wrap strapping round them.

POSITION FOR OPERATING Lie the patient on his back with his arm on a side table over a bucket. Operate sitting in a good light. Wash and prepare his arm up to his elbow. His forearm will then be ready for taking a skin graft if necessary. Ask your assistant to hold the patient's hand as required while you operate.

TOURNIQUETS Start by exsanguinating the patient's hand with an Esmarch bandage and a tourniquet (3.8). Then scrub up yourself and paint and drape him. For most wounds leave the tourniquet on throughout the operation, but don't exceed 1½ hours which is the maximum safe time for an adult with an average arm. If there is much tissue damage, remove it when you want to see what tissue is viable and what is not.

OPERATING ON A HAND INJURY

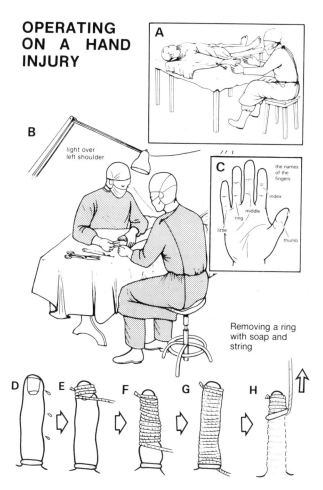

A

B

light over left shoulder

C

the names of the fingers

index

middle

ring

little

thumb

Removing a ring with soap and string

D   E   F   G   H

Fig. 75-5 OPERATING ON A HAND INJURY. A, and B, sit down, make yourself comfortable, and extend the patient's arm on a side table. C, the names of the fingers. D, how to remove a ring by lubricating a finger with soap and then using a piece of string. A, and C, kindly contributed by Peter Bewes. B, after Allen A.S. and Crenshaw. A.H. Campbell's Operative Orthopaedics' (6th edn) Fig. 3-1, The CV Mosby Company (1980), with kind permission.

273

You can wind a catheter round an injured finger and hold it with a haemostat.

CAUTION! Wherever you apply a tourniquet, remember that it is your responsibility to remove it.

WOUND TOILET In minor injuries the patient can help do this himself. The wound toilet must be thorough (54.1). Use plenty of soap and water. The skin of the hand is very precious, so excise much less skin than you would, say, in the leg. If his wound is clean cut, don't excise any skin. But, if any tissue is dead, don't try to preserve it. Remove any prolapsed fatty tissue from the palm of his hand.

INCISIONS FOR EXPLORING HAND INJURIES

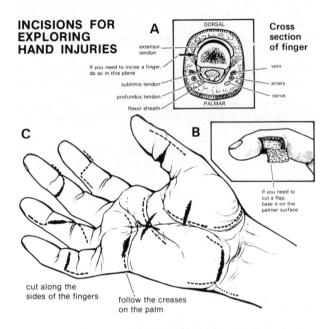

Cross section of finger

cut along the sides of the fingers

follow the creases on the palm

Fig. 75-6 INCISIONS FOR EXPLORING HAND INJURIES. A, if you have to incise a patient's finger, do so in its mid lateral line. **B,** if you have to turn down a flap, do so towards his palm. **C,** avoid extending an incision across a flexor crease. If you have to do this because of the position of the wound, 'snake' the incision across his hand, or extend it each way from the ends of the wound in the form of a 'Z'. *Kindly contributed by Peter Weston.*

INCISIONS In more severe injuries open up the wound, if necessary, in the directions shown in Fig. 75-6, so that you can see and clean the structures underneath. In the palm do this parallel to the creases, not across them.

If a wound crosses a crease and needs to be extended, make additional crease line incisions at the ends of the original incision, so as to make a 'Z'.

If you need to extend an incision on a finger, make it: (1) on the side of the finger in the mid–axial line, (2) obliquely across a finger, or (3) along a crease line on a finger.

CAUTION ! Avoid cutting at right angles to a crease in the patient's hand or fingers, because a contracture may follow.

If you have to reflect a flap on the sides of a finger, reflect it towards the palmar surface, as in B, Fig. 75-6.

Penetrating hand wounds Open these up carefully and explore their depths for injured structures.

NERVE AND TENDON INJURIES Do your utmost to do a primary repair on cut nerves as described in Sections 55.9 and 75.22.

If a patient's wound is severely contaminated, toilet it, and close it by delayed primary suture. Fix cut tendons and nerves with stay sutures to the surrounding tissues. This will stop his tendons retracting and his nerves rotating. Refer him for secondary suture at 3 weeks (55.10).

GRAFTING A HAND INJURY If there is skin loss, and you are in doubt about the completeness of the wound toilet, delayed primary or secondary grafting will be safer (57.2). A patient must have good quality skin at the tips of his fingers. Shortening his finger so that you can use a palmar flap over a finger tip is likely to be better than a graft (Fig. 75-27). On the sides or back of his fingers, a split skin graft is good enough.

The front of the forearm is usually the most convenient place to take split skin for grafting.

INTERNAL FIXATION WITH KIRSCHNER WIRE In closed fractures you will probably get better results with closed methods, which are enough for at least 95% of fractures you will see. In some open fractures, and especially in severe hand injuries, thin Kirschner wire is useful (70.13). In expert hands and under ideal conditions, this is indicated for: (1) Displaced fractures of phalangeal shafts, where closed reduction has failed. (2) Displaced fractures close to or involving a joint. (3) Major unstable injuries.

FOREIGN BODIES are difficult to remove unless you can feel them. When you X-ray a patient, cross two pieces of wire and put them over the entry hole as a marker. Fuse wire is very useful for this purpose.

CLOSING A HAND INJURY

CONTROL BLEEDING Release the tourniquet, apply a firm pack, and wait 5 minutes. If any bleeders remain, catch them in a fine haemostat and twist them, or tie them with fine catgut or monofiliament.

If an ooze persists, insert a small drain, but don't forget to remove it after 48 hours.

CAUTION ! (1) Don't use diathermy. (2) When you clamp vessels, do so under direct vision. Don't clamp blindly.

SUTURE MATERIALS Use 3/0 or 4/0 monofilament on fine needles, use fine stitches, and don't make them too tight. A common mistake is to use coarse catgut in huge needles. Don't try to bring the skin edges together down the whole length of the patient's wound, a few small gaps will allow it to drain.

CAUTION ! Don't stitch unnecessarily. Leave unstitched: (1) Transverse wounds in the line of the creases. (2) Linear wounds which do not gape.

IMMEDIATE PRIMARY SUTURE is more often indicated in the hand than it is elsewhere (54.2). Even so, it is only indicated if a wound: (1) Is less than 12 hours old. (2) Is really clean, and 'tidy', as in incised or penetrating wounds. (3) Allows you to bring the skin edges together without tension.

DELAYED PRIMARY SUTURE is safer in all but the cleanest and most recent wounds, especially if the wounds overlie joints or fractures. It is also best in 'untidy', burst, or severely bruised wounds. Don't delay suture beyond 3 days, and if the third day is a holiday, don't defer it a further day. It is still part of the primary suture, and therefore still an emergency.

ANALGESICS are necessary because hand injuries are painful, so make sure the patient is given pethidine.

ANTIBIOTICS are not nearly as important as a careful would toilet. Surgeons who do this and follow it by delayed primary suture usually get better results than those who use immediate primary suture and antibiotics (54.1).

RINGS can seriously impede the circulation in an injured hand. So remove all rings with either: (1) soap and water or (2) a ring saw. Or, (3) wind string closely round the finger from its tip towards the ring. Thread the string under the ring, and use it to help pull the ring off, as in D, to H, Fig. 75-5.

TETANUS TOXOID Don't forget this (54.12).

DRESSINGS Use these special dressing methods for the hand.

Thumb Bandage the patient's thumb well anteriorly and in abduction. Place a roll of bandage between his thumb and his palm, so that it opposes his fingers and does not lie in the plane of his palm.

Severe injuries Try to get uniform, firm compression. Pack plenty of dry gauze around a severely injured hand. If adjacent fingers are injured, pack plenty of gauze between them to prevent them sticking together. Don't bind them to one another.

CAUTION! If possible, keep the tips of the patient's fingers showing, so that you can check their circulation.

SPLINTS When necessary, splint the patient's hand in the position of safety (Fig. 75-8), except when his tendons have been injured. Leave the splint on until the wound has healed. (2) Splint IP joints extended. Splint MP joints flexed, unless it is absolutely necessary to splint them extended, as in an extensor tendon injury. (3) Splint his thumb in opposition.

CAUTION ! Don't forget to elevate his hand. If he is ambulant, raise his arm across his chest with a St John's sling (Fig. 75-1).

POSTOPERATIVE CARE IN A HAND INJURY

Watch the circulation in the patient's fingers, his temperature, and his regional nodes. If there are no signs of infection, leave the dressing and the splint for 7 days. Then remove the sutures.

If necessary, do a secondary repair of any cut nerves or tendons at 3 weeks.

EXERCISES IN A HAND INJURY

If a patient has a serious injury, *exercises are absolutely critical if he is ever to use his hand normally again! Start them as soon as traumatic oedema has subsided.* Explain that they are necessary to prevent his hand becoming stiff and make sure he understands. Tell him that he must start to move his hand, even if it hurts. Demonstrate the movements you wish him to make, and then get him to do them, actively, or, *gently,* passively many times a day. The range of movement should slowly increase until each joint goes through its *full range.* This means: (1) Flexion and extension of all his fingers and his thumb. (2) Adduction and abduction of all his fingers to and from the midline. (3) Abduction, adduction, and circumduction of his thumb, and its opposition to each of his fingers. Most adults can do these exercises on their own. Children usually recover so quickly that they hardly need them. Provided patients do their exercises, they need not come for physiotherapy. If they cannot be trusted to do their exercises by themselves, they must come every day.

CAUTION ! Explaining a patient's exercises to him is the most valuable thing you can do.

THE FURTHER MANAGEMENT OF A HAND INJURY

If a patient has a serious hand injury, refer him. Read on for injuries of his nails (75.5), finger fractures (75.6), fractures of his distal phalanx (75.7), mallet finger (75.8), fractures of his middle phalanx (75.9), angulated phalangeal fractures (75.10), open comminuted fractures of his fingers (75.11), fractures of his last four metacarpals (75.12), injuries of his thumb (75.13), fractures of the base of his first metacarpal (75.14), Bennett's fracture (75.15), transverse and T– or Y–shaped fractures of the base of his first metacarpal (75.16), dislocation of his fingers or thumbs (75.17), injuries of his volar plate (75.18), injuries of his collateral ligaments (75.19), extensor tendon injuries (75.20), flexor tendon injuries (75.21), repairing a digital nerve (75.22), accidental amputations (75.23), planned finger amputations (75.24), multiple fractures and the severely injured hand (75.25), degloving injuries (75.26), a groin flap for the back of an injured hand (75.27), and more difficulties with injured hands (75.28).

NEVER IMMOBILIZE AN MP JOINT IN EXTENSION

75.2 Stiffness in hand injuries

Stiffness is *the* great enemy in hand injuries. The bones of a patient's injured hand almost always unite, but if he is an adult, his finger joints easily become stiff as the result of oedema, infection, and immobility. Stiffness is fortunately seldom a problem in children. You can minimize stiffness if you: (1) Reduce oedema

THE POSITION OF SAFETY

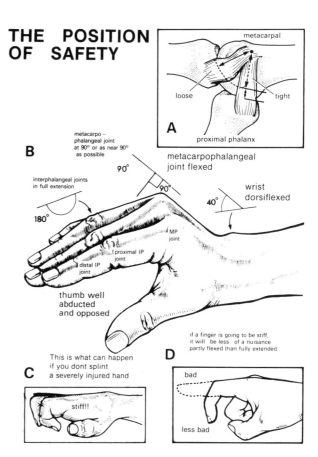

Fig. 75-8 THE POSITION OF SAFETY. A, shows that the collateral ligaments of a patient's MP joints are tense in the flexed position, and slack in the extended position (the reverse is the case with his IP joints). B, shows the position of safety. Note that the MP joints of his fingers are flexed, to as near 90° as they will go, but that his IP joints are in full extension. Both the joints of his thumb are extended, and his thumb is forward of his palm. C, shows the what will happen to his hand if you don't position it properly—his MP joints will extend, and his IP joints will flex. D, shows the least unsatisfactory position for a stiff finger. *A, after Campbell, with kind permission. B, C, and D, kindly contributed by Peter Bewes.*

by elevating an acutely injured hand (Fig. 75-1). A firm compression dressing with plenty of cotton wool will also help. (2) Minimize infection by paying particular attention to the principles of wound management, and never suture an injured hand or any of its fingers tightly. (3) Never immobilize a finger unnecessarily. (4) When immobilization is necessary, *don't do it for longer than 3 weeks.* Then start exercises immediately, whatever the condition of the patient's finger. If you break this rule, he may have a stiff finger forever. Many finger fractures don't need immobilising, and like most long bones, will unite as well or better without it. (4) Don't immobilize any neighbouring normal fingers, because they too will become stiff. (5) Dress a patient's injured hand in the position of safety described below. (6) Start movements early. From the very beginning, exercise all joints that have not been splinted, including his wrist, his elbow, and his shoulder. This will prevent his being left with a good hand, but a stiff shoulder.

Never try to bend fingers forcibly, or to stretch them passively. Instead, start active movements early, and if the injury is severe, make sure the patient has some occupational therapy. Encouraging him to do or make something is better than merely telling him to move his fingers.

CONTROL TRAUMATIC OEDEMA BY ELEVATION

FINGER SPLINTS

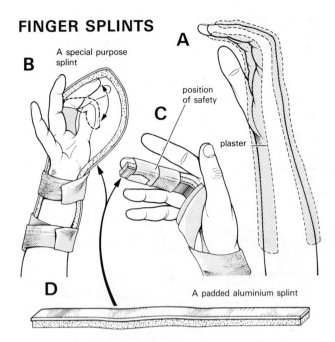

Fig. 75-9 SPLINTING AN INJURED HAND. A, dorsal and palmar plaster slabs in the position of function. B, padded aluminium splints can be used for many purposes. In this case the splint is for a fracture of the anterior lip of the patient's middle phalanx. It will allow his PIP joint to flex but not extend. C, a finger correctly splinted with its MP joint flexed and its IP joint extended. *Partly after Watson Jones with kind permission.*

75.3 Positions and splints for an injured hand, the position of safety (the James position)

If the ligaments of a finger joint which is not being used lie slack, they shorten, so that the joint becomes stiff. MP joints stiffen if they are left in the extended position, and IP joints stiffen if they are left flexed. The best way to prevent stiffness is to rest injured fingers in the position in which their ligaments are stretched. This is the position of safety in Fig. 75-8. It is the position from which a patient is most easily rehabilitated.

If you must splint a patient's injured hand, splint it in the position of safety. (1) Flex his MP joints to 90°, or as near to 90° as they will go. The collateral ligaments of these joints are attached eccentrically to the bones, so that they are slack at full extension, and are stretched in full flexion. (2) Keep his IP joints in full extension, because this is the position in which their ligaments are fully stretched. (3) His thumb is different, so keep its MP and IP joint extended. Also, keep it abducted and well forward of the plane of his palm, so that he can grasp with it. A stiff thumb in the plane of his palm will be useless. (4) Dorsiflex his wrist to 40°. The only exceptions are nerve and tendon injuries in which the positions for relaxing injured tendons take precedence over the position of safety.

The position of safety has been a great advance, but it is not an easy one to maintain. There are several ways of doing it. Adapt whatever method you choose to the needs of the injury. The only part which needs to be in the position of safety is the injured part. The rest of a patient's hand can be in any position—provided it is allowed to move.

The position of function is the most useful position for a finger or hand which will not move, and is different from the position of safety. The worst position for a permanently stiff or ankylosed finger is full extension. If a finger is going to become stiff permanently, it will be much less of a nuisance if it is partly flexed. It may be even less of a nuisance if you amputate

it (75.24). If several fingers are stiff, they should be partly flexed, as if the hand were grasping something.

POSITIONING AN INJURED HAND

THE POSITION OF SAFETY The patient's wrist is the key joint. If you hold it moderately extended, his fingers will tend to fall into the position of safety. Often, all you need do is to dorsiflex his wrist with a plaster cock-up splint (Fig. 69-2), and the rest of his hand will fall into position.

ALUMINIUM SPLINTS FOR FINGER INJURIES

Bend the splint to 90°, and strap it to the patient's palm with its angle just proximal to his *proximal* transverse palmar crease for his index and middle finger, or his *distal* palmar crease for his ring and little fingers. These are the positions of his MP joints—compare them with your own by looking at your own hand from the side.

Reduce his fracture, and lay it on the splint so that his MP joint is flexed to 90°, and his IP joints are extended. The splint need not cross his wrist. Don't double it back over the dorsum of his finger.

CAUTION ! (1) Look at his finger end on to check rotation. (2) Warn him not to meddle with his splint. He can easily alter its position, or take it off. If he is uneducated or uncooperative, a plaster slab will be wiser.

If you don't have aluminium splints, you can usually use a garter splint. Many surgeons use Kirschner wire for injuries for which an aluminium splint is indicated in the text.

A VOLAR SLAB FOR FINGER INJURIES

INDICATIONS (1) Fractures of single fingers in uncooperative, uneducated patients who might interfere with an aluminium finger splint. (2) Multiple fractures. (3) Some fractures of the thumb. (4) If necessary, you can use a volar slab for almost any fracture or wound of the hand. (5) Burns (58.29). (6) Infections involving joints or tendons.

Apply a volar slab with the patient's wrist dorsiflexed, his MP joints flexed, and his IP joints extended, as when using an aluminium splint. When the volar slab has set, add a dorsal one to maintain the position of his fingers against the volar slab. If necessary, add longitudinal ridges to the volar slab to give it greater strength.

CAUTION ! (1) If possible, leave the patient's thumb free. If you have to include it, bring it forward of his palm. (2) A hand which has been properly immobilized is bulky. Don't try to make a tidy parcel out of it. (3) Don't immobilize normal fingers—keep them moving.

DIFFICULTIES WITH SPLINTS FOR THE HAND

If you are IN DOUBT AS TO WHEN TO REMOVE A SPLINT, err on the side of removing it a little too soon, especially if a finger is not in a position of safety. Remove all splints at 3 weeks or earlier (the mallet splint is an exception, 75.8).

REHABILITATION IS EASIEST FROM THE POSITION OF SAFETY

75.4 Fixing fractures with Kirschner wire

A useful way of fixing some unstable fractures is to use Kirschner wire. If you can insert two wires which cross one another, you will immobilize a fracture very satisfactorily. See also Sections 70.13 and 75.25.

KIRSCHNER WIRE FIXATION

INDICATIONS Unstable fractures which you cannot immobilize in any other way, especially if they are open, and multiple.

KIRSCHNER WIRE

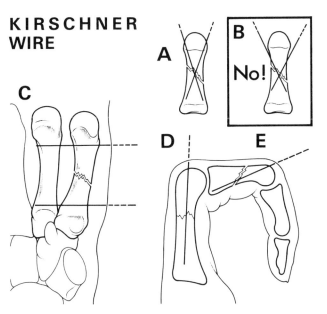

Fig. 75-9a FIXING FINGERS WITH KIRSCHNER WIRE. A, drill the wires through the sides of a condyle, which will be easier than drilling them through the side of the neck (B). C, fixing the shaft of the fifth metacarpal with Kirschner wire. D, longitudinal fixation for a metacarpal. E, is the same injury as in A, but is viewed from the side.
Kindly contributed by James Cairns.

EQUIPMENT A bone drill, a Kirschner wire plier cutter, and some 8 cm lengths of 0.75 mm Kirschner wire. If you don't have a drill, you may be able to put the wire in with a Steinmann pin introducer. These wires are usually supplied with sharp points; if you want to sharpen a cut end, do so with a stone. If possible use wire with a bevelled end slightly wider than the rest of the wire. This will overdrill the bone through which it passes and avoid distraction of the fragments.

METHOD Drill the wire in with a hand drill. Cut the wires short just under the skin, and leave them in for 12 to 21 days, or until the bone has united. To remove a wire, make a nick in the skin under local anaesthesia and extract it with pliers.

For the shaft of a phalanx, enter the lateral aspect of a condyle, and drill through the shaft, into but not through its base. Drill from the dorsal aspect of the condyle, towards the volar aspect of the base. Going through the sides of a condyle will be easier than trying to go through the sides of the neck of the shaft. The bone is harder here and it is difficult for the drill to enter the bone obliquely.

For fractures of the neck of a metacarpal, enter the condyle in a similar manner. Many of these fractures don't need Kirschner wire, so see Section 75.12.

For a severely injured hand, see Section 75.25.

75.5 Nail injuries

Splinters below the nail If you cannot remove a splinter with forceps, use scissors to excise a V—shaped area of the patient's nail under local anaesthesia, as in Fig. 75-10.

Subungual haematoma. A blow on the end of a patient's finger may cause blood to collect under his nail. You can easily relieve the severe pain that this causes without an anaesthetic: (1) Open out a paper clip, heat its end red hot, and push this into the nail over the haematoma. It will burn a hole in his nail, and the blood will flow out. Or, (2) use a large sterile hypodermic needle to drill a hole in his nail over the haematoma. In either case put a dressing over the hole and ask him to keep his finger dry.

TWO NAIL INJURIES

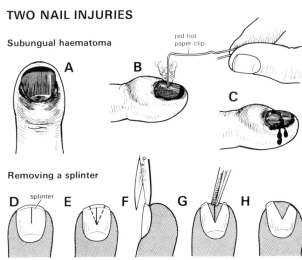

Fig. 75-10 TWO NAIL INJURIES. A, to C, trephining a subungual haematoma with a red hot paper clip. D, to H, removing a splinter.
Partly after Rutherford, Nelson, Weston, and Wilson with kind permission.

Avulsion of the fingernail A more severe injury to the tip of a patient's finger may remove his nail, completely or partly; it may also fracture his terminal phalanx or displace its epiphysis. If you don't treat him adequately, his finger may be disfigured permanently, or he may develop osteomyelitis. Clean his wound, remove the base of his nail, and replace his nail or his nail bed under his nail fold. Hold his nail in place with a mattress suture, and give him an antibiotic.

75.6 Finger fractures

Any of the bones in a patient's hand can break, so there are many possible fractures he can have. Some, such as those which enter joints, are serious, while others, such as undisplaced fractures of the phalanges, are not. Fig. 75-11 will help you to decide how to treat him.

You have several methods to choose from. (1) Active movements. (2) The garter splint, shown in Fig. 75-14, which will support an injured finger and yet allow it to move. If these two methods are appropriate, they are much the best. (3) An aluminium splint, or, failing this, (4) plaster slabs, as shown in Fig. 75-9. (5) The splint in Fig. 75-15, which holds a patient's fractured finger over a roll of bandage in his palm. (6) Kirschner wire internal fixation. We don't generally advise this for phalanges, but you may find it useful for severely injured metacarpals. (8) You may be able to refer a patient for expert internal fixation.

As stressed earlier (75.2), stiffness is the great enemy. The wrong treatment can easily stiffen a patient's hand—*an unnecessary splint is much worse than no treatment!* If you are wise, you will disregard many fractures and concentrate on helping the patient to regain movement. *The common error is to overtreat hand fractures, so avoid doing this!* The common disability that follows incorrect treatment is a flexion contracture of the IP joints.

Most phalangeal fractures are not displaced and so don't need reduction, but in those which do it is critically important. When phalangeal fragments angulate, the fragments are usually convex towards the palm, whereas those of the metacarpals are usually concave.

Undisplaced fractures are usualy stable, so are most fractures of the metacarpals, because they splint one another.

FINGER FRACTURES

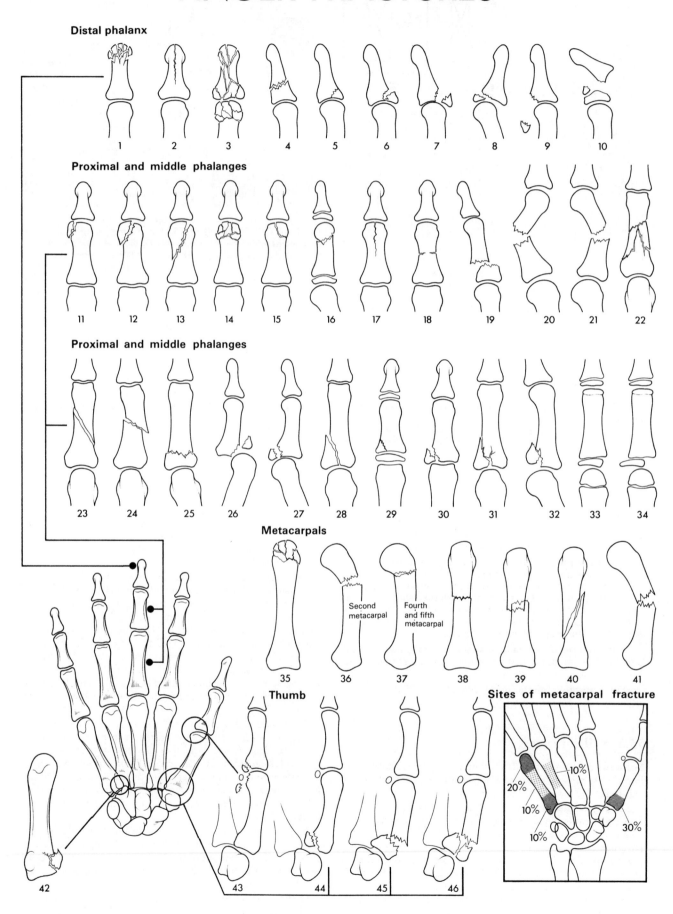

Distal phalanx

Proximal and middle phalanges

Proximal and middle phalanges

Metacarpals

Second metacarpal

Fourth and fifth metacarpal

Thumb

Sites of metacarpal fracture

Any joint which is subluxed must be reduced. As a general rule, any fracture which needs reduction also needs splinting, preferably with an aluminium splint.

Try to avoid two dangers:

(1) To prevent stiffness, don't immobilize injured fingers unless you have to. When you do immobilize them, do so in the correct position, and then don't immobilize them for too long. If a patient's proximal or middle phalanges are fractured, mobility is more important than *mild* anterior or moderate posterior angulation, so don't risk stiffness by trying to get perfect reduction.

(2) In fractures of the phalanges and metacarpals, avoid rotation, because this will make an injured finger overlap its neighbour as it flexes, as in Fig. 7-12. Prevent this serious disability by making sure that a finger always points to point 'X' in this figure. It is slightly to the lateral side of the wrist crease.

Fortunately, most fractures unite readily and seldom form callus, so there is no point in checking for radiological union. If after 3 weeks there is clinical union, you can assume that a fracture has united.

A child's epiphyses are easily displaced, especially those of a proximal phalanx close to its MP joint, sometimes with considerable rotation at the line of separation. Try to reduce these displacements as best you can.

AVOID ROTATION IN FINGER FRACTURES

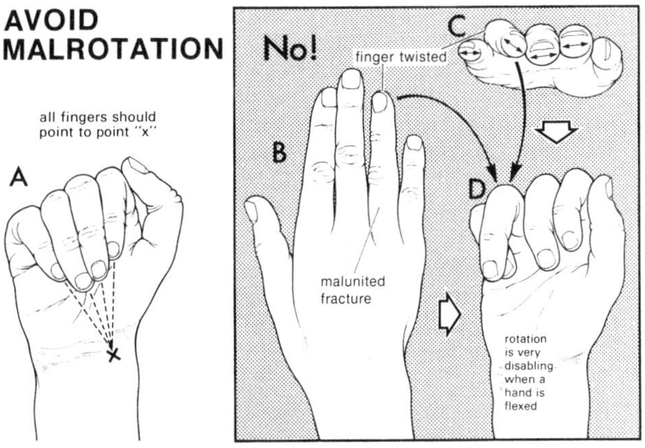

75.7 Injuries of the distal phalanx and distal IP joint

The tips of the three longest fingers are often crushed in a door, or hit with a hammer. Their distal phalanges may be small bones, but they are particularly important ones—especially if the patient is a typist or a violinist. In most injuries of a distal phalanx you can ignore injuries to the bone and the nail, and treat the patient as if he had only a soft tissue injury.

Injuries of the distal phalanges in children are different. In a child's finger, the tendon of flexor digitorum profundus is inserted into the metaphysis of a phalanx, and his long extensor tendon into the epiphysis. A combined angulating and crushing injury, such as crushing in a door, as in A, Fig. 75-13, can cause a mallet finger. Take a lateral X-ray to distinguish this from rupture of the extensor tendon which is rare.

FRACTURES OF THE DISTAL PHALANGES

CRUSH FRACTURES OF THE DISTAL PHALANGES

If a patient has a crush fracture (1, 2, or 3 in Fig. 75-11), don't suture his wound. Instead, mould the fragments

---

Fig. 75-11 FINGER FRACTURES. **Which diagram best matches the fracture your patient has? The numbered injuries are referred to in the following sections of the text. The box shows the commonest sites of metacarpal fractures and their approximate relative frequencies.**

Here is a summary of the treatment these fractures need.

Early active movements, where appropriate in a garter splint: 1, 2, 3, 4, 5, 11, 12*, 13*, 14*, 15, 16*, 17, 18, 22, 29, 31, 35, 37, 40, 42, 44 (optional), and 45. Fractures marked with an asterisk (*) should ideally have other treatment or be referred, but if this is impractical active movements are acceptable.

Mallet finger splint: 6 and 7.

Difficult surgery early: 8, 9, 26, 27, 28, 30 and 43.

Reduction and some kind of splint: 10, 19, 20, 21, 23, 24, 25, 32, 33, 34, 36, 37, 38, 39, 40, and 41. *Adapted from Watson Jones with kind permission. Treatment methods kindly summarized by Peter Bewes.*

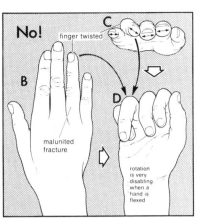

Fig. 75-12 AVOID MALROTATION. **All a patient's fingers should point to the place marked 'X'. If they don't, they will cause severe disability when they flex. You can easily miss a rotation deformity, so check the alignment of his nails by looking at them end on, as in C.**

---

together, apply a dry dressing, plenty of cotton wool, and a firm bandage or plaster cast round his distal phalanx only.

CAUTION ! (a) If possible, avoid including his terminal IP joint in the bandage or cast, because immobilization may stiffen it. Keep it moving. If you have to include it, make sure that if it does stiffen, it does so slightly flexed. (b) Don't splint his finger.

If there are no signs of infection, leave the cast on for 3 weeks. Warn him that his finger will remain tender for 6 weeks, and may continue to improve its shape for 6 months.

If he has a painful subungual haematoma, trephine his nail if this seems necessary (Fig. 75-10), leave it in place, and dress it with vaseline gauze. It may regrow abnormally; if it is a sufficient nuisance, he can have it removed later.

If his nail is loose, remove it. Reconstitute his nail bed and repair it with a single mattress suture which will draw it under his nail fold.

If the bone of his terminal phalanx is exposed, don't amputate it, or remove any bone if you can avoid doing so, because much of his finger tip may still be alive. If you remove the distal fragment, he will be left with a floppy finger tip. The distal phalanx has great capacity for repair, particularly in children. If necessary, trim the exposed bone.

If the injury includes the patient's distal IP joint (3), consider amputating through his middle phalanx, leaving enough of its shaft to include the attachment of his flexor tendons.

TRANSVERSE FRACTURES OF THE DISTAL PHALANGES

If a patient has an undisplaced transverse fracture (4), treat him with active movements as for a crush fracture (see above).

BASAL FRACTURES OF THE DISTAL PHALANGES

If the patient has a fracture of the dorsum of the base of his distal phalanx, treat him with active movements if it is not displaced (5), and as you would a mallet fracture (75.8) if it is displaced (6, and 7).

If a chip is displaced from the volar surface of the base of his distal phalanx (8, and 9), refer him early for difficult surgery. If you cannot refer him, treat him as for an avulsion injury of his profundus tendon. Suture or fix the bone fragment in place with a pull out suture, as in Fig. 75-26.

DISPLACED EPIPHYSES OF THE DISTAL PHALANGES

If the distal fragment is forced out through the nail bed (10 in Fig. 75-11, and A, Fig. 75-13), reduce the fracture by the open method, and insert the proximal end of the patient's nail into his nail fold where it will act as a splint. Splint his distal IP joint in extension (like a mallet finger) for 2 weeks. These are serious, difficult injuries, and a mallet deformity often follows.

75.8 Mallet finger

The extensor mechanism of the fingers is liable to two similar injuries—the distal IP joint to a 'mallet finger' (D, Fig. 75-13), and the proximal IP joint to the 'boutonniere injury' (75.20).

A mallet deformity is a distal IP joint which cannot be fully extended. A mallet finger in a child is often the result of an open injury; in an adult it is usually caused by a closed one. One of the patient's extensor tendons tears away from the base of his distal phalanx. In doing so it may remove a small fragment of bone. He cannot extend his distal phalanx actively, so that it remains permanently bent. This, however, is no disability, unless he is engaged in fine work. If you apply a cast in the first fortnight, you may succeed in preventing this deformity.

If a mallet cast is too tight, it will cause a pressure sore, and if it is too loose, it will be useless, so try to get it just right. Pressure sores and stiff fingers are common and the results of treatment are not good.

MALLET FINGER

If a patient has a mallet finger (5, 6, and 7, in Fig. 75-11), disregard it if he is a labourer, and encourage active movements. Many patients will accept the mild disability of a slightly bent finger tip. But, if a patient does fine work, apply a mallet splint or cast, especially if his index finger is involved. Treat him like this:

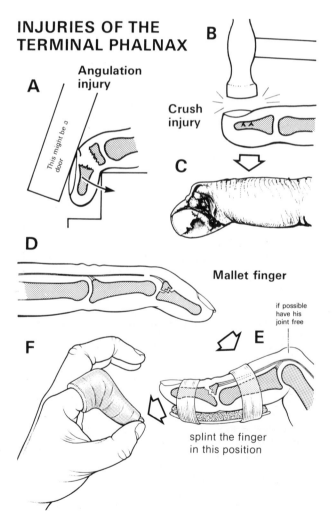

Fig. 75-13 INJURIES OF THE DISTAL PHALANX. A, an angulation injury fractures an adult's terminal phalanx, or displaces a child's epiphysis. **B,** and **C,** a crush injury. **D,** the typical deformity of a mallet finger. **E,** the position for splinting held with a metal splint. **F,** a plaster splint hardening in position. *Partly from Rutherford, Nelson, Weston, and Wilson. With kind permission.*

If a chip of bone is displaced (6, or 7), refer him for internal fixation. If this is impractical, do nothing, because a mallet cast will make him worse.

If there is no bony fragment, or there is one but it is not displaced (5), apply a special metal or plastic mallet splint, or failing this, a mallet cast.

A MALLET CAST Wind five turns of 7 cm dry plaster bandage round the end of the patient's finger, to include his flexed proximal IP joint. If you don't do this it will slip off. Wet the bandage and quickly mould it round his finger without including any bubbles. While the plaster sets, ask him to hold his distal IP joint in hyperextension, and his proximal joint flexed, by pressing his fingertip with his thumb, as in F, Fig. 75-13.

Leave the cast on for 6 weeks. When you remove it, full active extension of his distal IP joint is usually limited by about 25°. If he is unwilling to accept this deformity, reapply a mallet cast for a further 8 weeks. If necessary, his extensor tendon can later be shortened operatively.

75.9 Injuries common to a middle or proximal phalanx

You can treat many fractures of the proximal and middle phalanges in a garter splint. This has the great advantage of keeping the patient's injured finger moving and does not impair the movement of his adjacent normal fingers. Be sure to correct any rotational deformity first.

INJURIES COMMON TO A MIDDLE OR PROXIMAL PHALANX

INJURIES OF THE HEAD AND CONDYLES OF THE PROXIMAL AND MIDDLE PHALANGES

If a tiny chip of bone has been pulled away from the condyle of a phalanx by a collateral ligament (or by the capsule or volar plate), the patient has a sprain fracture (11, in Fig. 75-11). If there is no instability or subluxation, treat him by early active movements in a garter splint which joins his injured finger to the normal finger from which it is most displaced. If there is considerable instability, refer him for repair of his collateral ligaments, or repair them yourself with Kirschner wire (75.4). If his finger is not treated correctly, it will remain permanently bent, as in Fig. 75-14. Warn him that his injured joint will be permanently swollen.

If the joint is unstable, or a large fragment of a condyle is displaced (12), his injury is probably serious, especially if a PIP joint is involved. Refer him for the repair of his injured collateral ligament, or fixation of the fragment with Kirschner wire. If you cannot refer him, treat him in a garter splint.

If a condylar fracture line is oblique (13), the fragment is likely to displace longitudinally. This is a serious unstable injury, especially if it involves a proximal phalanx. If the fragment is undisplaced (rare), splint the patient's finger in a garter splint. If the fragment is displaced, refer him for a difficult internal fixation. If you cannot refer him, try to correct any displacement on an aluminium splint or plaster slab. The results are likely to be bad, and his finger may well be stiff and crooked permanently. Some surgeons would treat this injury with early active movements.

If a condylar fracture is comminuted or T−shaped (14), the future function of the finger is likely to be poor. If you cannot do an immediate arthrodesis, consider amputation. Alternatively, treat him with early active movements.

If the proximal part of the fracture line is transverse (15), the injury is stable, so treat the patient in a garter splint.

INJURIES OF THE NECK OF A PHALANX

If the neck of a phalanx is fractured, and the distal fragment is rotated (16), refer the patient for internal reduction. This is a common injury in children. It must be reduced and held in place with Kirschner wire, because it will not remodel. If you fail to reduce it, permanent loss of flexion may result. If you cannot reduce it, treat him with early active movements.

INJURIES OF THE SHAFT OF A PHALANX

If a fracture of the shaft is longitudinal (17), treat the patient with active movements.

If a fracture of the shaft is transverse, either complete or incomplete, and is undisplaced (18), apply a garter splint.

If the fragments of a transverse fracture are displaced end to end (19), reduce them by applying traction in the length of the patient's finger, and then apply a garter splint.

If a fracture of the shaft is transverse and angulated so that its fragments are convex anteriorly (common) (20), reduce it accurately as in Section 75.10.

If a fracture of the shaft is transverse and angulated so that its fragments are convex posteriorly (rare) (21), reduce it as in Section 75.10.

If a fracture of the shaft is comminuted and is not obviously unstable (22), aim for early mobilization in a garter splint. If it is obviously unstable, splint it with an aluminium or plaster splint (Fig. 75-9). Treatment is the same, whether or not it involves a joint. For open comminuted fractures, see Section 75.11.

If a fracture of the shaft is spiral (23), correct any rotation and apply a garter splint.

If a shaft fracture is oblique (24), try to reduce it on an aluminium splint. If this fails, refer the patient for internal fixation. This is a serious injury.

CAUTION ! The distinction between spiral fractures (23) and oblique ones (24) is important.

INJURIES OF THE BASE OF A PHALANX

If a patient has a transverse fracture at the base of a proximal phalanx (25), he is likely to be old. Be careful not to overlook marked angulation. You may mistake it for hyperextension of his MP joint. On the X-ray the overlap by his other fingers may obscure it. Reduce the angulation and splint his finger for 3 weeks with his MP joint flexed and his IP joints extended.

If he has a chip off the dorsal (26) or volar (27) surfaces of his phalanx, refer him for difficult surgery. If this is impossible, reduce any displacement by applying traction, and treat him by early mobilization. See also injury 32.

IF A FRACTURE ENTERS A FINGER JOINT

If the joint is subluxed, you must reduce it.

If the fragment is large (28), and facilities for internal fixation are available, refer the patient, especially if the fracture involves his proximal or middle IP joint. If you cannot refer him, treat him with early active movments.

If a patient has an undisplaced marginal fracture (29), treat him with early active movements.

If he has a displaced marginal fracture (30), be sure to reduce any subluxation or dislocation. If you cannot refer him, treat him in a garter splint.

If the articular surfaces of a joint are comminuted (31), treat the patient by early active movements in a garter splint.

If the anterior lip of the base of a middle phalanx is displaced (32), the joint is probably also subluxed, and the injury is serious. Don't treat the patient by unrestricted movements. Reduce the subluxation and try to keep it reduced. Extension is the unstable position. Splint it as in B, Fig. 75-9 (Dobyns' splint). Carefully strap an aluminium splint to the patient's hand and proximal phalanx, so as to prevent extension of his PIP joint, but to allow it to flex. X-ray him in the splint, if this shows any persistent subluxation, refer him for internal fixation.

EPIPHYSEAL INJURIES OF A FINGER

If an epiphysis is minimally displaced (33, in Fig. 75-11), no reduction is needed. Treat the child with early active movements.

If an epiphysis is more than minimally displaced, and especially if there is any rotation deformity (34), be sure to correct it, so that the injured finger is in the proper relation to its neighbours in both flexion and extension, and is not rotated. Then splint it, preferably with an aluminium splint. Most displaced epiphyses are in the proximal phalanx close to the MP joint. This is not a true hinge because it allows some sideways movement. Thus it remodels readily in both planes. If the epiphysis of a middle phalanx (a true hinge joint) is displaced, it will remodel in the plane of flexion and extension, but lateral and rotational deformities will not be corrected. So reduce this injury accurately.

A GARTER SPLINT FOR FINGER INJURIES

As soon as the immediate swelling is reduced, bind the patient's injured finger to one of its neighbours with adhesive strapping, as shown in Fig. 75-14. If there is the choice of two adjacent fingers, strap it to the finger which best corrects any deformity. A garter splint is more comfortable if you put a little padding between the two fingers.

If more than one phalanx is fractured, you may be able to apply more than one garter splint.

CAUTION ! (a) Be sure you correct any rotation deformity. (b) Be careful how you apply a garter splint during the acute phase, or the strapping may obstruct the circulation of the injured finger. (c) Don't let the strapping cross a joint, or it will prevent the movement that it is designed to encourage.

Remove a garter splint at 3 weeks, except for fractures of the middle phalanx, where you may need to leave it on longer. Rely on clinical union, and don't wait for radiological union.

If a garter splint fails to achieve good reduction of an oblique fracture, refer the patient for internal fixation.

CORRECT ANY ROTATIONAL DEFORMITY IN AN INJURED FINGER

A GARTER SPLINT

(or "buddy splint")

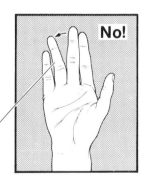

A garter splint lets an injured finger move, and so prevents stiffness. It also prevents angulation like this

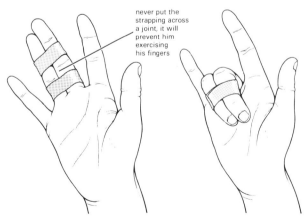

never put the strapping across a joint, it will prevent him exercising his fingers

Fig. 75-14 A GARTER SPLINT. This is also called a 'buddy' splint, because the injured finger is splinted by its 'buddy' (friend). The great advantage of a garter splint is that it keeps an injured finger moving. Never put strapping across a joint, because this will prevent the movement that the joint is designed to achieve. *Kindly contributed by Peter Bewes.*

75.10 Angulated phalangeal fractures

There is a common type of finger injury in which the fracture line runs transversely across the shaft of a patient's proximal or middle phalanx. The fragments are usually convex towards his palm so that they press on his flexor tendons. *If you don't correct this displacement, particularly in a fracture of his proximal phalanx, his tendons cannot work normally.* Although these fractures are easy to reduce, they easily displace again, unless you hold his MP joint flexed until the fragments have united. This is also the position of safety for this joint. At the same time, be sure to correct any rotation. Although closed methods are not perfect, they are likely to be better in your hands than the alternative, which is to fix the fragments with crossed Kirschner wires under X-ray control. The most practical closed method is to strap the patient's fractured finger over a firm roll of bandage in his palm.

ANGULATED PHALANGEAL FRACTURES

If a fracture is transverse and convex anteriorly (common) (20), pull (1) on the patient's finger to correct the angulation and disimpact the fragments, as in C, Fig. 75-15. Increase the angulation to get the fragments to hitch (2). Then flex the fragments forward (3) over the index finger of your other hand. Then, use adhesive strapping to hold the patient's injured finger flexed over a firm roll of bandage in his palm. Make sure his injured finger points to the point 'X' in Fig. 75-12. Hold it there with adhesive strapping for 10 days—not longer. Finally, protect it for another 10 days with a garter splint.

Alternatively, use an aluminium splint.

CAUTION! (a) Try to get good reduction. If closed reduction is not perfect, refer the patient for internal fixation. (b) Avoid rotation when you strap his fingers. (c) Unfortunately, this method immobilizes an injured finger, and is not a method to be used indiscriminately for all fractures. If a garter splint is practical, use it.

If a fracture is transverse, but concave towards the palm (rare) (21), reduce it and apply a dorsal plaster slab extending from the patient's lower forearm to the tip of his injured finger. Keep his MP joints flexed, and his IP joints extended. Keep the slab on for 10 days and encourage active movements of his other fingers meanwhile. Then apply a garter splint for a further 10 days.

75.11 Open comminuted crush fractures of the proximal or middle phalanges

When a patient crushes his fingers, he usually crushes several of them at the same time. The open comminuted crush fractures he receives are disappointing to treat, because there is usually much soft tissue injury, and both his flexor and extensor tendons may be badly bruised. If only one of his fingers is severely injured, and he is wise, he will probably agree to let you amputate it, especially if it is his ring or little finger, or even his index or middle finger. Preserve even a stump of an injured thumb.

OPEN FINGER AND THUMB FRACTURES

If the patient has multiple fractures and a severely injured hand, goto Section 75.25. His fracture is likely to become infected, so toilet his wound carefully. Remove detached fragments and any dead fatty tissue. Trim any grossly contaminated bone ends.

If the skin edges come together easily, suture them immediately with the minimum number of fine sutures. The hand is very vascular, so immediate primary closure is usually worth the risk. If the skin edges do not come together easily, or the injury is more than 12 hours old, leave the wound open for delayed primary suture, or apply a split skin graft.

If the patient's fracture is stable (as is usually the case) (22) and the next finger is normal, splint it in a garter splint. If there are no adjacent normal fingers, find the position that best holds the fragments reduced, close his wound, and then

FRACTURES OF THE PROXIMAL AND MIDDLE PHALANGES

(with forward angulation only)

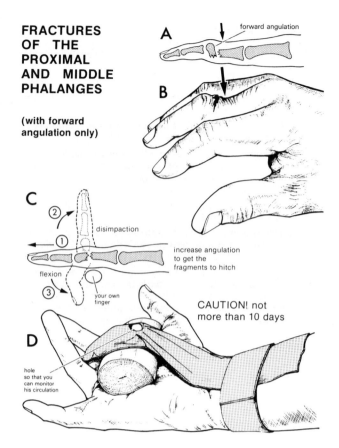

Fig. 75-15 FRACTURES OF THE PROXIMAL AND MIDDLE PHALANGES WITH FORWARD ANGULATION. A, and B, a fractured proximal phalanx with forward angulation. C, the movements of traction for disimpaction (1), posterior angulation for hitching (2), and flexion (3). D, the completed splint with the patient's finger flexed forwards in his palm over a roll of bandage.

devise an aluminium or plaster splint that will hold this position. Leave his normal fingers unsplinted and encourage him to move them. Elevate his hand.

If a severe open injury is unstable, you will have use Kirschner wire. Apply it in the position of safety. Drill it in through the head of a phalanx to one side of the midline (Fig. 75-9a). Pass it down to but not through the base of the phalanx. Cut it off under the skin over his proximal IP joint. Supplement this with an external splint.

If a fracture is unstable and you have no Kirschner wire, splint it with plaster slabs with the patient's MP joints flexed, and his IP joints just short of full extension.

If his finger is grossly injured, consider amputating it (75.24).

75.12 Fractures of the last four metacarpals

These common fractures usually follow a blow to someone else's jaw in which the patient breaks one or more of his metacarpals, usually the base of the first, the neck of the fifth, or the mid–shafts of the others. The fracture lines run either transversely across their shafts, or necks, or else spirally. If a fracture is transverse the fragments are usually concave towards his palm; if it is spiral they may overlap.

Typically, the back of the patient's hand is painful and swollen. When he clenches his fist, the normal contour of his knuckles is lost. X-rays are not essential, and may fail to show the fractures, unless you take several views.

Reduction in the anteroposterior plane is much less important than with fractures of the phalanges. The bowing of a transverse fracture and the overlap of a spiral one usually cause little disability. You can leave many of these fractures unreduced. There may be no need to splint them, except temporarily for comfort. *The main danger is a stiff hand, so early movement is more important than accurate reduction of the fragments.*

THE EARLY RETURN OF FUNCTION TAKES PRECEDENCE OVER THE ACCURATE REDUCTION OF FRAGMENTS

FRACTURED METACARPALS

METACARPAL HEAD FRACTURES

If the head of a metacarpal is comminuted (35, in Fig. 75-11), treat the patient by early active movements.

If a small chip of bone has been torn of the side off the head of a metacarpal (avulsion fracture, rare, not illustrated), apply a garter splint for 3 weeks. It is likely to be the result of a twisting injury.

METACARPAL NECK FRACTURES

If the neck of the patient's second metacarpal has broken so that its head angles forwards (36), you will have to reduce it because the shaft is immobile and does not allow any compensatory extension. If you cannot refer him, reduce the fracture by pushing the *proximal* fragment forwards. Maintain reduction by passing Kirschner wires transversely through the fractured metacarpal and on into its intact neighbour, as in C, Fig. 75-9a. Pass one wire through each fragment, cut the wires off subcutaneously, and remove them 3 weeks later. No cast is needed.

If the neck of his third metacarpal fractures, leave it.

If the necks of his fifth or fourth and fifth metacarpals have fractured, so that the heads have bowed forwards, and the fragments are impacted on one another (37, common), leave them. These metacarpals are mobile and can extend to compensate for the deformity. Treat him with active movements. Warn him that although his hand will probably work perfectly, it will have a lump on the back. This injury is usually the result of a fight with a closed fist.

CAUTION! Don't try to disimpact and splint these fractures because stiffness will result.

METACARPAL SHAFT FRACTURES

You can treat most of these fractures by rest and elevation for 10 to 14 days, with or without a protective bandage. Follow this with active finger and wrist movements. The patient can often use his hand fairly comfortably within a week. Explain that he may feel crepitus for some days and that he may have a lump on the back of his hand permanently. A transverse fracture takes 5 weeks to unite, and a spiral one only 3 weeks.

If his metacarpal shafts are fractured with little displacement (38), apply a plaster cockup splint as above. Mould his palm to it, so as to maintain his metacarpal arch. Bandage his hand to the splint and leave his fingers free.

CAUTION ! Encourage him to start exercising his fingers as soon as he can. They can easily become stiff.

If there is considerable overlap (39) use traction and pressure to reduce it. Try to correct any rotational deformity.

If the fracture is spiral (40), look carefully for any rotation deformity. If you find it, correct it by manipulation, and then apply a garter splint. Apply this in such a way as to rotate the injured finger towards its neighbour and restore the correct rotation.

If a fracture of the shaft of the fifth metacarpal is concave anteriorly (41), consider reducing it. Check for angulation by taking a lateral X-ray which superimposes all the metacarpals. Accept angulaton of up to 30°. If there is more than 30° of angulation, apply Kirschner wire fixation, as in

C, Fig. 25-9a, or apply the method of 3 point fixation in Fig. 75-16.

METACARPAL BASE FRACTURES

If the bases of the patient's second, third, and fourth metacarpals have been displaced posteriorly (not illustrated), the line of his knuckles will be flat instead of tracing a normal curve. This is a rare unstable and disabling injury, because he cannot dorsiflex his wrist, with the result that he cannot use his fingers normally. Reduce his metatacarpals by asking an assistant to exert traction on his fingers. Press firmly with your thenar eminence on the back of the patient's hand, while exerting counter pressure on the front of his carpus. Even a closely moulded cast often fails to maintain reduction, so drill some Kirschner wires obliquely through his metacarpals into his carpus, apply a cast, and remove the wires 4 weeks later.

If he has fractured the base of his fifth metacarpal (42, Fig. 75-11), treat him with early active movements. This is the equivalent of a Bennett's fracture on the other side of his hand.

75.13 Injuries of the thumb

Most thumb injuries are like those of the fingers, and you can treat most of them in the same way. Although the first metacarpal is more mobile and more like a phalanx than the other metacarpals, stability is also important. Try to keep a patient's injured thumb mobile and to maintain palmar (anterior) abduction, and radial abduction (less important). *Try, especially, to avoid an adduction contracture.*

The thumb also has some injuries of its own. One of them is a sprain. In this injury a violent lateral movement of the patient's thumb tears its medial MP ligament, or pulls a bony fragment from the base of its proximal phalanx. Unless this serious injury is successfully treated, he loses his pinch grip, so that he cannot write or open a door.

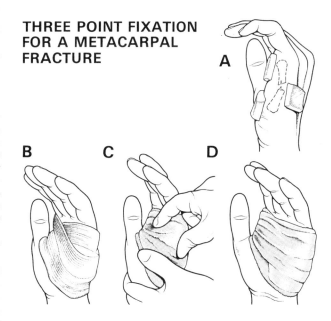

THREE POINT FIXATION FOR A METACARPAL FRACTURE

Fig. 75-16 MAINTAINING REDUCTION IN A TRANSVERSE FRACTURE OF A METACARPAL SHAFT. **This is an alternative to Kirschner wire for a fracture of the shaft of the fifth metacarpal. Don't use it for fractures of the neck. A, apply padding (preferably orthopaedic felt) ready for 3 point pressure. B, apply adhesive strapping to the patient's hand. C, apply an 8 cm plaster bandage to his hand and mould it by firm pressure to provide 3 point fixation. D, the completed cast.** *After Watson Jones, with kind permission.*

THUMB INJURIES

CRUSH INJURIES **If a patient's thumb has been crushed (not illustrated),** immobilize it with a dorsal aluminium splint, or scaphoid type of cast (Fig. 74-10), which leaves his fingers free and brings his thumb forward into a position in which it opposes his other fingers.

SPRAINED THUMB Hold the patient's first metacarpal steady, and try to move his thumb from side to side. Compare the movement you get with that on the normal side.

Examine his X-ray carefully for a small chip of bone off the ulnar corner of the base of his proximal phalanx (injury 43, in Fig. 75-11, see also Fig. 75-17).

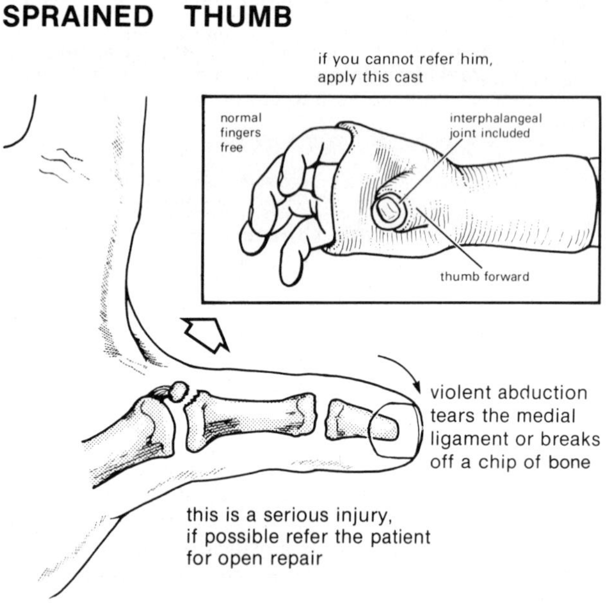

SPRAINED THUMB

if you cannot refer him, apply this cast

normal fingers free

interphalangeal joint included

thumb forward

violent abduction tears the medial ligament or breaks off a chip of bone

this is a serious injury, if possible refer the patient for open repair

Fig. 75-17 SPRAINED THUMB. If you cannot refer the patient for a difficult open repair, fit him with this cast. Just before it sets, try to move the shaft of his proximal phalanx into the reduced position.

If you are in doubt about the diagnosis, inject local anaesthetic into the site of the fracture, and take a stress X-ray with his thumb abducted, and with his other thumb, also abducted, included for comparison.

If there is abnormal movement, if the ligament is torn, or if the fracture is displaced (43), refer him for a difficult open repair. This can be done as late as 4 months.

CAUTION ! Note that there is normally a rounded sesamoid bone opposite the head of the metacarpal of the thumb. Don't interpret this as a fracture.

If you cannot refer the patient, fit him with the cast in Fig. 75-17. Make sure that: (a) His thumb is forward of his palm in the grasp position. (b) The IP joint of his thumb is free. (c) His normal fingers are free. (d) The cast goes above his wrist. Just before it sets, try to move the shaft of his proximal phalanx into the reduced position. Leave the cast on for 4 weeks.

75.14 Fractures of the base of the first metacarpal

The base of the first metacarpal is often injured. If there is no abnormal movement between a patient's thumb and his carpus, he has a sprain or an undisplaced fracture. Fit him with the cast described below. If there is abnormal movement, he has broken the base of his first metacarpal in one of the three ways shown in Fig. 75-18. (a) He can break off a chip, so that the joint with

the trapezium subluxes (Bennett's fracture, injury 44 Fig. 75-11). (b) He can fracture the base of his first metacarpal transversely (injury 45). (c) He may have a T−shaped or Y−shaped fracture into the joint (injury 46). You can, if necessary, treat all three fractures by early active movements, but warn him to expect a lump. Provided he really does do early active movements, the results are probably at least as good as with the other methods. If he neglects them, the results will be bad.

75.15 Bennett's fracture

In Bennett's fracture an oblique fracture line runs proximally into the joint from the ulnar border of the shaft of the patient's first metacarpal, about 1 cm from its base. The proximal fragment remains attached to his trapezium, and the long distal fragment which is most of his first metacarpal, displaces radially and dorsally, as in fracture 44, Fig. 75-11, and Fig. 75-18.

The base of the patient's thumb swells, moving it is painful, and the swelling obscures the displacement. This is one of the few fractures where you may examine for crepitus, so pull his thumb gently. It will elongate, and you will feel the two fragments grating together, after which his thumb will spring back. This distinguishes Bennett's fracture both from a dislocation, and from an impacted transverse fracture.

You have three choices; many surgeons would say the first is the best: (1) You can encourage early, active movements. (2) You can reduce the fracture and apply a Bennett's cast. Reducing it is easy, but holding it reduced while the cast hardens is not. This is an exacting method, so follow the instructions below carefully. (3) You can refer the patient for a difficult internal fixation.

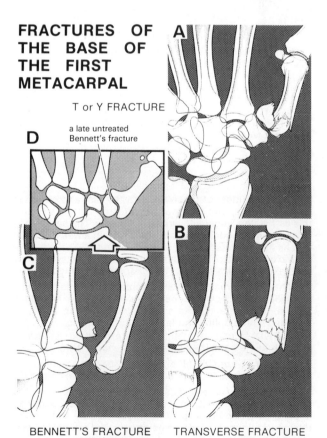

FRACTURES OF THE BASE OF THE FIRST METACARPAL

T or Y FRACTURE

a late untreated Bennett's fracture

BENNETT'S FRACTURE   TRANSVERSE FRACTURE

Fig. 75-18 FRACTURES OF THE BASE OF THE FIRST METACAR-PAL. A, a T−shaped or Y−shaped fracture. B, a transverse fracture. C, Bennett's fracture. If you don't treat this, it causes the characteristic deformity, D, which may, however, cause few symptoms. *Kindly contributed by Peter Bewes.*

TREATING BENNETT'S FRACTURE

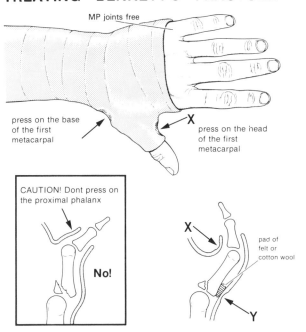

Fig. 75-19 BENNETT'S FRACTURE. Pad the base of the patient's first metacarpal. While the cast is setting, apply pressure to its head and base. Apply the cast with care so as to avoid a pressure sore. *After Sir John Charnley with kind permission.*

BENNETT'S FRACTURE

EARLY ACTIVE MOVEMENTS Bandage the patient's wrist in a crepe bandage for 4 days, and encourage him to use it. If he has a light job, send him back to work. The long term result is a stable fracture with the characteristic X-ray deformity shown in D Fig. 75-18.

BENNETT'S CAST

EXPLORING THE MOBILITY OF THE FRACTURE Under local anaesthesia press the palmar surface of the head of the patient's first metacarpal. At the same time press the dorsal surface of its base. This will extend his thumb, but take care not to extend it too much. The best position is just short of full forced extension. If you feel carefully as you do this, you may feel reduction taking place. If you now let go and allow his metacarpal to flex, you will see the base of his thumb riding up and out of the joint. Repeat the movements of reduction several times until you can feel the sensation of reduction by touch alone, without having to see it.

CAUTION ! Stick pads of adhesive felt or cotton wool over the base of the metacarpal and over its head. Rehearse reduction again. The sensation will now be muffled.

When you are confident that you can feel the position of reduction, apply the cast.

APPLYING THE CAST You must complete the whole cast while it is still soft. Rapidly apply a plaster bandage to the patient's hand and thumb without trying to hold the fracture reduced. Apply it from just below his elbow to the heads of his metacarpals. Bring it half-way up the proximal phalanx of his thumb.

While the plaster is still soft and wet, feel again for the sensation of reduction that you have already rehearsed. Recognize this through the wet plaster, and hold it while the plaster sets. Press against the palmar surface of the head of his first metacarpal ('X' in Fig. 75-19), and the dorsal surface of its base ('Y'). The hardened plaster should show where your fingers have pressed.

CAUTION ! (1) Press on the palmar surface of the head of his first metacarpal, not on the palmar surface of his prox-

imal phalanx. This hyperextends his MP joint without extending his first metacarpal. (2) Don't overextend his first metacarpal. This will redisplace the fragments. (3) Don't forget the padding!

Immediately take an X-ray to confirm reduction. If this is unsatisfactory, try once more. If this fails, or you are unable to maintain reduction without excessive pressure, refer him for internal fixation. If this is impossible, encourage early active movements. Leave the cast on for 6 weeks.

DIFFICULTIES WITH A BENNETT'S CAST

If the patient complains of SEVERE PAIN, remove and reapply the cast. It may be pressing on the base of his first metacarpal, and eroding the skin down to the tendon. Prevent this by: (1) Careful padding. (2) Achieving reduction more by judicious extension of his first metacarpal than by pressure over its base.

If the REDUCTION SLIPS, remove the cast and start active movements. Two years later most movement will have returned.

75.16 Transverse and T– or Y–shaped fractures of the base of the first metacarpal

A transverse fracture breaks the base of the patient's first metacarpal about a centimetre from the joint, but the fracture line does not enter it. The fragments impact and bow outwards as in fracture 45, Fig. 75-11, and A, Fig. 75-18. Although the base of his thumb is swollen and tender, moving it does not hurt him. When you pull it gently, you cannot feel crepitus. Both these signs distinguish this fracture from Bennett's. Even if you fail to correct gross angulation, he will not lose much thumb movement, and will only be mildly disabled. Treat him with early active movements.

A T– or Y–shaped fracture, enters the joint and is more serious. Ideally, these fractures need open reduction. If this is impractical, treat the patient with early active movements.

75.17 Dislocations of fingers and thumbs

These injuries are usually the result of severe hyperextension of the patient's fingers or thumb. The base of his dislocated phalanx comes to lie dorsal to the head of the bone proximal to it. IP dislocations are more common and more easily reduced than MP ones. Be sure to: (1) Hyperextend an MP joint first because this is a position in which the collateral ligaments are slack, and in which you can more easily push the base of the dislocated phalanx forwards into place. (2) Treat the injury early. These are acute emergencies; the longer you leave a dislocated finger, the more difficult will it be to reduce. After 4 days, reduction may be impossible.

DISLOCATED FINGERS AND THUMBS ARE ACUTE EMERGENCIES

DISLOCATIONS OF FINGERS AND THUMBS

In principle, you can reduce any IP or MP joint in the same way.

Reduce the patient's dislocation as in Fig. 75-20. Grasp his finger. Pull in the long axis of his dislocated phalanx (1), not his metacarpal. Hyperextend his finger (2). While maintaining traction, push the base of his dislocated phalanx forwards over the head of his metacarpal (3). Finally, flex his MP joint (4), and his finger will snap into position.

Test his finger for stability. Hold the proximal bone of the joint you are testing steady, and move the distal one from side to side. Does it give? Do this with an IP joint extended and

REDUCING A DISLOCATION OF A METACARPO-PHALANGEAL JOINT

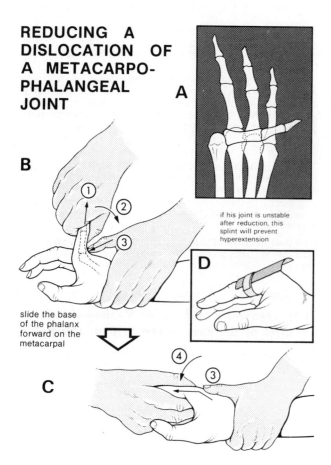

A

B

① ② ③

if his joint is unstable after reduction, this splint will prevent hyperextension

D

slide the base of the phalanx forward on the metacarpal

C

④ ③

Fig. 75-20 REDUCING A DISLOCATED MP JOINT. You can reduce fractures of a patient's proximal IP joint in the same way. If his finger is unstable after reduction, fit the guard in D. *After de Palma and Peter Bewes with kind permission.*

an MP joint flexed. These are the positions in which their ligaments should be taut.

If the reduction is stable, only immobilize the patient's finger long enough to let swelling and pain improve. Flex his injured finger over a roll of crepe bandage for 7 days as in Fig. 75-15, then apply a garter splint and start exercises.

If reduction is unstable, because the joint hyperextends: (1) Immobilize his finger in the position of safety with a splint (Fig. 75-9). Or, (2) strap a piece of stiff card or plastic to his proximal phalanx as in D, Fig. 75-20.

If closed reduction fails: (1) The anterior ligament may have become detached and gone into the joint. (2) The head of the phalanx may have buttonholed through the anterior capsule, so that the more you pull the tighter it becomes. (3) There may be an avulsion fracture of the base of the phalanx. Don't make more than two attempts at reduction, because you may damage the capsule and the collateral ligaments. If you tear them, the patient's finger will deviate to one side and cause him much disability. Refer him. If this is impossible, consider amputating a finger, but not a thumb.

DIFFICULTIES WITH A DISLOCATED FINGER

If, after a mild injury, a patient CANNOT EXTEND HIS FINGER at its MP joint, but the X-ray is normal, try manipulating his finger under anaesthesia—it may suddenly click into place.

75.18 Injuries of the volar plate

The volar plate is a piece of fibrocartilage over the volar surface of the MP and IP joints. A severe extension injury can tear it.

A PROXIMAL INTERPHALANGEAL JOINT

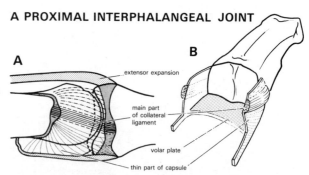

A

B

extensor expansion

main part of collateral ligament

volar plate

thin part of capsule

Fig. 75-21 THE ANATOMY OF A PROXIMAL IP JOINT. A, the main part of the collateral ligament is a strong narrow band. Anteriorly and posteriorly the capsule is thinner. The volar plate is a piece of cartilage on its anterior surface. B, the thick ligamentous structures round the joint form a closed box–like structure (shown here open) in which the head of the proximal phalanx rests. *After Campbell with kind permission.*

The front of the patient's injured joint is tender, but its collateral ligaments are stable when you stress them. Centre a good lateral X-ray on the joint and you may see that a small chip of bone has been displaced—a volar plate avulsion fracture (injury 27 in Fig. 75-11). Immobilize the patient's finger in flexion for a few days, then start active movements. The swelling may take weeks to heal. A flexion contracture, or a hyperextension deformity sometimes follows.

75.19 Injuries of the collateral ligaments

A violent sideways movement can tear the collateral ligaments of a patient's fingers. His IP joints have less sideways 'give' in them than his MP joints, and his proximal IP joint is the most likely to be injured. Be sure to examine his injured finger carefully to distinguish a strain from a tear.

INJURED COLLATERAL LIGAMENTS

Take a careful history to decide how force was applied to the patient's finger—end on, laterally, or in some other way.

Localize the tenderness and swelling exactly. Ask him to move his joint through its full range, from full flexion to full extension. If he cannot do this, expect a significant injury.

Stress his collateral ligaments by holding the proximal bone still and angulating the distal one. If stressing the joint is merely painful, but there is no abnormal mobility, it is only sprained. If there is abnormal mobility compared with his normal side, his collateral ligament is completely torn. If you are in doubt, do a ring block and test it again. X-ray him, and be sure to get a good lateral view.

SPRAINS Apply a garter splint. Warn him that his finger may be painful for 6 months and swollen for up to 2 years.

TEARS Reduce any displacement and splint his IP joint in extension. X-ray it. If you have been able to reduce the displacement, leave it splinted for 3 weeks. If you have been unable to reduce the displacement, refer him to have his joint explored and any interposed soft tissues extracted.

75.20 Extensor tendon injuries

Injuries to a patient's extensor tendons are easier to treat than those to his flexors: (1) The extensor tendons have only short sheaths, so that adhesion to them is not the problem that it is with flexor tendons. (2) They are joined to one another so that their cut ends do not retract. Any suture method which will bring their cut ends securely together is likely to be adequate.

286

THE BOUTONNIERE INJURY

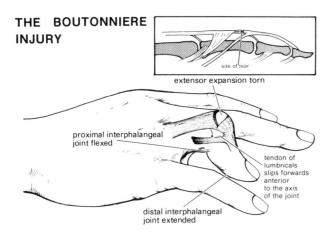

site of tear

extensor expansion torn

proximal interphalangeal joint flexed

tendon of lumbricals slips forwards anterior to the axis of the joint

distal interphalangeal joint extended

Fig. 75-22 THE BOUTONNIERE INJURY is a tear in the extensor expansion of a proximal IP joint in which the combined tendon of the lumbricals and interossei slips forwards anterior to the axis of the joint, so that the lumbricals and interossei flex the middle phalanx instead of extending it, as they do normally. The patient's distal IP joint is extended. If he is not treated correctly, a disabling flexor deformity will result.

The boutonniere deformity is the result of a wound on the dorsum of a patient's IP joint which destroys the central slip of his extensor tendon, so that he cannot extend the joint actively through its last 30°, although he still has a full range of passive movement. Such a wound may look minor when you first see it, and the skin over it may be only bruised, but it is potentially serious. If you don't treat him adequately, the deformity in Fig. 75-22 may follow. His proximal interphalangeal joint is acutely flexed, and his distal one extended. The tear in the central slip of his extensor expansion: (1) prevents extension of his middle phalanx, and (2) enables the combined tendons of his lumbricals and interossei to slip forwards and flex his proximal IP joint, instead of extending it in the normal way. Treat a boutonniere injury like any other injury of the extensor tendons, but the results will not be good.

EXTENSOR TENDON INJURIES

INDICATIONS FOR PRIMARY SUTURE (1) The injury occurred less than 24 hours ago. (2) There is no crushed or dead tissue. (3) The patient's wound is not badly contaminated. In all other cases delayed primary suture of the skin and secondary repair is wiser.

If there is severe loss of the skin of the back of the patient's hand, consider the groin flap in Section 75.27.

REPAIR Apply a tourniquet and do a thorough wound toilet. Splint the patient's hand and wrist in hyperextension while you operate. Toilet his wound (54.1), excise the skin edges, and extend the wound if necessary to expose the tendon ends. Trim them. Draw the proximal and the distal ends into the wound and hold them in place with needles which pass through the patient's skin, his tendon, and then his skin again. Dorsiflex his finger to bring the distal tendon into view. Suture the flat ends of the tendon with 3/0 or 4/0 wire or monofilament, using the 'X' suture in H, Fig. 75-23.

Splint his hand for 3 weeks with his wrist hyperextended (if possible), his MP joints flexed 15°, and his IP joints extended.

CAUTION ! Don't let him flex his injured hand until the period of splinting is complete.

DIFFICULTIES WITH EXTENSOR TENDON INJURIES

If you have repaired a BOUTONNIERE INJURY and the patient cannot extend his proximal IP joint when you take off the splint, refer him for a further attempt at open repair.

EXTENSOR TENDON INJURIES OF THE FINGER

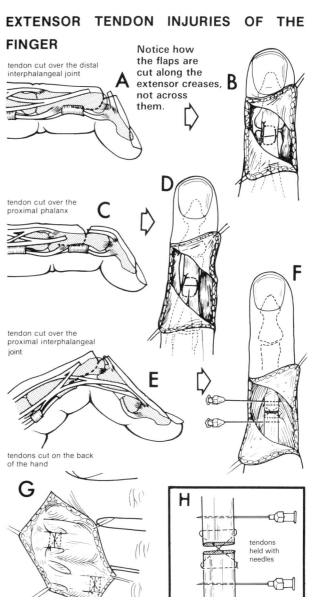

tendon cut over the distal interphalangeal joint

A

Notice how the flaps are cut along the extensor creases, not across them.

B

tendon cut over the proximal phalanx

C

D

F

tendon cut over the proximal interphalangeal joint

E

tendons cut on the back of the hand

G

H

tendons held with needles

Fig. 75-23 EXTENSOR TENDON INJURIES. A, and B, a tendon cut over the distal interphalangeal joint. The flaps to repair this injury have been cut along the extensor creases, not across them. C, and D, a similar injury, this time over the middle phalanx. E, and F, an injury over the proximal interphalangeal joint has been held with needles to make it easier to suture. It is often more convenient for these needles to go in through the skin on one side and out through the skin on the other side. G, cut extensor tendons over the back of the hend. *From Heim and Baltensweiler, with kind permission.*

If the EXTENSOR TENDONS TO A SINGLE FINGER ARE DESTROYED, he may be better with his useless finger amputated.

If his RADIUS HAS BEEN FRACTURED at the same time that his extensor tendons have been injured, they take precedence in repair. You may be able to lever the bone ends into place through his open wound. Use a tourniquet so that you are operating in a bloodless field.

75.21 Flexor tendon injuries

These are difficult injuries. On the anterior surface of the wrist there are 14 tendons, two main nerves, and two arteries, all of

THE STRUCTURES ON THE FRONT OF THE LEFT WRIST

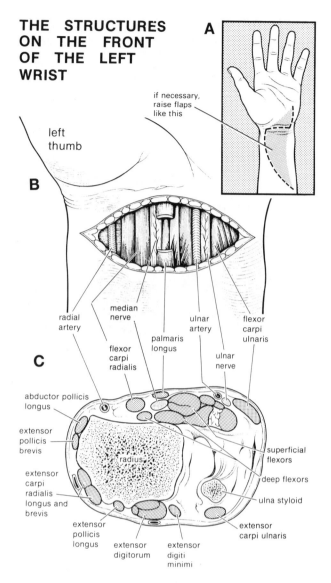

left thumb

if necessary, raise flaps like this

A

B

radial artery

median nerve

flexor carpi radialis

palmaris longus

ulnar artery

ulnar nerve

flexor carpi ulnaris

C

abductor pollicis longus

extensor pollicis brevis

extensor carpi radialis longus and brevis

radius

superficial flexors

deep flexors

ulna styloid

extensor carpi ulnaris

extensor pollicis longus

extensor digitorum

extensor digiti minimi

Fig. 75-24 STRUCTURES ON THE FRONT OF THE WRIST. A, if flaps are necessary, make them like this. B, the structures exposed through an incision in the flexor crease of the wrist. C, a cross section of the wrist.

which can be cut. Exposing and finding them is not easy, thus repairing them takes a long time.

Diagnosing that a patient has a flexor tendon injury is usually easy. His hand at rest should look like a normal hand at rest. However, if one of his fingers lies extended out of line with the others, it has probably been pulled into that position by the unopposed action of its extensor tendon. This enables you to decide which of his flexor tendons have been cut, as in Fig. 75-2.

For the purposes of repairing flexor tendon injuries, there are four zones:

Zone One, the tendons at the wrist which you must repair immediately because they retract rapidly.

Zone Two, the palm between the wrist and the distal palmar crease where repair is not too difficult. If you are moderately skilled, try to repair the profundus tendon(s) and disregard or remove sublimis. If you are unskilled, treat this zone as Zone Three.

Zone Three, an intermediate zone between the distal palmar crease and the proximal IP crease, where repair is very difficult because the superficial and deep flexor tendons are so closely packed and run in the same sheath. This zone used

to be called a 'no man's land' where even experienced surgeons got bad results. Recently, hand surgery has advanced so much that the the concept of a 'no man's land' is now outmoded—but only among real experts who can achieve good results in this zone by by primary repair. For the unskilled, and for the moderately skilled, the concept of 'no man's land' is still very relevant. If you are unskilled and you try to operate in this zone, you may injure a patient's normal fingers, or infect his hand. You will be wiser not to try. Instead, toilet his wound, and close his skin. There are then several possibilities: (1) You can refer him for a formal repair, but unless you can send him to a real expert the result is likely to be bad. (2) You can teach him the trick movements described below. A finger which can only be passively flexed by its neighbours is better than a stiff one which

FLEXOR TENDON INJURIES

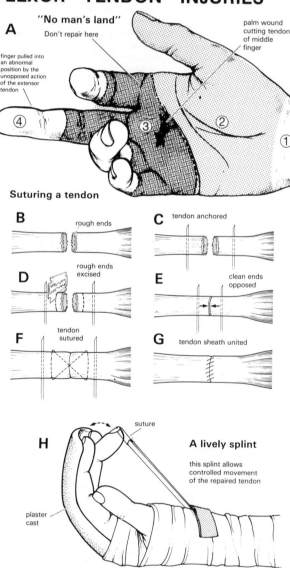

A

"No man's land"

Don't repair here

finger pulled into an abnormal position by the unopposed action of the extensor tendon

palm wound cutting tendon of middle finger

④ ③ ② ①

Suturing a tendon

B rough ends

C tendon anchored

D rough ends excised

E clean ends opposed

F tendon sutured

G tendon sheath united

H

suture

A lively splint

this splint allows controlled movement of the repaired tendon

plaster cast

Fig. 75-25 FLEXOR TENDON INJURIES. A, there are four zones for the repair of these injuries. Those in Zone One, at the wrist, are not too difficult. Zone Two is fairly difficult. Zone Three is a 'no man's land' that even experts find difficult. Zone Four is somewhat easier and is about as difficult as Zone Two.

B, the rough ends of a cut tendon. In real life injured tendons never look as tidy as this! C, the tendon anchored with intramuscular needles. D, its ends trimmed. E, its clean ends opposed. F, the suturing complete. G, the sheath united. H, after you have sutured a tendon, use this splint. Apply a plaster backslab and curve it as shown. Pass a suture through the patient's nail and tie a rubber band (or a 1.5 cm piece of surgical glove) from this to a piece of strapping in his proximal palm.

will not straighten. This is common even after supposedly expert repair. (3) You can amputate his injured finger. If referral is impossible, this may be the wisest course. A useless finger which gets in the way is likely to be worse than no finger. Discuss these possibilities with him and be completely frank. He will probably be wise to accept amputation.

'No man's land' does not extend to the thumb, so that if a patient's thumb tendons are injured, you can consider repairing them. Flexor policis longus is difficult to repair with good results, even if it is the only flexor tendon.

Zone Four, distal to the proximal IP crease, where repair is easier, because there is only the profundus tendon to be sutured. One difficulty is that the profundus tendon usually retracts. A flail DIP joint is a nuisance, but a stiff DIP joint after a repair is only a minor handicap.

One of the dangers in any flexor injury is that if a patient tries to clench his fist, he may pull the proximal end of a flexor tendon too far proximally in its sheath, especially in Zones Three and Four. If this happens, the blood vessels on the vinculae which nourish the sheath's cut end will be torn, and it will be deprived of its blood supply and die, so that when it is finally repaired, dense adhesions will form. The first principle in caring for such an injury is to prevent a patient's flexor tendons retracting by keeping his wrist flexed.

FLEXOR TENDON INJURIES

EMERGENCY TREATMENT Toilet the patient's wound. Put his arm in a sling, with his wrist and fingers flexed so that they form a 'C' (Fig. 75-1). This will keep his cut tendons in their sheaths with their blood supply intact. Toilet his wound, suture his skin only, and refer him to an expert hand surgeon. If you cannot refer him, proceed as follows.

AMPUTATION When the flexor tendons to a single finger have been cut and you cannot refer the patient, there are good arguments for amputation.

TRICK MOVEMENTS FOR FINGER INJURIES

LITTLE FINGER Teach the patient to adduct his little finger against his ring finger, so that his ring finger slightly overlaps it. When he flexes his ring finger, his little finger will flex with it.

ONE OF THE CENTRAL FINGERS Teach him to bring the fingers on either side of the injured one together and use them to flex it.

THE REPAIR OF FLEXOR TENDONS

INDICATIONS You must repair tendons in Zone One in Fig. 75-25. If you are reasonably skilled try repairing those in Zone Two. Zone Three is for experts only. You can attempt repair in Zone Four. Close the wound by primary suture if: (1) it occurred less than 8 hours ago, (2) there is no crushed or dead tissue, and (3) it is not badly contaminated. Otherwise, secondary closure would be wiser.

TOURNIQUET Don't forget this!

FINDING THE ENDS OF THE TENDONS If the proximal end of a cut tendon disappears into a wound, try squeezing the muscles of the patient's forearm to make it reappear. If the distal end of a tendon disappears, try curling his finger to make the distal end show itself. If necessary, open up his wound proximally and raise flaps as in Fig. 75-24.

If you are not sure what finger a tendon goes to, put a suture through the tendon and pull on this to see which finger moves.

ZONE ONE TENDON INJURIES

If the patient's wounded wrist is reasonably clean, do a primary repair. If necessary, enlarge the incision with flaps at either end, but don't angle the flaps too sharply. Never make a longitudinal incision down the centre of his wrist.

First find his median or ulnar nerves by the criteria in Fig. 55-7; it is seldom that both are involved. Then find his injured tendons—*beware, the median nerve looks very like a tendon!* Suture his nerves (55.9) and tendons (55.11).

If one artery has been cut, tie it. If both arteries have been cut, the collateral circulation may be enough to keep his hand alive, but ideally at least one should be repaired (55.6), especially if he is old.

Try to suture all tendons, except palmaris longus. If you have difficulty, a patient's deep flexors are the important ones to suture.

ZONE TWO TENDON INJURIES

If you are moderately skilled, proceed as in Zone One. Disregard sublimis and suture only profundus. Otherwise, proceed as in Zone Three.

ZONE THREE TENDON INJURIES ('no man's land')

Do a wound toilet, close the skin, and refer the patient for immediate primary repair, or if this is not possible, for secondary repair later, when the results will not be so good. *Keep his finger mobile until you can refer him.* If you cannot refer him, teach him trick movements or amputate his injured finger(s).

SUTURING THE DISTAL END OF A DEEP FLEXOR TENDON

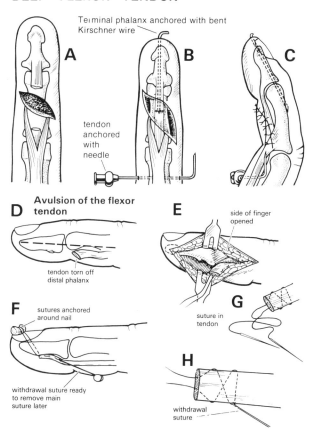

Fig. 75-26 FLEXOR TENDON INJURIES IN ZONE FOUR. A, an injury over the middle phalanx. B, the terminal phalanx has been anchored with Kirschner wire, and the profundus tendon brought into the wound and anchored with a needle. C, repair is complete. D, a tendon has been torn off a distal phalanx. E, open the patient's finger from the side and place a suture in the end of his deep flexor tendon. F, with a withdrawal suture in place, anchor the tendon with sutures round his nail. H, how the withdrawal suture is anchored. An alternative in these injuries is to persuade the patient to accept his deformity and teach him trick movements. *After Heim, Baltensweiler, and James Cairns.*

ZONE FOUR TENDON INJURIES

If a patient's deep flexor tendon has been cut over his middle phalanx, and his wound is reasonably clean, do a primary repair. Try to repair his profundus tendon beyond the fibrous flexor sheath. Squeeze it up into the wound and anchor it with a needle as in B, Fig. 75-26. Flex his terminal IP joint and anchor it with a Kirschner wire. Suture the tendon and then close the skin.

Alternatively, pass a suture through the proximal tendon, and fasten it to a button near the distal end of his finger. This will prevent the strong pull on the tendon pulling the repair apart. With an anchoring suture like this there is no need for Kirschner wire.

If his profundus tendon becomes detached from his terminal phalanx, perhaps with a fragment of bone (injuries 8 and 9 in Fig. 75-11), he has the volar equivalent of a mallet injury (75.8). Refer him. If you cannot refer him, open his finger from the side (E, Fig. 75-26), and pass a suture through the torn end of the tendon. Pass the suture round his terminal phalanx and tie it. In order to be able to remove this suture later, leave a removal suture in place.

Alternatively, if you think this is too difficult, start early active movements.

THUMB TENDON INJURIES Attempt primary repair.

POSTOPERATIVE CARE (ALL ZONES)

Immobilize the patient's wrist in flexion for 3 weeks, in the splint in Fig. 75-25. This allows an injured tendon to move in its sheath, and in doing so to minimize adhesions. It allows limited active extension, while the rubber band does the flexion without straining the suture.

The critical period for rupture of the suture line is immediately after you remove the splint, so start movements gradually, and try to devise some form of check strap to prevent sudden movements which may rupture the splint. The patient's hand will be stiff and painful after the injury, but if he perserveres, it should improve steadily for several months.

75.22 Repairing a digital nerve

If you can repair a patient's digital nerves so that his injured finger has sensation on both sides, it will be much more useful to him. It should have sensation on at least one side. Secondary suture is unsatisfactory, so do a primary repair if you can. The digital nerves are quite large and are entirely sensory, so they recover well.

REPAIRING A DIGITAL NERVE

INDICATIONS Transection of a digital nerve proximal to a patient's DIP joint; beyond this the nerve is too small for repair.

METHOD Apply a tourniquet so that you are operating in a bloodless field. Use fine instruments, 6/0 or 8/0 atraumatic monofilament sutures, and a magnifying loup, as in Section 55.9. If you have difficulty finding the patient's injured nerve, look for his digital vessels. His nerves lie near them, on their volar aspect. Place one suture on each side of the nerve.

After repair, immobilize his finger round a roll of bandage in his palm for 3 weeks. Injuries in the distal part of his hand will take 4 months to recover, and those proximal to his wrist at least a year.

FINGER STUMPS

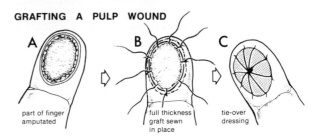

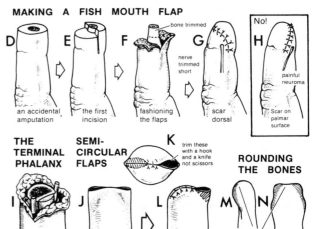

Fig. 75-27 FINGER STUMPS. A, B, and C show the stages in applying a full thickness skin graft to a patient's injured finger tip. D, to H, show you how to cover the end of his injured finger with a fish mouth flap. Note that the bone is trimmed and the dorsal flap is cut shorter so that the final scar lies dorsally (G). The digital nerves are trimmed so that if a neuroma forms, it is out of the way of the scar. I, shows the position of the structures in a cross–section of the finger, and J, K, and L, show the construction of semicircular flaps. M, and N, show you how to round the bones in a stump. *With the kind permission of Peter London.*

75.23 Accidental amputations

When a patient has cut off a piece of his finger, the treatment he needs depends on the completeness of the slice, and the size of the piece. Treatment also depends on how clean the cut is—a butcher's knife and a power saw cause very different injuries. If you allow an adult's entire fingertip to granulate without covering it with skin, he may be left with a painful deformed finger.

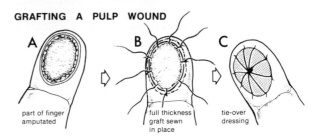

A DIGITAL NERVE INJURY

this operation is being done under a tourniquet

The cut ends of this nerve will have to be sutured

Fig. 75-26a A DIGITAL NERVE INJURY. If you can repair a patient's digital nerves so that his injured finger has sensation on both sides, it will be much more useful to him. Use the methods in Section 55.9. *After Rutherford, Nelson, Weston, and Wilson with kind permission.*

ACCIDENTAL AMPUTATIONS

INCOMPLETE ACCIDENTAL AMPUTATIONS

If the partly detached slice is still bleeding, showing that it is still alive, toilet it and sew it back, even if it is quite large. Apply the minimum of dressings, keep the patient's finger cool, and elevate his hand.

If the partly detached piece is not bleeding, or if its tendons or nerves have been cut, it is probably better amputated completely.

COMPLETE ACCIDENTAL AMPUTATIONS

If the piece is smaller than 1 square cm, it is not worth grafting. Apply vaseline gauze and let it granulate.

If the piece is larger than 1 square cm, you have 4 choices.

(1) You can shorten the bone so as to cover the stump with a good flap of palmar skin as in Fig. 75-27. Either cut fish mouth flaps as in D, to G, or semicircular ones as in J, to L. A shortened finger is often best, so the patients say.

(2) In a child under 10, you can leave the stump to granulate while it is covered with vaseline dressing. Change the dressing weekly. A child's finger can regenerate remarkably, so this method is only acceptable in children. An adult's finger tip may take 6 weeks to heal by this method and leave an ugly, tender stump.

(3) You can apply a full thickness graft (57.10). You may be able to take this from the amputated piece of finger, but only if it has been sliced off cleanly. Thin it by removing its pulp and apply it as a full thickness graft, as in A, B, and C, Fig. 75-27. Sew it in place and apply a dressing by the tieover method (Fig. 57-8).

(4) You can apply a split skin graft. If this takes, and provides a useful finger, good. If it fails to provide a useful finger, you will at least have preserved the length of the stump, and covered it with skin while it healed, so that a further operation can be done later. This is the easiest alternative.

75.24 Planned finger amputations

The common indication for amputating a patient's finger is an injury which is so severe that you cannot save it, or which if you can save it, is likely to be stiff permanently. There are no sites of election, so consider the needs of each patient carefully. You have several decisions to make.

Should you amputate? The indications depend partly on your skills. With sufficiently skilled microsurgery, almost any injured finger can be saved. Where skill is less, the indications for amputation are greater. *Most district hospitals make the mistake of not amputating early enough or often enough.*

A stiff, painful, useless finger is often worse than no finger. If the nerves and tendons of an injured finger have been cut, *it is usually better amputated immediately.* If elaborate procedures are done to save it, not only is it is likely to become stiff, but the patient's neighbouring normal fingers are likely to become stiff too. If, however, you amputate his injured finger, make sure he exercises his other fingers so that they have a greater chance of remaining supple. Many patients (particularly labourers and even some surgeons) hardly miss an injured finger.

If you decide to amputate, discuss the decision with the patient, before you premedicate him. If his hand is going to take a long time to recover, tell him so. Discuss any alternatives, and if a difficult decision has to be made, let him share it. If he helps to make the decision, he is much more likely to be enthusiastic about subsequent rehabilitation. If he decides against your advice, and finds the disadvantages of not following it, he will realize that he was responsible for them.

INDICATIONS FOR AMPUTATION Amputate regardless of surgical skills and facilities for: (1) Gross crush injuries. (2) Malignant neoplasms. (3) Infection which has made a finger useless and is in danger of spreading.

If skills and facilities are excellent, amputate a patient's finger only if: (1) The bone is fractured and both his flexor and extensor tendons are cut. (2) The bone is fractured and his flexor tendons and nerves have been cut.

If skills and facilities are not so good, consider amputation if the finger is likely to become stiff and useless permanently.

MOST DISTRICT HOSPITALS DO NOT AMPUTATE FINGERS OFTEN ENOUGH OR EARLY ENOUGH

How long should you leave the stump? Which would the patient prefer? A shorter finger covered with good skin, or a longer one covered with poorer skin? This is a common problem. Most patients are likely to prefer a shorter finger covered

AMPUTATING FINGERS

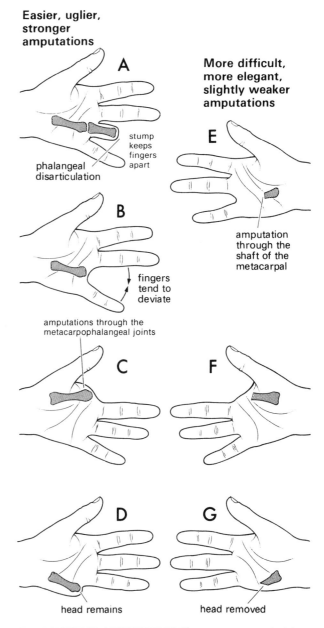

Easier, uglier, stronger amputations

More difficult, more elegant, slightly weaker amputations

Fig. 75-28 FINGER AMPUTATIONS. The amputations on the left are easier, uglier, and stronger than those on the right. Amputating through a joint is easier than cutting through a metacarpal. *Partly after Farquharson with kind permission*

291

with good skin. The old surgical axiom that length is all important, whatever the quality of the skin on the fingertip, is now being doubted. This applies even to the thumb, where length is normally considered paramount. A flap from the volar surface of the finger is thus usually better than a graft. But, if making a flap means sacrificing too much length, a graft may be necessary. If possible, use full thickness skin, although a split skin graft does sometimes hypertrophy and stand up to pressure remarkably. The sides and back of a finger are less important, so that a split skin graft is good enough here.

If you are amputating through the middle phalanx, try to retain the midddle of its shaft, because flexor superficialis is inserted into it. If you amputate more proximally than this, the patient will have no strength in his finger, although it will help to stop things falling out of his palm. If you are in doubt as to where to amputate, choose the more distal site. His amputation can be revised later.

PROVIDE GOOD SKIN OVER AN INJURED FINGERTIP

Should you leave the metacarpal head? Which would the patient like? An ugly amputation through his MP joint which preserves his metacarpal head, but leaves a gap through which beans, rice or money can slip? Or, a more elegant one, through the shaft of a metacarpal which removes its head? Opinions differ, but it is usually said that leaving the metacarpal head (preferably with a stump of phalanx) makes a stronger hand; it is certainly an easier operation. What does he do with his fingers? Most of your patients will be labourers who need a strong hand, so disarticulation through an MP joint is the common finger amputation in district hospitals. Retaining the stump of a phalanx as in amputation A, Fig. 75-28 further strengthens a patient's hand by keeping his fingers apart and preventing them from deviating towards one another as can happen in amputation B, in this figure. The stump will also help to stop small objects falling through his hand.

Removing an index finger causes less of disability than you might expect, and even a surgeon can operate quite satisfactorily without his left index finger (amputation F), provided the head of its metacarpal has been removed obliquely from the shaft. The middle finger soon learns to take over from it. A finger missing from one edge of the hand (amputations F, and G) is seldom noticed, provided the head of its metacarpal is removed, so this is an elegant amputation. If great strength not important, it is likely to be the best one.

The disadvantage of removing the metacarpal head is that it is a more difficult operation. If you are unskilled and you injure or infect a patient's hand, it may become stiff. *So, if you are in doubt, leave the metacarpal head.* He can always have an amputation through the shaft later.

IF IN DOUBT LEAVE THE METACARPAL HEAD

Should you amputate a patient's injured finger now or later? If an amputation is necessary, it is necessary immediately. Opinions vary, but many surgeons favour early amputation, because the patient is less likely to agree to amputation later, and more anxious to keep his useless finger.

How should you cut the flaps? If possible, use fish mouth flaps as in D, to G, Fig. 75-27 and in C, and D, Fig. 75-30. Plan them carefully in relation to the ends of the bones, and close them without tension, even if the finger has to be shorter. A shorter amputation with loose flaps is better than a longer one with tight shiny ones. The skin creases are important landmarks, but they are more proximal than you think. So study Fig. 75-30 carefully, and compare it with the patient's hand.

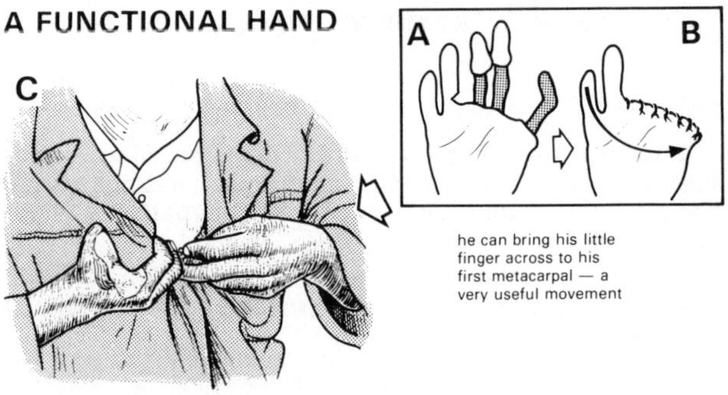

A FUNCTIONAL HAND

he can bring his little finger across to his first metacarpal — a very useful movement

Fig. 75-29 A FUNCTIONAL HAND AFTER A SEVERE INJURY. A, immediately after the accident. B, after the operation. C, some months later. This is the wood chopper Kalim, whose story is given in the text.
Kindly contributed by Peter Bewes

If possible, make the palmar flap a little longer than the dorsal one, as in this figure, because this will bring the scar dorsally, where it will not be pressed on.

CHANG (36), an amateur guitarist, amputated his index finger through its middle phalanx, and severely injured his middle, ring, and little fingers in a machine at work. They were hanging on only by some crushed soft tissue and were cold and without sensation or movement. The possibility of microsurgery and the many months of rehabilitation it would require was discussed. He wished to be back at work quickly because there was much unemployment, so he opted for amputation. After intensive physiotherapy involving heavy metalwork, he was soon back at work and still plays his guitar—but with a plectrum to pluck the strings.

KALIM (39) the wood chopper in Fig. 75-29, degloved his index, midddle finger, and thumb in a machine at work. His ring and little fingers were less severely injured. But he could still move them all normally—their tendons were undamaged. The possibility of burying them in an abdominal skin pouch was discussed, but it was not considered practical to restore sensation with a neurovascular island transfer, since this would have required months of physiotherapy. He was in danger of losing his job, so he chose to have his thumb, index, and middle fingers amputated. A few weeks of physiotherapy restored movement to his ring and little fingers and he was soon back at work; he can even do up his own buttons. LESSONS (1) All the surviving parts of his hand were covered with good skin. (2) It was possible to preserve the whole of his first metacarpal. (3) Active physiotherapy started almost immediately. (4) Early amputation can leave a very functional hand.

CONSIDER THE NEEDS OF EACH PATIENT

PLANNED FINGER AMPUTATIONS

INDICATIONS This extends Section 75.1 on the general method for a hand injury.

CAUTION ! With all amputations: (1) If in doubt, make all flaps a bit longer than you think you will need. You can always trim them. (2) Ask yourself if the skin of the finger you are amputating could help to close a nearby wound. (3) Don't forget the instructions at the end of this section about closing the wound.

AMPUTATING THROUGH A DISTAL PHALANX

If possible, preserve the base of the patient's distal phalanx, because of the tendons which are inserted into it. If less than a quarter of the length of his nail remains, he may be troubled later by the irregular hooked remnant, so excise his whole nail bed.

Flex his terminal joint and make a transverse incision across its dorsal surface 6 mm distal to the joint, as in A, Fig. 75-30. Continue the incision as far as the sides of his phalanx, and deepen it down to the bone. Cut a long rectangular (not pointed) palmar flap almost to the tip of his finger. Dissect the flap off the front of his phalanx and reflect it forwards.

INCISIONS FOR FINGER AMPUTATIONS

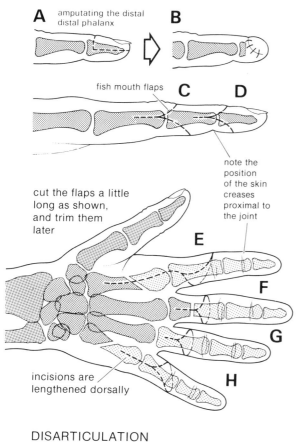

A amputating the distal distal phalanx

B

fish mouth flaps C D

note the position of the skin creases proximal to the joint

cut the flaps a little long as shown, and trim them later

E

F

G

H

incisions are lengthened dorsally

DISARTICULATION

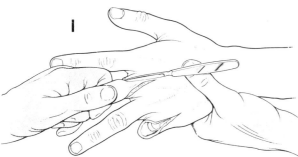

I

Fig. 75-30 INCISIONS FOR FINGER AMPUTATIONS. Cut the flaps long, you can always shorten them later if necessary. A, and B, amputating through the distal phalanx. C, and D, flaps for amputations through the interphalangeal joints. E, F, G, and H, more proximal amputations. *Partly after Farquharson with kind permission.*

Cut his phalanx with bone nibblers close to its base, then fold the flap and suture it (B).

AMPUTATING THROUGH A DISTAL IP JOINT

Incise the skin in the mid-lateral lines on either side of the neck of the patient's middle phalanx. Join these two incisions to make a dorsal flap at the level of the joint, and a palmar one 1 cm distal to the flexor crease as in D, Fig. 75-30.

Dissect back the fibro-fatty tissue to find his digital vessels and nerves, his extensor expansion, and his flexor tendon in its sheath. Divide both tendons at the neck of his middle phalanx.

Separate the nerves from the vessels, and divide the nerves proximal to the vessels. Tie the vessels without including the nerves. Complete the amputation by cutting the capsule and

the collateral ligaments. Pare away the articular cartilage, and close his wound as described below.

AMPUTATING THROUGH A MIDDLE PHALANX

Proceed as above, but amputate through the mid-shaft of the patient's middle phalanx, because this retains the attachment of the superficial flexor tendon to the sides of the phalanx. Some surgeons prefer to amputate through the proximal IP joint, as described below.

AMPUTATING THROUGH A PROXIMAL IP JOINT

Do this as for a distal joint, but cut flaps as in C, Fig. 75-30.

AMPUTATING THROUGH A PROXIMAL PHALANX

Try to amputate through the neck of a proximal phalanx. *If possible, preserve even a small stump of it.* This is easier than amputating through an MP joint. Cut flaps as in F, Fig. 75-30.

AMPUTATING THE INDEX FINGER THROUGH ITS METACARPO-PHALANGEAL JOINT

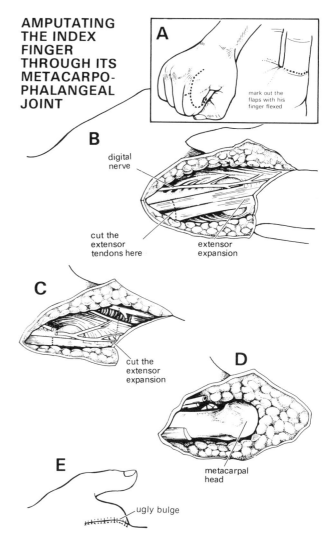

A

mark out the flaps with his finger flexed

B

digital nerve

cut the extensor tendons here

extensor expansion

C

cut the extensor expansion

D

metacarpal head

E

ugly bulge

Fig. 75-31 AMPUTATING AN INDEX FINGER THROUGH ITS MP JOINT. This operation preserves the head of a patient's metacarpal. It leaves an ugly though strong hand, is easier than amputating through the shaft of a metacarpal, and is more suited to the less exerienced surgeon. *With the kind permission of Peter London.*

AMPUTATING AN INDEX FINGER THROUGH ITS MP JOINT

This operation preserves the head of the patient's metacarpal. Flex his index finger and mark out the incision on its knuckle, as in A, Fig. 75-31, so that the lateral flap is larger and extends nearly half-way down the shaft of his proximal phalanx. It must be long enough to meet the web of the next finger without tension. Deepen the incision dorsally until you can see his extensor tendon, then cut it and turn it distally.

Separate the extensor expansion round the base of his proximal phalanx (B). Cut the collateral ligaments. Cut his flexor tendons as far proximally as you can (C). Cut the rest of the soft tissues, tie the vessels, shorten the digital nerves, and remove his finger.

Reduce the bulk of the scar by trimming away the ligaments around his metacarpal head (D), his volar plate, his collateral ligaments, and his flexor sheath. Close the flaps, trimming them where necessary.

Ring finger. **The procedure is almost identical to that above.**

Middle and index finger. **When you cut flaps through the webs, use a complete web on one side and no web on the other side. Don't use two half webs each side.**

AMPUTATING AN INDEX FINGER THROUGH ITS
METACARPAL SHAFT (Ray amputation)

CAUTION ! This is *not* an easy amputation, avoid it if you are unskilled.

Make a dorsal racquet incision as in A, Fig. 75-32. Preserve the subcutaneous tissue with the flap, cut the extensor tendon (B), and turn it distally. Cut the radial side of the flap long. You may need every millimetre.

Separate the patient's interossei from the shaft of his metacarpal. Deepen the palmar incision, and cut his vessels, nerves, and tendons. Reflect the periosteum with an elevator, and cut the metacarpal across with a Gigli saw at the junction of its proximal and middle thirds (C), then bevel it dorsally and radially. Or, use an osteotome and a mallet. Turn the palmar flap medially. Tie and shorten the vessels; shorten the nerves. Remove the flexor tendon sheath and shorten the flexor tendons as deep in his palm as you can. As you do so remove his lumbrical muscles.

Proximally, try to suture the sheaths of the patient's first and second dorsal interosseous muscles, so as to cover the cut end of the bone. Distally, suture the attachment of his first dorsal interosseous muscle to the extensor expansion of his middle finger. This will restore his pinch grip (D).

AMPUTATING A MIDDLE OR RING FINGER
THROUGH ITS METACARPAL SHAFT (Ray amputation)

This again is not an easy operation. Proceed as above. Be sure to: (1) Leave the base of the metacarpal. (2) Suture the deep transverse carpal ligaments on either side of the missing metacarpal. Failure to do this will result in a weak grip.

CLOSING THE WOUND AFTER ANY FINGER AMPUTATION

Don't suture the flexor and extensor tendons together over the bone. They will find their own attachments.

Find the patient's digital nerves and separate them from the vessels. This will be easier if you use a tourniquet. The nerves lie palmar to the vessels, as in I, Fig. 75-27. Divide the nerves cleanly 1 cm proximal to the volar flap. Don't include them in the ligature of a vessel. If possible, bury them in muscle or fat. Neuromas are sure to develop, but if you do this they will be away from the scar and the finger tip, as in G, Fig. 75-27, and not under them as in H.

When you amputate through a joint, pare down the condyles (where necessary) as in M, and N, in Fig. 75-27, so as to avoid making a bulbous stump. Tie the patient's digital arteries with catgut not monofilament, which will later be painful under his skin. Release the tourniquet and control all bleeding before you suture the flap. This will minimize the risk of subsequent infection. If oozing continues, leave part of the wound open for drainage.

If you are amputating for chronic sepsis, close the wound by delayed primary suture (54.4).

Don't close the finger stump under tension, because it will certainly break down. If necessary, reduce the bulk of the fibro-fatty tissue, so as to allow the skin edges to cover the stump without tension. Don't excise 'dog ears', they will later resolve and remould. If you decide to trim them, use a knife and a hook, not scissors which will crush the skin edges and impair healing.

Use fine sutures taking small bites of the skin about every

5 mm. Don't suture the edges tightly, but only lightly approximate them.

Apply a firm dressing, and raise the patient's hand as in Fig. 75-1. Change the dressings at 3 days, and remove the stitches at 10 days.

CAUTION ! Don't bandage the patient's other fingers with the amputated one or they may become stiff. He should be able to start moving them a day or two after the amputation. Use any convenient occupational therapy, such as rolling bandages, to make sure he starts using his fingers soon.

DIFFICULTIES AMPUTATING FINGERS

If the patient's FINGER STUMP IS PAINFUL, the causes are similar to those in other amputations: (1) You may not have cut the nerves proximally enough, so that a neuroma has formed and stuck to the scar. (2) You may have left the bone too long in relation to the flap. (3) There may be a fragment of the nail bed remaining. (4) An epidermoid cyst may be forming. Refer him for a revision amputation.

DON'T SUTURE A FINGER STUMP UNDER TENSION

AMPUTATING THROUGH
THE METACARPAL SHAFT

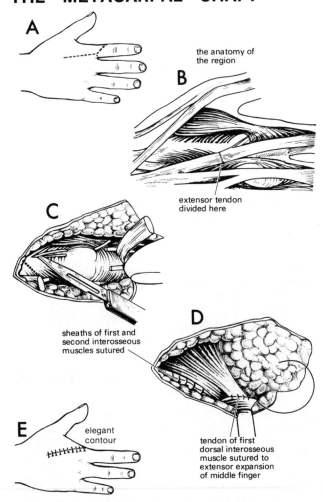

the anatomy of the region

extensor tendon divided here

sheaths of first and second interosseous muscles sutured

elegant contour

tendon of first dorsal interosseous muscle sutured to extensor expansion of middle finger

Fig. 75-32 AMPUTATING AN INDEX FINGER THROUGH ITS METACARPAL SHAFT. If conditions are difficult and you are inexperienced, avoid this operation, and amputate through the MP joint instead. *With the kind permission of Peter London.*

SOME SEVERE HAND INJURIES

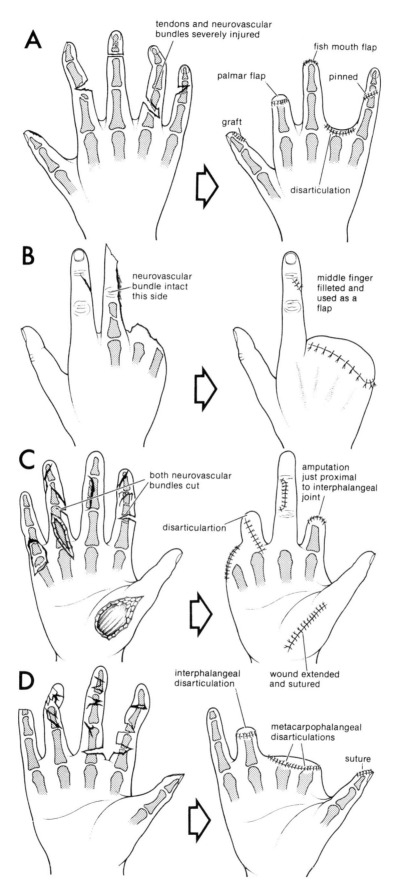

Fig. 75-33 SOME SEVERE HAND INJURIES. You may have to cope with any of these. One of your most difficult decisions will be whether to splint an injured hand or to mobilize it. *With the kind permission of Peter London.*

75.25 Multiple fractures and the severely injured hand

A patient with multiple fractures is difficult to manage because: (1) Some of the methods which are suitable for single fractures will not work with multiple ones. (2) His soft tissues are likely to be severely injured, causing much swelling and stiffness. (3) He may have other even more serious injuries elsewhere. He can usually tolerate one stiff finger, but two or more will be a serious disability. One of your most difficult decisions will be whether to splint his hand or to try to mobilize it.

A SEVERE HAND INJURY WITH MULTIPLE FRACTURES

GENERAL METHOD Carefully toilet the patient's hand by the method in Section 75.1. Don't suture it. Apply a wet dressing with plenty of cotton wool. His hand will swell severely, so admit him and elevate it. While you do so, keep it in the position of safety with a volar plaster slab. If any part of it is likely to become gangrenous, keep it cold with ice packs until you have made the decision to amputate it or leave it. Give him an antibiotic and an analgesic.

If possible, refer him. If you have to treat him yourself, apply the specific methods described below. Try to decide if more will be gained by splinting his hand or by mobilizing it. If you decide to mobilize it, start exercises after about 5 days, but reapply the volar slabs between exercises for a further 2 to 3 weeks.

SPECIFIC METHODS FOR A SEVERELY INJURED HAND

If you can refer a patient for expert internal fixation, do so. This is one of its main indications.

If he has fractures of his middle and ring fingers, you may be able to strap them to their normal neighbours. If this is impractical, support his injured fingers with a plaster slab.

If he has multiple phalangeal fractures, early active movements are likely to work well. They are less likely to work if his metacarpals are fractured. Here internal fixation, using longitudinal or oblique Kirschner wires, is more effective.

If a single finger is badly damaged, consider amputating it, especially if his other fingers are normal.

If several metacarpals are fractured and severely deviated, consider correcting the deformity with skin traction, or Kirschner wire traction; this may be useful if he has multiple injuries elsewhere. Apply gentle traction to a Kirschner wire which has been passed through a distal phalanx. If convenient, incorporate it in a cast which is immobilizing his wrist.

If several of his fingers are badly damaged, conserve as much function as you can using the examples described below.

THE 'KEBAB METHOD' USING KIRSCHNER WIRE

Mould what remains of the patient's hand into the best position you can. Splint his fractured metacarpals with pieces of Kirschner wire, as in Section 75.4. If necessary, insert them longitudinally down his fractured bones and transversely across his hand. Hold the ends of the wires together with epoxy resin, plaster, or string. Leave the wound open for the first few days. Close it by secondary suture, or with skin grafts as appropriate. Remove all Kirschner wires after 12 days.

Here are some examples of what you may have to do.

Hand A in Fig. 75-33. The tendons and the neurovascular bundles of this patient's index and ring finger have been so severely injured that you will have to amputate them. You can close the end of his index finger with a palmar flap, and his ring finger by removing the stump of its proximal phalanx. Close his middle finger with a fish mouth flap (Fig. 75-27), so as to save as much length as you can. The ulnar neurovascular bundle of his little finger is intact, so you can pin its middle phalanx with Kirschner wire. Graft the wound on the tip of his thumb with skin taken from the amputated tip of his index finger.

Hand B. Half of this patient's middle finger is intact, so you can fillet it by removing the bone to make a flap that will cover the stumps of his amputated fourth and fifth fingers. When you make this flap, take care not to damage its blood supply, including its dorsal veins. Remove his injured phalanges, pull his flexor and extensor tendons distally, cut them off cleanly, and allow them to retract. Cut back the digital nerves of his amputated fingers so that their cut ends lie deep in his palm. Leave all the fat in the flap, suture it in place without tension, and evert the suture line. If there is any excess skin, remove it from the back rather than the front of the flap, but don't make it too narrow.

Hand C. There is a soft tissue wound round the base of this patient's thumb. Close it without tension by slightly increasing its length. Both the neurovascular bundles in his index finger have been cut, so amputate it just proximal to his IP joint. Sew the small flap on his middle finger into place. His ring finger is so severely injured that you can only save its proximal phalanx. His little finger is also severely damaged, so amputate it through the head of its metacarpal. When you have done all this, he will still be able to grip things between his thumb and index finger, so he still has a useful hand.

Hand D. You can repair this patient's thumb by simple suture. Both his index and his middle fingers are so severely damaged that you will have to amputate them through their MP joints. More of his index finger remains, so you can amputate it through its proximal IP joint, and turn up a flap. After you have done this he will still have a powerful grip across his hand.

If a patient's hand is so severely injured that you cannot save any of his fingers, try to save as much of his metacarpus as you can. If his thumb remains, this will give it something it can grip against.

YVONNE (26) and her husband had been driving all night when he wandered into the fast lane on the motorway. He was killed instantly and severely injured their two daughters. She sustained multiple open dislocations of the MP joints of her right hand, its dorsum was degloved, and several of its metacarpals and proximal phalanges were fractured, as in Fig. 75-34. Amputation was considered, but the circulation and sensation in her fingers was good, and she was, moreover, a typist. Her wound was toileted under general anaesthesia and a tourniquet. Her metacarpals were repaired by threading Kirschner wire down their marrow cavities, and further stabilized with transverse wires held with epoxy resin. Her wound was covered with split skin (fortunately most of her extensor tendons were still covered with paratenon), and her hand was bandaged in the position of safety (75.3). She later returned to typing, and was kind enough to send her surgeon a colour photograph of her suprisingly normal hand.

KIRSCHNER WIRE FIXATION FOR A GROSSLY INJURED HAND

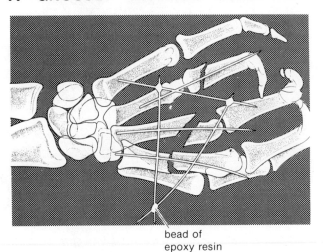

bead of epoxy resin

Fig. 75-34 THE 'KEBAB METHOD' FOR A GROSSLY INJURED HAND. This is the patient 'Yvonne' in the text, who was later able to return to typing, despite the severity of her injury. *Kindly contributed by Peter Bewes.*

A FINGER FLAP

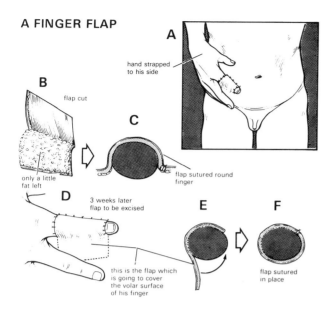

Fig. 75-35 AN ABDOMINAL FLAP FOR A FINGER is an alternative to amputation in degloving injuries. It needs care! *Kindly contributed by Mamdur Tahir.*

75.26 Degloving injuries of a finger

This injury removes the skin from a patient's finger. The skin can be pulled off if he catches his ring in something, or if he has a rope round his finger, and the cow on the other end of it decides to run away. An alternative to amputating his degloved finger is to cover it with an abdominal flap. *This is a method for the careful, caring operator.* It is easy to start this procedure, but difficult to see it through to a successful result. Too often the result is a stiff hand.

AN ABDOMINAL FLAP FOR A FINGER

Give the patient a general anaesthetic. Measure the size of flap that his degloved finger needs by wrapping a piece of vaseline gauze round it.

Lay the piece of vaseline gauze on his lower abdomen in the position that his hand might be in if it were in his pocket. Cut a flap the size and shape of the gauze with its base downwards, as in Fig. 75-35 (in this part of the body the blood supply is from below upwards), *leaving only a little* fat under the skin.

Make holes in the proximal end of his nail with a strong cutting needle. Wrap the flap round his degloved finger, leaving the nail outside it. Sew the base of his finger and his nail to the flap. Leave its upper border free.

Dress the flap and hold his hand in position with plaster bandages round his trunk.

At 3 weeks, the flap will have vascularized from his finger. Excise it from his abdomen, taking care to leave a further flap which will be wide enough to cover the volar surface of his finger. Sew this in place to leave a scar running along the side of his finger.

CAUTION ! Start active exercises as soon as you can!

75.27 A groin flap for the back of the hand

If a patient has a severe injury of the back of his hand, like that in Fig. 51-5, perhaps involving his extensor tendons, management will depend on whether or not the tendons still have a thin filmy pink sheath of paratenon over them. If they do, primary repair of the tendons and primary split skin grafting is much the best, and allows you to put the patient's hand into the position of safety (Fig. 75-8). If there is no paratenon over his extensor tendons, a split skin graft will not take. One way

A GROIN FLAP

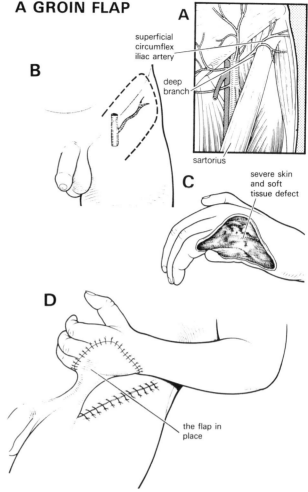

Fig. 75-36 A GROIN FLAP for an injury on the back of the hand. A, the anatomy of the superficial circumflex iliac artery. B, the anatomy of the flap. C, the defect in the hand. D, the graft sewn in place, the pedicle tubed, and the defect closed by suture with the patient's hip flexed. *Kindly contributed by Ian McGregor.*

to cover the exposed tendons on the back of his hand is to use the groin flap in Fig. 75-36. This uses the skin supplied by the superficial circumflex iliac artery. This arises 2 or 3 cm below the inguinal ligament, usually from the femoral artery, and runs laterally parallel to the inguinal ligament and below it. At the medial border of sartorius it gives off a deep branch. From that point it becomes more superficial and passes into the tissue that you can use as a flap. The artery divides into finer branches lateral to the anterior superior iliac spine and cannot be traced. The corresponding vein accompanies it and ends at the saphenous opening.

The skin of the groin is so loose that you can usually close the defect you took the flap from by direct suture, so that grafting is unnecessary. *This is another method which is only for the careful, caring operator.*

A GROIN FLAP FOR THE BACK OF THE HAND

INDICATIONS **(1) To resurface the hand. (2) As a local flap or a tube pedicle (not described here).**

THE HAND INJURY Do a careful wound toilet. Excise a small margin of tissue from the edge of the wound to make sure that the skin to which you suture the flap is viable and uninjured. If the wound is granulating, excise its edges radically, down to sound tissue. Where possible, place the junction between the flap and the hand along elective lines for scars. To achieve this, you may have to bring the flap beyond the obvious defect.

THE FLAP Mark out the patient's anterior superior iliac spine, his pubic tubercle, and his inguinal ligament running between them. Palpate the line of his femoral artery. Mark on it the origin of his superficial epigastric artery 2.5 cm below the mid–point of his his inguinal ligament. Draw the line of his superficial circumflex iliac artery parallel to his inguinal ligament and mark its point of entry into the flap where it crosses the medial border of sartorius.

Raise the flap to include the artery, which need not necessarily lie along its axis. The usual width is 10 cm, but extremes of 6 cm and 19 cm in an adult and 14 cm in a child have been used successfully. The maximum length of the flap is uncertain, but if you extend it beyond the anterior superior iliac spine, make the part beyond it square with a length to breadth ratio of 1:1.

Raise the flap at the level of the deep fascia starting laterally. When you make its upper margin, divide the superficial epigastric vessels. If you raise the flap in a plane deep to these vessels you are sure to include the superficial circumflex artery and vein, since they lie in the same plane. The key point in raising the flap is the virtually constant branching of the artery at the medial border of sartorius. When you reach sartorius, incise the fascia over it, and strip the muscle bare to just short of its medial border, preserving the deep branch of the artery. Then stop, knowing that the main part of the artery is safely out of the way in the flap.

Sew the edges of the flap to the defect in the patient's hand. Try to sew the edges of the bridge segment together into a tube.

CAUTION ! Make sure that the patient exercises his fingers as much as he can, so as to prevent stiffness and oedema.

CLOSING THE DEFECT Flex the patient's hip and try to close the defect in his groin by suture. If this is impracticable, graft the exposed area. If the flap overlies the area to be grafted, use primary split skin grafting with a tie–over dressing (Fig. 57-8). If the flap does not overlie the area to be grafted, exposed grafting is possible and easier.

75.28 More difficulties with hand injuries

You will meet many difficulties with hand injuries, which will cause you much trouble. Grease gun injuries and human bites are some of the worst. Many serious hand infections start with injuries, sometimes quite minor ones. These are described in Chapter 8.

MORE DIFFICULTIES WITH HAND INJURIES

If the patient's THENAR MUSCLES ARE SEVERELY CRUSHED, pressure may build up within the firm fascia that covers them and cause severe pain and paralysis. Pain on passively stretching his muscles is a sign of impending ischaemic contracture, so be prepared to do a surgical decompression (73.7). Make an incision over his thenar eminence parallel to the skin crease at its base. Cut the underlying fascia taking care not to go too far medially or proximally, and so injure the recurrent branch of his median nerve that supplies his thenar muscles.

If an industrial gun or pump has INJECTED GREASE, DIESEL OIL, PAINT, COMPRESSED AIR, OR ABRASIVES into a patient's hand, refer him rapidly. Guns or pumps can inject these materials under high pressure deeply among the tissue planes of the hand, and even up into the forearm. Although a patient's skin wound may be small and his initial injury almost painless, the tissues underneath are grossly injured. Soon his hand starts to swell and becomes very painful. This is an acute surgical emergency and an extensive wound toilet is essential. Neglect may lead to amputation.

If you cannot refer him, explore the injury under general anaesthesia and a tourniquet. Consult an anatomy book to show you where the important structures are and lay open his hand wherever you find foreign material. Spare his nerves, arteries, and tendons. Leaving foreign material in his tissues is more dangerous than opening up his hand fully. When you have removed all the foreign material, apply a firm dressing and take the tourniquet off. After 5 to 10 minutes remove the dressing and control bleeding. Then dress his wound without suturing it. Finally, leave his hand in the position of safety, inspect it daily, and remove more foreign material if necessary. His hand will be stiff, but if you don't treat him radically like this, it is likely to need amputating.

If a patient's HAND HAS BEEN BITTEN, the risk of infection, particularly after a human bite, is great. Osteomyelitis may follow. So toilet his wound thoroughly and leave it open. Admit him and elevate his hand in a roller towel. Give him chloramphenicol and metronidazole. Watch him carefully!

THERE IS NO SUCH THING AS A TRIVIAL HAND WOUND

---

76 The pelvis

76.1 Pelvic injuries

A patient's pelvis can be crushed, or it can be broken by a force transmitted to it through his femur. These are common injuries, and after a serious road accident, you may have to care for several patients with them. Pelvic injuries are of two kinds.

(1) Minor fractures in which a piece of a patient's pelvis breaks off, as in A, Fig. 76-1, while the ring itself remains intact. Apart from the associated soft tissue injuries, these minor fractures are of little importance and need no treatment.

(2) Major fractures which open a patient's pelvic ring as in C, D, E, and F, in Fig. 76-1. If the ring is to open, either he must have two fractures, or a single fracture must be combined with displacement of his sacro–iliac joint or his pubic symphysis. By themselves these fractures are much less important than the injuries to the organs inside his pelvis, and the massive bleeding that often follows. A patient with a fractured pelvis is particularly likely to injure his membranous urethra (68.3) or his bladder (68.2). A spicule of bone can also tear his femoral artery. Paralytic ileus sometimes follows the massive retroperitoneal haematoma that a pelvic fracture may cause, so watch for it (10.14).

ASSUME THAT ALL PATIENTS WITH A FRACTURED PELVIS HAVE COMPLICATIONS UNTIL YOU HAVE PROVED OTHERWISE

HAS THE PATIENT BROKEN HIS PELVIS?

Wherever a patient has had a history of a crush injury, suspect that he may have fractured his pelvis. Look for bruising and local tenderness in his groin, perineum, pubic area, and posteriorly over his sacro–iliac joints.

Grasp his pelvis firmly with your thumbs over its anterior superior iliac spines. Compress it from side to side. Then try to pull its two sides apart. Finally, press it firmly backwards, on to the couch. If you can feel movement or crepitus between its two parts, or, these procedures cause him great pain, he has fractured his pelvic ring.

Press over his pubic symphysis. If his pelvis is fractured, he may be tender locally, or he may feel pain over his sacro–iliac joints. Marked suprapubic tenderness suggests urinogenital damage. In a hinge fracture you may be able to feel a gap at his pubic symphysis.

Start at his anterior superior iliac spines and palpate each of his iliac crests for tenderness, irregularity, and crepitus. Palpate his pubic bones in his genitocrural folds, and around his obturator foramina. Palpate his ischial tuberosities.

Look for signs of rupture of his bladder, and injury to his urethra, as described in Section 68.1. Look particularly for urethral bleeding, perineal bruising, and extravasation of urine.

Examine his rectum to feel if a bony fragment has injured its wall. Is there blood on your glove? Feel for fractures of his sacrum and coccyx. If the head of his femur has dislocated centrally through his acetabulum, you may be able to feel the wall of his pelvis deviated medially, or the head of his femur moving when you rotate his thigh.

FRACTURES OF THE PELVIS

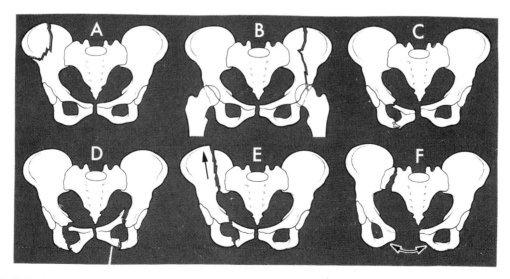

Fig. 76-1 FRACTURES OF THE PELVIS. Only the ilium of pelvis A, is fractured; in B, the fracture extends into the acetabulum. The ischio–pubic rami are fractured on one side in pelvis C, and the pubic symphysis slightly displaced. Pelvis D, has a compression butterfly fracture' of both ischio–pubic rami. Pelvis E, has a vertical fracture with upward displacement of its right half. Pelvis F, has a hinge fracture.

Look for injuries to his sciatic nerves (55.8), and particularly for a dropped foot.

CAUTION! If he has broken his pelvis, he may bleed severely, become shocked, and need several units of blood.

X-RAYS Take an AP and a lateral film of his pelvis and hips. If he has a fracture of his pelvic ring, look carefully for subluxation of his sacro—iliac joints. You can easily miss these.

FRACTURES OF THE PELVIS MAY CAUSE MASSIVE BLEEDING

76.2 Fractures which open the pelvic ring

Most pelvic fractures heal well. When the fragments of a patient's pelvis are seriously displaced, there are two ways in which you can reduce them: (1) When the two halves of his pelvis have hinged apart, you can try to bring them together. (2) If half of his pelvis has been pushed vertically upwards, you can apply skeletal traction to his leg and pull it down. You can leave most other fractures to heal themselves. Don't apply a Thomas splint because it is useless.

Compression fractures are those, such as C, and D, in Fig. 76-1, in which there is no marked hinging or upward displacement of the fragments. Reduction is impossible and unnecessary, so splinting is unnecessary also.

Hinge fractures are the result of a strong force applied to one of the patient's anterior superior iliac spines pushing his ilium backwards and outwards. His symphysis separates, so that the two halves of his pelvis open like a book, hinging on one of his sacro—iliac joints, like Pelvis F, in Fig. 76-1.

Vertical fractures follow an accident in which a force applied through a patient's femur pushes one side of his pelvis several centimetres upwards, as in pelvis E, Fig. 76-1. The fracture lines run vertically through his pubic bone and his ischium. On the same side his ilium splits vertically, just lateral to one of his sacro—iliac joints. Reduce these fractures by applying strong traction to his leg on the injured side. You can apply this more easily through the upper end of his tibia than through the lower end of his femur, which is the alternative site.

PELVIC FRACTURES

COMPRESSION FRACTURES Leave the patient in bed and encourage him to move his hips and spine. After 3 weeks if displacement is mild, or 6 weeks if it is severe, get him up on crutches.

HINGE SUBLUXATION FRACTURES Use the first method where possible, and the others as necessary.

(1) Lie the patient on his most comfortable side on a soft bed, and the fracture will probably reduce itself naturally. Bind his pelvis with a tight girth. This is all that most patients need.

(2) Sling his pelvis from a beam for 2 weeks, as in Fig. 76-3. Use heavy weights which will lift it just clear of his bed. The disadvantage with this method is that the sling has to be taken down for toilet purposes.

(3) Anaesthetize him, reduce the fracture by compressing the two sides of his pelvis, apply a hip spica, split it down the front, remove a strip a few centimetres wide, then bind it together with an Esmarch bandage.

(4) If the above methods are not practicable because of some other injuries, apply '90–90' traction to both legs (Fig. 77-11).

Leave the patient in bed for 3 weeks, and then get him up on crutches. Don't encourage him to bear weight for 6 weeks. Warn him that his sacro—iliac joints will be painful for some months.

DISPLACED VERTICAL FRACTURES Put a Steinmann or Denham pin through the patient's tibia, as for extension traction (Fig. 78-3), apply 10 to 15 kg of traction for 4 to 6 weeks, and then allow him up on crutches. The injured side of his pelvis can no longer support his weight, so he must not try to bear weight on it for another 6 weeks.

Warn him that his injured leg may be a little short, and that his hip may be painful for 18 months or more. If he wears shoes, the shoe on his short side can be raised.

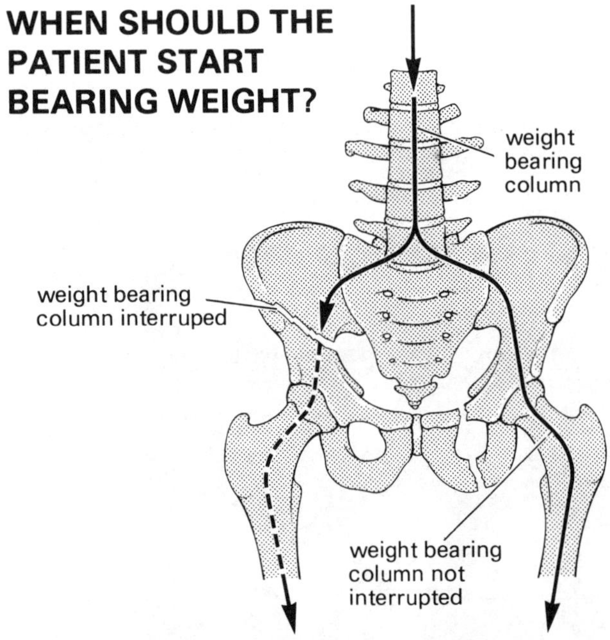

WHEN SHOULD THE PATIENT START BEARING WEIGHT?

weight bearing column

weight bearing column interruped

weight bearing column not interrupted

Fig. 76-2 HOW SOON SHOULD A PATIENT WITH A FRACTURED PELVIS BEAR WEIGHT? His weight is transmitted from his spine to his sacrum, then through his acetabulae to his femora. If this weight bearing column is fractured, he should be in bed for at least 3 weeks, and not bear weight until 6 weeks. But if the weight bearing parts of his pelvis are intact, he can start weight bearing in a few days, if his other injuries allow it. *Kindly contributed by John Jellis.*

A SLING FOR THE PELVIS

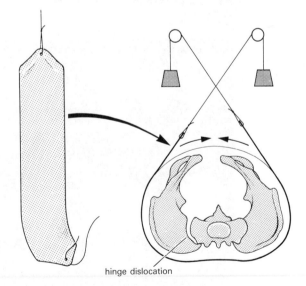

hinge dislocation

Fig. 76-3 A SLING FOR HINGE FRACTURES OF THE PELVIS. Use heavy weights which just lift a patient's pelvis clear of the bed. The disadvantage with this method is that the sling has to be taken down for toilet purposes.

76.3 Acetabular fractures

The outlook for a patient with an acetabular fracture depends mostly on whether or not the head of his femur has destroyed the upper part of his acetabulum. This is the part which bears his weight, and if enough of it remains unbroken, his outlook is good. Otherwise severe degenerative arthritis is likely to follow.

Fracture of the posterior rim of the acetabulum is one of the results of a car accident in which the patient's knee hits the dashboard. The head of his femur is driven backwards, and breaks off a piece of the rim of his acetabulum. At the same time, his hip may dislocate posteriorly, and his sciatic nerve may be injured. Provided his hip has not been dislocated, the attitude of his leg is normal, and there is no shortening. These fractures are often missed and their late effects are underestimated.

Fracture of the floor of the acetabulum is the result of the patient's falling from a height onto his greater trochanter and forcing the head of his femur against the floor of his acetabulum. Or, he may be struck on the hip in a car accident. The head may remain in its socket as in A, Fig. 76-4, or it may dislocate centrally through the broken floor of his acetabulum into his pelvis, so that he has a central dislocation of his hip as in B, in this figure.

He cannot move his leg or lift his foot off the couch. His foot is in its normal position showing that his hip is in its normal attitude. Unless displacement is gross, his leg is not shortened. Although the X-ray is characteristic, fractures of the acetabular floor are often overlooked.

Traction combined with gentle movements gives suprisingly good results. Don't treat him in a Thomas splint.

FRACTURES OF THE ACETABULUM

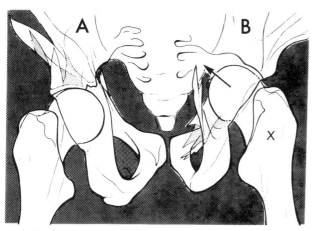

fracture of the floor of the acetabulum

central dislocation of the hip

Fig. 76-4 A FRACTURE OF THE FLOOR OF THE ACETABULUM can leave the head of a patient's femur in its normal place (A), or it can dislocate it centrally into his pelvis (B). 'X' shows the point at which you can insert a Steinmann pin to extract the head of his femur from his pelvis.

ACETABULAR FRACTURES

FRACTURE OF THE POSTERIOR RIM

If the patient's hip is dislocated, reduce it (77.4). When you have reduced it, check it for stability. Flex his thigh to 90°, then push it posteriorly to see if it is stable or easily redislocates.

If it is stable, keep him in bed until he is comfortable, perhaps within a week. Then let him walk on crutches with partial weight bearing.

If the head of his femur will not stay in the acetabulum, refer him immediately to have the posterior lip of his acetabulum screwed back. The longer you delay the more difficult this will become. If you cannot refer him, put him in '90-90 traction' for 6 weeks as in Section 77.12.

If a fragment of bone is trapped inside the joint, it must be removed at open operation, so refer him.

FRACTURES OF THE FLOOR OF THE ACETABULUM

WITHOUT CENTRAL DISLOCATION Encourage the patient to move his hip actively and then get him up on crutches as soon as pain will allow.

WITH CENTRAL DISLOCATION This is a severe injury and the patient is likely to need a blood transfusion. Anaesthetize him; thiopentone (A 8.6) or ketamine (A 8.2) is suitable.

When he is lying on his back, his leg rotates laterally. Correct this by rotating his leg so that his patella faces anteriorly. Flex his hip a little and feel for his greater trochanter. Insert a Steinmann pin, or, better a Denham pin antero–posteriorly at point 'X' in Fig. 76-4. It will go in more easily if you hammer it first, before using the handle.

CAUTION ! Don't put the pin too far medially or you may injure his sciatic nerve!

Insert another pin in his upper tibia, and apply 7 to 10 kg of longitudinal traction. Put a stirrup on the vertical pin and apply 15 kg for 15 minutes. If you can pull the head of his femur out, it will usually stay out. So remove the vertical pin and send him back to the ward with a tibial pin in for extension traction (Fig. 78-3).

Alternatively, try forcibly flexing and abducting his thigh. Or, try adducting it using your foot as a fulcrum. Or, put a block between his thighs and try to bring his knees together.

X-ray him to check reduction.

If reduction is satisfactory, continue to apply 5 to 10 kg of extension traction to his tibia, and exert countertraction by raising the foot of his bed 25 cm. This will make him more comfortable, but it will not by itself reduce the dislocation. Put a sling under his thigh and pass the cord from this over a pulley to let him exercise his hip.

Keep him in traction for at least 6 weeks. Encourage him to exercise as much as he can. Then get him walking. Allow him up with crutches with gradually increasing weight bearing (77.1). Remove his crutches as soon as he can stand normally on his injured leg.

If reduction is still unsatisfactory, refer him for open reduction.

77 The hip

Rehabilitating a patient with an injured lower limb

Your ultimate objective after any lower limb injury is to get a patient walking again without a limp. There are three stages in doing this, and in the first two of these he needs crutches: (1) a non−weight bearing stage in which he does not put his foot to the ground, (2) a stage of partial weight bearing, and (3) a stage of full weight bearing in which he has no help, except perhaps from a stick.

If an injured patient learns to walk normally, he uses all his muscles, and stabilizes his injured limb. But if he limps, some of his muscles remain unused, with the result that he may limp permanently, and quite unnecessarily. So try to interest your ward staff in the way their patients walk, and make them into active physiotherapists.

HELP WITH WALKING

If a patient has a forearm fracture, he can use a crutch with an arm support like this

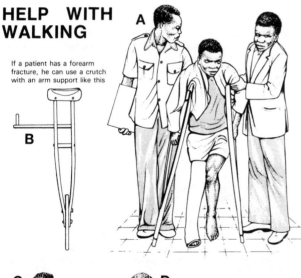

Weight born on the arm rest, not his axilla

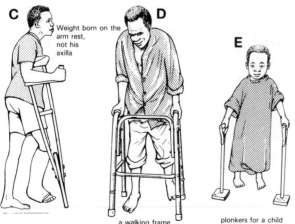

a walking frame   plonkers for a child

Fig. 77-1 HELP IN WALKING. A, a patient being taught to walk. B, a crutch with an arm support. C, the same crutch in use. D, a walking frame. E, 'plonkers' for a child.

REHABILITATING A PATIENT WITH AN INJURED LEG

The time at which a patient should be mobilized without weight bearing, and the time when he should start partial or full weight bearing depend mostly on the kind of injury he has, and are described later for each injury.

CRUTCHES FOR AN INJURED LEG

A plentiful supply of crutches is essential. Some hospitals find it convenient to ask the patient to leave a small deposit for them. Ask the hospital carpenter to make well padded axillary crutches with rubber tips, adjustable for height, and for the position of the hand grips, which should be about one third of the way down the crutches.

Fit crutches carefully so that when a patient is standing, his crutches are just short of his axillae. When his hands are on the hand grips, his elbows should be slightly flexed. A crutch which is slightly too short is better than one which is too long.

CAUTION! (1) A patient must bear weight on his hand rests, not his axillae, or he may get a crutch paralysis. Any of the nerves of his brachial plexus may be injured, usually his radial nerve, which may take 6 months to recover. (2) A comfortable crutch will do much to reduce the burden of his disability.

Stand behind him, tell him to put his crutches close to his side slightly in front of his feet, and to look straight ahead. Ask him to take his weight on his hands, to lean forwards, so that his weight is over his crutches, and then to transfer his weight to one crutch before moving the other one.

NON−WEIGHT BEARING Ask the patient to hop on his normal leg while steadying himself with his crutches.

PARTIAL WEIGHT BEARING Ideally, you should use bathroom scales to measure how much weight a patient is putting on his injured leg. You will probably not have suitable scales, so encourage him to bear as much weight as he can without causing pain.

'Three point walking' Ask him to bring his crutches and his injured leg forward together, taking some weight on each.

'Four point walking' Ask him to advance his right crutch followed by his left leg, and then his left crutch followed by his right leg. This is slow at first, but is more like normal walking.

STICKS FOR LEARNING TO WALK

Two sticks are better than one, and less likely to cause a limp. Use the four point gait described above. Flat pieces of wood on the bottom of two sticks ('plonkers') will make them easier for a child to use.

WALKING IN A CAST

If a patient is in a cast, he should, if possible, start walking normally right from the start, erect and looking ahead. Teach him to lift his heel, to transfer his weight to his forefoot, to bend his knee, to move his leg forward, and to put his forefoot on the ground, to lower his heel, and to move his body forward, repeating these movements with both legs until he is walking normally.

After his cast has been removed, teach him to walk without a limp, using crutches at first to minimize the pain. Teach him to balance on his two feet. Let him start by holding with both hands on to the foot of his bed, then teach him to balance on one foot. This is the most important part of his training. Stand in front of him and let him put his hands on your shoulders. Ask him to hold tight and lift his injured leg first, then his good one. To start with, he may be unable to balance his body over his injured leg, but he soon learns to do so by abducting his hip on the injured side.

As soon as he can balance on one leg, ask him to bend his opposite knee to a right angle. This makes balancing more difficult.

Next, make him lift first one leg then the other, while standing in the same place. When he can do this, ask him to take short steps, putting his good foot down 10 cm in front of his bad one, and then his bad foot the same distance in front of his good foot. Like this, he learns to put equal weight on both legs to avoid a limp.

TURN YOUR WARD STAFF INTO PHYSIOTHERAPISTS

INJURIES OF THE HIP AND FEMUR

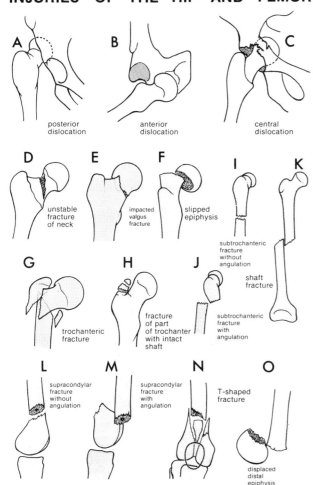

Fig. 77-2 INJURIES TO THE HIP AND FEMUR classified according to the methods you might use to treat them in a district hospital. A, B, and C, posterior, anterior (rare), and central dislocations of the hip. D, and E, unstable and impacted valgus fractures of the neck of the femur. F, slipped upper epiphysis. G, a trochanteric fracture. H, fracture of part of the trochanter with an intact shaft. I, and J, subtrochanteric and trochanteric fractures both with and without angulation. K, one of many possible fractures of the shaft. L, and M, supracondylar fractures with and without angulation. N, a T–shaped fracture is only one of several fractures that occur around the knee (79.13). O, displacement of the distal femoral epiphysis.

77.2 An overview of injuries to the hip joint and femur

Working from above downwards, and using the methods of treatment that are practical in a district hospital as the main guide in classifying them, you will encounter the injuries of the hip and femur shown in Fig. 77-2.

Dislocations are usually posterior (A), and occasionally anterior (B), or central through the acetabulum (C).

Fractures of the neck of the femur are of two kinds: the common unstable ones (D), which may be complete in that the fracture line runs all the way across the bone, or incomplete, in that it only runs part of the way across. There is also the rarer stable impacted valgus fracture (E). Fractures here unite badly, and conservative treatment is generally unsatisfactory, so that most of these fractures need internal fixation, if this is possible.

Slipping of the upper femoral epiphysis (F) occurs spontaneously in teenagers, either slowly or suddenly.

Intertrochanteric fractures (G) occur between the two trochanters. Fractures here unite well, so that conservative treatment is usually satisfactory.

Fractures of the greater trochanter are rare and not serious. A patient falls on his hip and breaks off his greater trochanter without breaking the shaft of his femur (H). Get him walking on crutches until he is free from pain. No other treatment is necessary.

Subtrochanteric fractures occur a few centimetres below the trochanters. The important distinction is between those fractures in which the fragments are approximately aligned, so that you can treat a patient in Perkins traction (I), and those fractures in which the proximal fragment has been so sharply flexed by his iliopsoas that he has to be treated by '90–90 traction' (J).

Fractures of the central part of the shaft of the femur are common (K). Treatment varies with the patient's age: (1) At birth no treatment is strictly necessary, although some may be advisable. (2) From birth to 3 years use gallows traction or a plaster spica. (3) Between 3 and 18 years use extension traction. (4) If he is over 18 years use Perkins traction.

Supracondylar fractures occur just above the condyles. Their treatment parallels that for fractures just below the trochanters: (1) If the fragments are more or less aligned, you can treat a patient in Perkins traction, as for a fracture of the shaft of his femur (L). (2) If his gastrocnemius has flexed the distal fragment (M), you will have to treat him with his knee sharply flexed.

Fractures around the knee are of several kinds, only one of which (N) is shown. They are discussed in Section 79.13. You can treat some of them by Perkins traction.

Displacement of the distal femoral epiphysis follows a violent injury in a teenager (O), or osteomyelitis (7.10).

IF A PATIENT'S FEMUR IS FRACTURED, MAKE SURE HIS HIP IS NOT DISLOCATED ALSO

EXAMINING THE HIP

As always, modify the methods which follow to suit your patient's needs. Some of them are not indicated in an acute injury. You will find them particularly useful if you don't have an X-ray.

Remove his clothes. If he can walk, watch him do so. Does he limp? If he can walk, he is unlikely to have a serious leg injury, but he can however have an impacted fracture of the neck of his femur.

Ask him to stand on one leg. When a normal person does this, his pelvis tilts so that his opposite hip lifts. This can only happen if the hip on which he is standing is normal. If his opposite hip falls, the hip mechanism of the leg he is standing on is abnormal. His gait may be abnormal in a similar way (Trendelenburg sign and gait).

WHAT IS THE ATTITUDE OF HIS HIP?

When a normal patient lies on his back, his legs rotate externally a little. If his leg is abnormally externally rotated after an injury, he has probably fractured the neck of his femur. If it is rotated 90° the fracture is probably low in the neck. If it is rotated only 45° it is likely to be high in the neck where it is partly retained by the capsule.

Is his hip flexed, adducted, and internally rotated after a violent injury? (posterior dislocation).

Is his hip flexed, abducted and externally rotated? (anterior dislocation, rare).

DOES HIS HIP MOVE NORMALLY?

Rotation in extension—testing for spasm. (1) Lie the patient flat with his pelvis level. With your hands on his thigh, gently rock his leg from side to side. Compare both sides. Any painful limitation of movement indicates muscle spasm. This is such a sensitive test that if it is acutely painful, you may have to modify the remaining tests.

(2) Lie the patient on his front, bend his knee, grasp his foot, and rotate his leg from side to side.

Can he extend his hip normally? A patient can compensate for being unable to extend his hip by extending his lumbar spine. First exclude this. Lie him on his back. Put one hand palm upwards under his lumbar spine. With your other hand flex his normal hip. This will flatten the normal curve in his lumbar spine, and force it against the couch. If his other hip is able to extend normally, it will remain flat on the couch as you do this. If his other hip is unable to extend, it will flex.

Flexion Flex his knee on the affected side, and then carefully flex his hip as far as possible. If it rotates externally as it comes up in flexion, this is a sign of slipping of his femoral epiphysis.

Rotation in flexion While his hip and knee are flexed to 90° rotate his hip externally and internally, and compare its range with the opposite side. Any 'crunchy feeling' in this or any other movement is a sign that his hip joint is abnormal. It may indicate an acute massive slip of the head of his femur.

Abduction (1) Flex his normal knee and hook his normal leg over the edge of the couch. This will lock his pelvis and prevent it tilting. Now, keeping his other knee straight, grasp his ankle and then abduct his leg as far as it will go.

(2) As you abduct his leg, put one hand on the opposite anterior superior iliac spine to detect if his pelvis rotates. In a child, put one hand across both his anterior superior iliac spines.

Adduction. Still steadying his pelvis, bring one thigh as far as it will go over the other one. It should be able to cross the middle third of his other thigh.

WHERE ARE HIS GREATER TROCHANTERS? **Stand over him, face his head, place your thumbs on his anterior superior iliac spines, and put your middle fingers on his trochanters. Compare both sides, and feel if the trochanter on the affected side is displaced.**

Is his trochanter displaced upwards towards his anterior superior iliac spine? (posterior dislocation). Or, away from it? (fractured neck of femur, or slipped epiphysis, or anterior dislocation).

Has his greater trochanter moved medially towards his pelvis? (central dislocation of his hip).

WHERE IS THE HEAD OF HIS FEMUR? If a patient is very thin, you may be able to feel it. If the position of his leg suggests that the head of his femur might be displaced, feel for it in his perineum, in his groin, or on the back of his ilium. Make sure that what you feel really is the head of his femur by feeling it move when you rotate the shaft. Remember that, provided the neck of his femur is intact, its head points in the same direction as its medial condyle.

Feel the base of his femoral triangle. If his hip has been dislocated posteriorly, this will feel soft, his femoral artery will be difficult to palpate, and there may even be a hollow.

WHERE IS THE POINT OF MAXIMUM TENDERNESS? In front of his hip joint? (fractured neck of femur). Over his greater trochanter? (trochanteric fracture).

IS HIS LEG SHORT? The measurement of true shortening is useful in many hip and leg conditions. Method (1) is essential for adjusting Perkins traction if you have no X-rays. Method (2) is not applicable to an acute injury.

(1) Put the patient's injured leg into exactly the same position as his normal one and compare measurements from each side. For example, if he has an abduction deformity, abduct the normal leg before you measure them both. If you don't measure both legs in the same position, you will make big errors. Use a tape measure to measure the distance between these three points: (a) The inferior edge of his anterior superior iliac spine. (b) The joint line of his knee. You can find this most easily when his leg is flexed, but take the measurement with his leg straight. (c) The tip of his medial malleolus.

(2) Sit, and ask him to stand in front of you. Put your thumbs on his anterior superior iliac spines. One may be higher than the other. You will be able to observe a centimetre or more of shortening.

SCIATIC NERVE Test this. Can he dorsiflex his foot?

MEASURING SHORTENING

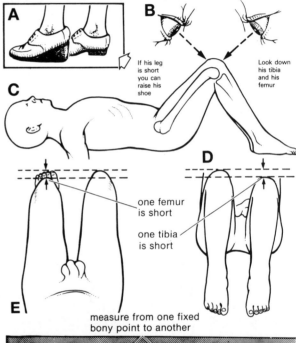

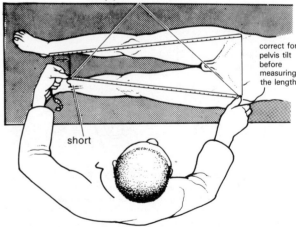

Fig. 77-3 MEASURING TRUE SHORTENING is useful in many hip and leg conditions. Method E, is essential for adjusting Perkins traction if you have no X-rays. Method B, to D, is not applicable to an acute injury. A, if a patient's leg is short enough to cause him discomfort or disability, you can raise his shoe.

X-RAYS

Always X-ray a patient's hip if he complains of pain on weight bearing after a fall. Take the AP film *with his hip in as much internal rotation as possible,* even if you have to hold his leg in this position yourself. Don't take it in external rotation which is the natural position of a resting injured hip. Also take a lateral view to see if the head of his femur has been displaced posteriorly. This should be a horizontal view with the tube in his groin and the plate pressed well into him above his iliac crest.

If the films are difficult to interpret, compare both sides.

If you suspect a slipped upper femoral epiphysis in a teenager, take an AP 'frog leg' view to include both his hips on the same film, as in Fig. 77-9.

If you suspect he has broken the neck of his femur, take an AP view and a lateral view with his leg extended, the tube pointing along his groin on the inside of his leg, and the X-ray cassette pressed firmly into his flank and perpendicular to the axis of the tube.

CAUTION ! You can easily miss a fracture of the neck, especially if it is close to the head (subcapital). If you are in doubt, look all around the cortex for small breaks in continuity, a step, or an angular deformity.

THE MAJOR FEATURES OF SOME COMMON INJURIES

An unstable fracture of the neck of the femur The patient is in severe pain and cannot walk or lift his foot off the bed. His leg is externally rotated with 1 cm or more of shortening.

A stable impacted valgus fracture of the neck of the femur The patient has little pain, he can lift his foot off the bed and he may be able to walk. His leg is not rotated and there is no shortening.

An intertrochanteric fracture He is in severe pain. He cannot walk or lift his foot off the bed. His leg is externally rotated with shortening. Maximum tenderness is over his greater trochanter.

Posterior dislocation His hip is flexed, adducted, and internally rotated, and his leg is shortened.

Anterior dislocation His hip is flexed, abducted, and externally rotated, and his leg is shortened.

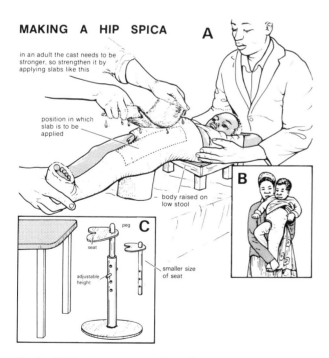

Fig. 77-4 MAKING A HIP SPICA. You will need to support the patient's buttocks. You can use a low stool as in a A. Better, get the support C made. This has a metal base, an adjustable stem made of two sliding tubes, and a seat of two sizes, with a peg to support the patient's groin. Rest his back on a table, and put the seat under his sacrum. *Kindly contributed by John Stewart.*

Central dislocation His trochanter is displaced medially. You may be able to feel the head of his femur rectally. There is no shortening.

77.3 A hip spica

You will sometimes find a plaster spica (figure of 8 bandage) useful to immobilise a patient's hip, or more often, his femur. Unfortunately, hip spicas are expensive because they need a lot of plaster. Also, they are inconvenient, because a patient has to be lifted on to a bedpan. But, provided a family is capable of this much nursing, you can use a spica to treat some patients, particularly children with fractures of the femur, at home or in a health centre for at least part of their illness, whereas they would otherwise need a hospital bed.

A HIP SPICA

INDICATIONS (1) Fractured femurs in children, preferably after union has occurred in gallows or extension traction. (2) Postoperatively following the relief of a flexion contracture of the hip. (3) Septic arthritis of the hip.

CONTRAINDICATIONS (1) Fractures of the femoral neck in old people, in whom a spica may be lethal. (2) As the sole method of treatment of fractures of the femur in adults.

EQUIPMENT You will need to support the patient on the special support in Fig. 77-4, or on a low stool.

APPLYING THE SPICA Support the patient and pad his leg and trunk. Put extra padding over his bony points, particularly his sacrum.

Wrap several wide bandages around his trunk. Put a folded towel on his abdomen, and remove this when the cast is completed. This will leave a space into which his abdomen can expand after a full meal.

Pass bandages in a figure of eight round his trunk and upper leg.

If you are trying to fuse his hip, as in TB, take the spica down as far as his ankle, or if this is not advisable, insert a pin through the lower end of his femur and incorporate this in the cast. It will allow him to move his knee and stop his femur rotating at his hip.

If he has a fracture of his femur, continue the spica to his ankle.

Lay a slab from his thigh to his iliac fossa to strengthen the spica in his groin where it is most likely to break. Turn up the free edge of the padding in his other groin and bind it into the cast with another plaster bandage.

Remove the supports, turn him over, and inspect the back edge of the cast carefully to make sure it is comfortable and not pressing into him.

CAUTION ! (1) A hip spica must engage his lower ribs on each side. (2) There must be space for his stomach to expand, or ileus may follow. (3) Enough of his buttocks must be free to enable him to sit on a bedpan.

If his hip spica is too tight, cut a large hole out of it over his abdomen when it has dried.

Alternatively, you can apply a long leg cast first and then convert it into a spica.

77.4 Posterior dislocation of the hip

Fortunately, dislocation of a patient's hip is much less common than dislocation of his shoulder or elbow. His car has a head—on collision, his knee hits the dashboard and drives the head of his femur out of his acetabulum. At first the head lies behind his acetabulum, but it soon rides up on to the dorsum of his ilium. He usually has other serious injuries also, especially a fracture of the shaft of his femur, so that his dislocated hip is often missed.

305

POSTERIOR DISLOCATION OF THE HIP

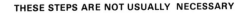

THESE STEPS ARE NOT USUALLY NECESSARY

they are for a dislocation of his left leg

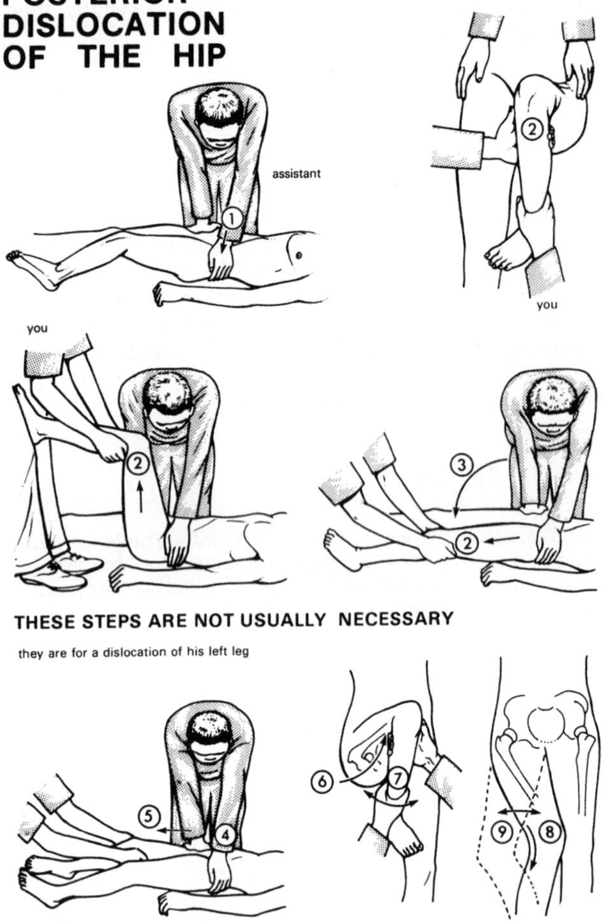

Fig. 77-5 POSTERIOR DISLOCATION OF THE HIP—FIRST METHOD. You will need a strong assistant. *After de Palma with kind permission.*

He is likely to be severely shocked, and cannot stand. His leg lies in a highly characteristic position, with his thigh flexed, adducted, and internally rotated. His leg is shorter than on the other side. His knee rests on his opposite thigh and his greater trochanter and buttocks are abnormally prominent.

If your anaesthetist is not expert, use the first of the two methods described below in which the patient lies on the floor. If he is expert enough to prevent a tracheal tube falling out while the patient is lying on his face, the alternative method is likely to be best, because it uses gravity and the weight of the patient's leg to achieve reduction. It is also the least traumatic.

POSTERIOR DISLOCATION OF THE HIP

Reduce this injury early, because every hour's delay makes reduction more difficult and avascular necrosis of the head of the patient's femur more likely. Look for other fractures, especially a fracture of the posterior rim of his acetabulum. Check the function of his sciatic nerve before and after reduction (55.8), and examine his dorsalis pedis pulse.

You can reduce his dislocation by: (1) having him supine on the floor (Fig. 77-5), or (2) prone on the table (Fig. 77-6). A subarachnoid anaesthetic is suitable for either method. If he is prone on the table after a general anaesthetic, he must be intubated. Good relaxation is essential, ketamine is not enough.

THE FIRST METHOD FOR A POSTERIOR DISLOCATION OF THE HIP

Place the patient on the floor, as in Fig. 77-5. Stand over him and ask an assistant to push downwards on his anterior superior iliac spines (1).

Flex the patient's knee and his hip, and rotate his leg into a neutral position. Pull his leg upwards steadily and gently (2). While still pulling in the line of his femur, lower his leg to the floor (3). Reduction is usually obvious, but X-ray him to make sure.

If the above method fails to reduce the dislocation, ask your assistant to continue pressing firmly on the patient's anterior superior iliac spines (4).

With his knee partly flexed, pull on his leg in the line of the deformity (5).

Slowly bring his hip to 90° of flexion (6) and gently rotate it internally and externally (7) to disengage the head from the structures which are holding it.

Put the head back in place by further internal rotation and extension (8), or external rotation and extension (9).

While he is still anaesthetized, examine his knee for rupture of his posterior cruciate ligament (79.6).

AN ALTERNATIVE METHOD FOR A POSTERIOR DISLOCATION OF THE HIP

As soon as the patient is anaesthetized, place him face downwards on a table, as in Fig. 77-6, so that his injured thigh hangs downward with his knee at 90° and his foot resting on your knee. Ask an assistant to hold his normal thigh horizontally. This will prevent his pelvis tilting.

Press steadily downwards on his flexed knee until his muscles relax and the head of his femur drops into his acetabulum. If necessary, rock his knee slightly.

If reduction fails, refer him for open reduction.

TEST FOR STABILITY (both methods)
While the patient is still anaesthetized, flex his hip to 90° and check to see if the head of his femur easily slips out of his acetabulum posteriorly, or if it stays in place. If it slips out easily, suspect a fracture of the posterior rim of his acetabulum (76.3).

POSTOPERATIVE CARE FOR A POSTERIOR DISLOCATION OF THE HIP

IF THE DISLOCATION IS STABLE
management depends on whether or not movement is pain-free.

If movement is pain-free, there is no need for traction, so start active movemets in bed, and after 10 days get the patient up on crutches with partial weight bearing.

POSTERIOR DISLOCATION OF THE HIP (alternative method)

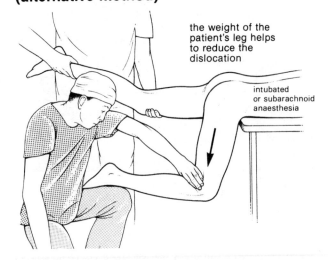

the weight of the patient's leg helps to reduce the dislocation

intubated or subarachnoid anaesthesia

Fig. 77-6 AN ALTERNATIVE METHOD FOR REDUCING A POSTERIOR DISLOCATION OF THE HIP. This is the best method to use if you have a good anaesthetist who can intubate a patient and prevent a tracheal tube slipping out while he is prone. *After de Palma with kind permission.*

If movement is painful, put him in extension traction until the pain has gone, then get him up on crutches, progressing from partial to full weight bearing.

IF REDUCTION IS UNSTABLE, so that the head of the patient's femur slips out of his acetabulum, X-ray him. If this shows that a large chip has broken off the rim of his acetabulum, refer him to have it repaired. Otherwise, try extension traction with a tibial pin. If this controls the reduction, continue to apply it for at least 6 weeks.

If extension traction fails to control his unstable hip, it is probably because the posterior rim of his acetabulum has been shattered. Put him up in '90-90 traction' (77.12), with a pin through the upper end of his tibia, and treat him as for a fracture of the posterior rim of his acetabulum (76.3). Take an AP and a lateral X-ray to make sure the reduction is satisfactory. Take them while he is in bed in traction. After his hip has been held like this for 6 weeks, there will be enough scar tissue in his posterior acetabulum to hold it. Provided the range of movement in his hip and his ability to control it increase each day, allow him to move it as he wishes.

Explain that late complications may occur, and follow him up for 2 years.

DIFFICULTIES WITH DISLOCATED HIPS

If the patient's HIP IS PARTICULARLY PAINFUL immediately after reduction, consider aspirating it (7.17) if you are expert and can be sure not to infect it.

If he CANNOT DORSIFLEX HIS FOOT, test the sensation on its dorsum. If this is absent, he has a sciatic nerve palsy. A palsy is common, but fortunately it usually recovers. If he fractured the rim of his acetabulum, the displaced fragment may have impaled his sciatic nerve. Refer him so that his hip can be explored and the fragment fixed.

If his FOOT IS COLD, BLUE, AND SWOLLEN, his femoral artery or vein has thrombosed, so reduce his dislocation urgently. If his foot is swollen, raise his leg. If his artery is thrombosed, keep his leg cool. Refer him urgently for vascular surgery. If this is to be effective the operation must be done within 2 hours.

If he has DISLOCATED HIS HIP AND FRACTURED THE HEAD OF HIS FEMUR, there may be a loose fragment inside the joint. Refer him so that it can be removed. A chip can break off the head of his femur, instead of the rim of his acetabulum.

If he has DISLOCATED HIS HIP AND FRACTURED THE SHAFT OF HIS FEMUR, his dislocation can only be reduced at open operation, so refer him. With this combination of injuries a dislocated hip is often missed. *So, always X-ray a patient's hip whenever his femur is fractured.*

If the posterior DISLOCATION OF HIS HIP HAS BEEN MISSED, try to reduce it by closed methods up to 2 weeks after the injury. If you fail, refer him. Older dislocations are usually impossible to reduce by closed methods.

If his HIP BECOMES PROGRESSIVELY MORE PAINFUL some months or years after a dislocation, this is probably due to avascular necrosis and the osteoarthritis that follows it. Avascular necrosis shows itself on the X-ray as an increase in the density of the head of his femur. You may see this at 6 weeks but it usually occurs much later. If pain is unbearable, the patient's only hope is referral for the excision of the head of his femur or an arthroplasty.

REDUCE DISLOCATED HIPS IMMEDIATELY

77.5 Anterior dislocation of the hip

In this rare injury the patient falls from a height and displaces the head of his femur in front of his acetabulum. The earlier steps in this method convert an anterior dislocation into a posterior one.

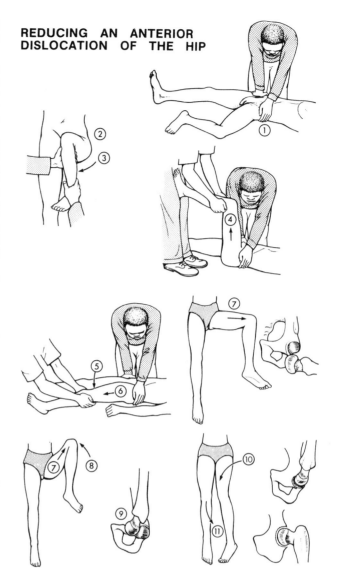

Fig. 77-7 REDUCING AN ANTERIOR DISLOCATION OF THE HIP. In this rare injury the patient falls from a height and displaces the head of his femur in front of his acetabulum. The earlier steps in the method of reduction convert an anterior dislocation into a posterior one. *After de Palma with kind permission.*

ANTERIOR DISLOCATION OF THE HIP

Lie the patient on his back on the floor, and anaesthetize him as for a posterior dislocation.

Stand over him and ask a strong assistant to hold his pelvis firmly throughout the manoeuvre by its anterior superior iliac spines (1). Hold the patient's leg and bend his hip and his knee to 90° (2).

Rotate his leg into a neutral position (3). This will convert an anterior dislocation into a posterior one. Pull the patient's leg steadily upwards (4) so as to lift the head of his femur into his acetabulum.

If his hip is not reduced, lower his leg to the floor (5) while still maintaining traction (6).

If his hip is still not reduced, apply traction (7) in the direction of the deformity (flexion and abduction). While maintaining traction, lift his leg (8) into vertical position so as to bring the head of his femur on to the anterior rim of his acetabulum (9).

Now, still maintaining traction, rotate his leg internally (10), and lower his thigh into an extended position (11).

If his hip is even now not reduced, ask one assistant to continue holding his pelvis firmly. Ask a second assistant to stand over him and pull very hard in the line of his femur. Abduct his normal hip and put your unbooted heel where you think the head of his femur is. Then press posterolaterally until the head goes 'clunk' into its socket.

If you fail to reduce his dislocation, refer him for open reduction.

POSTOPERATIVE CARE Keep the patient in bed until he has regained control of his hip. Then allow him up and let him bear weight. Watch the head of his femur for aseptic necrosis, as with a posterior dislocation. Provided he is lucky enough to avoid this, he should recover well.

77.6 Fractures of the neck of the femur

These are difficult fractures. The nearer they are to the head of a patient's femur, the less likely they are to unite (except in the case of a stable impacted valgus fracture), and the more likely the head is to undergo avascular necrosis. There are no satisfactory closed methods for most of these fractures, and no open ones that are practical in the district hospitals for which we write. The blood supply of the head of the femur is precarious, little callus is formed, and rigid internal fixation provides the only hope of union. Almost all such injuries should be treated by early internal fixation. If you cannot refer a patient to have this done, there is a chance that he will benefit from Perkins traction, but he will probably have to be content with crutches. Suprisingly, these fractures are often missed.

For the purposes of management in a district hospital, there are three kinds of fractures of the neck of the femur: (1) The common complete, unstable ones. (2) The rare incomplete unstable ones. (3) The less common, stable impacted valgus fractures. These are all shown in Fig. 77-8.

THREE FRACTURES OF THE FEMORAL NECK

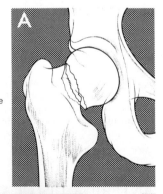

unstable incomplete fracture

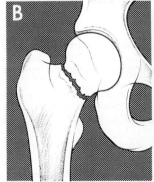

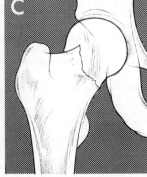

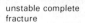
unstable complete fracture

impacted valgus

Fig. 77-8 THREE FRACTURES OF THE FEMORAL NECK. A, the rare incomplete unstable fracture. Note that the fracture line has not gone completely through the neck. B, the common complete unstable fracture. C, the uncommon impacted valgus fracture. *Kindly contributed by John Stewart.*

77.7 Unstable fractures of the neck of the femur (adults)

Most fractures of the femoral neck are unstable and complete. The patient is either a young adult who has sustained a severe injury, or an old person who has fallen and injured his hip.

The patient cannot stand or lift his foot off the bed; moving his hip gives him great pain. His leg is externaly rotated so that his foot points laterally, and his leg is shortened about a centimetre. This is less shortening than with intertrochanteric fractures, so it is a useful point of differential diagnosis. Sometimes, his injury may seem to be trivial. Occasionally, he complains of pain in his knee, rather than in his hip.

Any patient who cannot walk after a fall must have his hip X-rayed, with his leg held in maximal internal rotation in order to get the best view of the neck of his femur. External rotation makes the neck look foreshortened. If his hip is not X-rayed, and you allow him to walk about, he can easily convert an incomplete fracture into a complete one. If the films are hard to interpret and the fracture line difficult to see, compare his injured hip with his normal one.

If possible, refer all patients with incomplete fractures for internal fixation or for the fitting of a prosthesis. If you cannot do this, put the patient into extension traction for 12 weeks.

If a patient has an unstable fracture and you cannot refer him for internal fixation, or a prosthesis, you have two choices: (1) You can do Girdlestone's operation. (2) You can get him up and around on crutches as best he can. A false joint will develop, and the final result will resemble that after a Girdlestone's operation, except that it may be somewhat less satisfactory. He will probably limp and need crutches always, or at the very least a walking stick, but he may do suprisingly well. There is no indication for excising the head of the femur immediately, and traction is useless. A hip spica in an old villager is likely to be a certain prescription for a slow and painful death.

UNSTABLE FRACTURES OF THE NECK OF THE FEMUR

If possible, refer the patient immediately for internal fixation or prosthetic replacement, especially if he is young. A Smith–Petersen nail should be inserted as soon as possible, but an Austin–Moore prosthesis can be inserted at any time, although it is not indicated in the young. If you can refer the patient, he will be more comfortable with his legs bandaged gently together with cotton wool between them.

If you cannot refer him, proceed as follows.

If he has an incomplete unstable fracture (rare), it may become complete at any moment. There is no way of testing for clinical union, so apply Perkins traction or extension traction for at least 12 weeks, but without the vigorous exercises that are so necessary for fractures of the shaft of the femur.

If his unstable fracture is complete, keep him in bed for a week, until the pain is less, then sit him up daily. As soon as he can tolerate it, get him walking on crutches with very little weight bearing at first. If he is lucky, he will get a comparatively painless pseudoarthrosis, need a stick, and perhaps a raised shoe, and adapt his life style to his disability. If pain is a problem later, you may be able to refer him for prosthetic replacement of the head of his femur or a Girdlestone femoral head resection.

77.8 Stable impacted valgus fractures of the neck of the femur (adults)

The fracture line runs across the proximal part of the neck of the patient's femur, the fragments are firmly impacted on one another, with the head in valgus. This makes the fracture stable and is a useful point in recognizing this particular fracture.

The patient is usually an old person. He may be able to walk after the accident, and with a little encouragement can lift his leg off the bed. There is no rotational deformity and no shortening.

Because the fracture line is mainly horizontal, there is little shearing stress across it, and a good chance that the head will not disimpact. Bearing a little weight on it is beneficial because it maintains the impaction. It is a useful rule that if a patient can walk into the hospital, his fracture is probably stable. If he is lucky it will remain so.

STABLE, IMPACTED VALGUS FRACTURES OF THE NECK OF THE FEMUR

If there is any doubt about the stability of the impaction and you can refer the patient immediately for internal fixation, do so. There is no case for the application of a hip spica, the complications are too great.

CAUTION ! Don't apply traction, because it will destroy the impaction.

If the patient is already walking, let him continue, with partial weight bearing and crutches. The head is at its softest and most liable to displacement 10 to 14 days after the fracture. Supervise his walking carefully for the first 2 or 3 weeks before discharging him. Warn him that he must not trip or stumble.

If he cannot walk, keep him in bed, while doing vigorous quadriceps exercises, until the pain has subsided enough to let him walk on crutches, with partial weight bearing while he is careful supervised. He must walk with crutches for 3 to 4 weeks, but as the pain lessens he can bear progressively more weight on his injured leg. He must be very careful of it for at least 2 months.

Supervise him carefully as an out–patient.

DIFFICULTIES WITH IMPACTED FRACTURES OF THE NECK OF THE FEMUR

If a patient has been walking satisfactorily on an impacted valgus fracture, and his LEG NOW SUDDENLY BECOMES PAINFUL, so that he can no longer bear weight on it, the fragments have probably disimpacted. If internal fixation is impossible, treat him as if he had an unstable fracture, and get him up on crutches.

77.9 Fractures of the neck of the femur in children

Fractures of the neck of a child's femur are rare but serious. Subsequent moulding will not correct the femur's deformities. Changes in its angle persist, so if the fracture produces coxa vara (lessening of the angle between the neck of the femur and its shaft), this deformity will become worse and be permanent. Apply extension traction and try to get the angle of the neck of his femur correct. Overlapping and anteroposterior angulation are less important. Correct the deformity and then apply a plaster spica.

77.10 Separation of the upper femoral epiphysis

This is quite a common disease of middle to late teenagers, usually boys. It is an epiphyseal injury (Salter Harris Type 1, 69.6a) in which the patient's upper femoral epiphysis slips spontaneously backwards and downwards through the epiphyseal line, either gradually or suddenly, often after only a minor injury. In 20% of of cases, the other epiphysis slips too, even while the patient is in bed being treated for the first one. Try to diagnose and refer these patients for internal fixation early, because the results will be good. If you leave an epiphysis which has started to slip, it may slip completely, so that extensive and often unsuccessful major surgery is needed.

Gradual slipping A teenager complains of pain in his hip or knee, and starts to limp. Examine him carefuly, using the methods in Section 77.2, and compare his abnormal leg with his normal one, because the signs are not obvious. Look for:

SLIPPED UPPER FEMORAL EPIPHYSIS

The "frog leg" view

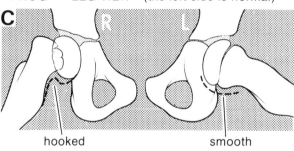

A

AP VIEW   Smooth line   angulated

B

FROG   LEG VIEW   (the left side is normal)

C

hooked   smooth

Fig. 77-9 SLIPPED UPPER FEMORAL EPIPHYSIS. A, this shows you how to take a frog leg view. This is essential for diagnosing a minimally slipped upper femoral epiphysis. The patient's lower legs are horizontal and parallel with the edge of the table. B, and C, his upper femoral epiphysis has slipped on the right side. In the AP view the upper border of the neck continues on smoothly into the head whereas it normally angulates sharply. In the frog leg view the lower border of the neck is sharply hooked, instead of being smooth. *Kindly contributed by John Stewart.*

(1) limitation of abduction, (2) loss of internal rotation, and (3) external rotation of his hip while you are flexing it, as in Fig. 7-17.

Rapid slipping The patient may not have had symptoms of gradual slipping before. He falls to the ground with a severe pain in his leg, which is externally rotated and short. He cannot move his leg off the couch, and finds passive movements acutely painful.

Although the physical signs may be minimal, a suitable X-ray is diagnostic—if you examine it carefully. You should be able to recognize an acute slip in an ordinary AP view, but an early slip is harder to recognize. So if you suspect an early slipped epiphysis, always take a frog leg view, as in Fig. 77-9. The epiphyseal line is widened and fluffy, and the epiphysis is displaced downwards. Normally, in an AP view the upper border of the femoral neck angulates sharply where it joins the head, but if the epiphysis has slipped, it continues on smoothly without a step. In a frog leg view the epiphysis projects below the neck as a sharp hook.

SEPARATION OF THE UPPER FEMORAL EPIPHYSIS

If you cannot refer the patient, try to rest his hip in internal rotation and abduction, either in a hip spica or in extension skin traction (Fig. 78-3). A hip spica needs less supervision and is more convenient, especially in younger children.

HIP SPICA Flex the child's knee about 15°. This will enable you rotate his leg internally and abduct it. Then apply a spica to just above his ankle. Keep it on for not more than 6 weeks. Then keep him on crutches until there are X-ray signs that his epiphyses have fused, or there is no further slipping. His epiphyses may unite earlier, but he may need to be on crutches for a long time. If there are any signs of further slipping, do your best to refer him for internal fixation.

TRACTION Apply extension traction for 8 to 12 weeks, as in Fig. 78-3, but with his leg in abduction.

If neither form of treatment is practical, at least avoid further slipping by preventing him from bearing weight on his leg. Give him crutches.

IF A PATIENT BETWEEN 10 AND 15 LIMPS, OR HAS PAIN IN HIS HIP OR KNEE, THINK OF A SLIPPED EPIPHYSIS

77.11 Intertrochanteric fractures of the femur

In these common fractures the patient's femur breaks between its two trochanters. The lesser one sometimes separates as a third fragment, or there may be multiple fragments. Angulation reduces the normal 145° varus angulation of the neck of his femur on its shaft to 90°, and shortens his leg. Sometimes, there is little displacement when you look at the fracture from the front, and yet there may be considerable displacement in a lateral view.

Although the patient is commonly an old person who trips and falls, a more severe injury can cause this fracture in a young person. Typically, an old lady cannot walk after a fall. She lies in bed unable to lift her leg, with her foot turned outwards, and her leg as much as 3 cm short. The outer side of her thigh is painful, and moving her hip gives her great pain. After a few days, blood from the fracture site spreads to cause a bruise at the back of her thigh.

Although internal fixation greatly shortens the time in bed and reduces morbidity, these fractures usually unite with non—operative treatment. You can treat them with Perkins traction, or less successfully, with extension traction. The advantage of Perkins traction is that, unlike extension traction, it allows the patient to sit up and exercise, and so reduces the incidence of pneumonia and bedsores. Even so, it is more than some very old patients can bear, so that an occasional one stops eating and dies.

Surgeons vary as to how long they keep a patient in bed. The critical milestone is the patient's ability to lift his leg off the bed. This may occur as early as 6 weeks, or not for 12 weeks. Most patients are partly weight bearing with two sticks or a walking frame by 12 weeks. If a patient bears weight on the fractured femur too soon, it may angulate or refracture.

Refracture and non—union will be much less likely if you displace the lower fragment medially under the head of the patient's femur. This sometimes happens spontaneously at the time of the injury, but if it does not, you can produce it.

MEDIAL DISPLACEMENT OF THE SHAFT OF THE FEMUR

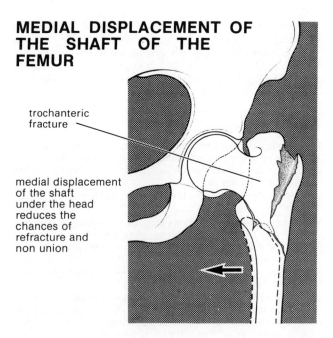

trochanteric fracture

medial displacement of the shaft under the head reduces the chances of refracture and non union

Fig. 77-10 MEDIAL DISPLACEMENT OF THE SHAFT OF THE FEMUR after a intertrochanteric fracture. If the shaft is displaced medially, it is better able to support the neck and head. *Kindly contributed by John Stewart.*

INTERTROCHANTERIC FRACTURES OF THE FEMUR

If displacement is minimal, and the patient elderly, keep him in bed for 3 weeks, then get him up with partial weight bearing for another 2 weeks.

If the fracture is more than minimally displaced and is not comminuted, apply Perkins traction in abduction.

If the fracture is more than minimally displaced and is comminuted, as in Types 2c and 2d in Fig. 78-5, displace the shaft of the femur medially under the head, as in Fig. 77-10, and then apply Perkins traction.

DISPLACING THE SHAFT OF THE FEMUR UNDER THE HEAD If the shaft of his femur is not already displaced medially under the neck, anaesthetize the patient, lie him on his normal side, and ask an assistant to abduct his leg a little and exert some traction. Put both your hands on his thigh just below the fracture site. With one good push using your full weight, move the lower fragment medially. You cannot push it too far or too hard.

PERKINS TRACTION Put a Denham nail, or, less satisfactorily, a Steinmann pin through the patient's tibia 3 cm below his tibial tubercle, as described in Sections 70.11 and 78.4. If you don't have a Steinmann pin, and so cannot put him into Perkins traction, put him into extension traction.

Apply traction equal to one seventh of the patient's body weight (10 kg for a 70 kg patient), and raise the foot of his bed 40 cm. Make sure the pin is horizontal when his patella faces the ceiling.

Make sure he does breathing exercises and quadriceps exercises. If the pin holes become sore, remove the pin, and either put it in again 3 cm further down his tibia, or apply skin traction instead. Pin track infection is such a common problem in old people that some surgeons always incorporate the pin in a short leg cast (81.3). Skin traction is not a good first choice, because the skin of old people tolerates it badly (70.10).

Keep the patient in bed for 6 to 12 weeks with daily exercises until he can lift his leg off the bed with his knee straight. His fracture will now have united, but will not have consolidated. X-ray him and if this confirms union, remove the traction.

If X-rays show that the distal fragment is still medially displaced, partial weight bearing in crutches can start immediately.

If medial displacement has not occurred or been maintained, or if the fragments have displaced into a varus position, he must bear very little weight indeed. So ask him to walk in crutches using only the heel and toe of his injured leg.

After 5 to 6 months of partial weight bearing his fracture will have consolidated. This is difficult to evaluate clinically, so evaluate it from the X-ray.

Alternatively, you can apply Russell traction; this is not described here.

CHILDREN WITH INTERTROCHANTERIC FRACTURES

A HIP SPICA is suitable for a young child. With his hip in wide abduction, apply a plaster hip spica for 8 to 10 weeks.

GALLOWS TRACTION is described in Section 78.2 and is suitable for children up to about 3 years, or at the most 5 years if the child is thin.

77.12 Subtrochanteric fractures

Fractures of the shaft of the femur just below the trochanters can occur at any age if the force is severe enough. Provided the fragments remain more or less aligned, you can treat the patient in Perkins traction. If however his iliopasoas muscle flexes the proximal fragment, and his gluteal muscles abduct it, so that it no longer lies in line with the shaft, you will have to use some other method which will flex the shaft of his femur, and bring it into line with the proximal fragment. In young children gallows traction does this very well. Put an older patient into '90–90 traction' with his knee flexed to 90°. A merit of his method is that it also corrects rotation.

This is a part of the femur in which non–union is particularly likely to occur. It is even more likely to occur if you use extension traction, or traction in a Böhler–Braun frame.

'90–90 TRACTION'

INDICATIONS Fractures of the subtrochanteric part of the femur in which the upper fragment is flexed.

METHOD Insert a Steinmann pin through the supracondylar region of the patient's femur or the upper end of his tibia (70.11, 78.3). Both have their disadvantages. A femoral pin is better placed mechanically, but tends to tear the soft tissues. A tibial pin loosens up his knee joint. Arrange traction so that his knee and hip are flexed to 90°. If convenient, support his lower leg in a light cast, and support this in a sling.

X-ray him, and if this shows that union is progressing, take the '90–90 traction' down after 4 to 5 weeks, and put him into Perkins traction.

Alternatively, you can apply Russell traction.

77.13 Girdlestone's operation for an ununited neck of the femur

If an arthrodesis or a prosthesis is impractical, Girdlestone's procedure can be done, either as the definitive operation, or as a temporary one before a prosthesis is fitted. There are two ways of doing it: (1) The method to be used following infection is described in Section 7.19. (2) The method following an ununited fracture of the neck of the femur is described here. This is not an easy operation, and is for more experienced operators only. Refer the patient if you can.

GIRDLESTONE'S OPERATION

INDICATIONS A patient who is walking painfully as the result of : (1) An ununited fracture of the neck of his femur. (2) Osteoarthritis with a femoral neck which is too osteoporotic to allow a prosthesis to be fitted. (3) Avascular necrosis following the insertion of a pin or plate in sickle cell disease.

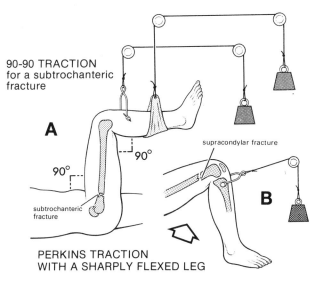

TRACTION WHEN THE PROXIMAL OR DISTAL FRAGMENT IS FLEXED

90-90 TRACTION for a subtrochanteric fracture

A

90°

90°

subtrochanteric fracture

supracondylar fracture

B

PERKINS TRACTION WITH A SHARPLY FLEXED LEG

Fig. 77-11 IF A FRAGMENT AT EITHER END OF THE FEMUR IS MORE THAN MILDLY FLEXED, ordinary Perkins traction is not satisfactory, and special methods have to be used. A, if the proximal fragment of a subtrochanteric fracture is sharply flexed, you can align it with the shaft using '90–90 traction'. B, if the distal fragment of a supracondylar fracture is moderately flexed you can align it with the shaft using Perkins traction with the knee flexed. This is only satisfactory with moderate flexion; with severe flexion internal fixation is necessary—see Section 79.13. *Kindly contributed by John Stewart.*

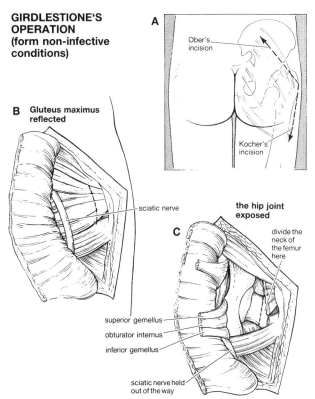

GIRDLESTIONE'S OPERATION (form non-infective conditions)

A

Ober's incision

Kocher's incision

B Gluteus maximus reflected

sciatic nerve

the hip joint exposed

C

divide the neck of the femur here

superior gemellus

obturator internus

inferior gemellus

sciatic nerve held out of the way

Fig. 77-12 GIRDLESTONE'S OPERATION FOR NON–INFECTIVE CONDITIONS. A, Ober's and Kocher's incisions. B, the patient's gluteal muscles have been reflected and the next incision marked. C, pyriformis, obturator internus, and the gemelli have been reflected and his sciatic nerve has been pulled out of the way. *Kindly contributed by Peter Bewes.*

METHOD If you cannot refer the patient, start exactly as for Ober's incision (7.18), but extend the incision upwards almost to the iliac crest and downwards in a vertical incision through skin and fascia lata down to the bone on the outer surface of the patient's femur. This is Kocher's incision.

Use a periosteal elevator to detach the gluteal muscles from the femur so as to reflect an inferomedial flap of gluteal muscles and expose the patient's obturator internus, his two gemelli, and the upper fibres of quadratus. Divide these about 1 cm from their insertion into his femur, and swing them medially where they will protect his sciatic nerve.

Approach his hip joint from behind. Open it and check that it really is the hip joint by asking an assistant to move the patient's leg and seeing the head of his femur move too.

Dislocate the head of the patient's femur from his acetabulum, by asking your assistant to adduct his leg and forcibly rotate it internally, while you divide the remaining fibres of the capsule and the ligamentum teres. If necessary, use a sharpened spoon to divide these.

Cut the neck of his femur flush with the shaft using an osteotome or Gigli saw. Remove the head. If the neck is already fractured, trim it back with a rasp.

Wash out the the joint thoroughly to remove chips of bone. Control bleeding. Close the wound without drainage, and apply skin traction as above.

If you have difficulty removing the head of his femur, try to get a Gigli saw under the neck of his femur. If you don't have the special retractors, use a pair of curved haemostats to help you do this. If this is difficult, use an osteotome to remove the head and neck of his femur piece by piece. The lower border of its neck will be the hardest piece to cut through.

78 Fractures of the shaft of the femur

78.1 How serious are shortening and distraction?

When the femur is fractured, the fragments sometimes overlap, so that the patient's leg is short. How serious is this and how much trouble should you take to prevent it? Traction can usually correct shortening, but it may not be convenient or desirable to do so, because *moderate shortening (up to 4 cm in an adult) is harmless.* So treat the patient, not his X-ray, and don't worry too much about the position of the fragments of his femur. Moderate overlap is acceptable and may even be beneficial. A patient's legs can vary in length by up to 1.5 cm, even before they are broken, and he can compensate for up to 4 cm by tilting his pelvis. If he does complain of shortening, you can easily raise the heel of his shoe. Always do this if his leg is more than 4 cm short, because backache can complicate a short leg, and this will lessen the risk of it.

Up to 1.5 cm of shortening can even be an advantage in a child, because a fracture is often followed by this degree of bony overgrowth at the epiphyseal lines. This is useful because it will allow you to treat a child's fractured femur in a hip spica without causing permanent shortening.

Distraction is much more serious than shortening, and although a fractured femur may unite even if the ends of the fragments do not touch, it will unite more quickly if they do. Sometimes, even 2 mm of distraction between the bone ends will prevent union, so make sure that nobody adds extra weights to the traction apparatus by mistake!

A CENTIMETRE OF OVERLAP IS IDEAL IN A FRACTURED FEMUR

78.2 Fractures of the shaft of the femur in younger children—gallows traction.

At birth fractures of the femur are common injuries, and heal themselves. Massive callus forms quickly, and a year later all signs of the fracture will have gone. Bandage the baby's thigh to his abdomen as in the foetal position for 10 days. Don't apply traction.

Under 3 years you have two alternatives—gallows traction or a plaster spica. Gallows traction: (1) does not need plaster and (2) makes nursing easier. But (3) it may cause ischaemia and later Volkmann's contracture in the injured leg *or the normal one,* especially in larger children (70.4). It can also cause gangrene. Don't send a child home in a gallows traction, because many families find nursing a child in them difficult, and a child's mother is less likely than the ward staff to diagnose ischaemia early. A plaster spica avoids this risk, and makes home treatment more practical, but even with a spica, nursing is not easy, and the spica soon becomes soiled. You can combine these methods, and it may be convenient for treatment to start in gallows and end in a spica.

LAXMAN (3 years) fractured the shaft of his femur. He was put in gallows traction and the longitudinal strips of strapping were held in place with several circular turns. In the interests of tidiness, a sheet was put over his legs. He cried loudly during the night. Next morning BOTH his feet were cold and had later to be amputated. LESSONS: (1) Never put circular strapping around any leg in traction. If you want to hold longitudinal strips in place, apply figure of eight strapping as in Fig. 78-1. (2) Don't cover the legs of a child in gallows traction.

FRACTURED FEMURS IN CHILDREN UNDER 3

GALLOWS TRACTION

INDICATIONS (1) Fractures of the shaft of the femur from soon after birth until the child weighs 15 kg at 1 to 3 years. Don't use gallows traction in larger children. (2) Prolapse of the rectum.

EQUIPMENT (1) Use a beam above a cot or bed. Or, put a bar across the sides of a cot. If necessary, you can hang several children from the same beam. (2) Ask a carpenter to make several gallows in a range of sizes. The base and the gallows should be the same length.

SETTING UP GALLOWS TRACTION Apply traction to both the child's legs. Pad his malleoli and the head of his fibulae. Paint his legs with compound tincture of benzoin (optional). Wait until this is tacky, and then apply adhesive strapping directly to his skin, and not over encircling bandages. Keep the knots away from his malleoli. Wind a crepe bandage around the strapping. Suspend his legs so that his pelvis is just clear of the bed, and you can slip your hand under his buttocks. The weight of his pelvis will reduce the fracture, and hold the fragments in position.

If you do not have any crepe bandage, and have to use adhesive strapping, apply it as two figure of eight spirals, one clockwise, and the other anticlockwise, as on the right leg of the child in Fig. 78-1.

If his fracture is subtrochanteric, avoid an adduction deformity by keeping his legs well apart.

CAUTION ! (1) Don't apply circular strapping around his leg, for it will be likely to impair its circulation. (2) Watch to make sure the strapping does not slip. (3) Check the circulation in his toes *on both sides,* especially during the first 3 days. Feel his dorsalis pedis pulses. (4) Don't cover his legs with a sheet, because this will make his circulation less easy to monitor. (5) Don't apply traction to one leg only—it makes him much too mobile.

Crying is the first sign of ischaemia, so if he cries, examine him carefully. Pain on stretching his calf muscles is another early sign. Test the movement of his toes, and check sensation over his foot. If you fail to relieve his circulation early enough, Volkmann's contracture and perhaps gangrene may follow (70.4). Watch for pressure sores, especially on his heels, and over his Achilles tendon.

Keep him in traction for 3 weeks. By the second week the strapping will be showing signs of strain, and by 3 weeks it will be wearing out, he will want to be set free, and he can go home. Gentle weight bearing can start at 6 weeks.

Alternatively, when the first few days are over, you can, if necessary, send a child home in a spica (77.3).

A GALLOWS TRACTION FRAME

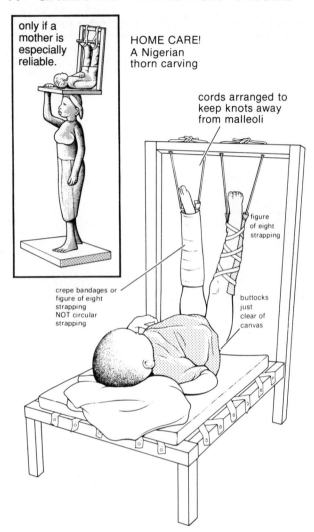

only if a mother is especially reliable.

HOME CARE!
A Nigerian thorn carving

cords arranged to keep knots away from malleoli

figure of eight strapping

crepe bandages or figure of eight strapping NOT circular strapping

buttocks just clear of canvas

Fig. 78-1 GALLOWS TRACTION IN A FRAME. A, a traction frame is not suitable for home treatment, unless the child's mother is unusually reliable. B, if you don't have a crepe bandage, use two turns of 2 cm strapping in a figure of eight. NEVER put circular strapping around a leg. *Kindly contributed by Andrew Pearson, John Stewart, and Richard Batten*

A PLASTER SPICA FOR A FRACTURED FEMUR

Apply a plaster spica for 6 to 10 weeks, depending on the child's age (77.3). Take care to make this strong enough. Apply extra plaster at the hip.

CATASTROPHES WITH GALLOWS TRACTION

If THE CHILD'S FOOT GOES COLD AND BLUE, it is a sign of ischaemia. This can be the result of: (1) too tight a bandage, (2) suspending too much of him—only his pelvis should be suspended, or, (3) using gallows traction when he is too old. A conscious child will begin screaming as soon as ischaemia starts. But if he is unconscious from a head injury, for example, he cannot scream, so that a head injury with a fractured femur is particularly dangerous—he should not be on gallows traction!

Ischaemia is particularly likely to occur if gallows are used to treat children weighing more than 15 kg, because more traction is needed with heavier children. So treat these children in extension traction as in the next method.

MONITOR THE CIRCULATION IN HIS TOES CONSTANTLY

GALLOWS TRACTION FROM A BEAM

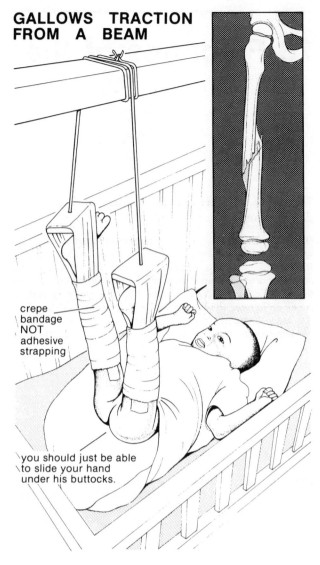

crepe bandage NOT adhesive strapping

you should just be able to slide your hand under his buttocks.

Fig. 78-2 GALLOWS TRACTION FROM A BEAM. If necessary, you can suspend several children from the same beam—watch the circulation in their toes! Ischaemia is particularly likely to occur if you use gallows to treat children weighing more than 15 kg, because more traction is needed with heavier children. So treat these children in extension traction as in the next method.

78.3 Fractures of the shaft of the femur in older children—extension traction

A child over 3 years is too heavy for gallows traction so he has to be treated by applying traction to his extended lower leg. The traction cord passes over a pulley at the foot of his bed which is raised to apply counter–traction. Use extension traction for patients from the age of 3 until the age of 18 when the proximal tibial epiphysis fuses with the shaft. If you use a pin in a patient who is under 18, you may damage his epiphysis. Extension traction keeps a patient's leg extended so that he cannot exercise it. This is less important in children and teenagers because their immobilized joints are much less apt to stiffen. The great value of Perkins traction in preventing knee stiffness in older patients is thus unnecessary in younger ones.

A fracture of the femur in an older child is usually spiral. Extension traction corrects angulation, rotation, and lateral shift. It also usually corrects overlap too, but if some persists, this is not important, because subsequent growth soon corrects shortening. The danger of extension traction is that it does occasionally cause Volkmann's ischaemic contracture. An alternative is a hip spica. Don't use a Thomas splint or a Böhler–Braun frame.

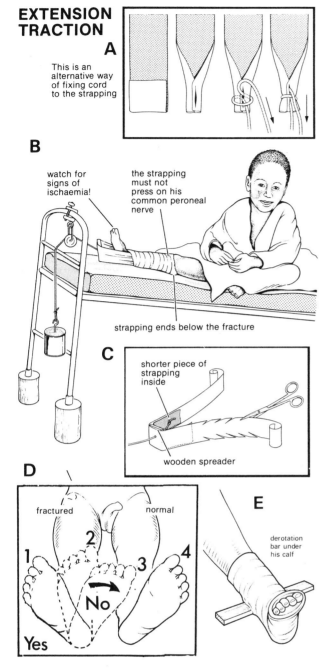

EXTENSION TRACTION

A

This is an alternative way of fixing cord to the strapping

B

watch for signs of ischaemia!

the strapping must not press on his common peroneal nerve

strapping ends below the fracture

C

shorter piece of strapping inside

wooden spreader

D

fractured   normal

1   2   3   4

No

Yes

E

derotation bar under his calf

Fig. 78-3 EXTENSION TRACTION. A, one method of fixing the cord to the strapping. B, skin extension traction in action. C, fixing a spreader to the strapping. D, try to make the patient's injured leg (1) match his normal one (4). If you put it in position 2 it will rotate internally into position 3 when he walks (as shown by the arrow) and will cause severe disability. His anterior superior iliac spine, his patella, and the space between his first and second toes normally lie in a straight line. E, a derotation bar in use. Note that it lies under the patient's ankle, not his heel. Don't fit a derotation bar to a damp cast, or it may cause a pressure sore. *Kindly contributed by Richard Batten, Andrew Pearson, and John Stewart.*

Controlling rotation in fractures of the femur. One of the beauties of Perkins traction is that the patient's bent knee controls the rotation of the fragments of his femur when he sits up and exercises it. But with extension traction you need to watch rotation of the fragments carefully.

At rest, the external rotators of the leg at the hip are stronger than the internal rotators, *so they externally rotate the upper fragment* This means that you have to rotate the lower fragment externally to match it. The important thing *not* to do, therefore,

is to rotate the lower fragment *internally* in the position of rest. If you do this, for example by making a patient's patella point to the ceiling (foot 2 in Fig. 78-3), he will end up with a considerable degree (20 or 30°) of internal rotation (as shown by the arrow in this figure) and will walk pigeon toed on the injured side (as in foot 3). This will be a considerable disability, and he may need a corrective osteotomy. The position of rest of a normal leg in bed is 30 to 45° of external rotation (foot 4), so if you make his injured foot (foot 1) match his normal one, the degree of rotation will probably be about right. Increased external rotation is little disability, so this is the side to err on. If you want to check the degree of rotation of the upper fragment, take a film to show both a patient's lesser trochanters and to compare their position.

EXTENSION TRACTION

EXTENSION SKIN TRACTION

INDICATIONS (1) Fractures of the shaft of the femur between the ages of 3 and 18. (2) Intertrochanteric fractures in adults when you have no Steinmann pin. (3) Separation of the upper femoral epiphysis. (4) An unstable hip after the reduction of a dislocation.

METHOD Apply compound tincture of benzoin (optional) to the child's skin and then apply a long length of broad adhesive strapping from just distal to the fracture down to his lower leg. Pass it around a block of wood to act as a spreader, and then up the outer side of his leg as far as the fracture but not beyond it. Prevent the longer length of strapping sticking to his ankle by sticking a shorter piece to it. Pass this around the other surface of the spreader.

If necessary, make small cuts in the strapping to make it fit more closely to his leg. Pass a cord through the hole in the spreader and fix it to the foot of his bed. Raise the foot of his bed 40 to 50 cm, or use a weight as in Fig. 78-3.

Start with traction equal to one seventh of his body weight, and compare the lengths of his legs with a tape measure (Fig. 77-3) to make sure you have not distracted the fragments.

Encourage him to move about in bed.

Wait 6 weeks for clinical union (Fig. 69-4) and then take a check X-ray. If union is satisfactory, get him up on crutches.

CAUTION ! (1) Watch carefully for signs of ischaemia, especially calf pain and pain on dorsiflexing his foot. (2) Make sure the strapping does not press on his common peroneal nerve as it winds around the head of his fibula.

EXTENSION PIN TRACTION

INDICATIONS An adult who cannot sit up and exercise his knee, for example if he has a dislocated hip, or has some internal injury. This form of traction is contraindicated in anyone young enough for his upper tibial epiphysis not to have united, because a pin might damage it.

Insert the pin as for Perkin's traction (78.4), but don't sit the patient up, and don't remove the lower part of the mattress.

CONTROLLING ROTATION (both forms of extension traction)

Make sure that the rotation of the patient's injured leg matches his normal one. If necessary, fit a derotation bar: (1) Fit it to his ankle, not to his heel, where it may cause pressure sores. (2) Wait for the cast to harden before you fit it, or this too may cause a pressure sore.

DIFFICULTIES WITH EXTENSION TRACTION

If there is OUTWARD BOWING of the patient's femur to begin with, put both his legs in traction, and keep them wide apart.

If there is OUTWARD BOWING LATER, correct it with a spica. If necessary, bend his leg straight under anaesthesia, then apply the spica. You may be able to do this as late as 6 weeks.

PERKINS TRACTION

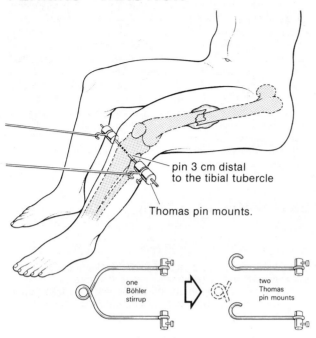

pin 3 cm distal
to the tibial tubercle

Thomas pin mounts.

one
Böhler
stirrup

two
Thomas
pin mounts

Fig. 78-4 PERKINS TRACTION. Thomas pin mounts are better than a Böhler stirrup. If necessary, you can cut a Böhler stirrup and make two pin mounts from it.

78.4 Perkins traction

Your aim in treating an adult's fractured femur should be to make his bone unite in a good position without his knee becoming stiff. Perkins traction does this admirably using the principles discussed in Section 69.3. Put a pin through the upper end of his tibia, and apply enough traction to it to keep the fragments in place, to pull his leg to its normal length, and to correct any angulation or rotation. Meanwhile, *sit him up in bed, and see that he exercises his knee as actively as possible, and as soon as he can* so that: (1) controlled movement and compression of the bone ends encourages union, (2) his knee does not become stiff, (3) the tone of his quadriceps muscle is maintained, and (4) the exercises he does keep him fit and free from thrombosis and hypostatic pneumonia.

Perkins traction differs from extension traction in that in the latter a patient's leg is held straight and he does not sit up and exercise it. Except for the few special indications for extension traction in Section 73.3, Perkins traction is much the most useful method.

Perkins traction uses the same simple equipment for all sizes of patient, it prevents knee stiffness more effectively than other methods, and it gives a patient a wide range of knee movement, which is important in societies where people squat. Excessive shortening is rare, and as soon as the end of the patient's bed has been dropped, and he is flexing his knee, malrotation of the lower fragment is impossible. Physiotherapy and nursing care are easy, and after a few days he can lift himself on to a bedpan. Most patients spend 6 to 8 weeks in traction, followed by 2 weeks, exercising their legs over the end of the bed, and then 2 more on partial weight bearing. They are out of hospital in 8 to 10 weeks with at least 90° of knee movement, and without noticing that their injured legs are a centimetre or two short. Finally, if a patient's tibia has also been fractured, you can treat this at the same time that his femur is in traction.

There are several less satisfactory alternatives to Perkins traction. They are:

(1) Some form of internal rod or plate fixation which requires a wide range of nails or plates as well as reamers, guide wires,

and extractors, all of which are seldom available in district hospitals. Many tragedies have followed attempts to fix these fractures in hospitals with limited equipment and expertise (69.3). Although modern methods of closed rodding, when done under ideal circumstances, enable a patient to be walking in 10 days, if you attempt them with inadequate equipment in a theatre of questionable sterility, there will be too many complications. This is a method for experts working under ideal conditions.

(2) Böhler–Braun traction (Fig. 79-10) takes longer to achieve union, and because it does not allow active knee exercises, a patient's quadriceps atrophies, and his knee usually stiffens, unless it is carefully exercised daily. Böhler–Braun traction is so much less satisfactory, that it should now be used only for the few special indications in Section 79.13. *One of the most important changes that is needed in the orthopaedic practice of many hospitals is to change from traction in a Böhler–Braun frame to Perkins traction for fractured femurs.*

(3) Thomas splints are excellent for first aid, and for treatment during the first few days, but not for definitive treatment. They too will stiffen a patient's knee, and may cause pressure sores in his groin. They also make nursing more difficult.

(4) A hip spica enables a patient to be discharged in a few days, but it causes prolonged disability and seriously stiffens an adult's knee. It may also cause excessive shortening. A hip spica is much more satisfactory in a child, whose knee does not stiffen, and whose femur will grow and compensate for shortening.

It is sometimes said that Perkins traction lengthens a patient's stay in hospital, and increases the pressure on scarce beds. Admittedly, internal fixation gets most patients up quicker, but some of them develop such serious complications of non–union and infection that they may remain in hospital 2 years or more, so greatly extending the average stay of patients treated by this method.

Although cast bracing is an excellent method, we have not described it here. It allows you to discharge a patient 3 weeks earlier, but under your circumstances it is probably not worth the extra trouble.

DON'T TRY INTERNAL FIXATION FOR FRACTURED FEMURS

WHEN IS PERKINS TRACTION INDICATED?

INDICATIONS As you will see in Fig. 78-5, Perkins traction can be used for some fractures of the pelvis, and for most fractures of the femur. The line AB in Fig. 78-5 is approximately that of the attachment of the capsule. Fractures proximal to it on the avascular neck of the femur are not suited to Perkins traction (with the rare exception of incomplete fractures of the neck), whereas most fractures on line AB or distal to it are suitable.

Vertical fractures of the pelvis with upward displacement of one fragment (76.2). (1) Undisplaced incomplete fractures of the neck of the femur (77.7). (2) All intertrochanteric fractures (77.11). (3) Those subtrochanteric fractures in which the contraction of the iliopsoas has not flexed the upper fragment so much as to bring it seriously out of line with the shaft (77.12). (4) All fractures of the shaft of the femur in patients over 18, including overlapped, double, spiral, comminuted and open fractures, and fractures with severe soft tissue injury. Perkins traction is particularly well suited to comminuted fractures. (5) Those supracondylar fractures in which the lower fragment has not been too severely flexed by the contraction of gastrocnemius (79.13). (6) All condylar fractures of the femur, except those in which a condyle has rotated completely (79.15).

CONTRAINDICATIONS TO PERKINS TRACTION (7) All complete fractures of the neck of the femur (77.7). (8) Displace-

PERKINS TRACTION

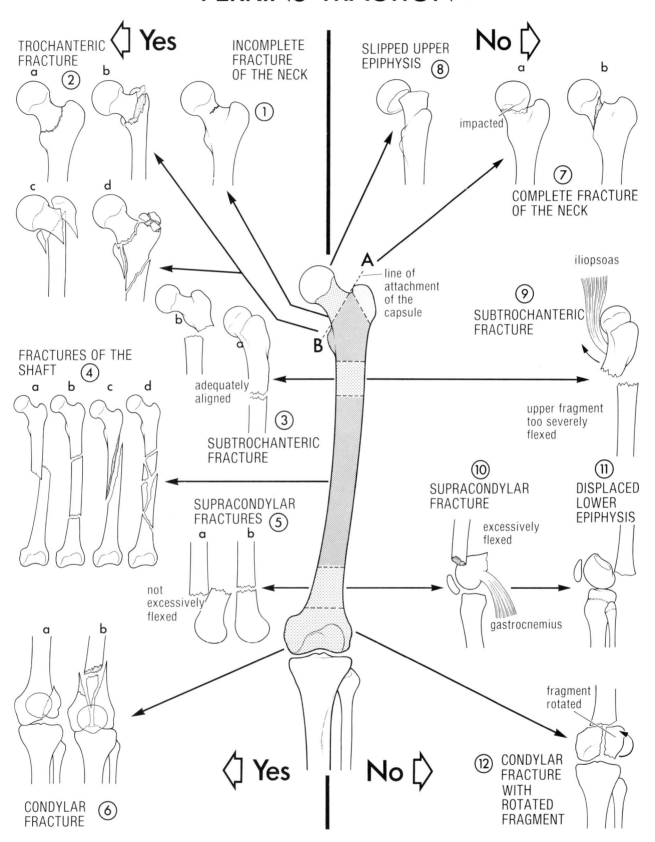

Fig.78-5 THE INDICATIONS AND CONTRAINDICATIONS FOR PERKINS TRACTION. The indications are on the left and the contraindications are on the right. *Kindly contributed by Peter Bewes and John Stewart.*

ment of the proximal femoral epiphys1s (77.10). (9) Subtrochanteric fractures with severe flexion of the proximal fragment (77.12). (10) Supracondylar fractures with marked flexion of the distal fragment (79.13). (11) Displacement of the distal femoral epiphysis (79.16). (12) Fractures of the condyles in which a fragment has rotated completely (79.15).

Other contraindications include: (a) All patients under 18. Their epiphyses will not have united and the pin may damage the epiphyseal plate. (b) Arthritis of the knee, or a stiff knee from any cause, which will make exercise impossible without moving the fragments too much. (c) Non−union in fractures treated by other methods.

ADAPT AN ORDINARY BED

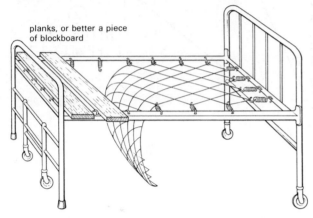

planks, or better a piece of blockboard

Fig. 78-6 CONVERT AN ORDINARY BED FOR PERKINS TRACTION. You may find it convenient to convert several beds like this. *Kindly contributed by Peter Bewes.*

Perkins traction only gives good results if you persist with it, and follow the details carefully. *The secret of success is to start periods of 10 to 30 minutes of active exercise several times a day from the third day onwards.* This early movement is critical. It is the callus formed during the first 10 days that determines the outcome. Most supposed failures are due to not starting exercise early enough, or not doing it vigorously enough. Patients need to be coaxed into exercising their knees. Let them do their exercises together, so that they can encourage one another. Quadriceps exercises by themselves are not enough to achieve satisfactory union.

There are many important points of nursing, so teach your staff about them, and make sure they understand the principles of Perkins traction. Setting up and managing Perkins traction is not difficult and medical assistants soon learn to manage it most competently.

EXERCISES IN THE FIRST 10 DAYS ARE CRITICAL

78.5 Applying Perkins traction

After a severe accident the patient is shocked and cannot walk. He has a painful, deformed, and very swollen thigh, and sometimes also a dislocated hip (77.4). So palpate his buttocks and trochanters and look at the position of his hip on the X-ray. Suspect that his hip might be dislocated if the proximal fragment of his femur is strongly adducted.

PERKINS TRACTION FOR FRACTURES OF THE SHAFT OF THE FEMUR

INDICATIONS AND CONTRAINDICATIONS See Section 78.4, and Fig. 78-5.

SHOCK If the patient is severely shocked, he may need 2 to 4 units of blood or intravenous fluid, particularly if his fracture is comminuted. Careful splinting (51.2) on the way to hospital will minimize blood loss.

PERIPHERAL PULSES Have you checked these?

INITIAL X-RAY Take an AP and a lateral view and X-ray his hip.

EQUIPMENT FOR PERKINS TRACTION (1) An ordinary hospital bed from which the lower springs have been removed or tied back. You may have some broken beds you can use, and you may find it convenient to convert several beds for Perkins traction permanently. Ideally, these beds should have large casters so that you can wheel a patient to the X-ray department in traction. (2) You can use a mattress in two parts, or let the lower half of an ordinary mattress hang down. (3) Fracture boards to go across the lower half of his bed. (4) Blocks to raise the foot of the bed 25 to 50 cm. (5) A sharp, thick (4 mm) Steinmann or Denham pin. Sharpen it on a grindstone regularly. (6) Thomas pin mounts or a Böhler stirrup. If you use an unmodified Böhler stirrup, it will rub on the patient's skin, or the rope will get in the way of his skin, so convert it into two Thomas pin mounts by cutting and bending it, as in Fig. 78-4. (7) Picture cord, or orthopaedic traction cord. (8) Weights of 2 and 5 kg. These can be bags of sand, or bricks. (9) A set of pulleys to fix to the foot of the bed. These are not essential, and the cords can, if necessary, pass directly over the rail at the end of the bed, preferably over a cylinder of old X-ray film rolled round the rail. If the lower rail is too low, consider reversing the bed, and using the rail at its head.

INSERTING THE PIN Do this in the theatre, or in a treatment room off the ward, using local anaesthesia, as in Section 70.11.

SETTING UP PERKINS TRACTION Apply weights to each end of the pin. Apply traction equal to one seventh of the patient's weight. A man needs 10 to 14 kg (5 to 7 kg on each end of the nail) and a small woman only perhaps 7 kg. Raise the foot of the bed 4 cm for each kilo. You will find 25 cm blocks useful. If possible, pass the cords over pulleys, and make sure they clear his toes.

CAUTION ! The cords must pull equally on each end of the pin, see Fig. 70-14.

Put a folded towel or small pillow under the fracture to give his femur the correct degree of anterior bow.

ALIGN THE PIN AT 90° IN BOTH AXES

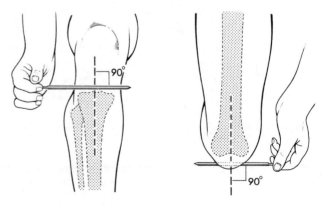

Fig. 78-7 ALIGN A STEINMANN PIN so that it is at 90° to the shaft in both planes. *Kindly contributed by Peter Bewes.*

X-RAYS FOR PERKINS TRACTION The need for X-rays to adjust traction varies with the site of the fracture. Take them while the patient is in traction.

In a fracture of the proximal third of the femur, take a lateral X-ray while he is in traction. Face the X-ray tube into his inner thigh, with the cassette above the crest of his ilium. If the proximal fragment is sharply flexed, '90–90 traction' (77.12) will be more appropriate than Perkins traction.

In fractures of the distal third, including supracondylar fractures, take an X-ray to make sure the distal fragment is not excessively flexed. If it is goto Section 79.13.

If the fracture is elsewhere in his femur, a lateral X-ray is not essential, but a AP one is useful to see if you have corrected any excessive overlap, or if you have applied so much traction so that there is a gap between the bone ends.

If you cannot X-ray a patient, measure both his legs from his anterior superior iliac spines to his medial malleoli, to make sure they are the same length (77-3). If necessary, adjust the traction weights, and the elevation of the foot of his bed, so as to let the bony fragments overlap about 1 cm. *A little overlap is safer than a little distraction.* Up to 2 cm of overlap is acceptable. Check his leg length daily for 2 weeks, and adjust the traction as necessary. After 2 weeks the fragments will have started to stick together so that further adjustment will be more difficult, and need more weight. After a month it may be impossible.

If his fracture is comminuted, a little overlap is even more important.

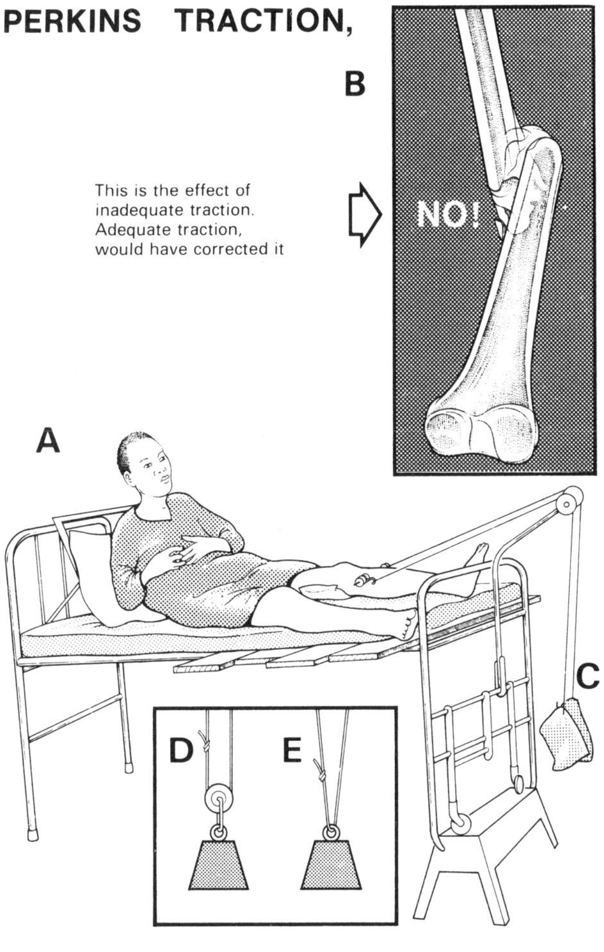

PERKINS   TRACTION,

B

This is the effect of inadequate traction. Adequate traction, would have corrected it

NO!

A

C

D   **E**

Fig. 78-8 PERKINS TRACTION during the first 2 days. A, on the third day the fracture boards should be removed and the patient must start exercising. B, shows the effect of incorrect traction. Insufficient weight was applied and the foot of the bed was not raised. C, D, and E, show various methods of arranging the weights. If you don't have a pulley, pass the cord through the ring of the weight to equalize the pull on each side. *Kindly contributed by Peter Bewes and John Stewart.*

CAUTION ! (1) Don't apply excessive traction, because bone ends far apart cannot unite. This is particularly important if there are multiple fragments. (2) Less traction is needed after the first 2 weeks, so reduce it as necessary.

EXERCISES FOR PERKINS TRACTION

Start these as soon as possible, preferably by the third day. Remove the fracture boards from the lower half of the patient's bed, push down his mattress, and let him flex his knee. Replace the boards when he has completed his exercises.

Encourage him to bend and straighten his knee. To begin with this will be painful. You can minimize his pain in two ways: (1) Give him a mild analgesic for the first few days. (2) Hold his heel and let him flex his knee against resistance, then let him extend his leg freely. He will need help, but at the end of a week he should be able to flex and extend his knee unassisted. Encourage him by telling him that his exercises will soon be painless.

To begin with let him exercise for 10 to 30 minutes at least three times a day. Encourage him to exercise his leg longer and more vigorously each day. He should soon be exercising it at least 2 hours a day.

CAUTION ! (1) Make sure the nurses understand that these regular periods of exercise are an important nursing routine. (2) Check his leg length daily for 2 weeks, and then weekly until union is complete. Reduce traction as necessary.

Measure his legs soon after traction has been set up, and adjust it accordingly. Rotation will correct itself as soon as he can flex his leg to 90°. Check the knots daily.

TESTING FEMUR FRACTURES FOR CLINICAL UNION Each week, examine the fracture site for palpable callus, and look for the signs of union. These are: (1) No tenderness over the fracture. (2) The bone cannot be angled at the fracture site. (3) Trying to angulate the fracture site does not hurt. (4) The patient can exercise and lift his flexed leg fully without support.

CAUTION ! (1) Don't test for union by asking him to lift his straightened leg from his hip, because it angulates the fracture site. (2) Resist the temptation to apply a cast in order to discharge him early.

In fractures of the upper third of the femur, you may have to X-ray him to confirm adequate union. Elsewhere, X-rays are not really necessary. Often, clinical union will seem well advanced, when there is only a mass of callus on the X-ray.

X-ray him at 4 weeks, 6 weeks and 12 weeks.

If there is no callus on the X-ray at 4 weeks, suspect that union is going to be delayed. Check his X-ray to make sure that: (1) there is no distraction (if so, reduce the weights), (2) there are no fragments of avascular bone (if so, he will need to be in traction much longer), and (3) there is no interposed soft tissue. Fortunately non–union is rare—*if he exercises as he should!*

ENCOURAGE   HIM TO   EXERCISE   HIS LEGS

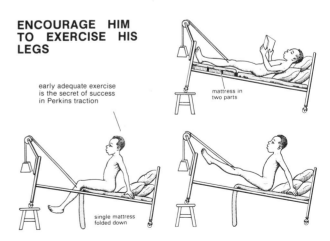

early adequate exercise is the secret of success in Perkins traction

mattress in two parts

single mattress folded down

Fig. 78-9 ENCOURAGE HIM TO EXERCISE HIS LEG. Early exercises are the secret of success with Perkins traction. *Kindly contributed by Peter Bewes.*

Removing traction too early is worse than leaving it on too long. Don't decide in advance, or fix a day to remove it. Instead, give him the joy of suddenly finding it gone.

When there are definite signs of clinical union, usually at 6 to 10 weeks, remove the weights and continue exercises with his knees over the side of his bed, and the pin still in his tibia. If you were right, and his femur has united, his range of movement will increase progressively. But, if he gets pain at the fracture site and his range of movement decreases, his femur is not yet adequately united, so put him back in traction. If pain or bowing of his femur occurs, keep him in traction longer, until his fracture is stable and his pain disappears.

If you are uncertain if union is satisfactory, continue traction, but with reduced weight.

If you are happy that union is far advanced, remove the pin. Keep him in bed for 2 more weeks while he exercises his legs over the side of his bed. When he can flex his leg to 90°, lie him on his abdomen and encourage him to flex it further.

WEIGHT BEARING AFTER PERKINS TRACTION After two weeks of exercises without traction, examine the patient again. If possible X-ray him with a portable X-ray, or take his bed to the X-ray department, because his leg may refracture on the way there if he walks there and it has not united. If you are happy that his femur has united, and his range of knee flexion is good, start protected weight bearing with crutches, as in Section 77.1, but at first *he must only put his leg to the ground to balance with.*

CAUTION ! Help him out of bed carefully. If union is weak his leg may refracture when he first starts to walk.

When he can walk safely on crutches send him home. Ask him to continue his exercises there. Most patients can be discharged with their fractures clinically united at 8 weeks. The period is shorter in younger patients and longer in older ones. Transverse and oblique fractures take longer than spiral ones.

When the time taken to achieve clinical union has doubled, he can discard his crutches and bear his full weight on his leg. For example, if clinical union took 8 weeks, he must keep his crutches for a further 8 weeks before discarding them. Usually, an X-ray is unnecessary at this stage and shows only massive callus.

Tell him to avoid violent exercise for a year. Teenagers are particularly likely to refracture their femurs.

DISTRACTION IS MORE SERIOUS THAN OVERLAP

78.6 Difficulties with a fractured femur

Don't be put off by this long list. Fractured femurs are common and most of these difficulties are rare. You will meet them less often with Perkins traction than with other methods. If you are careful you can avoid most of them.

DIFFICULTIES WITH A FRACTURED FEMUR

If a patient's femur FRACTURE IS OPEN, treat him as for any other open fracture (69.7). Do a wound toilet (54.1), and get the fragments into the best position you can. Unless a fragment is completely loose, leave it in place. Provided the periosteum remains, the bone will reform. Keep his leg out to approximately its normal length in traction. Don't close his wound for 3 to 5 days. Either close if by delayed primary closure, or by delayed skin grafting. Then start Perkins' exercises.

If his LEG IS PULSELESS AND COLD, the fragments of his femur have probably injured his femoral artery, so explore it and, if necessary, attempt to repair it (55.6). Alternatively, apply traction and hope that his circulation will return when his fracture is reduced. If it does not, you may have to amputate his leg later.

If the BONE ENDS ARE MORE THAN 1 cm APART, they may be separated end to end, or side to side.

If the fragments are separated end to end, **they may fail to unite.** If the patient is traction you are probably applying too much weight, so reduce it. Or, there may be soft tissue between the bone ends. If you cannot reduce end to end separation, try manipulation.

If the fragments are separated side by side, **this is less dangerous,** and at least 1 cm of such separation is acceptable. Early active movements may promote callus formation across a gap of 2 cm, but if there is more than 1 cm of side by side separation, manipulate the fragments under anaesthesia until you can feel them grating.

If the SITE IN THE TIBIA WHERE THE PIN IS NORMALLY INSERTED IS INJURED OR INFECTED, insert the pin at the lower end of the patient's tibia (70.11), or through the lower end of his femur, as in 90–90 traction' (77.12).

The movement of a pin in the bone promotes infection. If you can stop it moving, infection will be less likely. So use low friction swivels, and, if possible, a Denham pin which you can screw into the tibia, rather than a Steinmann pin. Another precaution is to make sure that traction is applied equally and at right angles to the pin. Make sure the cords join through a pulley or a ring attached to the weight.

Another way of preventing movement of the pin is to incorporate it in a below–knee cast. Watch carefully for pain, but only if the patient complains should you window the cast, and look at the skin round the pin. Once a pin has become loose, a cast is useless.

If a STEINMANN PIN BECOMES LOOSE AND ITS TRACK INFECTED, you may have inserted it in an unsterile manner, or allowed the drill to get too hot, so that it has killed the bone around it and formed a ring sequestrum. Infection is usually not serious—if you diagnose it early and don't neglect it. But

AN OPEN FRACTURE OF THE FEMUR

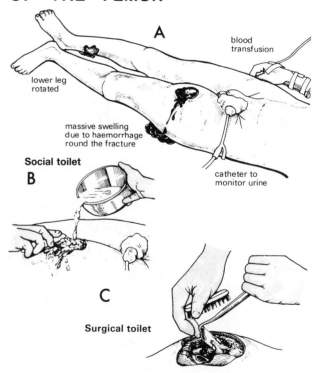

Fig. 78-10 TOILETING AN OPEN FRACTURE OF THE FEMUR. Treat an open fracture of the femur in the same way as any other open fracture. Do a wound toilet and get the fragments into the best position you can. Unless a fragment is completely loose, leave it in place. Provided the periosteum remains, the bone will reform. Keep the leg out to approximately its normal length in traction. *Kindly contributed by Peter Bewes.*

it can be a catastrophe, because osteomyelitis may result and infect the patient's knee. This is more common in old patients with soft bones, because the pin pulls through the bone. Prevent this by incorporating the pin in a short leg cast to prevent movement.

Prevent this disaster by inspecting the pin track daily, and removing the pin if there is pain or any sign of redness or loosening. Either put the pin in again lower down, through healthy skin, or apply skin traction, or traction on a Böhler–Braun frame with the pin through the lower end of the patient's tibia, or his calcaneus (70.11).

If the whole of the proximal end of his lower leg becomes inflamed, you cannot reintroduce the pin. Don't put it in higher up, because you will infect his knee joint.

If an infected pin track heals over but his bone remains tender, open up the track and curette it.

If a pin track infection lasts more than a month, x-ray his tibia and look for a ring sequestrum round the track of the pin. If you find one, remove it.

CAUTION ! Remove a pin immediately it becomes loose.

If a PIN TRACK INFECTION HAS ALREADY INFECTED THE PATIENT'S KNEE JOINT, immediately incise and drain his knee through incisions on either side of his patella. Irrigate the joint (7.16), give him antibiotics and splint his knee in a plaster cylinder until the infection is quiescent. Infection can easily follow a neglected pin track infection. You should be able to prevent it by the methods described above.

If, during the first 2 or 3 days after a patient has fractured his femur, he becomes DISORIENTATED, DROWSY or COMATOSE, or he has a cough, shortness of breath and haemoptysis, suspect that he is suffering from FAT EMBOLISM. This is the result of globules of fat escaping from the injured marrow of his femur and entering the capillaries of his lung and brain. Look for petechiae over his chest, in his mouth and in his conjunctivae. Fat in his urine is useful confirmatory evidence if you find it. About 15% of patients die, usually from respiratory failure, due to the accumulation of fluid in their lungs. Give him oxygen, restrict his fluids, and give him diuretics.

If you DON'T HAVE A STEINMANN PIN or a Denham pin, you can use skin traction (70.10), with a plaster backslab to maintain the forward bow of his femur, but this is far from ideal. It is difficult to apply enough traction through his skin, he cannot exercise his knee, and the fracture takes longer to unite. Less callus is formed, so it should be followed by a walking caliper. There is a greater risk of non–union with skin traction and more physiotherapy is needed.

If he has FRACTURED HIS FEMUR AND THE SHAFT OF HIS TIBIA in the same leg, anaesthetize him, put in the Denham pin, and then reduce his tibial fracture. Apply a below–knee cast to maintain reduction of his tibial fracture and incorporate the nail in the cast. Leave enough space behind his knee for it to flex, then treat him as a fractured femur. Two fractures will divide his leg into three pieces, so make sure they are all correctly aligned, as in D, Fig. 78-3. His femur will probably unite before his tibia, so discharge him in a patellar weight bearing short leg walking cast (81.5).

If his fractured tibia needs calcaneal traction to reduce it, apply this for a few days first, then insert a Steinmann pin and put him into Perkins traction.

If he is unruly and PULLS DOWN HIS TRACTION, consider applying a hip spica (77.3).

If, after 16 weeks in traction, a patient's FRACTURED FEMUR HAS NOT UNITED, or union is poor, this may be due to: (1) Distraction of the bone ends, caused by too much traction. (2) Interposed soft tissue. (3) Exercises that were inadequate or started too late, or quadriceps exercises that you hoped would be enough. Consider referring him.

If his FEMUR FRACTURES AGAIN AT THE SAME SITE, apply Perkins traction again, and it will re-unite rapidly. Don't try internal fixation. Refracture is rare and usually follows a fall, particularly in a patient who is allowed up too early, or in a youth who plays football too soon.

CAUTION ! Don't stop traction too early.

If a patient's KNEE IS VERY STIFF, and the fracture was at or above the lower third of his femur, and is solidly united, stiffness may be due to adhesions around his knee joint. Firm, *gentle* manipulation under anaesthesia may restore movement. If the fracture is in the lower third, especially in the immediate supracondylar region, you will probably be unable to free the adhesions by a single manipulation. Refer him for a possible quadriceps plasty.

If a patient's KNEE BECOMES PAINFUL some years after a fractured femur, one cause is angulation of his femur, which disturbs the normal mechanics of his knee. Prevent it by correcting angulation early on during treatment. Late correction requires an osteotomy.

If, a year after a fracture, a patient returns with SEVERE BOWING OF HIS FEMUR, this is the result of discharging him before his fracture has adequately consolidated. Prevent this by warning him when you discharge him that his femur may angulate, and ask him to return immediately if it does. Be especially careful if he lives many kilometres away and cannot easily return. Once a severely angulated fracture has united, the only treatment is an osteotomy.

BILATERAL FRACTURES OF THE FEMUR AND TIBIA

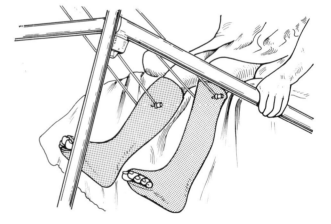

Fig. 78-11 FRACTURES OF THE FEMUR AND TIBIA on both sides can readily be treated by Perkins traction. Below–knee casts have been used which enable the patient to exercise his knee. *Kindly contributed by Peter Bewes.*

79 The knee

79.1 The general method for the knee

The mildest knee injury is a bruise accompanied by an effusion. More severe ones can tear its menisci, or its collateral or cruciate ligaments, or break its bones. As with the ankle, ligamentous injuries are often missed and cause prolonged disability. Occasionally, a patient's patella or his knee dislocates. An injury which would tear the ligaments of an adult can displace the epiphyses of a child, who can also displace his tibial spine, or his tibial tuberosity.

A severe injury makes the knee swell so much that you cannot tell where the fractures are until you have taken an x-ray. Fortunately, there are adequate closed methods for most knee fractures, and for most soft tissue injuries. Don't try to operate inside the knee.

This chapter describes soft tissue injuries and fractures of the patella and lower femur. The next one describes fractures of the upper tibia which involve the knee.

Most surgeons evolve their own examination routine for particular circumstances or parts of the body. As an example, here is one such routine for the knee, followed by the special methods for particular structures.

GENERAL METHOD FOR AN INJURED KNEE

HISTORY

This is vital. If the patient received a blow to his knee, his history is straightforward. If, however, nothing touched it, but instead, his foot locked on the ground and his knee twisted inwards in flexion, and is now acutely painful, ask him these questions:

How soon did your knee swell? If it swelled immediately, it is probably full of blood as the result of the rupture of a larger vessel. If it swelled more slowly over 6 or 8 hours, a smaller vessel has ruptured, or he has a sympathetic effusion.

If he was engaged in some violent activity, such as playing football, could he continue the game? If he could continue, he probably has only a minor injury.

If: (1) he felt a snap or a pop, or (2) he has had previous episodes, or (3) he has locking and pain on weight bearing, he has probably injured a meniscus.

Where is the pain?

A ROUTINE EXAMINATION FOR AN INJURED KNEE

Sit the patient on the couch with his knees over the edge of it, and his trousers and his shoes off. Look at and feel the muscles of his thighs. Look for atrophy, and compare the two sides. If necessary, compare their circumferences with a tape measure.

Extend his leg, place it on your knee, and examine it for fluid as in Section 79.3.

With his knee extended, grasp his ankle between your arm and your chest, on your right side for his right knee, and on your left side for his left knee.

Now, with his knee flexed a degree or two, to unlock his cruciate ligaments, put both your hands just below his knee and try to move it from side to side. This will test the integrity of its collateral ligaments. There is very little movement in a normal knee.

With his knee flexed, use both your thumbs to palpate his medial and lateral joint lines. Feel for tenderness anteriorly (anterior meniscus injury), in the mid–joint line (ligament or meniscus injury), and posteriorly (posterior meniscus injury, or lesions of his hamstring tendons).

Feel for the origins and insertions of the medial and lateral collateral ligaments above and below the joint lines.

Now lie him flat on the couch. Flex and extend his knee fully. His injured knee should extend and flex as much as his normal knee, and touch or nearly touch his buttocks.

Flex his thigh and his knee. Grasp his ankle and rotate it internally and externally. Finally, lie him on his face, with his knee extended, and feel the back of his popliteal fossa.

CAUTION ! (1) If a child has spontaneous knee pain, examine his hip. His upper femoral epiphysis may have slipped (77.10). (2) In any severe knee injury, always examine a patient's hip.

SPECIAL METHODS FOR AN INJURED KNEE

Apply the appropriate special tests for the following lesions: effusions (79.3), injuries of the patient's collateral ligaments (79.5), tears of his cruciate ligaments (79.6), injuries of his menisci (79.7), and injuries of his quadriceps mechanism (79.11).

X-RAYS Take an AP and a lateral view of his knee.

NERVES AND PULSES Have you remembered to examine his common peroneal nerve (55.8), and his dorsalis pedis and posterior tibial pulses? This is especially important if his tibial condyles have been fractured.

DIFFICULTIES WITH AN INJURED KNEE

If a patient has VARUS OR VALGUS INSTABILITY with his knee fully extended, he has probably torn his collateral ligaments, the posterior capsule of his knee, or perhaps his posterior cruciate ligament.

79.2 A plaster cylinder for the knee

This is the standard treatment for a soft tissue injury, and for some fractures. It will protect a patient's injured knee until the pain and swelling have gone, and it may allow him to walk. If you are not careful, it will slip down his leg and press on his Achilles tendon, or on the dorsum of his foot. You can prevent this happening by compressing the cast from side to side above the flare of his femoral condyles, and by holding it in place with pieces of strapping.

A plaster cylinder is usually applied with a patient's knee just short of full extension, or occasionally in 30° or 60° of flexion. If you apply it in full extension, it will be very painful indeed. Even if you have applied it correctly, his knee is sure to be stiff and extension will be limited when you remove it, so warn him about this, and show him how to do extension exercises. Cycling is excellent exercise for a stiff knee.

A PLASTER CYLINDER

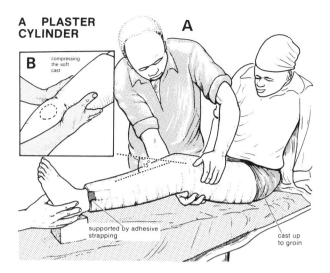

Fig. 79-1 A PLASTER CYLINDER FOR THE KNEE. A, the patient's knee is in 15° of flexion. B, make sure the cylinder will stay in place by compressing it from side to side just above the flare of his femoral condyles before the plaster sets. *Kindly contributed by John Stewart.*

A PLASTER CYLINDER TO IMMOBILIZE THE KNEE

INDICATIONS (1) Soft tissue injuries of the knee. (2) Postoperative immobilization. (3) Some fractures.

METHOD Stick a piece of adhesive strapping down the medial and lateral sides of the patient's lower leg, as for a plaster gaiter (81.6). Let them hang loose below his malleoli.

Apply a cast from his groin to about 3 cm above his malleoli with his knee *in 10° of flexion*. While the cast sets, compress it between the palms and heels of your hands from side to side (not from front to back) just above the flare of his femoral condyles, as in Fig. 79-1.

Pull the strips of strapping tight up over the cast and bind them into it with a few more turns of plaster bandage. Start quadriceps exercises as soon as the cast is dry.

CAUTION ! Never apply a plaster cylinder in full extension—his knee will be very painful and osteoarthritis may follow later.

79.3 Fluid in the knee

If a fracture enters a patient's knee, it rapidly fills with blood which remains liquid for about 2 weeks. Aspirating his tensely swollen knee will greatly relieve his pain and make moving it much easier. Aspiration is also useful in diagnosing less obvious effusions, and especially in distinguishing between infection (7.18) and haemorrhage. Careless aspiration can infect a sterile effusion, *so take the strictest aseptic precautions.*

ASPIRATE ALL KNEE EFFUSIONS

FLUID IN THE KNEE

TESTING FOR AN EFFUSION The first sign of an effusion is the obliteration of the natural hollow on either side of a patient's patella. Press the fluid from one of these hollows into other parts of his knee, and then, in a good light, slowly watch the empty hollow refill.

Can you ballot the patient's patella? Grasp his thigh between your fingers and thumb just above his knee. Press the

FLUID IN THE KNEE

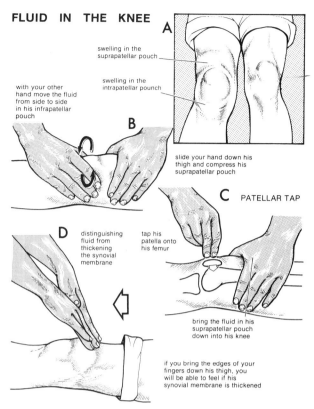

Fig. 79-2 FLUID IN THE KNEE. A, inspection. The first sign of an effusion is the obliteration of the natural hollow on either side of a patient's patella. B, moving fluid from one side of his knee to the other. C, ballotting the patella on the femur. D, distinghishing fluid from thickening of the synovial membrane. *Kindly contributed by John Stewart.*

effusion distally towards his patella, so as to drive fluid from his suprapatellar pouch down into his knee. Press his patella sharply. If fluid is present, you can feel his patella tapping on his femur. This sign is absent if there is very little fluid present, or so much that his patella cannot reach his femur. Compare his injured knee with his normal one.

If his knee is hugely distended and fixed in flexion, aspirate it. When you have done so, examine it again.

ASPIRATING THE KNEE

EQUIPMENT A sterile 20 ml syringe, a large (1.2 mm) needle, iodine, swabs, adhesive strapping, and a receiver.

CAUTION ! Make quite sure that the equipment has been properly sterilized. Never aspirate a knee in a minor theatre used for septic cases. This is a procedure for the main theatre, or a clean treatment room with full aseptic precautions.

ASPIRATION Introduce the needle into the patient's infrapatellar pouch from the medial side laterally. Aspirate the effusion.

If the effusion is bloody, let it settle for 5 minutes and then look at its surface. If fat from an injured marrow cavity is floating on the top, a fracture has entered his knee.

THE FLUID Examine this carefully.
Blood with fat floating on the top—a fracture.
Blood or blood stained fluid—synovial or capsular tears.
Clear amber fluid—torn menisci, osteoarthritis, loose bodies, or synovitis.
Cloudy fluid—septic arthritis, or rheumatoid arthritis. If there are 'rice bodies' he probably has a tuberculous arthritis. If it is frank pus, he probably has septic arthritis.
If possible, send the fluid for culture.

79.4 A swollen knee after a minor injury

When a knee swells after a minor injury the cause can be: (1) a minor fracture, (2) a synovial or capsular tear, (3) a loose body, (4) a torn cartilage, or (5) synovitis of obscure origin. Take a careful history. If the patient has had previous episodes, he may have a chronic ligamentous injury, a loose body, or a torn cartilage. A history of locking suggests a loose body, or a torn cartilage. An abduction or adduction injury suggests a torn ligament, and a rotational one suggests a torn cartilage. The absence of any history of force suggests a loose body or 'synovitis' This has many causes, including rheumatoid arthritis, gonococcal disease, etc. If the swelling appeared slowly over 6 to 12 hours before producing acute pain, it is probably a haemarthrosis, perhaps from quite a minor injury. Examine his knee (79.1), aspirate it (79.3), and look at the fluid. Remember that repeated haemarthroses may be the first indication of a bleeding disorder.

TREATMENT FOR A MINOR KNEE INJURY

Minor fractures, and synovial and capsular tears Aspirate the patient's knee as necessary. Apply a well padded dressing, and mobilize it as pain subsides.

Loose bodies Refer him, removing a loose body from the knee is a specialist task.

'Synovitis' Rheumatoid arthritis is responsible for half the cases. Treat the underlying cause and make sure you exclude TB.

STRESS X-RAYS OF THE KNEE

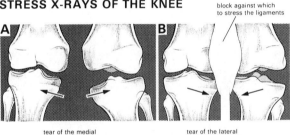

block against which to stress the ligaments

tear of the medial collateral ligament

tear of the lateral collateral ligament

Fig. 79-3 STRESS X-RAYS OF THE KNEE. A, shows a tear of the medial and B, a tear of the lateral collateral ligament. The anterior cruciate ligaments of both these patients were torn. *From Apley, with kind permission.*

79.5 Tears and sprains of the collateral ligaments

A patient can injure his knee while it is extended, or flexed (as when his knee hits the dashboard), and sustain a variety of complex injuries to his collateral ligaments, his cruciate ligaments, and his menisci. Sprains (partial tears) of his collateral ligaments are usually obvious, but you can miss a complete tear because: (1) It causes less pain than a sprain, so that he may even be able to walk, and you may be able to move his knee. (2) Blood can escape through the capsule in a complete tear, so that swelling is less. Distinguishing between a sprain and a complete tear is important, because a complete tear needs primary repair whereas a sprain will heal with closed treatment. Both sprains and tears make a collateral ligament painful and tender, thus the only sure way to distinguish between them is to examine the patient under general anaesthesia. A sprain is only a minor injury, but a tear can cause prolonged disability.

COLLATERAL LIGAMENT INJURIES OF THE KNEE

EXAMINATION Tenderness is a good indication as to where a patient's ligament has been injured, so feel for it carefully. His collateral ligaments may be tender over their femoral or tibial origins. Narrowly localized tenderness (usually about 2 cm above the joint line) indicates a partial tear. Severe diffuse tenderness suggests a complete one.

If his medial ligament is tender at the joint line, his medial meniscus may be injured also.

If you suspect that a collateral ligament may have been ruptured, test the stability of his knee like this.

Hold his leg with one of your hands just above his injured knee, and the other one just above his ankle. With his knee just short of full extension move his lower leg from side to side. If either of his collateral ligaments is grossly torn, his tibia will wobble on his femur.

CAUTION ! (1) His knee must be just a little flexed when you do this test. If it is fully extended, his cruciate ligaments will stabilize it and mask tears in his collateral ligaments. (2) A fracture of his tibial plateau can also make his knee unstable and resemble a torn collateral ligament.

Alternatively, sit him on a table. Sit on a chair in front of him. Hold his foot and ankle firmly in your axilla. With both hands, grasp his upper tibia with his knee flexed 5°. Try to angle his leg on his knee.

X-RAYS If you suspect torn medial collateral ligaments, sedate the patient, put a pillow between his ankles, bind his knees together, and take an AP view to compare the joint space between his femoral and tibial condyles on either side, as in Fig. 79-3. Or, using a lead glove, stress his injured knee as the X-ray is taken.

EXAMINATION UNDER ANAESTHESIA If you want to distinguish between a sprain and a tear, examine him under anaesthesia, in full extension and 15° of flexion. His cruciate ligaments can make his leg appear to be stable, even when his collateral ligaments have been torn. With a few degrees of flexion his cruciates are relaxed and the tears of his collateral ligaments will become more obvious.

THE TREATMENT OF TEARS OF THE MEDIAL AND LATERAL COLLATERAL LIGAMENTS

If there is no medial or lateral angulation when you examine a patient under anaesthesia, his injured collateral ligament is probably only sprained and not torn. So fit a plaster cylinder (79.2) to relieve pain and protect his sprained ligament. If he is walking easily without pain at 2 weeks, remove it, otherwise leave it on for 2 more weeks, then start active knee exercises.

If lateral angulation causes an opening of less than 1 cm on the side of the knee joint, proceed as above, but apply the cylinder in 30° of flexion (to relax his torn ligament) and continue immobilization for 6 to 8 weeks. Warn him that extension will be slow to return, and tell him to do progressively increasing extension exercises. This may give as good results as attempts at secondary repair.

If lateral angulation causes an opening of more than 1 cm on one side of the knee joint, the collateral ligament on that side is torn, and perhaps the patient's meniscus is injured also. Refer him immediately for primary repair. This gives only fair results in most cases. If you cannot refer him, fit a plaster cylinder as described below.

If you see a patient after the first week, primary repair is more difficult and less satisfactory. So fit a plaster cylinder with his knee just short of full extension in the position of abduction or adduction that will best close up the torn ligament. Leave it on for 6 weeks.

If he presents late with an unstable knee, refer him for secondary repair, this has about a 50% chance of a good result.

79.6 Torn cruciate ligaments

A patient's posterior cruciate ligament is attached posteriorly on the proximal surface of his tibia, and anteriorly on his femur. It tightens when his tibia is pushed backwards on his femur. He can tear it when his tibia hits the dashboard of his car and is driven back on his femur. Less often his anterior cruciate is

THE DRAW SIGN FOR TORN CRUCIATE LIGAMENTS

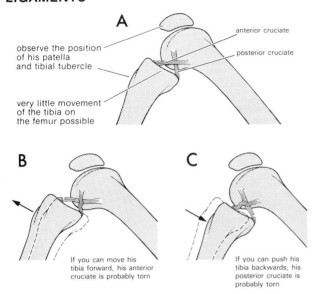

A

observe the position of his patella and tibial tubercle

anterior cruciate

posterior cruciate

very little movement of the tibia on the femur possible

B

If you can move his tibia forward, his anterior cruciate is probably torn

C

If you can push his tibia backwards, his posterior cruciate is probably torn

Fig. 79-4 SIGNS FOR TORN CRUCIATE LIGAMENTS. A patient's posterior cruciate ligament is attached posteriorly on the proximal surface of his tibia, and anteriorly on his femur. It tightens when his tibia is pushed backwards on his femur. If you can push his tibia backwards, his posterior cruciate is torn. *Kindly contributed by John Jellis.*

injured if his foot remains on the ground, and his femur is driven backwards by some twisting injury. Satisfactory repairs are seldom possible on either of these ligaments.

INJURIES TO THE CRUCIATE LIGAMENTS

EXAMINATION If the patient's knee injury is very recent, and the following test is likely to be painful, examine him under anaesthesia. Otherwise, ask him to sit up, bend his knee to 90°, and put his foot on the couch. Sit on his foot, then take hold of the proximal end of his tibia with both hands, and move it forcibly backwards and forwards. There should be very little movement.

Now with his normal knee in the same position, look at the outline of both his knees from the side. Observe especially the relative positions of his tibial tuberosities and his patellae, as in A, Fig. 79-4. Compare his normal with his injured knee.

If you can move his tibia forwards, his anterior cruciate is probably torn. This is rare.

If you can push his tibia backwards, his posterior cruciate is probably torn.

THE TREATMENT OF INJURED CRUCIATE LIGAMENTS

If the patient's anterior cruciate ligament is torn, rest him in bed until most of the pain has gone in about 5 days. Then start active quadriceps exercises. Hypertrophy of his quadriceps can compensate for a tear of his anterior cruciate with complete return of function. Some surgeons advise an operative repair.

If his posterior cruciate is torn, immobilize his knee in 60° of flexion for 6 weeks. Injuries of this ligament are not worth referring.

79.7 Torn menisci

A footballer playing on hard ground can easily injure his menisci. The pressure of his femoral condyle against his tibia may split one of them, so that a piece becomes loose at one end and may

lock his knee. A history of injury to a flexed loaded knee is highly suggestive, especially if he also says that it sometimes locks. When you see him, his quadriceps will already have started to waste, he may have an effusion, and he will be tender over the joint line of his knee. Most patients learn how to move their knees so as to unlock them. If a patient has repeated episodes of locking with effusion, refer him for meniscectomy. This suggests the presence of a large tear which will eventually cause osteoarthritis.

INJURIES TO THE MENISCI

EXAMINATION Tests for injuries to a patient's menisci are not reliable, so place great importance on the history of the injury (flexion of a loaded knee) and a history of locking.

(1) Sit him down and extend his knee. With the tip of your fingers press firmly over the joint line just medial to his patellar tendon. Now, still pressing hard, flex his knee and at the same time rotate his tibia to and fro on his femur several times. You may feel the torn meniscus click and move under your finger, or roll against the head of his tibia, showing that it is displaced.

(2) Press with your thumb close beside his patellar tendon over the anterior horn of his medial meniscus. Flex and extend his knee passively. Do the same thing with the anterior horn of his lateral meniscus. Compare the tenderness with that of his normal leg. Significant tenderness in one place suggests that the meniscus under it is injured.

(3) Lie him on his face. Hold his foot, and flex his knee, until his heel almost reaches his buttock. Rotate his foot externally as far as it will go and then extend it. If you feel a 'click' while you do this, the posterior horn of his medial meniscus is probably torn.

TREATMENT Refer him early, because the result of late meniscectomy is likely to be bad.

If his knee is locked, and you cannot refer him, give him a general anaesthetic and manipulate his knee. Use combinations of flexion, extension, rotation, abduction, and adduction. You may be able to unlock it, temporarily at least.

79.8 Dislocation of the knee

A violent injury such as a road accident can dislocate a patient's knee. At the same time it may tear his cruciate ligaments, and one or both of his collateral ligaments. It may also obstruct his popliteal vessels, and impair the circulation to his lower leg. Reduction is usually easy, but the easier it is, the more likely his knee is to be unstable afterwards. If his knee is completely dislocated, it is unlikely to function normally again. An injury severe enough to dislocate his knee may also injure his hip, so check that too.

A DISLOCATED KNEE Check the circulation in the patient's leg. Reduce his dislocation, and, if necessary, aspirate his knee. If he has a skin wound, toilet it. If possible, suture the torn ligaments back in place with catgut.

Apply a plaster cylinder with his knee flexed to 90°, and split it to allow for swelling. Leave it on for 3 to 4 weeks. Remove it and start gradual extension exercises. He will take several months to regain his normal movements.

Start quadriceps exercises from the begining. Let him start weight bearing in his cast as soon as he can lift his leg.

If reducing his dislocation does not restore the circulation to his leg, his popliteal artery is probably injured. You will not have time to refer him, so get what help you can and explore his popliteal space (3.7). If you cannot restore his circulation, he will probably lose his leg at his knee.

79.9 Dislocation of the patella

There are two varieties of this injury: (1) Some sudden uncoordinated movement of a patient's leg dislocates his patella outwards, and rotates it so that its articular surface lies against the outer side of his femur. The fibres of his vastus internus tear, and his knee fills with blood. He is in great pain, his knee is flexed and he cannot move it. His knee has an abnormal shape, and you can feel that his patella is not in its normal place. Provided you remember that dislocation is a possibility, the diagnosis should not be difficult. (2) Partial dislocation can follow a much less serious injury, and is more common in women.

A DISLOCATED PATELLA If you see the patient within a few hours of the injury, you may be able to reduce his dislocation without an anaesthetic. His knee will probably be flexed. If you extend it slowly, his patella will probably reduce spontaneously. If it does not, ask your assistant to extend the patient's knee. While he does so, place both your thumbs on the outer side of the patient's patella and suddenly flick it back into the midline while he is relaxed and unaware. If this fails, anaesthetize or sedate him. As soon as his muscles relax, glide his patella back into place.

If possible, take skyline X-ray views and look for displaced bony fragments free in his joint.

The medial attachment of his quadriceps to his patella may be torn, so fit him with a plaster cylinder (9.2) for 2 or 3 weeks, and encourage him to do straight leg raising and quadriceps exercises. Recurrence is rare. If his dislocation does recur, or if he gives a history of recurrence since childhood, refer him for reconstructive surgery.

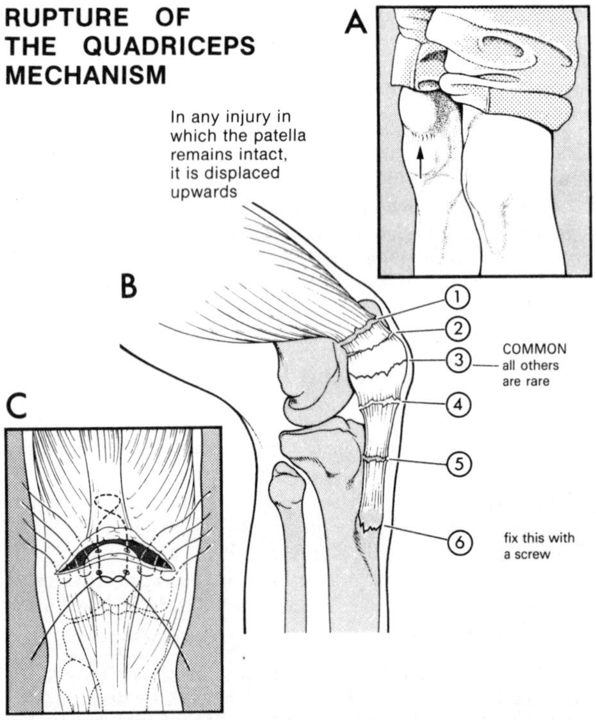

his leg as he walks, and he has difficulty climbing stairs, or going up a slope. Apart from fracture of the patella, all these other injuries are rare. Repairing them involves open joint surgery, with the risk of infection, so refer the patient if you can.

As with the olecranon (72.18), the proper management of these injuries, especially fractures of the patella, depends on whether a patient's quadriceps mechanism is intact or not. This is the mechanism which extends his knee.

TESTING THE QUADRICEPS MECHANISM Feel his patellar tendon between the lower margin of his patella and his tibial tuberosity and ask him to gently lift his leg off the couch. Pain may prevent him from doing this, but if you can feel his patellar tendon tightening, you can be sure his quadriceps extension is sufficiently intact to justify closed treatment. This test may be difficult.

Palpate his quadriceps tendon, his patella, his patellar tendon, and its insertion. Feel for a transverse crack in his patella with your thumb nail.

Put your hand on his patella and ask him to flex and extend his knee. If the surfaces of his patella and femur are rough, you may feel crepitations as they slide over one another.

PATELLAR FRACTURES

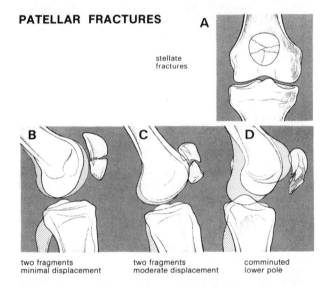

stellate fractures

two fragments minimal displacement

two fragments moderate displacement

comminuted lower pole

Fig. 79-6 SOME PATELLAR FRACTURES. A, a stellate fracture. B, lateral views of other fractures of the patella. In A, and B, the patient's quadriceps mechanism will probably be intact; if so, you will be able to treat him by closed methods. In C, you will probably have to sew up his extensor expansion, and in D, to excise his patella. The important factor in deciding when to operate is not the look of his X-ray, but whether his quadriceps mechanism is intact or not. *Kindly contributed by John Stewart.*

RUPTURE OF THE QUADRICEPS MECHANISM

In any injury in which the patella remains intact, it is displaced upwards

COMMON
all others are rare

fix this with a screw

Fig. 79-5 INJURIES OF THE QUADRICEPS MECHANISM. Injury 3, fracture of the patella, is much the most common of these injuries. The others involve open joint surgery, with the risk of infection if your operating conditions are not good, so refer the patient if you can.

79.10 Injuries of the quadriceps mechanism

If a patient falls on his leg at the same time as his quadriceps tendon is contracting, he can sustain any of the injuries shown in Fig. 79-5. He can rupture his extensor expansion (1), or he can pull it from the upper pole of his patella (2). He can also fracture his patella (3), as described in the next section. He can pull his patellar tendon away from his patella (4), he can rupture it (5), or he can pull it away from his tibia (6). But the result if always similar, he cannot extend his knee fully, he drags

79.11 Patellar fractures

Fractures of the patella resemble those of the olecranon, but are more often missed. A common mistake with disastrous results is to suture a cut knee which overlies a patellar fracture and an open knee injury. Such a patient needs a careful wound toilet and exploration of his knee under general anaesthesia.

A patient can fracture his patella in two ways: (1) He can receive a direct blow to his knee which fractures it directly; this usually causes a stellate fracture which leaves his quadriceps mechanism intact. In a fracture of this kind the fracture lines usually radiate out from a central point as in A, Fig. 79-6. (2) He can fall on his leg at the same time that his quadriceps are contracting. This typically happens in someone who is past middle age, who misses his step, who hears something snap in his knee, and who then falls to the ground. Afterwards, he has difficulty walking. The injury has split his patella horizontally into two halves, separated them, and torn his extensor expansion (more accurately, his patellar retinaculae). This is the tough fibrous capsule of the knee on either side of the quadriceps tendon, the patella, and the patellar tendon. In both kinds of fracture a patient's knee swells with blood and he cannot extend it.

If a patient's quadriceps mechanism is intact, you can treat him by closed methods. If it is not intact, you will have to repair it by one of the methods in the next section. If this is not done, he will not be able to extend his knee the final 20°, although he will be able to walk.

CLOSED METHODS FOR PATELLAR FRACTURES

INDICATIONS (1) The patient's quadriceps expansion must be intact as tested for in Section 79.10. (2) The fragments must not be widely separated. Provided these conditions hold, conservative treatment is indicated, particularly if he has a stellate fracture with many radiating fracture lines.

TREATMENT There will be blood in his painful swollen knee, so aspirate it.

If pain and swelling are mild, teach him to use crutches (77.1). No dressing is needed.

If pain and swelling are severe, fit him with a plaster cylinder (79.2).

Alternatively, bandage his leg from his ankle to his groin with alternate layers of cotton wool and crepe bandage, making four layers in all. Keep him in bed until he has regained control of his knee. Then allow him up. Encourage him to move his knee actively within the limits of the bandage.

After 2 weeks, remove the bandages and add knee flexion exercises to those he is already doing.

SUTURING THE EXTENSOR EXPANSION

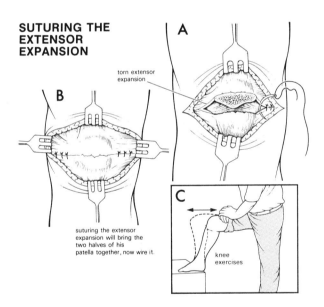

Fig. 79-7 SUTURING THE EXTENSOR EXPANSION. A, before, and B, after suture. C, shows a useful postoperative exercise. Ask the patient to put his foot on a step and gently bend it to and fro. *Kindly contributed by John Stewart.*

79.12 Operations on the quadriceps mechanism

If a patient's quadriceps mechanism is not working, you will have to repair it.

If his patella is in two pieces all you need do is to sew up his extensor expansion on either side of it. The tear can be opposite the middle of his patella, in which case it will be in two halves, or it can be at the top or bottom of his patella, in which case there may be one large fragment and one small one.

If his patella is in several widely comminuted fragments, excise them and pass a purse string suture around the hole where his patella was.

Although operations on the patella itself are possible, they are not always necessary, because the important part of the extensor mechanism is not the patella, but the quadriceps expansion around it. Rarely, the patella may be intact and only the patellar tendon or quadriceps tendon may be torn, and need suture.

When the patella is in two pieces, they should be fixed so that the posterior surface of the patella is smooth. Our contributors differ as to how you should do this. Some advise that you wire the patella round its circumference, and others suggest that you pass Kirschner wires through it.

OPERATIONS ON THE QUADRICEPS MECHANISM

If possible, refer the patient. If you cannot do this, proceed as follows.

INDICATIONS A patellar fracture with rupture of the quadriceps mechanism.

WHEN TO OPERATE ? If the skin over the patient's patella is normal, operate as soon as is practical. If it is bruised, operate immediately. If it is infected, wait for 7 to 10 days until infection subsides and treat the infection in the meanwhile.

ANAESTHESIA Give the patient a general or a subarachnoid anaesthetic (A 7.4). Apply a tourniquet (3.8).

INCISION Make a transverse skin incision passing across the top of the patient's patella. Be sure that the incision goes far enough around his knee to reach the ends of the tears. It may need to go half way round on each side. If an area of skin is bruised, avoid it, or excise it.

Reflect his skin proximally and distally to expose the whole anterior surface of his patella, his patellar tendon, and his quadriceps tendon.

Inspect his quadriceps tendon medially and laterally. Remove any small detached fragments of bone.

His knee will be full of blood; wash it out until all clots are gone. Use a 20 ml syringe to squirt saline under high pressure into all its recesses, until the fluid comes out clear. Alternatively, wash it out with a litre of intravenous saline.

SUTURING THE EXTENSOR EXPANSION

If the patient's patella is in two halves, and his extensor expansion is torn, sew it up from the sides towards the centre with strong monofilament sutures, or strong chromic catgut, as in A, and B, Fig. 79-7. Bring the fragments together accurately. If convenient, hold the two halves of his patella together with towel clips, while you sew up the expansion. You now have 5 alternatives, depending on your skill.

(1) You can leave the repair as it is.

(2) You can strengthen the repair by passing a figure of eight loop of strong catgut through the patient's quadriceps expansion above, cross it over his patella, and pass it through the attachment of his patellar tendon. To maintain a smooth undersurface to his patella, do this with his knee flexed about 30°.

(3) You can encircle his patella with 1 mm stainless steel wire, thick chromic catgut, or monofilament, preferably with a large Gallie needle. Alternatively, thread the wire through a large intravenous needle as in Fig.54-7. Pass the wire in and out of his quadriceps expansion, taking big bites very close to his patella. Go all around the superior border and lateral borders and pass the wire straight through the patellar tendon, close to his patella. Finally, bring the ends together and twist them tight. This circumferential wiring prevents the fragments separating. Place this wire superficially in his patella, so that when his knee flexes, the posterior aspects of the fragments are brought together in compression. The wire must lie close to his patella, particularly above and below, or it will cut out when his knee flexes.

(4) You can combine method (3) with passing 2 Kirschner wires through the two halves of the patella from above downwards. Cut them short and bend over their tips.

THE PRINCIPLES OF TENSION BAND WIRING

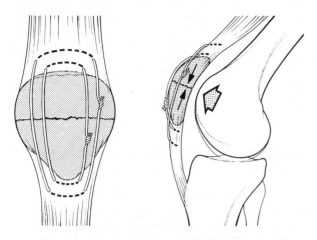

Fig. 79-8. THE PRINCIPLE OF TENSION BAND WIRING. Wires in the anterior part of the patella will bring its posterior part into compression when the knee is bent. Some surgeons keep the fragments aligned with Kirschner wires.

(5) If you have the experience and the equipment, apply tension band wiring as in Fig. 79-8.

EXCISING THE WHOLE PATELLA FOR COMMINUTED FRACTURES

If a patient's patella is in several widely separated fragments, use a very sharp scalpel to cut them out of the tendon. Keep the edge of the scalpel close to the bone all the time. Change the blade frequently as it blunts, and preserve the soft tissue coverings of the excised fragments.

Excise all fragments except for a small anterior chip in both proximal and distal tendons. Preserve as much tendon as you can. Repair the medial and lateral tears in his quadriceps expansion with interrupted sutures of thick catgut, beginning at the sides of his knee and working towards the gap created by removing his patella. Pass a purse string suture around the edges of this gap and pull them together. If one purse string does not seem to be enough, put in another one. Don't worry if you have a gap in the middle where his patella was.

If his quadriceps expansion is torn at the sides of his knee, be sure to repair it.

REPAIRING THE QUADRICEPS TENDON

This is open joint surgery, with the risk of infection, if your operating conditions are not good. Refer the patient if you can.

If you cannot refer him, join the ends of his quadriceps tendon with strong catgut.

If his quadriceps tendon has torn away from his patella (rare), drill some holes for sutures through its edge as in C, Fig. 79-5.

If his injury is an old one, and his quadriceps muscle has retracted, pass a Steinmann pin through his quadriceps tendon, apply traction, and when, after some days, the muscle has lengthened sufficiently, suture the tendon.

REPAIRING THE PATELLAR TENDON

This again is open joint surgery, so try to refer the patient. If you cannot refer him, suture the torn ends of his patellar tendon with strong catgut. If necessary, drill some holes through the lower pole of his patella to hold the sutures.

If the patient's patellar tendon has pulled away from his tibia, drill some holes in it to hold wire sutures, or hold his patellar tendon in place with a screw.

If his injury is an old one and his patella is much retracted, push his skin upwards and his patella downwards. Make two small nicks in his skin at either side of his patella tendon. Pass a Kirschner wire through it and exert traction for at least 2 weeks. Keep the wire in place and incorporate it (without its tensioner) in a long leg plaster cylinder (79.2). Then operate and repair the tendon.

POSTOPERATIVE CARE FOR OPERATIONS ON THE QUADRICEPS MECHANISM

Dress the patient's wound with gauze, cover this with plenty of cotton wool from 10 cm above his knee to 5 cm below it. Hold this firmly with two 15 cm crepe bandages. With his knee just short of full extension, apply medial and lateral plaster slabs from his groin to his ankle, pad them with cotton wool, and bandage them on firmly.

CAUTION ! These slabs must be strong enough to prevent him bending his knee as he awakes from the anaesthetic.

Encourage him to do regular quadriceps exercises and straight leg raising as soon as he can.

On about the twelfth day, remove his bandages and dressings. If his wound is clean and dry, take out the sutures. Protect his malleoli with padding and apply a plaster cylinder.

At 4 weeks bivalve his cast and let him start non-weight bearing extension exercises under supervision. Let him wear his bivalved cast for weight bearing. Abandon the cast: (1) when he can flex his knee to 90° and, (2) when he can extend it against resistance. This is usually at 6 to 8 weeks.

At 6 weeks start gentle active flexion exercises.

At 8 weeks, begin the passive flexion exercises shown in C, Fig. 79-7.

CAUTION ! He may refracture his patella and need a further operation if: (1) You let him walk too soon without his bivalved cast, and he accidentally stumbles. (2) He exceeds the exercise routine described above.

Gradually increase his exercises—provided he can fully extend his knee actively. If he ceases to be able to do this, don't allow him to flex his knee any further until he has regained active extension.

Expect the recovery of flexion to be slow. He will not be able to flex his knee fully for 4 to 6 months.

PERKINS TRACTION FOR A SUPRACONDYLAR FRACTURE

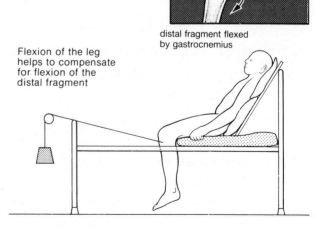

distal fragment flexed by gastrocnemius

Flexion of the leg helps to compensate for flexion of the distal fragment

Fig. 79-9 PERKINS TRACTION FOR A SUPRACONDYLAR FRACTURE. This is the most suitable treatment if the distal fragment is only mildly flexed. If it is severely flexed, he should be referred for internal fixation. If you cannot refer him, we describe some methods you can use. *Kindly contributed by Peter Bewes.*

If a patient's KNEE IS STIFF, continue progressive active movements. Don't try forcible manipulation under anaesthesia, or you may rupture the repair, tear his ligaments, or break the lower end of his femur.

79.13 Supracondylar fractures of the femur

The patient falls, strikes his knee, and breaks his femur above its condyles. Usually, there is little displacement, but it can be severe, as in A, Fig. 79-11. Occasionally, his gastrocnemius flexes the proximal end of the distal fragment, so that the shaft of his femur comes forward in front of it. When this happens, the distal fragment may press on his popliteal vessels and obstruct the circulation in his leg.

If the distal fragment is only mildly flexed, Perkins traction may be satisfactory. But if it is severely flexed, refer him for internal fixation, because this is a difficult fracture, even in the best hands, and permanent knee stiffness is common. If you cannot refer him, use traction in a Böhler–Braun frame, or Perkins traction with his knee hanging flexed for the first few days. Your hospital carpenter may be able to make a wooden Böhler–Braun frame as in Fig. 79-10.

SUPRACONDYLAR FRACTURES

If necessary, aspirate the patient's injured knee (79.3).

CHILDREN'S SUPRACONDYLAR FRACTURES

Anaesthetize the child, manipulate the fragments into position, and apply a long leg cast from his ischial tuberosity to his toes. Apply it with his knee in the position that best reduces the fracture. If necessary, flex it to 90°.

ADULT'S SUPRACONDYLAR FRACTURES

If you cannot refer the patient, proceed as follows.

MILD DISPLACEMENT If the fragments are in a reasonable position and the patient's peripheral pulses are normal, apply Perkins traction as in Section 78.4, but with his hip and knee flexed, as in B, Fig. 77-11, or as in Fig. 79-9. Encourage him to move his knee. Ignore lateral displacement on the x-ray, and flexion of the distal fragment. Concentrate on getting good antero–posterior alignment.

MORE SEVERE DISPLACEMENT Anaesthetize the patient, preferably using a relaxant (A 14.3). Insert a Steinmann or Denham pin through his upper tibia (70.11, 78.4).

If there is lateral displacement, apply the necessary side to side forces to reduce it. Then apply Perkins traction as below.

If there is overlap or severe angulation, ask one assistant to exert traction in the line of the patient's femur. This is movement 1 in Fig. 79-10. Ask another assistant to hold his iliac crests (2).

When your assistants have restored the length of the patient's femur, grasp its distal end with both hands, and bring it forwards (3). Either apply Perkins traction with the patient's knee flexed, as in Fig. 79-9, or leave him on a Böhler–Braun frame for 10 days, until the bone ends have become sticky, before starting Perkins traction, as for a fracture of the femoral shaft (78.4).

If the above method of reduction fails, pass a Kirschner wire or a Steinmann pin through the anterior margin of the distal fragment. Pull it anteriorly and distally so as to reduce the fracture. The disadvantage with this method is that the pin or wire has to be inserted through the patient's joint capsule with the risk of infecting his knee. So remove it as soon as the fracture is stable, usually at about 3 weeks, and continue with traction through his tibial tubercle, with his knee at 90°.

CAUTION! As always in fractures of the lower limb, correct rotation (78-3).

REDUCING A SUPRACONDYLAR FRACTURE

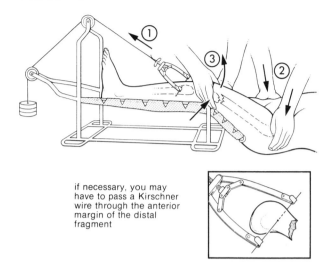

if necessary, you may have to pass a Kirschner wire through the anterior margin of the distal fragment

Fig. 79-10 REDUCING A SUPRACONDYLAR FRACTURE ON A BÖHLER–BRAUN FRAME is only necessary if there is very severe angulation. It is one of the few correct uses of this frame. *After de Palma, with kind permission.*

Alternatively: (1) Apply a period of skin traction to his lower leg first. (2) You may be able to get the lower fragment into a suitable position by putting a pillow under his lower thigh.

If you still cannot achieve satisfactory reduction, refer him for open reduction.

LATER CARE FOR A SUPRACONDYLAR FRACTURE

Maintain traction until there is clinical union, usually in about 8 weeks. Two weeks later allow the patient up on crutches without weight bearing, as in Section 77.1; then after 2 more weeks, and if X-rays show solid union, start protected weight bearing. Don't allow unprotected weight bearing until his fracture has consolidated. His knee is likely to be stiff for a long time, and he will need continued exercises to help him extend it.

Alternatively, at 4 to 6 weeks apply a long leg cast while he is standing, keep this on until the fracture has consolidated, usually after 2 to 4 more weeks. This is a poor alternative to continued Perkins traction, but it may be necessary to free a bed.

79.14 T–shaped fractures of the femur into the knee joint

An adult falls on his bent knee and breaks his femur transversely near its lower end, as in B, Fig. 79-11. Another fracture line runs proximally from the joint to meet the transverse fracture line and separates his two femoral condyles. At the transverse fracture the fragments are usually end on, but they may be angled or displaced. His condyles may be separated by a gap, or one condyle may be displaced on another. Perkins traction usually reduces the displacement satisfactorily. If one of the fragments has turned through 180° open reduction is essential, so refer him.

79.15 Fracture of a femoral condyle

When a patient's knee is struck from the side and forced medially, the lateral condyle of his tibia usually fractures. Occasionally, the lateral condyle of his femur fractures instead, as in C, Fig. 79-11. If it is only slightly displaced, and not completely

FRACTURES OF THE DISTAL END OF THE FEMUR

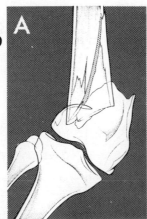

Supracondylar fracture with severe angulation

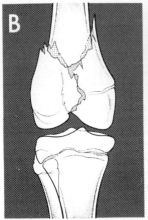

T-shaped fracture

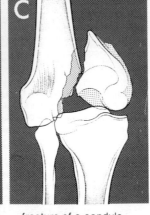

fracture of a condyle with rotation

Fig. 79-11 FRACTURES OF THE DISTAL END OF THE FEMUR. A, a supracondylar fracture with severe angulation. B, a T–shaped fracture. C, fracture of a condyle with rotation. *Kindly contributed by John Stewart.*

SEPARATION OF THE DISTAL FEMORAL EPIPHYSIS

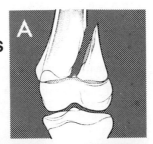

Type II injury, fracture line passes out through shaft

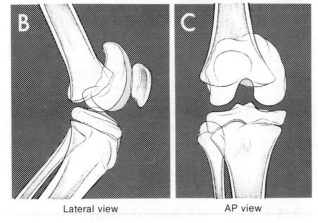

Lateral view

AP view

Type I injury, separation occurs along the epiphyseal line

Fig. 79-12 SEPARATION OF THE DISTAL FEMORAL EPIPHYSIS in a child is the result of the same kind of injury that would cause a supracondylar fracture in an adult.

rotated, treat him in Perkins traction. But if the detached femoral condyle has completely rotated, and you cannot reduce it, immediate operative After reduction and internal fixation are essential, so refer him.

79.16 Separation of the distal femoral epiphysis

A severe injury in an older child, which would cause a supracondylar fracture in an adult, produces a Salter Harris Type I epiphyseal injury (69.6a, Fig. 69-8) as in B and C, Fig. 79-12, or a Type II one as in A in this figure, or a Type IV injury. His distal epiphysis usually moves anteriorly, displacing the distal end of the shaft of his femur posteriorly where it may obstruct his popliteal vessels. His knee is swollen, he has a painful swelling immediately above it, and it may be unstable. Replace his epiphysis under anaesthesia, and hold his knee in flexion in a cast as described below. You can use Perkins traction if displacement is mild.

TOPO (18 years) was injured in a football match, and severely displaced his lower femoral epiphysis. No attempt at reduction was made, and a cast was applied. He was referred 6 weeks later by which time it was too late to try to attempt reduction. His severe angulation will have to be corrected later by osteotomy. LESSONS (1) Reduce epiphyseal injuries within 3 days. (2) Casts are not a universal treatment for all bony injuries.

REDUCING A SEPARATION OF THE DISTAL FEMORAL EPIPHYSIS

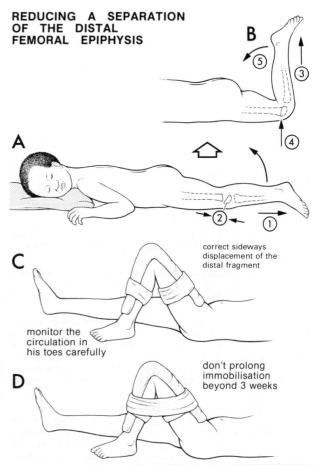

correct sideways displacement of the distal fragment

monitor the circulation in his toes carefully

don't prolong immobilisation beyond 3 weeks

Fig. 79-13 REDUCING A SEPARATION OF THE DISTAL FEMORAL EPIPHYSIS. This method assumes that the separation is of the more common Type I variety, with the distal fragment displaced anteriorly. If the circulation in the child's leg is impaired, reduction is urgent. *After Mercer Rang with kind permission.*

SEPARATED DISTAL FEMORAL EPIPHYSIS

DIAGNOSIS If you are not sure whether a child has ruptured his medial ligament, or displaced his epiphysis, take another film with his extended knee in a valgus position. This will show you the site of the abnormal movement.

MILD DISPLACEMENT Apply Perkins traction.

SEVERE DISPLACEMENT If possible, refer the child, especially if his injury is of the rarer Salter Harris Type IV variety (Fig. 69-8) in which the fracture line opens into his knee joint. The method which follows assumes it is of the more common Type I variety, with the distal fragment displaced anteriorly. If the circulation in his leg is impaired, reduction is urgent.

Anaesthetize him and lie him on his face, as in Fig. 79-13.

If the distal fragment is displaced sideways, apply traction (1) with his leg extended, and try to correct it (2).

Correct anterior displacement by applying traction to his partly flexed knee (3). Push the distal fragment posteriorly (4), and then increase the flexion of his knee to about 110° (5), just as you would if you were reducing a supracondylar fracture at the elbow (72.6).

If reduction is stable, apply an anterior plaster slab to his flexed leg (C), and secure the slab to his thigh with circular plaster bandages. Then put another plaster bandage around his thigh and his lower leg (D). Don't flex his thigh more than the degree of swelling will permit.

Ten days later reduce flexion to 60°. Remove the cast after a further 3 weeks. Movement will return slowly.

CAUTION ! (1) Monitor the circulation in his toes carefully during the early stages. (2) Don't prolong immobilization beyond 3 weeks, because the flexion contracture that results may be very difficult to treat. (3) Watch for loss of reduction, which may occur as late as the third week.

If reduction is unstable, refer him.

80 The proximal tibia

80.1 Infracondylar fractures of the tibia

An infracondylar fracture is the result of a blow to the patient's leg fracturing his tibia and fibula 5 cm below his knee, as in A, Fig. 80-1. Although his lower leg may bend in any direction, there is usually only slight lateral shift and no overlap or rotation. The fracture does not enter his knee. You can treat him in a long leg cast, just as you would if his fracture were more distal in his tibia. If the fragments are displaced, manipulate them into position, and apply a long leg cast (81.4) for 6 weeks. Then remove it and start protected weight bearing in crutches.

80.2 T–shaped fractures of the shaft of the tibia into the knee

An adult falls from a height, drives the shaft of his tibia up between the condyles of his femur, and injures the soft tissues of his knee severely. The condyles of his tibia may split apart, as in B Fig. 80-1, so that the shaft of his tibia rides up between them. Distal tibial traction (80.5) will often reduce these fractures adequately.

80.3 Fractures of a tibial condyle ('bumper fractures')

This fracture is usually the result of a blow to the outer side of the patient's knee from the bumper of a car, which fractures one of the condyles of his tibia, usually the lateral one. There are three varieties of this fracture: (1) His lateral condyle may split vertically and hinge outwards, as in C, Fig. 80-1, while his fibula remains intact. (2) The articular surface of his lateral condyle may be depressed or pulped without harming his fibula, as in D, in this figure. Minor varieties of this fracture may be difficult to see on an X-ray, so look carefully. (3) The lateral condyle of his tibia may be displaced downwards, leaving its articular surface unharmed, while breaking the neck of his fibula (E). Fortunately, you can usually neglect the displacement of most of these fractures. Distal tibial traction (80.5) with early knee movement will usually give a patient full movement in his knee.

80.4 Comminuted fractures of the upper tibia

In a comminuted fracture of the upper tibia the fragments are usually held in a sleeve of intact periosteum, as in F, Fig. 80-1. If so, you may be able to reduce them by strong traction, and then treat him in distal tibial traction (80.5).

80.5 Treating fractures of the proximal tibia—distal tibial traction

The treatment for fractures of the proximal tibia differs considerably from the treatment of those of its shaft. If the patient's knee joint is not involved you can treat him in a long leg cast, in the same way as you would if the fracture were more distal in his tibia. But if the fracture enters his knee joint and disturbs its articular surface, he will need early active movements to mould the articular surfaces of his disturbed knee joint into place. Perkins traction is not safe because a pin through his upper tibia would pass too close to the fracture line, or through it, and might cause osteomyelitis, or infect his knee. The alternative is to put the pin through his lower tibia—the middle of his tibia is unsuitable because it is much too hard.

If the articular surface of a patient's knee joint is disturbed, distal tibial traction is much better than a cast, because it reduces most of the displacement, it maintains reduction, and it provides early movement without weight bearing. Early movement helps the surfaces of his knee to slide over one another and minimizes stiffness.

FRACTURES OF THE UPPER TIBIA

If you are going to refer the patient for internal fixation, do so early, within the first week, because the cancellous bone of his tibia soon becomes soft and difficult to fix.

If he has a tense haemarthrosis, aspirate it.

If necessary, apply any of the following manoeuvres under anaesthesia, before applying distal tibial traction.

If his lateral tibial condyle is displaced, put a strong varus strain on his knee, while you try to mould the displaced fragments proximally into place.

If his tibial condyles are comminuted, flex and extend his knee a few times to mould the fragments into shape. If they are much displaced, ask an assistant to pull on the patient's leg while you try to squeeze them into place between your hands.

If the fragments are difficult to reduce, insert a distal tibial Steinmann pin. While the patient is still anaesthetized, apply 10 to 15 kg traction for a few minutes through this pin, and manipulate his knee as above. Send him back to the ward in bed with traction applied.

DISTAL TIBIAL TRACTION See Section 70.11. Use an ordinary bed with a pulley over the end. Apply 5 kg or one fourteenth of the patient's body weight. Place a pillow lengthwise under his lower leg.

CAUTION ! (1) Never put a pad directly under his heel, or pressure sores will form. Instead, support his lower leg to keep his heel off the bed. (2) Don't put a pillow under his knee where it may obstruct the vessels or press on his popliteal nerves.

Next day, encourage him to move his hip, his ankle, and the joints of his tarsus and toes. Exercise his leg gently at first, and then more vigorously.

Put a sling under his *lower thigh,* with a cord passing over an overhead pulley as in Fig. 80-2, and ending in a handle so that he can raise his thigh, and exercise his knee. He should eventually be able to bend it to 90°. Don't put a sling directly under his knee, because it may injure his common peroneal nerve. A sling is essential because you cannot lower the fracture boards and let him dangle his leg, as you can with Perkins traction.

FRACTURES OF THE UPPER TIBIA AND FIBULA

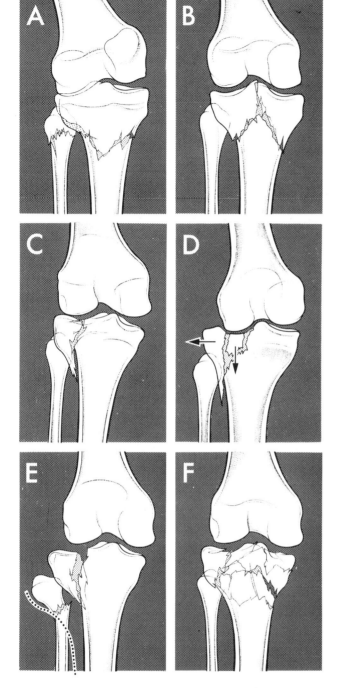

Fig. 80-1 FRACTURES OF THE UPPER TIBIA showing: A, an infracondylar fracture with angulation. B, a T–shaped fracture. C, a fracture of the lateral condyle. D, a fracture of the lateral condyle with depression of the central part of the tibial plateau. E, downward displacement of the lateral condyle with fracture of the neck of the fibula. Note the relation of the common peroneal nerve to the fracture. F, a comminuted fracture of the upper tibia. *Kindly contributed by John Stewart.*

LATER CARE He should have fully controlled flexion and extension of his knee of at least 90° by 4 weeks. Continue to apply traction for 6 weeks, then get him up and teach him to walk on crutches for another 6 weeks, as in Section 77.1, without weight bearing but following the normal movements of walking. Follow this by partial weight bearing with crutches for 6 more weeks.

EXERCISING AN INJURED KNEE DURING DISTAL TIBIAL TRACTION

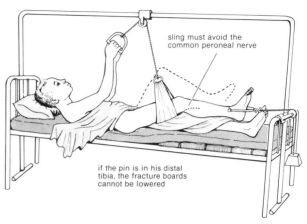

Fig. 80-2 DISTAL TIBIAL TRACTION WITH A SLING UNDER THE THIGH. If a patient has a fracture of his upper tibia which involves his knee joint, you will have to put a pin through his distal tibia and let him exercise his knee like this.

At 12 weeks he should be walking without a stick, unless he is old and frail. If traction is continued for too short a time, there is risk of lateral angulation. Most patients can move their injured knees and walk normally at 6 months.

80.6 Fractures of the tibial spine

In this uncommon injury a child falls on his bent knee, drives his femur posteriorly on his tibia, and pulls his anterior cruciate ligament away from its insertion into his tibia. As it comes away, it brings with it a wedge–shaped piece of his tibial plateau, which is usually called the 'tibial spine'. His knee fills with blood, either immediately, or not until the following day; it is tender all over, and he cannot move it. A lateral X-ray shows a thin flake of bone anteriorly between his tibia and his femur. *The AP view may look almost normal.* This injury is worse than it looks, because much translucent cartilage may be pulled up with the small bony fragment. The diagnosis is often missed. If the loose fragment remains caught in his knee, he will lose the last 10° of full extension.

FRACTURE OF THE TIBIAL SPINE

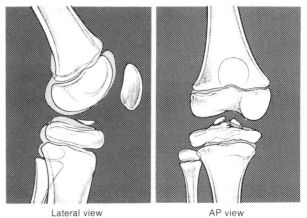

Lateral view   AP view

Fig. 80-3 A FRACTURE OF THE TIBIAL SPINE. In this uncommon injury a child pulls his anterior cruciate ligament away from its insertion in his tibial spine. *Kindly contributed by John Stewart.*

FRACTURES OF THE TIBIAL SPINE Aspirating blood from the child's tensely swollen knee joint will immediately relieve his pain. Anaesthetize him and try to extend his knee fully. This will not reduce the fracture completely, but you can usually reduce it enough to permit full extension.

If you cannot fully extend his knee, refer him.

If you can extend his knee, hold it in full extension (not overextended) and apply a plaster cylinder (79.2) from the upper part of his thigh to just above the heads of his metatarsals. Allow him up immediately, and teach him to walk as naturally as possible. Leave the cylinder on for 6 weeks. Knee movements will then return gradually as he uses his leg.

If he presents late, and you cannot extend his knee, even under anaesthesia, refer him for open reduction.

80.7 Avulsion of the tibial tuberosity

During childhood a projection of the proximal tibial epiphysis forms the tibial tuberosity and the attachment of the patellar tendon. At any age until early adult life when the epiphysis unites, sudden contraction of a child's quadriceps may tear his tibial tuberosity away from his tibia.

AVULSION OF THE TIBIAL TUBEROSITY Treatment depends on the degree of separation.

If separation is mild, immobilize the child's knee in extension in a plaster cylinder for 4 weeks.

If separation is severe, anaesthetize him, try to push his tuberosity back into place, then apply a plaster cylinder in extension.

If closed reduction fails, refer him for open reduction.

80.8 Displacement of the proximal tibial epiphysis

Treat this rare injury in the same way as displacement of the lower tibial epiphysis. Study the X-ray carefully, and try to push the child's displaced epiphysis back into place. If his epiphyseal line is crushed (a Salter Harris Type V lesion, Fig. 69-8), a severe deformity will develop that will later need osteotomy.

81 The tibial shaft

81.1 Introduction

The tibia is the most common major long bone to be injured. It has a long subcutaneous surface, so fractures of the tibia are the commonest open fractures. If you don't treat these fractures carefully, they cause much disability. As you see from the long list of 'difficulties' we give later (81.13), they really can be difficult.

EXAMINING THE LOWER LEG The patient's anterior superior iliac spine, the middle of his patella, and his big toe are usually in a straight line. Compare them with his uninjured leg. If he has had a leg injury, and they are not in line, suspect a fracture.

Feel the subcutaneous border of his tibia, and 'spring' his fibula on it, by squeezing them together. If either of them is fractured, this will be painful.

Have you examined his dorsalis pedis and his posterior tibial pulses? Test his peroneal nerve for power (Can he extend his toes?) and sensation (Can he feel a pin prick on the dorsum of his foot?). Record your findings before doing anything else.

X-RAYS Take an AP and a lateral view.

Raising an injured lower leg in a distal limb injury: (1) Eases the patient's pain. (2) Reduces the swelling. (3) Minimizes the stiffness that follows the organization of any oedema fluid. (4) Enables you to apply a cast to a limb from which most of the swelling has gone. This will make it less likely to become loose subsequently. *So splint and elevate all leg fractures before you manipulate them, operate on them, or put them in a cast.* Elevate a patient's injured leg during an operation, and in the ward afterwards. Elevate it from the moment you see him in casualty, until swelling is no longer a problem. Resting his leg on a chair or on pillows is not enough. His injured leg must be higher than his heart. So, raise the end of his bed on a stool or chair, or on 30 cm blocks for several days if necessary. Encourage him to move his foot and ankle actively, so as to improve the circulation in his calf muscles. Explain how important this is to all your ward staff.

RAISE ALL SEVERELY INJURED LEGS

81.2 The principles of treatment

Internal fixation is possible, but is never advisable under the conditions for which we write (69.1). External fixation is also possible, but the standard equipment for it is expensive ($2 000 for a single tibia), and you need special training to use it. Simpler methods of external fixation are being devised, and when these have been adequately evaluated, they may be described in later editions of this manual. The only method of external fixation we do describe is the incorporation of two Steinmann pins in a cast (81.12).

Fortunately, you can use the closed methods described in this chapter for all the fractures of a patient's lower leg. They avoid

an operation, and the simpler ones require only a few days admission to hospital. They do not always succeed, but your failures will be less awful than those of internal fixation. You will at least avoid the distress of seeing a metal plate firmly fixed in a dead ununited bone at the bottom of a wound pouring pus.

The fragments of a patient's broken tibia are much more likely to unite satisfactorily, if: (1) You get the fragments into an acceptable position to begin with. And (2) you *let him walk on his fracture inside a snug well fitting cast early, and continuously.* Start as soon as the swelling has subsided, during the first few days after the injury, and sometimes as early as the first day. Early weight bearing will not make infection worse, but it may shorten his leg 1 or 2 centimetres, particularly in oblique fractures, where one fragment can easily slip over another. Although this is not ideal, it is not important, because he can, if necessary, compensate for up to 4 cm of shortening by tilting his pelvis, or, if he wears shoes, by having one of them raised. You can, however, usually prevent excessive shortening by a short period of traction to start with. A little shortening (78.1) is a small price to pay for the much greater certainty of union. But there is no way in which he can compensate for the non–union which all too often complicates attempts to prevent shortening. Shortening is even less important in children, because a child's fractured tibia will grow faster than his normal one on the other side, and will compensate for some, if not all, of it.

Although traction for 6 weeks or more is very useful for treating fractures of the femur, *never apply it for more than 2 weeks for an uninfected fracture of the tibia,* because traction for longer than this encourages non–union. Sometimes, if a tibial fracture is open and infected, you may need to apply traction for as long as 3 weeks while you treat the patient's soft tissue injury. Apply traction from a Steinmann pin through his calcaneus (70.12),

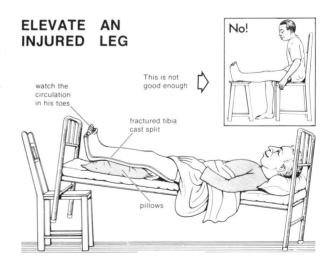

ELEVATE AN INJURED LEG

watch the circulation in his toes

This is not good enough

No!

fractured tibia cast split

pillows

Fig. 81-1 RAISING AN INJURED LEG: (1) Eases the patient's pain. (2) Reduces the swelling. (3) Minimizes the stiffness that follows the organization of oedema fluid. (4) Enables you to apply a cast to a limb from which most of the swelling has gone. *Kindly contributed by Peter Bewes.*

or his distal tibia (80.5). If his fracture is open or badly comminuted, his leg swollen, and his circulation poor, a week or two in traction will help to align the fragments while his soft tissues heal. Some surgeons apply traction to all but the easiest transverse tibial fractures. Others use it only for severely comminuted open ones. As with the femur (78.4), try not to distract the fragments.

Uncomplicated fractures of an adult's tibia take 16 weeks to heal. Children's fractures heal faster. Healing is delayed if the tibia is comminuted, if soft tissue injury is severe, or if a fracture is open or infected, union may take a year or more.

Dehne E. and Nitz et al. The treatment of Fractures by Direct Weight bearing. Journal of Trauma 1961;1:514-535.

GET THE FRAGMENTS INTO AN ACCEPTABLE
POSITION
GET THE PATIENT WALKING EARLY INSIDE A CAST

81.3 Casts for the lower leg

A patient can walk and bear weight in any of the following three casts. In order of decreasing stability, but increasing mobility and convenience, they are: (1) a long leg walking cast from his groin to the bases of his toes, (2) a short leg walking cast from just below his knee to the bases of his toes, and (3) a plaster gaiter from just below his knee to just above his ankle. A long leg cast is applied first, and renewed if necessary, followed by shorter ones as his fracture heals.

If a patient walks on the sole of his cast it soon becomes useless, and children, especially, rapidly wear through the soles of their casts. So the way in which a cast is made is important: (1) The patient's ankle should usually be in neutral. (2) His heel and his foot must also be in neutral and not be everted or inverted. (3) The sole of the cast should be strong enough to bear his weight. (4) He may have to walk several kilometres in the rain, so if it is likely to get wet, paint it with oil paint. (5) Fit his cast with a stirrup or, less satisfactorily, with a walking heel, which will raise it out of the mud and puddles. A stirrup will last longer because it is stronger and will distribute his weight

more evenly. You will get the stirrup back when you change his cast, so a stock of stirrups is a useful investment. If you fit a walking heel, the patient should be able to pivot on it. This means that: (a) it must be sufficiently narrow, which is why trying to mould a sandal to the sole of a cast is less satisfactory, (b) it must project about 2 cm below the sole of the cast to allow his foot to rock, and (c) it must be aligned with the anterior surface of his tibia.

There is no point in removing any leg cast, unless it is loose, until the patient is walking on it painlessly without a stick. If he is walking with pain or difficulty, the cast usually needs to be replaced with another one in which treatment can continue.

DON'T REMOVE A CAST UNTIL THE PATIENT IS
WALKING PAINLESSLY WITHOUT A STICK

81.4 A long leg walking cast

This is the first cast for an unstable fracture of the tibia. Its purpose is to immobilize the fragments and to get a patient walking as soon as he can.

(1) Make sure that a patient's foot points in the right direction to begin with, because a foot which points in the wrong direction is a great disability, especially if it points inwards. So, in all tibial and malleolar casts (82.6), *make sure that his foot points in the same direction in relation to his knee on the injured side as it does on the normal one.*

(2) The cast must stop the distal fragment rotating on the proximal one, and so delaying union. When union is well advanced, rotation is less likely, but the fragments can easily rotate in a recent fracture. Prevent the proximal fragment from rotating by applying a long leg cast with the patient's knee in 15° of flexion. Prevent the distal fragment from rotating by including his foot and ankle in the cast.

MAKE SURE THE PATIENT'S FEET ARE
SYMMETRICAL
PREVENT THE FRAGMENTS FROM ROTATING ON
ONE ANOTHER

MAKE SURE HIS FOOT POINTS IN THE RIGHT DIRECTION

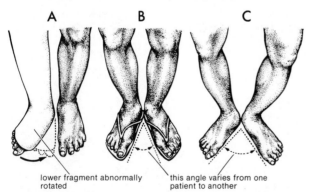

Fig. 81-2 MAKE SURE THE PATIENT'S FOOT POINTS IN THE RIGHT DIRECTION. **Some patients have feet which are almost parallel, like patient A. Others, like patient C, have markedly externally rotated feet. Symmetry is more important than making sure that a patient's feet always point in the same direction as his patella. Patient A's cast was applied with the lower fragment in too much external rotation. This is undesirable, but too much internal rotation would have been worse—see Fig. 78-3.** *Kindly contributed by John Stewart.*

A LONG LEG WALKING CAST

Let the patient's leg hang over the end of the table. If he is conscious, let him sit on the table. If he is anaesthetized, pull him down to the end of the table, and let his legs hang over it.

Pad his injured leg paying especial attention to his malleoli, the subcutaneous surface of his tibia, and the head and neck of his fibula.

CAUTION ! (1) If you neglect to pad the neck of the patient's fibula, the cast may compress his common peroneal nerve and cause foot drop. (2) Don't apply the cast with his leg horizontal, because controlling the position of the fragments will be more difficult. (3) If you fail to align the fragments, union will take longer and his leg will be crooked.

Make the cast in two parts.

First part. Use two 15 cm plaster bandages to make a thin below–knee cast which is just strong enough to control the fragments. This is easily done if the patient's knee is flexed over the end of the table so that gravity helps to align the fragments.

Second part. When the below–knee part of the cast has hardened, ask one assistant to hold the patient's lower leg, and another one to support his thigh. Cover the first part of the cast with a further layer of plaster from his toes to his groin, with his knee in 15° of flexion. If you apply it in full

A LONG LEG WALKING CAST

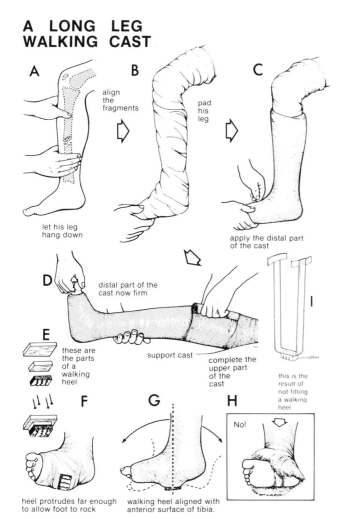

Fig. 81-3 MAKING A LONG LEG WALKING CAST. A, the patient's leg must hang down so that you can align the fragments more easily. B, applying the padding. C, applying the distal part of the cast. D, the distal part of the cast is now firm and the upper part is being completed. E, and F, a locally made walking heel. G, how a walking heel should be aligned with the tibia. H, what happens if you don't fit a walking heel. I, if possible, fit a stirrup like this. *Kindly contributed by John Stewart.*

extension, it will be less effective in controlling rotation, and his knee will be painful. Apply enough layers of plaster bandage for the upper part of the cast to grip the lower part. Incorporate medial and lateral slabs to strengthen the knee part of the cast. Finally, apply some more turns of bandage to make the upper part adequately strong.

CAUTION ! (1) While you are applying the cast, check the position of the patient's ankle carefully; it should be in neutral, and neither inverted nor everted. (2) Make sure that his foot has the same relation to his patella as on the uninjured side. (3) A normal tibia has a slight natural inward bow, so try to restore this. (4) Make a shelf of plaster under his toes, to protect them and prevent flexion contractures. (5) Take care to strengthen the knee, and the ankle parts of the cast, because these are its weakest places.

If the patient's fracture is very recent, split the cast from top to bottom that evening (70.4). Monitor the circulation in his feet meanwhile. Make sure you split the cast on the same day that you apply it, but don't split it immediately, because the junction of the top to bottom parts of the cast take an hour or two to become sufficiently firm to split.

If he has been in calcaneal traction for 2 weeks, any swelling will have gone, so there is less need to split the cast.

Don't worry about a little angulation in a recent fracture.

If necessary, correct this 2 or 3 weeks later, when the healing bone at the fracture site is still soft, and more stable. Either wedge the cast (70.7) or, preferably, replace it by another one with his leg in a better position. Replacing a cast is safer and less likely to cause pressure sores than wedging.

CAUTION ! (1) If possible, admit him, so that he does not walk on his cast until it is dry and hard. This may take 24 hours or more in wet weather. If he walks on a soft cast, it will soon become useless. (2) Be sure to tighten or renew the cast if his leg becomes loose within it. If you fail to do this, the fragments may displace.

CLOSING A CAST If you split it and the swelling has gone down, close it with a few turns of plaster bandage.

If it is loose, remove a small strip of plaster from the front of it, and then close it with with a few turns of plaster bandage. This is easily done with an electric cast cutter.

FIT A STIRRUP OR A WALKING HEEL Either fit them immediately, or later, when the patient's wound is no longer a problem and he can manage crutches. If possible, fit a metal stirrup. If you don't have one, fit a walking heel. There are several ways of making a heel. Even a piece of wood is better than nothing: (1) Nail a piece of car tyre to a wooden block, mould this to the cast with a plaster bandage, and bind it on with more bandages, as in Fig. 81-3. (2) Cut a piece from the tyre of a small car, put this around the cast, and hold it in place with laces.

ALTERNATIVELY: (1) Start the cast by applying medial and lateral slabs, or a posterior slab only. This will make a smoother cast. (2) Incorporate strips of bamboo in the cast, particularly across fracture lines and joints. This is a considerable economy in plaster.

DIFFICULTIES WITH LONG LEG CASTS

If the patient's ANKLE SWELLS when the cast is removed, treat it by raising his leg, asking him to do exercises, and compressing the swelling with a crepe bandage. Swelling is so common as to be normal, and soon improves.

If his KNEE IS STIFF when you remove the cast, one reason may be that you left it on too long.

DON'T LET A PATIENT WALK HOME IN A WET CAST

A SHORT LEG WALKING CAST

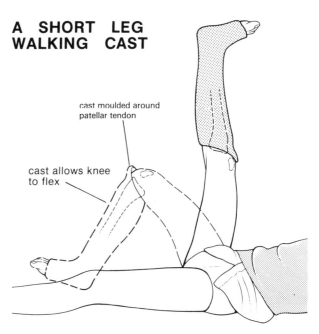

Fig. 81-4 A SARMIENTO TYPE SHORT LEG WALKING CAST is applied with the patient's knee flexed to 90°. It has an oblique upper edge, and is moulded by triangular compression, as in the next figure.

81.5 A short leg walking cast

You can use a shorter cast to protect a fracture of the middle or lower third of a patient's tibia as soon as the fracture has become stable and the swelling has gone. A shorter cast is not absolutely necessary, and some surgeons don't use them. The advantages of a short cast are that: (1) It allows a patient to move his knee earlier; if you fit him with a gaiter, as described in the next section, he can also use his ankle earlier. (2) A short cast uses less plaster than a long one.

As with a long leg cast, try to prevent the fragments from rotating. There are two ways you can do this: (1) You can mould the cast carefully to the patient's upper leg, using Sarmiento's total contact method of triangular compression, as described below. Or, (2) you can pass a Steinmann pin through the upper end of the patient's tibia and incorporate it in the cast. This is the most certain method, and is the one to use if he has a fracture of his femur in the same leg (78.6).

Sarmiento A, A functional below knee cast for tibial fractures. Journal of Bone Joint Surgery. 1967; 49A: 855.

Sarmiento A, Below the knee total contact cast. Clinical Orthopaedics. 1972;82:213

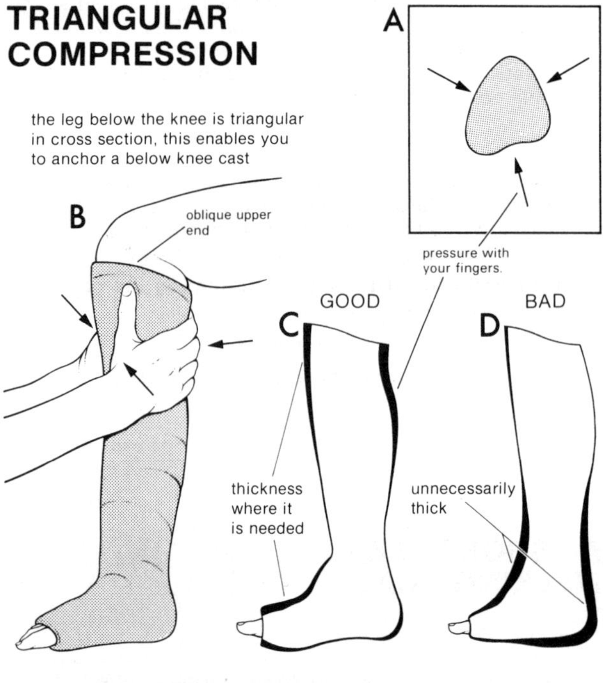

TRIANGULAR COMPRESSION

the leg below the knee is triangular in cross section, this enables you to anchor a below knee cast

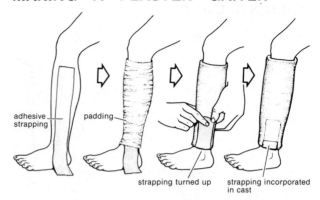

Fig. 81-5 TRIANGULAR COMPRESSION. While a short leg cast is setting, compress its upper end so as to mould it to the patient's leg. *After Sarmiento.*

A SARMIENTO SHORT LEG WALKING CAST Apply a cast from just proximal to the patient's toes, to as high as possible in his popliteal fossa with his leg bent to 90°. Bring the cast above his tibial tuberosity in front, and below his popliteal fossa behind, so that it has an oblique upper end as in Fig. 81-4.

As the cast hardens, apply compression between the patient's upper calf and the anterior surface of his leg, as in Fig. 81-5. This will give the cast a triangular cross-section, as in A in this figure, and help to prevent rotation.

CAUTION ! (1) Triangular compression is safe in a short leg cast, where muscular activity can relieve excessive pressure. But, don't apply it in a long leg cast, because pressure necrosis can occur. (2) Don't try to economize by cutting off a long leg cast below the knee. It is always loose and unstable.

MAKING A PLASTER GAITER

Fig. 81-6 MAKING A PLASTER GAITER. Use this for protecting fractures of the middle third of the tibia as it heals. *Kindly contributed by Peter Bewes.*

81.6 A plaster gaiter

This is the simplest and lightest leg cast; it is the easiest one to walk with, but it is also the least secure. Use it for protecting fractures of the middle third of the tibia, *after union has taken place.* It does not provide enough stability for fractures of the proximal or distal thirds. If you put it on immediately after a patient has been in a long leg cast, his foot and ankle will swell immediately. Some surgeons don't use gaiters.

MAKING A PLASTER GAITER Apply pieces of adhesive strapping to either side of the patient's leg, as if you were going to apply traction. Pad his leg and especially his Achilles tendon. Then apply the cast. Just as you apply the last layer of plaster bandage, fold up the two pieces of strapping and incorporate them in the cast. They will stop it slipping down his leg and rubbing against the top of his foot.

As the cast sets, mould it around the expanding upper and lower ends of his tibia, so that it grips them firmly. His knee, foot, and ankle should be free.

81.7 Closed fractures of the shaft of the tibia (alone) in adults

Two kinds of injury can break an adult's tibia without breaking his fibula: (1) If his leg is struck from the side, it may break transversely or obliquely, leaving his fibula intact, and thus able to splint the fragments, so that they shift very little. (2) A combination of compression and twisting can cause a long spiral oblique fracture with almost no displacement, and very little soft tissue injury. These fractures usually heal rapidly.

CLOSED FRACTURES OF THE SHAFT OF THE TIBIA IN ADULTS

REDUCTION If displacement is minimal, leave the fragments as they are. If displacement is significant, anaesthetize the patient and reduce them.

Apply a long leg cast or medial and lateral splints, held with a crepe bandage until the acute swelling has subsided. Close the cast, fit a walking heel, get the patient up as soon as he can bear weight with crutches, and make him bear weight on his leg.

If he has a long, spiral oblique fracture, discard the long leg walking cast in about 6 weeks, and apply a protective gaiter for another 2 weeks.

If he has a transverse fracture, it will probably take 12 to 16 weeks to heal. It will heal sooner if the fragments are nicely impacted and he starts weight bearing immediately.

If the fracture is in the middle third of his tibia *and has united*, fit a plaster gaiter (81.6). If the fracture is elsewhere, fit a short leg walking cast. Continue protection until he has no pain when you spring his tibia and fibula together. As soon as his tibia is solid and no longer springy, remove the cast or gaiter.

If he has a short oblique fracture, expect it to heal more slowly due to the shearing stress. Remove his long leg cast at 8 weeks, and test for clinical union (69-4).

If clinical union is not present, apply a close fitting short leg cast, as in Fig. 81-4, for another 6 weeks.

If clinical union is present, apply another long leg walking cast for 6 weeks, or a Sarmiento short leg walking cast (81.5).

FRACTURES OF A SINGLE BONE

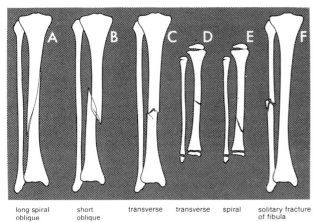

CHILDREN

long spiral oblique   short oblique   transverse   transverse   spiral   solitary fracture of fibula

Fig. 81-7 FRACTURES OF THE SHAFT OF A SINGLE BONE IN THE LOWER LEG. A, a long spiral oblique fracture heals readily. B, a short oblique fracture takes longest to heal. C, a transverse fracture. D, and E, transverse and spiral fractures of children. F, a fracture of the fibula only.

81.8 Fatigue fractures of the tibia

Bones need to get into training in the same ways as soft tissues. If they are repeatedly stressed without adequate training, they may break as 'fatigue fractures'. This can happen when an athlete starts sudden training, when a raw recruit starts marching, or when an invalid gets out of bed. Fatigue fractures start without any history of injury as microscopic lesions which steadily progress. The first symptoms are bone pain at night after heavy exercise, then pain after ordinary exercise, and finally bone pain during exercise. They are a common cause of undiagnosed pain in: (1) the tibia, (2) the metatarsals (especially the second and third), (3) the calcaneus, and (4) the neck of the femur.

The callus that forms presents as a tender bony lump, and the fracture may not be visible on X-rays for 5 weeks. When it does appear, the only signs may be slight periosteal elevation and increased density of the cancellous bone. The danger in these fractures is that they may be mistaken for tumours. No treatment is needed, apart from the protection of a plaster gaiter in the tibia.

81.9 Closed fractures of the shaft of the tibia in children

A child falls, and afterwards refuses to walk. He has few signs and you have to make the diagnosis from his history. X-rays usually show a long spiral fracture with little displacement, commonly in the lower half of his tibia. If the fracture is transverse it may be sufficiently displaced to need reducing.

INCOMPLETE FRACTURES Although neither reduction nor splinting is strictly necessary, apply a long leg walking cast (81.4), for 2 or 3 weeks, as described below, to relieve the child's pain and prevent his fracture from becoming complete.

COMPLETE FRACTURES **If there is no significant displacement,** apply a long leg walking cast. Anaesthesia is usually unnecessary. If he is too young to co-operate and is in much pain, give him ketamine.

If there is significant displacement, anaesthetize the child and reduce it.

Elevate the fracture above the level of his heart (Fig. 81-1), by raising his foot off his bed on pillows.

CAUTION ! Always split the cast, because nobody will watch the circulation in his foot carefully enough, especially during the night. There is no need to spread it (70-3), unless there are signs that the circulation in his leg is in danger.

As soon as the swelling has gone, renew or complete the cast by pulling its split edges together, and binding it round with a plaster bandage. Apply a walking heel, and allow him up with crutches. Let him bear his full weight on his leg as soon as pain allows.

Leave the cast on for 6 weeks. When you remove it, he will be unable to walk for the first few days, but full movements will then return quickly.

81.10 Closed fractures of the shaft of the fibula

A force applied to the outer side of the patient's leg can break his fibula transversely anywhere. His tibia remains intact, so there is either no displacement or only a little sideways shift. He is usually able to stand. The muscles of his leg cover the fracture, so that you need X-rays to confirm the diagnosis.

Reduction, splinting, and protection are unnecessary, so provided his ankle joint is normal (82.1), get him walking as soon as his soft tissue injury allows.

81.11 Closed fractures of both bones

In this fracture a patient twists his leg, and in doing so breaks both the bones in his lower leg obliquely, usually in their lower thirds. The fragments shift laterally, overlap, and rotate.

Treatment depends on whether or not there is shortening. If there is significant shortening, a week of calcaneal traction will reduce it. Many of the details described in the Section 81.12 on open fractures also apply to closed ones.

CLOSED FRACTURES OF THE TIBIA AND FIBULA
Admit the patient. He needs close observation, because his leg may swell severely.

WITHOUT SIGNIFICANT SHORTENING If there is swelling, or signs of threatened ischaemia, maintain the position of the fragments by applying: (1) Medial and lateral slabs from the patient's foot to his groin held on with crepe bandages. Or, (2) a temporary long leg cast split to allow swelling.

When the swelling has subsided, apply a long leg walking cast (81.4), or close the split in the cast he already has. If the fracture is oblique, take care to correct rotation. Then continue weight bearing on crutches. Review him and X-ray the fracture regularly. Wedge (70.7) and replace the cast as necessary. A closed transverse fracture should unite in 12 to 16 weeks. The last 8 weeks can be in a short leg cast, especially if it is a total contact one of the Sarmiento type (81.5).

WITH SIGNIFICANT SHORTENING The patient probably has an oblique fracture. Anaesthetize him. Apply medial and lateral slabs as above. Pass a Steinmann pin through his calcaneus (70.11) and rotate his leg to correct any external rotation.

Apply 5 kg traction, and raise the foot of his bed 25 cm to counteract it. Put a pillow longitudinally under his leg. This will hold his knee in a comfortable semiflexed position and prevent his heel from pressing on the bed uncomfortably.

Leave his leg in traction for a week, and treat its soft parts energetically meanwhile. Encourage him to move his toes, his ankle, and his knee. This period of traction will allow his soft tissues to heal.

After a week, remove the pin, apply a long leg cast, and encourage him to walk.

Leave the cast on for at least 8 weeks. Then remove it and examine his leg for signs of clinical union (Fig. 69-4).

If the fracture has united and is barely springy, apply a close fitting short leg cast (81.5) for 6 to 8 more weeks. Encourage him to walk normally.

If the fracture has not united, reapply a long leg cast and continue weight bearing for another 5 weeks, then apply a short leg cast.

81.12 Open fractures of both bones of the lower leg

Open fractures of the tibia and fibula are the commonest open fractures in man, and are one of the more unfortunate results of a traffic accident, particularly a motor cycle accident. They vary from a minor cut over a broken bone to the grossest mutilation, and displacement of the bony fragments. This is worst when the wheel of a car has run over a patient's leg, squashed his muscles, and torn his skin from the underlying fascia over a wide area (54.8). His fracture may be transverse or oblique, or comminuted into many widely scattered pieces.

These are dangerous fractures: (1) They are often infected and, if you allow gas gangrene to occur, they can be fatal. (2) They are often transverse, and pieces of bone may be lost, so that great care has to be taken to make them unite. (3) If treatment is prolonged, the patient may become very demoralized, and may be away from work so long that he loses his job. (4) Serious complications may occur later, including a stiff ankle, and foot drop.

Fortunately, the following method is satisfactory for most cases. A really thorough wound toilet is critical. After this, *you must leave the wound open unsutured until the danger of infection is over.* Never close it by immediate suture. As soon as it is safe to do so, apply a long leg cast and encourage the patient to walk. *The secret of success is early weight bearing while his leg is still in a cast, and while his skin wound is still incompletely healed.* Many severe injuries heal dramatically, even some of those which might at first seem to need a bone graft.

LEAVE THE PATIENT'S WOUND UNSUTURED UNTIL THE DANGER OF INFECTION IS OVER
NEVER ATTEMPT PRIMARY SUTURE OVER AN OPEN FRACTURE
EARLY WEIGHT BEARING IS ESSENTIAL

If a patient's skin and muscles have been widely damaged, his leg will swell severely. Applying a cast too soon is dangerous,

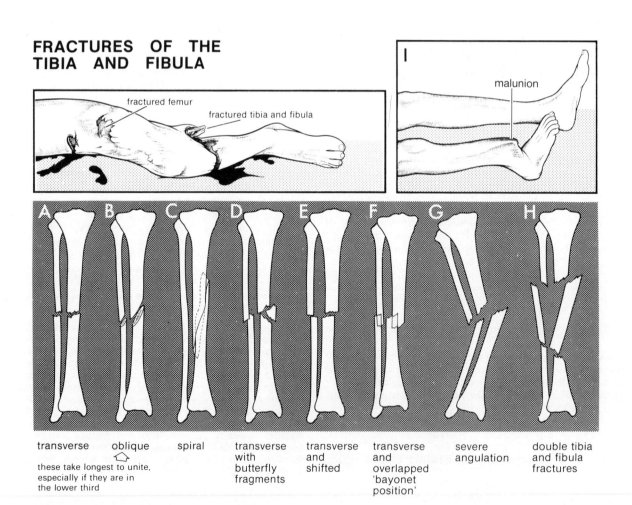

FRACTURES OF THE TIBIA AND FIBULA

fractured femur

fractured tibia and fibula

malunion

| A | B | C | D | E | F | G | H |

| transverse | oblique | spiral | transverse with butterfly fragments | transverse and shifted | transverse and overlapped 'bayonet position' | severe angulation | double tibia and fibula fractures |

these take longest to unite, especially if they are in the lower third

Fig. 81-8 FRACTURES OF THE SHAFTS OF BOTH THE BONES OF THE LOWER LEG. A, transverse, B, oblique and C, spiral fractures. D, a transverse fragment with a butterfly (triangular) fragment. E, a transverse shifted fracture. F, the fragments are in a bayonet position.

Never leave a fracture like this. H, double fractures of both bones. I, shows the malunion that may result if a fracture like G is inadequately treated.

so admit him to allow the swelling to subside, and his soft tissues to start healing, before you apply it. If you apply a cast immediately and discharge him, he may return in great pain 24 hours later with the compartment syndrome (73.7).

Two periods of treatment are necessary. The first is a period of *provisional treatment* during which the spread of infection is prevented by a thorough wound toilet. After this you can leave the patient's wound open to the air to allow drainage, to reduce the risk of sepsis, and to prevent gas gangrene. Antibiotics are no substitute for an adequate wound toilet. Close his wound a few days later by delayed primary suture or skin grafting. Apply a cast and start the period of *definitive treatment* as soon as: (1) the danger of gas gangrene is over, (2) most of the swelling has gone, and (3) most of his wound (not necessarily all of it) has been covered by skin. He is usually ready for a cast at 5 to 17 days; his skin wound will continue to heal while he is walking about in it. If his soft tissues have not been widely damaged, you can apply a long leg cast immediately, as described below, but this is not so easy, nor so safe.

The first step in reducing an open tibial fracture is to get the fragments into the best position you can through the open skin wound during the wound toilet. After that you can control their position in one of the two ways: (1) You can apply a temporary plaster and bivalve it (70.3), so that you can inspect and treat the patient's wound. Or, (2) you can apply traction with a Steinmann pin through his calcaneus, or just above his malleoli. A pin through his calcaneus: (a) corrects even severe displacement, (b) does not obstruct the circulation in his leg, (c) leaves his wound open for inspection and treatment, and (d) requires that the foot of his bed be raised. This is useful, because it helps to reduce swelling at the fracture site. The main disadvantage of a pin through the calcaneus is the remote possibility of osteomyelitis (7.13). There is less risk of this if you put the pin through his lower tibia, but traction there is less well placed mechanically, and it may pull the lower fragment of his tibia up into the wound, as in A, Fig. 81-9.

Treat the patient rather than his X-ray, and aim for a leg which works, rather than for a beautiful film. This method needs good plaster technique, and sometimes careful wedging (70.7). He may need much encouragement to make him walk in his cast, especially if he can feel his broken bones grating against one another with each step he takes. Persuade your nurses to encourage him to do this. If they fail, persuade him yourself.

**A THOROUGH WOUND TOILET IS CRITICAL
GET HIM WALKING EARLY IN A CAST**

Brown P.W. and Urban J.G. Early weight bearing the treatment of open fractures of the tibia. Journal of Bone Joint Surgery. 1969;51A:59-75

Nicoll E.A. Fractures of the Tibial Shaft. Journal of Bone and Joint Surgery, 1964;46B:373.

OPEN FRACTURES OF THE TIBIA AND FIBULA

This section applies to any fracture over which there is any skin wound, or skin which looks as if it might break down.

Have you felt the patient's dorsalis pedis and posterior tibial pulses and tested the sensation in his toes?

Admit him. He needs careful observation. Give him penicillin, and tetanus prophylaxis (54.11). For the use of broad spectrum antibiotics, see Sections 2.7 and 54.1.

PROVISIONAL TREATMENT FOR OPEN TIBIAL FRACTURES

Resuscitate and anaesthetize the patient, give him a general or a subarachnoid (spinal) anaesthetic (7.4), or ketamine (A 8.2).

TWO KINDS OF PROVISIONAL TRACTION

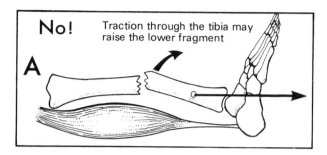

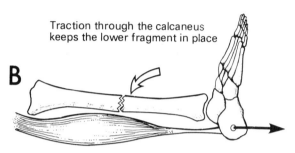

Fig. 81-9 TWO METHODS OF PROVISIONAL TRACTION FOR TIBIA FRACTURES. A, traction through the lower tibia may pull the lower fragment out of the wound. B, traction through the calcaneus keeps the lower fragment in place, but if osteomyelitis occurs it will be very troublesome. *After Charnley with kind permission.*

THE EARLY WOUND TOILET must be thorough (54.1). If necessary, apply a tourniquet.

Scrub the skin around the patient's wound with water, soap, and a soft nail brush, to remove all ingrained dirt. Sponge his wound clean. Pour plenty of water over it, and if it is severely contaminated, syringe it forcibly with saline.

Prepare the skin of his leg with an antiseptic solution, as for any surgical operation. Drape it and do a careful surgical toilet. If the tissue is tense, incise the fascial planes to prevent the compartment syndrome and minimise the risk of gas gangrene (54.13). Remove any dirt–encrusted fat and muscle. Excise a millimetre or two of skin from the edges of the wound.

If there are any loose bone fragments, leave them, especially if they have any attached periosteum. They may settle down and act as a bone graft. If the wound becomes infected, remove them at your next wound toilet.

When the whole of his wound is surgically clean, take off the tourniquet. Stop bleeding with packs (3.1), and the minimum number of the fine ligatures. Cover it with sterile gauze for delayed closure, or delayed skin grafting later. Some surgeons use hypochlorite pressure dressings.

CAUTION ! (1) Don't close his open wound by primary suture. (2) Avoid relaxing incisions, rotation flaps, and pedicle grafts as primary procedures.

EARLY TREATMENT OF THE FRACTURE Immediately the wound toilet is complete, and while the patient is still anaesthetized, reduce the fracture as best you can. Bringing the fragments into contact with one another is more important than correcting angulation, because you can correct this later while the bone ends are still sticky.

If his fracture is transverse, try to get as much as possible of the diameters of the fragments to touch one another. Even if they only touch over part of their circumference, this will be useful. Bringing them into contact can be difficult if there is soft tissue between them. Don't leave them in the bayonet position, as in F, Fig. 81-8. If reducing overlap is difficult, insert a periosteal elevator or some other suitable instrument between the bone ends, and lever them into position.

If you cannot get enough traction on the patient's foot to reduce the fragments, insert a Steinmann pin temporarily in his calcaneus and exert traction on this. Do this now while he is still in the theatre.

CAUTION ! In a transverse fracture avoid any end to end distraction, no matter how slight, it is the great enemy of union.

If his fracture is oblique or comminuted, calcaneal traction (see below) is particularly useful. You may be unable to prevent mild overlap. Some separation of the fragments is inevitable, but they will unite slowly.

If a pointed fragment of bone is sticking through the patient's skin and you cannot easily reduce it, nibble it away.

Dress his wound, then splint his leg with medial and lateral slabs, held on with crepe bandages. This will let you inspect and treat it by unwrapping them.

CAUTION ! (1) If his soft tissue injury is severe, remember the possibility of gas gangrene (54.13). Beware, especially, of fever, pain, a rising pulse, and a falling blood pressure. (2) Watch also for signs of the compartment syndrome (81.14)—severe pain, inability to move his toes, and numb toes.

THREE DAYS LATER Open up the dressings and look at the patient's wound; there are several possibilities.

If his wound looks clean, and you can close it without tension, consider delayed primary suture.

If his wound looks clean, but you cannot close it without tension, graft it with split skin (57.2). You may need to repeat this on about the eighth and if necessary again on the thirteenth day. Don't try grafting until there are good granulations to put the graft on. Don't let him start weight bearing until the graft has taken.

If his wound is very dirty, toilet it again surgically in the theatre.

DEFINITIVE TREATMENT FOR OPEN TIBIAL FRACTURES

FIT A LONG LEG WALKING CAST When the patient's wound is mostly closed by skin, or a graft is taking, usually at 14 to 17 days, fit him with a long leg walking cast (81.4). The swelling will have subsided, so there is no need to split it. Even so, watch the circulation in his foot carefully.

Put a dressing over his wound, but preferably don't window the cast (70.7). Inspect his wound when the cast needs changing.

Apply the cast with his ankle in 10° of dorsiflexion, unless this position causes posterior angulation of the fragments, as it may do in a lower third fracture when a piece of the tibia is comminuted anteriorly.

If dorsiflexion does cause posterior angulation, leave his foot in equinus, but fit a stirrup as in Fig 81-11, or a high enough walking heel (81.3). If possible, raise his opposite shoe. Make the cast strong enough to last 6 to 8 weeks.

Raise his leg for 12 hours after fitting the cast.

TEMPORARY CALCANEAL TRACTION

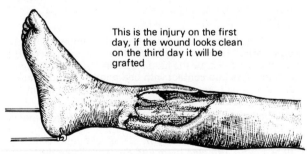

This is the injury on the first day, if the wound looks clean on the third day it will be grafted

fragments approximately aligned

Fig. 81-10 PROVISIONAL TRACTION FOR AN OPEN TIBIAL FRACTURE. This is useful if the bone is very comminuted, but don't apply it for more than 2 weeks. *Kindly contributed by Peter Bewes.*

EARLY WALKING FOR OPEN TIBIAL FRACTURES The next day allow the cast to rest on the floor. Give the patient crutches and encourage him to walk on his broken leg, bearing as much weight as he can tolerate. Let him gradually increase the weight he bears on his cast, but don't push him to the point of pain. If he feels crepitus, or he feels the fragments are moving, tell him to persist. Explain that this is normal and will help his bones to unite.

CAUTION ! Early walking is critical to the success of this method.

In the early days, when he is not walking, tell him to keep his leg raised. This will minimize swelling and make it more comfortable.

When he is bearing nearly all his weight on his injured leg, exchange his crutches for a stick. Most patients reach full weight bearing in a few weeks, and some within a few days.

Send him home when he is walking well. Review him in 3 weeks. Make sure he is walking properly, and his plaster is in good condition.

IF NECESSARY, CONTROL ANGULATION If an adult's fracture is angulated more than 5° in any direction, correct it by renewing the plaster or, less safely, if plaster bandages are scarce, by careful wedging (70.7). Don't do this immediately. The best time is usually at 3 to 4 weeks in an adult, and sooner in a child. Be sure you do it while the patient's bone ends are still sticky, and before they have united.

Use an opening wedge a little above the fracture, so that pressure does not increase over it. If his leg is angulated in two planes, you may be able to control it with one wedge, or you may need two. This may make the cast look ugly, but it will improve the final look of his leg.

CAUTION! Don't try to wedge a cast more than once—change it. The risk of pressure sores is too great.

DRESSINGS Change the dressings when you change the cast. This is better than repeatedly changing them through a window.

CHANGING A LONG LEG CAST IN AN OPEN TIBIAL FRACTURE If the cast is snug and comfortable, leave it for 5 to 8 weeks. Change it earlier if it becomes loose or uncomfortable, because the position of reduction is easily lost inside a loose cast. If plaster bandages are scarce, you may be able to cut a longitudinal strip out of a loose cast and close it up. Change it if pus or blood soaks through excessively and stinks unbearably. A patient may need as few as 3 casts or as many as 15. He will probably need about 6.

TEST FOR CLINICAL UNION At 5 to 8 weeks, remove the cast and examine the patient's fracture for signs of clinical union (Fig. 69-4). If you are in doubt, X-ray it and renew the cast. Don't discard a full length cast until: (1) The patient can walk without crutches, and (2) there are signs of clinical union as shown by: (a) no tenderness at the fracture site, and (b) mature bridging callus in the X-ray. The clinical signs are more important than the X-ray. Don't leave a long leg cast on too long, because it will prevent him from bending his knee, and make it stiff. Fit a short leg cast as soon as you can.

Spiral or transverse fractures reach clinical union more quickly, usually in about 12 weeks in adults, especially if a patient starts weight bearing early. A short oblique fracture usually takes 12 to 16 weeks to unite, but it may occasionally take a year or more, especially in the lower third of the leg where delayed union is a particular danger, *and particularly if you unwisely treated it in prolonged traction!*

A SHORTER CAST As soon as there is good clinical union, give the patient a shorter cast. If a middle third fracture of his tibia is now firm, give him a well padded plaster gaiter (81.6), or a Sarmiento total contact cast (81.5), because fractures here need less protection than they do elsewhere. If his fracture is anywhere else in his tibia, apply a Sarmiento cast which includes his foot. Keep him walking and gradually increase his range of activities.

CAUTION ! Pain and tenderness over a fracture site are signs that clinical union is not yet complete, so continue to protect his fracture in a short leg cast.

A STEINMANN PIN TO STOP A SHORT LEG CAST ROTATING
A long leg cast is heavy, and because it prevents a patient bending his knee, he cannot easily turn himself in bed, so it makes nursing difficult. A long leg cast is thus contraindicated: (1) if he is old, or (2) if he has other serious injuries, such as a femoral or malleolar fracture.

Under these conditions apply a short leg walking cast and prevent rotation by incorporating a Steinmann pin in it. Insert the pin *obliquely* 1.5 to 2 cm distal to his tibial tuberosity (70.11). Make sure the cast allows him to bend his knee. Don't allow him to bear weight on on the cast while the pin is in it, because the pin may break. Remove the pin as soon as is practical, so as to allow him to bear weight on the fragments of his tibia.

TEMPORARY CALCANEAL OR LOWER TIBIAL TRACTION TO ALIGN THE FRAGMENTS If a fracture is very comminuted, or a patient's wound needs repeated toileting, traction may be useful to hold the fragments approximately in place during the first week or two only.

Insert a Steinmann or a Denham pin through the patient's calcaneus, or his lower tibia just above his ankle; apply 5 to 7 kg traction, and raise the foot of his bed 25 cm. This will align his leg and make him comfortable. Don't leave the pin in for longer than is necessary, preferably not more than 2 weeks. Keep him exercising his foot while he is on traction; this will reduce oedema and minimize stiffness. When the fragments have become sticky enough to stay in place on their own, remove the traction, allow his leg to shorten to a stable position, and then apply a long leg cast.

CAUTION ! (1) Don't apply so much weight as to produce distraction at the fracture site or endanger the blood supply of the patient's leg. (2) Don't apply traction to a cast unless you have put a pin into his tibia and incorporated this in the cast, because it is almost certain to cause a slough on the dorsum of his foot.

USING A BOHLER–BRAUN FRAME This can be used for provisional treatment, and is shown in Fig. 79-10. After the first few days it is much less effective than early mobility in a long leg walking cast.

APPLYING A LONG LEG CAST IMMEDIATELY **If a patient's soft tissue injury is minimal,** some surgeons apply a long leg cast without a period of provisional treatment. If you are inexperienced, this is a method to be applied with extreme caution.

After the wound toilet, align the fragments with the patient's lower leg hanging over the end of the table. Sit, and rest his foot on your knee, adjusting the height of the table to make this possible. Study the X-ray and manipulate the fragments into position.

EXTERNAL FIXATION WITH TWO STEINMANN PINS If a patient has a severe soft tissue injury, you may be able to apply two Steinmann pins, one well above and one well below the fracture, and incorporate these in a cast, if necessary with a window, and get him walking. Later, you may be able to remove the bottom pin and mould the cast around his ankle. This will minimize shortening, but union may be slower than if you accept it, and treat him as above.

81.13 Difficulties with fractures of the tibia

If a piece of a patient's tibia is missing, treatment depends on how much is missing, and where. Try to make the broken ends of the tibia impact. *Making the bone ends touch is more important than maintaining length.*

DIFFICULTIES WITH OPEN TIBIAL FRACTURES

If a patient's FOOT IS SO SEVERELY INJURED that you are thinking about amputation, preserve it if it still has a pulse and normal sensation. Provided you do a thorough wound toilet and avoid the danger of gas gangrene, you can, if

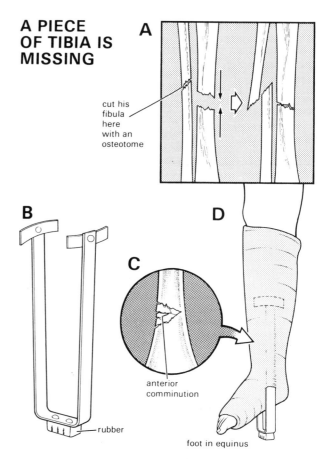

A PIECE OF TIBIA IS MISSING

cut his fibula here with an osteotome

anterior comminution

rubber

foot in equinus

Fig. 81-11 A PIECE OF TIBIA IS MISSING. A, if a piece of the patient's tibia is missing anteriorly, his fibula will probably be broken also, so you can let the fragments of his fibula over ride one another and push those of his tibia together. If his fibula is intact, cut it. B, C, and D, if his tibia is comminuted anteriorly, fit him with a stirrup with his foot in the equinus position. If you don't have a stirrup, fit a wooden block under his heel. *Kindly contributed by John Stewart.*

necessary, amputate later. Raise his leg, keep it cool, with ice if possible, and resuscitate him meanwhile. Even the severest bony injury is never by itself an indication for amputation.

If a small PIECE OF TIBIA IS MISSING, it will probably heal adequately.

If his tibia is intact posteriorly, but a PIECE OF TIBIA IS MISSING ANTERIORLY, the lower fragment is in danger of bending forwards, so refer him. If this is impossible, prevent forward angulation by putting his foot into plaster in equinus, as in Fig. 81-11, until the comminuted area has stabilized. Fit a metal stirrup on it instead of a walking heel. This will let him walk on his injured leg, even though his ankle is in equinus.

If LESS THAN 3 cm OF TIBIA IS MISSING, wait for the wound to heal, and for the patient's skin to become clean. If his fibula has not already been broken by the injury, make a separate lateral incision far enough above or below his tibial fracture to leave some stability at the fracture site. Cut his fibula obliquely with a sharp osteotome. Push the ends of his tibia together, so that the fragments of his fibula overlap. If absolutely necessary, you can remove a piece of fibula. Apply a long leg cast and get him walking and weight bearing as soon as possible. His tibia will unite, but it will take several months. If necessary, raise his shoe to compensate for shortening.

If MORE THAN 3 cm OF TIBIA IS MISSING, apply calcaneal traction, but don't try to maintain its full length. Traction will stabilize his leg and make a wound toilet easier. Refer him for an operation in which cancellous bone chips or part of his fibula is used to bridge the missing portion. When this is done, his fibula may hypertrophy surprisingly. If referral is impossible, you will have to treat him as above.

CAUTION ! Don't attempt any early bone nibbling to remove supposed dead or infected bone. Instead, encourage early weight bearing, and hope that the patient's tibia will unite posteriorly. Then, do any bone nibbling that is needed.

If PUS GATHERS IN HIS WOUND, it fails to heal, and his tibia fails to unite, open the wound widely so that it can drain. Remember that wounds drain by gravity so that the bottom of a pus pocket must be open. Infection may be caused by an inadequate wound toilet or by dead bone. Continue irrigating and toileting the wound as necessary. As soon as it is reasonably clean, put him into a long leg cast and get him walking.

If OSTEOMYELITIS occurs, X-ray the fracture and look for sequestra. If you find them, take the patient to the theatre, remove all pieces of dead bone, irrigate his wound, and provide dependant drainage, or, better, suction drainage. Alternatively, raise his leg on a Böhler–Braun splint, and apply calcaneal traction. Lay a catheter alongside the wound, or use the tube of a drip set with multiple holes cut in it. Irrigate his wound with saline (the addition of penicillin is optional), and let it drip into a basin underneath the splint. Sterile saline is expensive, so you may have to use clean tap water and salt. Irrigation needs much care and attention, and will require all the nursing skills you have. Later, reapply the cast, keep the patient walking, and change the cast when it becomes soft, or stinks excessively.

If GAS GANGRENE occurs, immediate amputation may be necessary to save the patient's life. Treat it as in Section 54.13. The way to prevent it is: (1) to explore and excise his wound properly, (2) to open up all the fascial spaces where pressure could build up, and (3) to lay his wound open without an encircling cast after you have explored it.

If there is DEAD BONE at the bottom of an infected wound, you may be able to remove it without anaesthesia, as in B Fig. 81-12, because bone is insensitive. Use a bone gauge or chisel, and hammer, to remove any bone which looks white and does not become pink or bleed, and especially any exposed bone, until you get to healthy bleeding bone. Later, when granulations have appeared, graft it, as in Section 57.2. Don't remove too much bone, or you will weaken the patient's tibia. Removing it to a depth of 1 or 2 mm is usually enough. Let the patient carry on walking, and look at his wound a week later. If any exposed bone remains, repeat the process. Go on doing this until healing is complete.

If a patient's TIBIA HAS NOT UNITED after 16 weeks, don't be alarmed. Fractures of the upper third of the tibia usually unite quite easily. It is fractures of the lower third that often don't. Even so, most of them unite by 16 weeks, but some take a year or even 2 years. Give him 6 months to unite in a *well fitted* short leg walking cast (81.5). If there is no union at 6

months consider referring him. If his tibia has not united in a year, he will probably need bone grafting. Here are some reasons for non–union. Faulty treatment may be to blame.

He did not exercise his broken leg enough. The fibula unites quickly, and may hold the two ends of his tibia apart, and so prevent them from uniting. Prevent this by teaching him to contract the muscles of his foot, and get him walking as soon as possible. Each step he makes will help his broken tibia to unite. Unfortunately, his other injuries may prevent early exercise.

His tibia was extensively injured. In severe open fractures, in which large bone fragments have protruded through the skin and been stripped of their periosteum, much of the injured bone dies. The callus that forms has to cross a wider gap, so that union and consolidation take longer, and the risk of non–union is greater.

You applied too much traction, or tried internal fixation under unsatisfactory conditions. Both of these errors will delay union, especially if a patient has been discouraged from walking early.

His wound has become infected. Infection delays union greatly, particularly if pus has accumulated because you have not opened up the patient's tissues and allowed it to drain freely through his open wound.

His ankle was immobilized in equinus without the application of a stirrup. When this has happened he cannot put his foot to the ground without bending the callus around his fracture, and causing hinging stresses which lead to healing with fibrous tissue, rather than with bone. Either immoblize his ankle in neutral, or if you have to immobilize it in equinus, fit the cast with a stirrup.

If there is MALUNION, it can take several forms:

(1) Shortening is usually minimal and unimportant (78.1). If the patient is fortunate enough to wear shoes, you can compensate for a loss of up to 4 cm by raising the heel of one of them, and lowering the heel of the other one.

(2) Angulation is serious and unnecessary. Prevent it by: (a) aligning the fragments carefully to begin with, (b) wedging or changing the patient's cast early (70.7), and (c) making sure that when he starts weight bearing, he does so in a cast which fully supports the fracture. It is not the weight bearing that causes the malunion, it is improper casting—not having a snug cast. Valgus or varus malunions are more serious than backward or forward bowing, because he can compensate for them less easily.

(3) Rotation deformities in which a patient's foot points inwards or outwards are also serious. Prevent them by making sure that his foot points in the same direction relative to his patella on the injured side as it does on the normal one (Fig. 81-2).

If his SKIN WILL NOT HEAL COMPLETELY over the front of his tibia, despite one or two skin grafts, forget this for the present, and keep him walking in a cast. Remove the cast after 5 to 6 weeks, and look at the wound. It will probably have healed.

If HIS FOOT SWELLS and he is in a cast, bring him into hospital overnight. Let him sleep with his foot raised. The following day *before you allow him out of bed* apply a new cast which fits properly.

If he has been in a cast for many weeks, his foot is sure to swell when it is removed. If necessary, compress it with an elastic bandage, elevate his leg at night, and continue to exercise it.

If a patient's FOOT IS STIFF AND PAINFUL, there is little you can do. There is always some stiffness, especially after a fracture of the lower third of the tibia, due to scar tissue forming around the extensor tendons. The preventable causes include the tragedy of Volkmann's contracture (70.4), or unnecessarily applying a cast with the patient's foot in equinus.

If he CANNOT DORSIFLEX HIS ANKLE (foot drop): (1) He might have injured his common peroneal nerve at the time of the accident, so when you first see him, ask him to dorsiflex his foot so that you can test the sensation on its dorsum, and record your findings. (2) His common peroneal nerve may also have been injured by a cast, especially if it was not

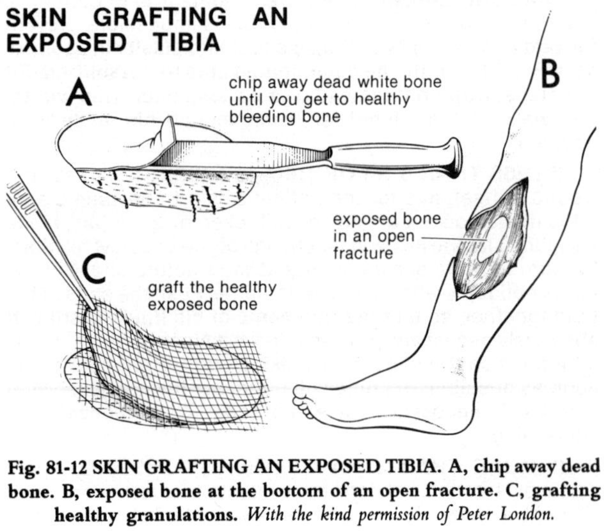

SKIN GRAFTING AN EXPOSED TIBIA

Fig. 81-12 SKIN GRAFTING AN EXPOSED TIBIA. A, chip away dead bone. B, exposed bone at the bottom of an open fracture. C, grafting healthy granulations. *With the kind permission of Peter London.*

padded around the neck of his fibula. If his paralysis persists, he will need a brace to support his foot. (3) In the early days pressure in the anterior compartment of his leg can prevent him from raising his foot. If this happens, decompress his leg urgently as described in Section 81.14.

DON'T LET A PATIENT WALK ABOUT IN A LOOSE CAST, OR THE FRAGMENTS WILL MOVE OUT OF POSITION

DON'T GIVE UP HOPE TOO EARLY

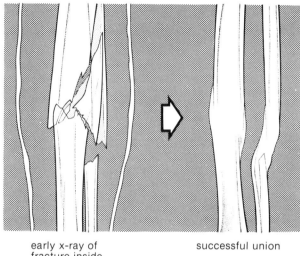

early x-ray of
fracture inside
a cast

successful union

Fig. 81-13 DON'T GIVE UP HOPE TOO EARLY; this comminuted fracture healed well after 28 weeks walking in a cast. *Kindly contributed by John Stewart.*

BRING THE ENDS OF THE PATIENT'S TIBIA TOGETHER

81.14 The compartment syndrome in the leg

If a patient with a lower leg injury: (1) has severe pain, (2) cannot move his toes, or (3) has numb toes, be careful. These are signs of the compartment syndrome which can be followed by Volkmann's ischaemic contracture, as in the arm (70.4). A normal pulse and apparently normal filling of his nail beds do not exclude it. When a patient's fracture is reduced his pain should become less. *Severe postoperative pain is thus the critical early sign.*

There are four musclar compartments in the lower leg, separated from one another by strong fascia: (1) The lateral compartment contains a patient's peroneal muscles. (2) The anterior compartment contains the extensor muscles of his ankle and toes. (3) The superficial part of the posterior compartment contains his gastrocnemius and soleus muscles. (4) The deep posterior compartment contains his deep flexors. After a fracture, or even after bruising of his lower leg, blood and oedema fluid may collect in all, or any, of these compartments under such pressure that the circulation to his foot is obstructed. Unless you immediately open up each compartment in turn through a

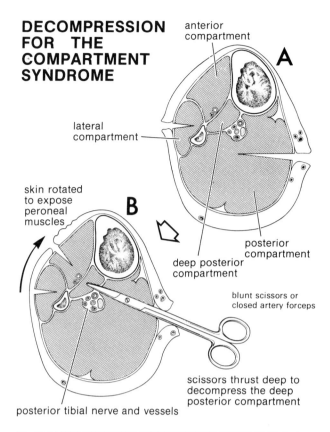

DECOMPRESSION FOR THE COMPARTMENT SYNDROME

Fig. 81-14 TREATING THE COMPARTMENT SYNDROME. A, incisions for the lateral and posterior compartments. B, opening up the deep posterior compartment. This diagram also shows how you can slide the skin incision you have used to open the lateral compartment forwards, so that you can also open the anterior compartment through it. *Kindly contributed by Peter Bewes.*

generous longitudinal incision, Volkmann's ischaemic contracture or gangrene may follow. The after effects of a fasciotomy are minimal, but ischaemic muscle never recovers.

THE COMPARTMENT SYNDROME

If a patient with an injured lower leg complains of severe pain, or cannot move his toes, believe him. If his leg is in a cast, split it, spread it, and elevate his leg. If this does not rapidly relieve his symptoms, remove the cast. If his symptoms persist, proceed urgently with fasciotomy.

WHICH COMPARTMENT ? Stretching an ischaemic muscle causes pain so:

If flexing his foot and toes causes pain, his anterior compartment is ischaemic.

If extending his foot and toes causes pain, his posterior compartment is ischaemic.

FASCIOTOMY FOR THE COMPARTMENT SYNDROME

Medial incision Make a longitudinal 15 cm incision on the medial side of the patient's leg. Cut through the deep fascia from his knee to his ankle. Incise the turgid, dark, reddish blue, ischaemic muscle of his posterior compartment.

Lateral incision Make a similar 15 cm longitudinal incision on the outer side of his leg. Incise the fascia and the muscle directly underneath it, and decompress his peroneal compartment.

Slide the skin incision anteriorly over the subcutaneous tissue, as shown by the arrow in B, Fig. 81-14, and incise the muscle under it so as to decompress his anterior tibial compartment. This will enable you to decompress both compartments through the same incision.

If the circulation returns to his foot, **no further incisions are necessary.**

If the circulation does not return to his foot in a few minutes, deepen the medial incision to open up his deep posterior compartment. Push scissors deeply into it and open the blades, as if you were exploring an abscess by Hilton's method (Fig. 5-3). Don't use a knife in the depths, or you may cut his posterior tibial artery, or his tibial nerve.

If he has a fracture, treat this by calcaneal traction until definitive treatment is possible later.

CAUTION ! Don't apply a cast until the swelling has subsided.

LATER TREATMENT The compartments cannot be closed after these incisions, so leave them wide open, covered with gauze. They will close as the swelling subsides. If necessary, close the wound with a skin graft, or delayed primary suture.

82 The ankle

82.1 Introduction and examination

Ankle injuries are common and commonly mismanaged. They include minor sprains, disabling tears of the collateral ligaments, usually the lateral one, serious malleolar fracture dislocations, and ruptures of the Achilles tendon. Occasionally, a child displaces his lower femoral epiphysis.

EXAMINING THE FOOT AND ANKLE

Is the patient's foot normally aligned with his leg? Is it internally or externally rotated, everted, inverted or swollen? Is one malleolus abnormally prominent, or his heel displaced backwards? (malleolar fracture). Is his heel abnormally broad? (fractured calcaneus).

Can he walk normally on his heels? This tests the power of his dorsiflexors. Can he walk on the balls of his feet (his metatarsal heads)? He can only do this if his calf muscles and his Achilles tendon are normal.

A NORMAL AND A SPRAINED ANKLE

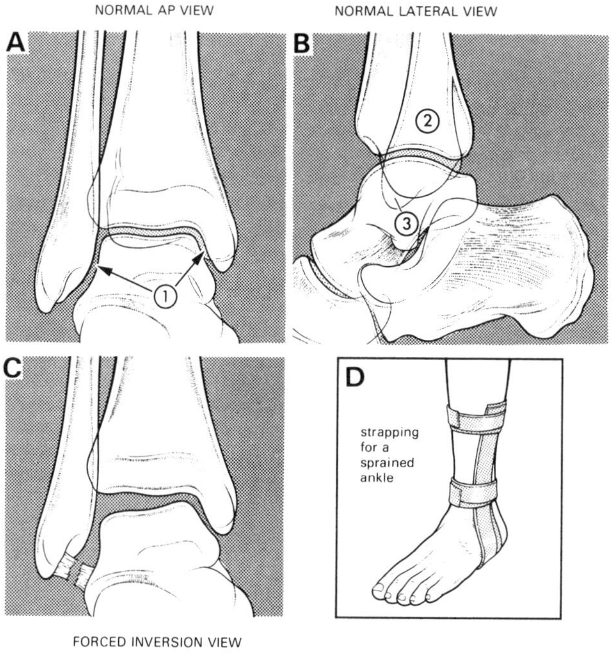

NORMAL AP VIEW   NORMAL LATERAL VIEW

FORCED INVERSION VIEW

Fig. 82-1 A NORMAL AND A FORCED INVERSION VIEW TO SHOW RUPTURE OF THE LATERAL COLLATERAL LIGAMENT. If a normal ankle has been X-rayed correctly: (1) you should be able to see the joint space between the patient's talus and both his malleoli simultaneously in the AP view. This will only be possible if it is taken in 20° of internal rotation. (2) In a lateral view his fibula should lie just within the posterior border of his tibia. (3) You should just be able to see the lower end of his fibula outlined against his talus. Note how even the normal joint space is, and how congruous the joint surfaces are in a normal ankle. A common error is not to take the X-ray in 20° of internal rotation. C, shows a forced inversion view showing a rupture of the lateral collateral ligament. D, shows how to apply strapping for a sprain. Kindly contributed by John Stewart.

Ask him to point to the site of the pain. Feel for the exact site of tenderness. Palpate his two malleoli, and the medial and lateral ligaments of his ankle. Abnormal inversion, and tenderness below his lateral ligament suggest that it is sprained or ruptured. If tenderness is maximal over a malleolus, it is probably fractured.

Feel his tarsal and metatarsal bones, and especially the base of the fifth. Feel his calcaneus between your fingers and thumb.

How far can the patient flex and extend his ankle? How far can you or he invert or evert his heel on his ankle? This tests the movement of his subtalar joint. Examine it further by grasping his heel with one hand and his lower tibia with the other. Move his injured ankle from side to side and compare it with the movement of his normal one.

Palpate the subcutaneous surface of his tibia, and 'spring' his fibula against it.

If he has no signs of an acute injury, and he can walk, watch him do so. Does he limp? Is his heel and toe strike normal? Remove his socks and shoes, and observe how his shoes are worn.

X-RAYS are unnecessary if he can walk normally bearing his full weight.

If you are going to X-ray him, decide if you want X-rays of his ankle or his foot.

If his ankle is injured, take an AP view in 20° of internal rotation to compensate for the external rotation of a normal ankle. Also take a true lateral view.

If you are worried about the integrity of one of his collateral ligaments, especially the lateral one, take forced inversion views.

If his foot is injured, take an AP, a lateral, and an oblique view of his foot.

If you suspect he might have injured his calcaneus, ask for a special axial view of it.

There are many variations in the structure of the foot, including many accessory ossicles, which you can confuse with fractures. His other foot will probably show the same anomaly, so, if you are in doubt, X-ray that too.

82.2 Sprained and torn ankle ligaments

A sprain tears only some of the fibres of a collateral ligament, usually the lateral one. A sprained ankle is swollen, and its collateral ligament is tender. Although a patient with a sprained ankle may walk with difficulty, his ankle will eventually recover, even if you do nothing. But if the lateral ligament of his ankle is completely torn, and is not correctly managed, his ankle will be unstable and cause difficulty when he walks on rough ground. Ruptures of the lateral ligament are often missed because the talus tilts over temporarily and then returns to its normal position, *so that the ordinary AP and lateral films look normal.* The critical test is to ask the patient to walk. If he cannot walk after an ankle injury, suspect some more serious injury than a minor sprain. X-ray his foot to exclude a fracture, and test the stability of the ligaments of his ankle. If the diagnosis is seriously in doubt, X-ray his ankle in the same position of forced inversion which caused the original injury. If you are still in doubt, over-treatment is probably better than undertreatment.

SPRAINS AND TEARS OF THE ANKLE LIGAMENTS

This section describes the care of the common injuries of the lateral collateral ligament. Treat the rarer injuries of the medial (deltoid) ligament in a similar way.

If you are not certain if one of a patient's collateral ligaments is sprained or torn, take a forced inversion (or ever-sion) X-ray. These are only rarely needed.

FORCED INVERSION X-RAY Give the patient an analgesic, such as pethidine. Some radiologists inject 2% lignocaine into the haematoma around the ankle. Forcibly invert his ankle while you take an AP X-ray. If his lateral ligament is completely ruptured, the joint will open up as shown in C, Fig. 82-1.

THE TREATMENT OF SPRAINED AND TORN ANKLE LIGAMENTS

If a patient's lateral ligament is not ruptured, and there is only minor swelling, apply adhesive strapping and encourage him to walk normally.

If his lateral ligament is not ruptured, but there is more severe swelling, apply a below–knee walking cast with his ankle in neutral and his foot in slight eversion. Encourage him to walk in the cast. As soon as he feels that his cast is loose when he gets up in the morning, ask him to come and have it changed. This must be done while the swelling is down. If necessary admit him for a night so that his leg can be elevated. Leave the cast on for 3 to 6 weeks.

If his lateral ligament is ruptured with wide opening of his ankle joint, treat him in a below–knee walking cast as above, but leave the cast on for 6 to 10 weeks, so that his torn liga-ment can unite.

After removing the cast, apply a crepe bandage or adhesive strapping, and encourage him to walk without a limp. By walk-ing normally he uses his muscles normally, which strengthens both them and his ankle (77.1). If he limps, he uses some muscles excessively and others not at all. The muscles which are not used waste, and this may make his ankle unstable permanently.

If his ankle becomes permanently unstable, repair may be possible, so refer him.

A NEGLECTED TORN LIGAMENT IS AS SERIOUS AS A FRACTURE

82.3 Malleolar fractures classified

Hippocrates had difficulty treating these fractures, so has everyone who has treated them ever since, and so will you. *Displaced malleolar fractures are major injuries, and are often not taken seriously enough.* If you don't treat a patient correctly, he will be disabled for life by a stiff, painful equinus ankle, like that in Fig. 82-2, and may need a difficult arthrodesis to give him a useful foot.

When a patient sustains one of these injuries, his foot remains fixed on the ground in an abnormal position, while his body continues onwards. The position of his foot and the movement of his body relative to it, determine how the bones of his ankle will break and its ligaments tear. This is the basis of the most meaningful classification of these fractures. The movements of the foot are complex, and similar to those in the hand. Supina-tion combines inward rotation of the forefoot with inversion of the hindfoot. Pronation combines outward rotation of the forefoot and eversion of the hindfoot. If a patient's foot locks, either in extreme supination, or in extreme pronation, it becomes a rigid inflexible structure, and readily breaks at his ankle when a force is applied between it and his leg.

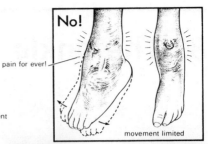

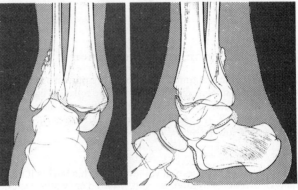

Fig. 82-2 A VERY BADLY MANAGED MALLEOLAR FRACTURE. The patient's foot is in equinus, and the little movement she has is about this position. This makes walking impossible, except with a crutch, and is a very great disability. Her fracture should have been reduced and put in a malleolar cast; instead, she was given a backslab and not prevented from walking on it.

There are four groups of fractures with several stages within each group.

Supination–external rotation fractures are the most com-mon. The patient's foot remains supinated on the ground, while his body and leg continue to move in such a way that his foot rotates externally on his leg. The first thing that happens is that his anterior tibio–fibular ligament ruptures (Stage I). His distal fibula then fractures spirally (Stage II). As the forces continue, the posterior part of his tibia fractures, to form a posterior tibial fragment, and, or, his posterior tibio–fibular ligament ruptures (Stage III). Next, his deltoid ligament ruptures, or his medial malleolus fractures. This is Stage IV and is the classical Potts fracture. Finally, his ankle may dislocate. The process may stop at any stage to produce injuries of varying severity. The distinguishing feature of this group of fractures is the spiral frac-ture of the distal fibula. Other varieties of this injury include fracture of the fibula several centimetres above the ankle, and sometimes even as high as its neck.

Supination–adduction fractures are caused by a patient's body moving laterally on his supinated foot. His lateral collateral ligament ruptures, or his fibula fractures transversely, and his medial malleolus fractures, usually vertically.

The remaining two groups of fractures (pronation–abduction and pronation–external rotation fractures) are less common, and will not be discussed further here.

One of the advantages of classifying these fractures by the force that caused them is that you can use the opposite force to reduce them. In practice, recognition of the exact type of fracture is not important. *The main principle is to recognize the incongruity between a patient's talus and his tibia, to replace them exactly in contact with one another, and then to immobilize his foot without weight bearing until his broken bones and torn ligaments have healed.* The mortice between his talus and his tibia is small, and transmits his whole weight, *so you must replace its joint surfaces exactly*—if you want his ankle to bear weight normally afterwards. Unfor-tunately, the ankle is not one of those joints which you can allow to mould itself by early active movements (69.4).

Lauge–Hansen. Acta Orthopaedica Scandinavica. 1978: 51;181–192

82.4 The early management of malleolar fractures

A patient's malleolar fracture can be treated by immediate internal fixation, preferably using AO methods, or by the closed methods describe later. Try closed methods first. If you succeed, good. If you fail, and you can refer him, subsequent internal fixation will be easier, because the fragments will at least be in nearly the right position. Meanwhile, here are some critical steps in his early management.

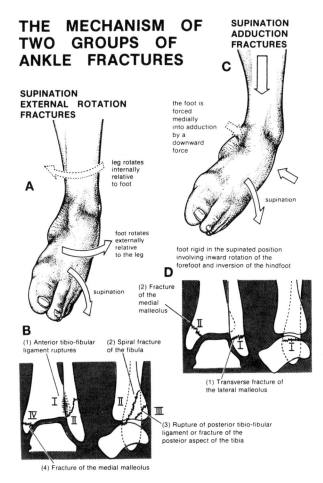

THE MECHANISM OF TWO GROUPS OF ANKLE FRACTURES

SUPINATION EXTERNAL ROTATION FRACTURES

A — leg rotates internally relative to foot

B — foot rotates externally relative to the leg — supination

(1) Anterior tibio-fibular ligament ruptures
(2) Spiral fracture of the fibula
(3) Rupture of posterior tibio-fibular ligament or fracture of the posteior aspect of the tibia
(4) Fracture of the medial malleolus

SUPINATION ADDUCTION FRACTURES

C — the foot is forced medially into adduction by a downward force — supination

D — foot rigid in the supinated position involving inward rotation of the forefoot and inversion of the hindfoot
(2) Fracture of the medial malleolus
(1) Transverse fracture of the lateral malleolus

Fig. 82-3 TWO COMMON GROUPS OF FRACTURES. A, and B, in supination–external fractures the patient's foot remains on the ground while his leg rotates internally on his foot which supinates. The four injuries of his foot occur in a characteristic order; the first with only mild trauma and all four if trauma is severe enough. C, and D, in supination–adduction fractures the patient's foot is forced medially into aduction by a downward force. His lateral collateral ligament ruptures, or his fibula fractures transversely, and his medial malleolus fractures, usually vertically. The exact pattern of these injuries is not important. What matters is getting his talus back under his tibia exactly. *Adapted from Lauge–Hansen*

EARLY MANAGEMENT FOR A MALLEOLAR FRACTURE

HOW URGENT IS REDUCTION ?

If the patient's talus has dislocated (is grossly out of place), reduce it immediately, whatever the swelling.

If his ankle is only subluxed (the fragments are more or less in their normal places), you can either reduce the fracture immediately, within a few hours, before it starts to swell, which is best, or 3 to 7 days later when the swelling is less.

Meanwhile, keep his ankle in stockinette traction (Quigley traction) as described below, to allow the swelling to subside and make reduction easier. Manipulating a very swollen ankle is not easy.

CAUTION ! Never let a malleolar fracture remain, even temporarily, in an undesirable position, particularly in equinus. The blood in the joint will organize, and the ligaments will tighten into undesirable positions, so that later reduction will be difficult or impossible.

STOCKINETTE TRACTION FOR THE EARLY MANAGEMENT OF MALLEOLAR FRACTURES

Thread the patient's leg through a tube of stockinette, and fix this to his thigh with several short pieces of zinc oxide strapping, as in Fig. 82-5. Don't put strapping around his thigh because it may obstruct his circulation. Suspend the loose end of the stockinette from a drip stand, so that his foot lies about 20 cm above his bed. Most fractures will reduce themselves automatically in 2 or 3 days, while the swelling subsides.

If you don't have stockinette, and the swelling is severe, reduce the fracture by the method to be described, and temporarily hold the best position with a long horse shoe plaster splint which extends down one side of the patient's leg, around his foot, and up the other side. Hold it with a crepe bandage. Keep him in bed with the foot of his bed raised until the swelling has subsided. Tighten the crepe bandages as swelling subsides, and then apply a cast as in Fig. 82-9.

MALLEOLAR FRACTURES

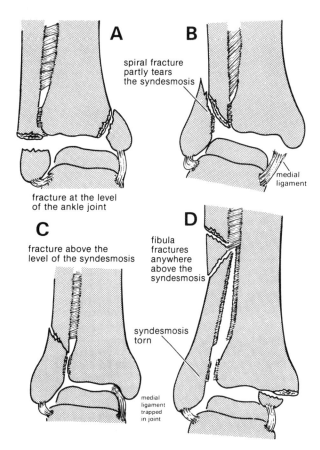

A — fracture at the level of the ankle joint

B — spiral fracture partly tears the syndesmosis — medial ligament

C — fracture above the level of the syndesmosis

D — fibula fractures anywhere above the syndesmosis — syndesmosis torn — medial ligament trapped in joint

Fig. 82-4 THE BONY AND LIGAMENTOUS INJURIES IN MALLEOLAR FRACTURES. A, is a supination–adduction fracture. B, and C, are a supination–external rotation fractures in which the patient's medial collateral (deltoid) has pulled off his medial malleolus. In C, it has gone inside his ankle joint and will make reduction difficult. In D, his fibula has fractured higher up. *Adapted from Weber.*

82.5 Is reduction good enough?

Before you reduce a fracture you will want to know if you have succeeded. This section tells you what to aim for; the next one tells you how to achieve it. *The purpose of reduction is to align a patient's talus with the anterior part of the joint surface of his tibia.* So look for congruity there. Gross displacement or widening of his ankle joint is easy to recognize, but minor degrees of non–congruity may be difficult to distinguish from a normal joint. When you reduce his fracture, take great care to obtain the highest possible degree of congruity. A common error is to accept an unnecessary degree of non–congruity.

STOCKINETTE TRACTION FOR MALLEOLAR FRACTURES

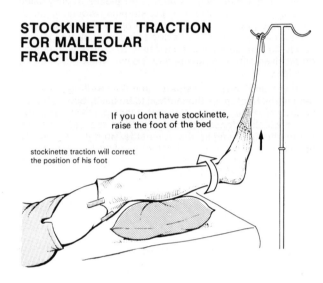

Fig. 82-5 STOCKINETTE TRACTION FOR A MALLEOLAR FRAC-TURE. If a patient's foot is held like this by the stockinette, his leg tends to rotate externally, and apply the forces necessary to reduce the common supination—external rotation fractures in which his foot rotates externally on his leg. *Kindly contributed by Peter Bewes and John Stewart.*

POST–REDUCTION X-RAYS FOR MALLEOLAR FRACTURES

ANTERO–POSTERIOR VIEW IN 20° OF INTERNAL ROTA-TION. This must be taken correctly, as in Fig. 82-1: (1) The gap between the patient's talus and his medial and lateral malleoli should be about the same as the gap between his talus and the lower surface of his tibia. (2) The saddle-shaped surfaces of his talus and his tibia should be congruous. (3) Close reduc-tion of his medial malleolus should show that there are no soft tissues between the fragments and indicate an excellent prognosis. (4) Compare the length of his two malleoli, and the congruity of his fibula to his talus. His lateral malleolus should project more distally than his medial one. If you cannot cor-rect proximal displacement or obvious incongruity, refer him for open reduction and internal fixation.

A TRUE LATERAL VIEW The anterior surface of a patient's tibia should be congruous with his talus.

If there is a posterior tibial fragment, it will almost cer-tainly be displaced upwards. This is less important, provided his talus is accurately aligned with the anterior part of his tibia, as in B, Fig. 82-6. Misalignment of the talus and the shaft of the tibia, as in C, produces a high spot on the joint sur-face so that osteoarthritis is sure to follow.

If his talus and tibia are misaligned, in the lateral view, you will have to remove the cast and try to improve reduction.

If a gap remains in the AP view between his medial malleolus and his talus, there is soft tissue in the joint. This is especially likely to happen if the patient's medial malleolus is intact, trapping his torn deltoid ligament in his ankle joint between his talus and his medial malleolus.

If in a lateral view, one third or more of the posterior lip of a patient's tibia has been fractured, his ankle will be

CONGRUITY IN A LATERAL X-RAY

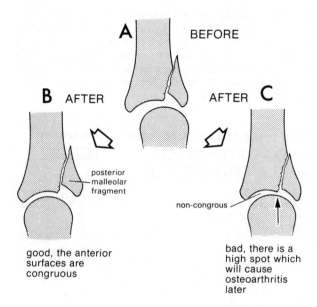

Fig. 82-6 CONGRUITY IN A LATERAL X-RAY. If a patient has a large posterior tibial fragment, try to make the anterior part of his ankle joint congruous. In B, it is congruous; in C, there is a high spot, which will lead to osteoarthritis later. *After Charnley, with kind permission.*

unstable in an AP plane, so try to refer him for open reduc-tion and screw fixation. If this is impossible, we describe a method later which may help you to replace the fragment—see 'If the posterior fragment is large. . .'.

82.6 Treating a malleolar fracture

This is one of the fractures in which *expert* internal fixation gives excellent results. If you cannot refer a patient for it, careful closed reduction by Charnley's method is satisfactory in most cases.

These are difficult fractures by any method. Be sure to admit the patient who will need 10 to 14 days of in–patient care. Your results will be better if you either reduce his fracture immediately before his ankle starts swelling, or if you allow the swelling to subside first. A malleolar fracture needs careful manipulation using three point fixation, several X-rays, some well applied casts, and, finally proper follow–up during several out–patient visits to make sure that the position of the fragments is not lost. The way the casts are applied is critical. *Always put them on yourself.* This is not an easy fracture to treat—it needs particular care.

Your main difficulty will be less in reducing a patient's frac-ture, than in making sure it stays reduced. In spite of the com-plexity of these fractures, in most of them *there are really only two fragments.* The shafts of his tibia and fibula form one frag-ment, while his foot and his malleoli form the other one. The fragments attached to his foot move as one piece because they are all firmly joined by ligaments. If you can put his talus back accurately under his tibia, the other fragments will usually reduce themselves. Align his foot on his leg by eye and by feel, and you will find you have reduced his fracture. If there is a posterior tibial fragment which is less than one third of the width of his tibia, you can usually leave it to look after itself, but if it is larger than this you may have to use the special method for it that we describe later.

You will be able to feel that a patient's talus is back under his tibia more easily when there is no plaster on his foot. So explore the mobility of his foot before you apply it. Start by getting the feel of where his talus should be. Then apply plaster, fit his talus back in position, and hold it there until the plaster has set, as in B, Fig. 82-9.

The common supination–external rotation fracture is caused by external rotation of a patient's ankle on his leg, so you will need moderate internal rotation of his foot to correct it. Use one of your hands to support his heel and nudge his lateral malleolus medially, while your other hand presses his tibia laterally. Meanwhile, ask your assistant to steady his knee. Between you, you will be able to apply three point fixation.

After reduction the patient's foot must not rotate on his leg, if it does, reduction will certainly be lost. So, the cast must extend above his knee, and his knee must be gently flexed.

There are no short cuts. Be sure to: (1) Apply the cast as described. (2) X-ray the patient at least once before 2 weeks have elapsed, so that you can have another attempt to reduce his fracture before it is too late. Most reductions are lost during this period. (3) Prevent him from walking on his cast too early—this is a very common error.

THERE ARE TWO FRAGMENTS IN A MALLEOLAR FRACTURE

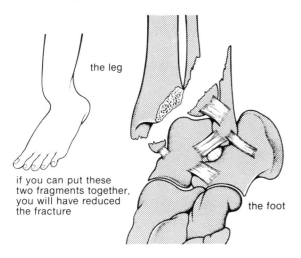

the leg

if you can put these two fragments together, you will have reduced the fracture

the foot

Fig. 82-7 MOST MALLEOLAR FRACTURES HAVE ONLY TWO PARTS. One part is the patient's leg, and the other part is his foot. If you can put these together, you will have reduced his fracture. *From Charnley, with kind permission.*

MOST MALLEOLAR FRACTURES HAVE ONLY TWO
PARTS
SUCCESS DEPENDS ON GETTING THE DETAILS
RIGHT

CHARNLEY'S METHOD FOR MALLEOLAR FRACTURES

MANAGEMENT

INITIAL X-RAYS Study these carefully. Order all the X-rays when you first see the patient, make sure they are taken on the right days, look at them within hours of their being taken, and act on them that day. If you forget to do this, nobody will bother to see they are taken.

If there is only a hairline crack in a patient's lateral malleolus, firm strapping may be enough.

If there is more than a hairline crack, but no incongruity in the joint surfaces, apply a short leg walking cast (not a malleolar cast) for 2 weeks. If a forced inversion X-ray shows that his lateral ligament has been ruptured, leave it on for 8 to 10 weeks. Encourage him to walk without a limp as soon as he comfortably can.

If there is any incongruity of the joint space, admit him and treat him by closed reduction as described below.

If there is a large upwardly displaced posterior tibial fragment, expect difficulty, and try to reduce it by the special method described later.

CAUTION ! (1) A severe malleolar fracture is not suitable for out–patient treatment. (2) If he cannot walk, even a few steps on the night of admission, suspect a serious ankle injury. If X-rays show no fracture, he may have ruptured his lateral ligament. If clinical signs are inconclusive, take a forced inversion X-ray (Fig. 82-1). If you delay treatment, your chances of success will be much less.

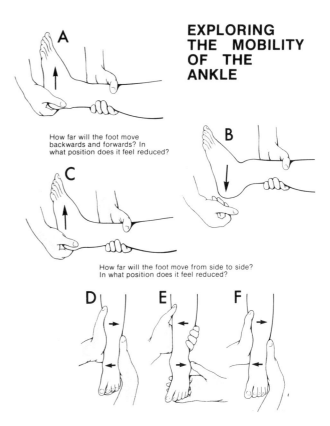

EXPLORING
THE MOBILITY
OF THE
ANKLE

How far will the foot move backwards and forwards? In what position does it feel reduced?

How far will the foot move from side to side? In what position does it feel reduced?

Fig. 82-8 EXPLORING THE MOBILITY OF A MALLEOLAR FRACTURE. If you hold the patient's leg by his calf and his heel (A), his heel will fall when you remove your hand (B). Remember how far you have to lift it in order to replace it (C). Similarly, remember how far you have to move it sideways (D, E, and F) to reduce it. *From Charnley with kind permission.*

CLOSED REDUCTION

CONTRAINDICATIONS If the patient has a severe open or comminuted malleolar fracture, treat him as in the next section. If possible, refer him for internal fixation if he has: (1) Shortening of his fibular malleolus. (2) Impaction of his tibial plateau. (3) A posterior fragment more than one third of the width of his tibia. If you cannot refer him, do what you can by closed methods.

ANAESTHESIA Give him a general anaesthetic, or ketamine (A 8.2).

EXPLORING THE MOBILITY OF A MALLEOLAR FRACTURE
The following description applies to the common severe Stage III or IV supination–external rotation trimalleolar fractures,

in which a patient's talus and his foot together are displaced posteriorly. In other fractures, and particularly the rarer ones in which his talus is displaced anteriorly, adjust your manipulations appropriately.

Lie him with his legs over the end of the table. Find an assistant.

Finding the position of reduction Explore the up and down and side to side mobility of the patient's ankle joint, as in Fig. 82-8, while you try to find the best position of reduction.

If you hold his heel in the palm of your hand, with his leg horizontal and in slight external rotation, as in A, Fig. 82-9, the fracture will probably reduce itself.

If it is not reduced, rotate his foot internally a little, and fit his talus back into the lower end of his tibia. Align his patella carefully with his toes, so that it is the same on the fractured side as on the normal one. In this position the fracture should stay reduced. Ask an assistant to hold the patient's leg, and see if you can improve the position by applying three point fixation, as in B, Fig. 82-9. Feel if there seems to be any danger of over–reduction. This is usually not possible.

Memorize the most stable position where you can most easily apply pressure to reduce the fracture. Remember carefully just how far forwards and how far medially you have to move his foot. You will need to return it to this same position while the plaster sets.

APPLYING THE FIRST MALLEOLAR CAST

Ask your assistant to *hold the patient's toes.*

Apply 1 cm of cotton wool padding to his foot, ankle, and calf. Bind the wool on tightly and smooth it carefully.

Use *cold* water to make the cast set slowly. Quickly wet and apply three 20 cm plaster bandages lightly from his MP joints to just below his knee. Three bandages will make the cast thick enough to hold his foot reduced, without obscuring the feel of reduction. At this stage disregard the reduction of the fracture, and the position of his foot.

As soon as the plaster is on, and *while it is still soft,* take his leg from your assistant. Massage the plaster thoroughly to remove air bubbles from between the layers of the bandage.

If the posterior tibial fragment is small, ignore it. Feel the fracture by moving his foot about inside the soft cast. Use

the experience you have already gained to reduce it. Apply three point fixation, as in B, Fig. 82-9. Ask your assistant to steady the patient's knee (1). With one of your hands press the lower end of his tibia laterally (2). With your other hand press his heel upwards and press his lateral malleolus medially (3), while you rotate his foot internally a little (4). His lateral malleolus is attached to his foot. So, the pressure of the palm of your hand medially on his ankle will restore it to its correct position. Very little force is necessary, and if you have placed his foot correctly, gravity alone should be almost enough.

CAUTION ! (1) Keep his foot absolutely still until the cast has set. Don't apply any finishing touches until it is hard. (2) Don't apply the cast with his ankle inverted. (3) As an additional check, make sure both his feet are similarly aligned in relation to his patellae. (4) Avoid the errors in Fig. 82-10.

If the posterior fragment is large, is displaced upwards, and does not come down on the usual manipulation, make use of the distal tibial origin of the patient's flexor hallucis longus muscle. Strongly plantar flex his ankle into equinus. Dorsiflex his big toe sharply. Then, holding his toe dorsiflexed, bring his foot into the neutral position. Hold his foot in this position and apply a cast as described above.

If the posterior fragment is large (more than 1/3 of the width of his tibia), and does not come down by this method, **refer him.**

THREE COMMON ERRORS

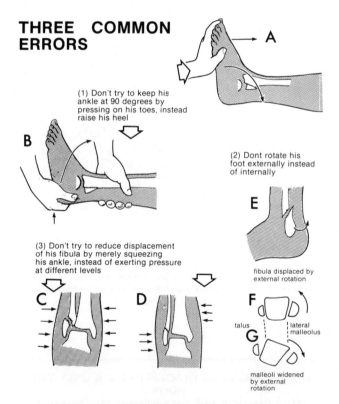

(1) Don't try to keep his ankle at 90 degrees by pressing on his toes, instead raise his heel

(2) Dont rotate his foot externally instead of internally

(3) Don't try to reduce displacement of his fibula by merely squeezing his ankle, instead of exerting pressure at different levels

fibula displaced by external rotation

talus   lateral malleolus

malleoli widened by external rotation

Fig. 82-10 THE THREE COMMON ERRORS IN REDUCING A MALLEOLAR FRACTURE. (1) Don't try to keep the patient's ankle at 90° by pressing on his toes (A); instead raise his heel (B). (2) Don't try to reduce the displacement of his fibula by squeezing his ankle from side to side (C). Instead, exert pressure at different levels (D). (3) Don't externally rotate his foot. His lateral malleolus is already displaced posteriorly (E). Further external rotation will separate his malleoli from their normal position (F) into position G. *From Charnley with kind permission.*

THREE POINT FIXATION

upper part of the cast completed later

your assistant

slight internal rotation

you

you

if you hold his heel like this the fracture will probably reduce itself

you

you

you support his heel

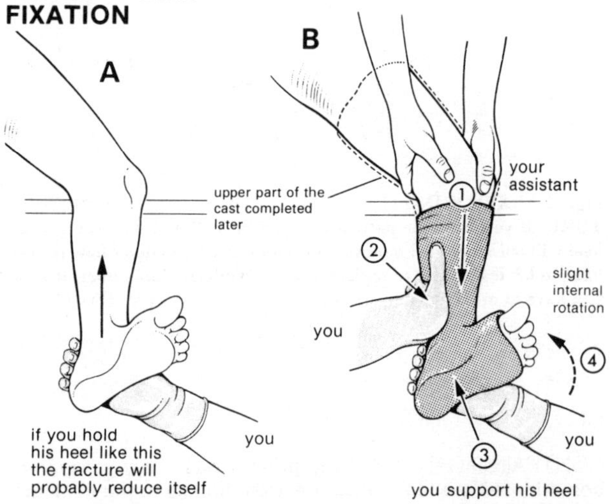

FIG. 82-9 THREE POINT FIXATION FOR A MALLEOLAR FRAC-TURE. A, if you hold a patient's foot like this, his fracture will probably reduce itself. B, if it is not reduced, rotate his foot internally a little, and fit his talus back into the lower end of his tibia. Align his patella carefully with his toes, so that it is the same on the fractured side as on the normal one. In this position the fracture should stay reduced. Ask an assistant to hold the patient's leg, and see if you can improve the position by applying three point fixation like this. When you have reduced his fracture, apply the cast below his knee. When this has set, extend it above his knee with his knee slightly flexed. *From Charnley, with kind permission.*

AFTER THE CAST AROUND HIS ANKLE HAS SET

When the first coating of plaster has set, and there is no danger of his fracture slipping, complete the cast up to his mid–thigh, with his knee flexed to 20°. Finish its top and bottom edges, and apply extra plaster bandages to strengthen it if necessary. *While it is still soft,* split the lower leg portion anteriorly down to his skin, *but don't spread it.*

CHECK X-RAYS Take an AP view in 20° of internal rotation and a lateral view immediately after reduction. If his talus is not in exactly its right place (Fig. 82-6), remove the foot and ankle part of the cast, have another try, and complete the cast once more, making sure that the junction of the new and old parts do not press on his skin.

POSTOPERATIVE CARE FOR A MALLEOLAR FRACTURE

Put the patient to bed, raise his leg to reduce swelling (81-1), and observe the circulation of his toes carefully for 24 hours. If it is impaired, or if he is in pain, spread or remove the cast, and reduce the fracture again later. Ask him to move his leg and toes inside the cast as much as he can. Keep him in bed for 2 weeks.

If the swelling was allowed to subside before you manipulated and reduced his fracture, keep him in bed for a few days, and then get him up on crutches.

One week after reduction, X-ray him to make sure the position has not been lost.

If reduction is satisfactory, **discharge him, on crutches without weight bearing.**

If reduction is not satisfactory, **have another attempt at closed reduction. If this fails, refer him for internal fixation, if you can.**

Two weeks after reduction, take another check X-ray. If reduction is not satisfactory, have a final attempt at reduction. If this fails, refer him for open reduction.

CAUTION ! If his fracture is severe, make sure he understands that he must not bear weight on his ankle until 6 weeks after the injury. Keep him on crutches. If his fracture is less severe, he can start to bear weight at 4 weeks.

Six weeks after reduction is the normal time for weight bearing to start.

Eight weeks after reduction, change his full length malleolar cast for a short leg walking cast (81.5). Carefully mould its upper end by triangular compression (Fig. 81-5) and fit it with a walking heel. Let him continue walking on crutches with increasing weight bearing to tolerance for 4 more weeks.

At 10 to 12 weeks, remove his short leg walking cast.

ALTERNATIVELY: (1) If necessary, you can end the cast below his knee and incorporate an oblique Steinmann pin in it (81.12). (2) The number of X-rays you take and casts you apply can, if absolutely necessary, be reduced. Always X-ray a patient immediately after reduction and at the end of the first week.

DIFFICULTIES WITH MALLEOLAR FRACTURES

If a patient's FOOT IS POSTERIORLY DISPLACED on his lower leg, pull his leg forwards and suspend the foot in stockinette until the swelling has gone. This is common when there is a large posterior tibial fragment.

If you CANNOT REDUCE AND HOLD THE FRACTURE by three point fixation, there are probably soft tissues between the fragments, or in the joint cavity, as in C, Fig. 82-4. If you rely on closed reduction, the fracture will probably slip later, so refer him for open reduction.

REDUCE THE PATIENT'S FRACTURE CAREFULLY
APPLY THE CAST PROPERLY
X-RAY HIM AT THE END OF THE FIRST WEEK
DON'T LET HIM BEAR ANY WEIGHT FOR 6 WEEKS

82.7 Open or comminuted malleolar fractures

Severe open or comminuted malleolar fractures are not suited to the method in the previous section. You will meet with various difficulties: (1) The end of the patient's tibia may be comminuted, and his talus driven up into it, as in Fig. 82-11. (2) One or other, or commonly both, the collateral ligaments of his ankle may

AN EXPLOSION FRACTURE OF THE ANKLE

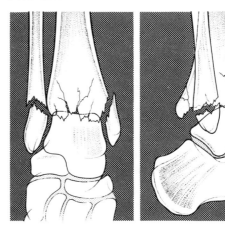

Fig. 82-11 AN EXPLOSION FRACTURE OF THE ANKLE. This patient has little hope of a pain—free, moveable ankle. Make sure that what little movement he will have will be about the neutral position (the position of function). A fixed equinus foot is a real disaster.

be stretched or ruptured completely. (3) His foot may be displaced posteriorly, and the lower end of his tibia may be sticking out of a dirty wound.

If there is an open wound over a malleolar fracture, do a thorough wound toilet, and reduce the fragments as best you can by closed methods. *Then leave it open.* If you fail to do an adequate wound toilet, or you close it by immediate primary suture, the patient's ankle joint is certain to become infected. He has little hope of a pain—free moveable, ankle, so make quite sure that what little movement he will have will be about the position of function in neutral. An ankle fixed in equinus, as in Fig. 82-2, is a real disaster. If pain becomes a major handicap, his ankle can be fused later.

AN OPEN OR GROSSLY DISORGANIZED ANKLE

If a patient's malleolar fracture fracture is open, take him to the theatre, anaesthetize him, and do a thorough wound toilet (54.1). Scrape the dirt out of his ankle, squirt saline into it, scrub his wound well, explore it, and enlarge it if necessary. Restore the position of his bones as best you can. Make a special point of trying to align his talus with his intact malleolus and his tibial plateau. If both his malleoli are fractured, line his talus up with his tibia as best you can.

CAUTION! Don't close his wound!

If possible, refer him at this stage, his fracture may be one of those in which skilled internal fixation can give him a useful ankle. If you cannot refer him, proceed as follows.

If there is serious damage to the weight bearing part of his ankle joint, as in Fig. 82-11, the best he can hope for is early spontaneous fusion. Start by applying medial and lateral splints until the swelling has subsided. Then apply a long leg cast, and start partial weight bearing with crutches as soon as pain will allow. If his ankle does not fuse, it may need to be fused surgically.

If the weight bearing part of his ankle is not seriously injured, try to preserve some function, and apply calcaneal traction (if his calcaneus has not been injured). Pass a Steinmann pin through his calcaneus (70.11), apply 5 kg traction, and raise the foot of his bed 25 cm. Cradle his leg on a pillow. On the day after the accident, encourage him to start moving his ankle. Maintain traction for 6 weeks. After that he can get up, but he must not bear weight for another 6 weeks.

If his foot is warm and sensation is present, don't amputate, however severe his injury is. Some sort of a foot is likely to be better than none. Only amputate if his foot is cold and without sensation, and if he can get a prosthesis.

CAUTION ! If movement is likely to be limited subsequently, it must be about the neutral position.

82.8 High spiral fractures of the fibula (Maisonneuve fracture)

This rare fracture is really a variety of malleolar fracture in which a patient's fibula, instead of breaking at his ankle, separates from his tibia at his ankle, twists, and breaks just below his knee. His lower tibio–fibular ligament ruptures, so does the whole of his interosseous membrane from top to bottom.

HIGH SPIRAL FRACTURES OF THE FIBULA Treat the patient as if he had a malleolar fracture (82.6).

If you can reduce the fracture satisfactorily, apply a long leg cast with his knee in a slight flexion. X-ray him weekly to make sure that reduction is maintained. If it is lost, correct it immediately before malunion occurs.

If you cannot reduce the fracture satisfactorily, refer him.

82.9 Separation of the distal tibial epiphysis

This is a child's equivalent of a malleolar fracture. You can usually manage Salter Harris type II epiphyseal injuries (69.6a), like those in Fig. 82-12, by closed reduction. Type III injuries, in which the fracture line opens into the joint, need open reduction to restore a smooth joint surface. This is also the most common site for the Type V injuries which crush the epiphyseal plate. Because there is no displacement, you may think that a child has only sprained his ankle, until growth deformities occur years later.

SEPARATION OF THE LOWER TIBIAL EPIPHYSIS Anaesthetize the child, exert strong traction on his foot and manipulate his ankle into position. Take great care to correct rotation. Apply a long leg walking cast for 6 weeks.

82.10 Injuries to the flexor mechanism of the ankle

Injuries of the flexor mechanism of the ankle can be open, as when cut by a kinfe, or closed. Closed injuries are the result of spontaneous rupture of flexor mechanism during violent or even moderate activity. They take two forms:

(1) Rupture of the plantaris tendon or a minor tear of the gastrocnemius muscle present as a sudden pain in the calf muscle, often during only minor exertion, accompanied by exquisite tenderness in the middle of the calf. This is a much less serious injury than rupture of the Achilles tendon. Distinguish it from rupture of the Achilles tendon by the 'kneeling on a chair test' in Fig. 82-13. It will recover spontaneously in a few days. A raised shoe will ease symptoms.

(2) Rupture of the Achilles tendon occurs during some violent sport. The patient hears a loud snap and cannot rise on the ball of his foot. You may be able to feel a gap just above his calcaneus. This injury is commonly missed, because nobody tests the integrity of his tendon as described below. Treat him conservatively—its frayed ends are difficult to repair.

An open injury, as by a knife, can be repaired without difficulty by the standard methods. Or, you can treat the patient conservatively in an equinus cast. If he has a ragged wound, an equinus cast is better, because the Achilles tendon has a poor blood supply and is easily infected. Some surgeons prefer it for all open Achilles tendon injuries, because the results are so good.

Although injuries (1) and (2) are usually considered to be distinct, there is probably a continuum between them. The important distinction as far as treatment is concerned is whether the 'kneeling on a chair test' is positive (indicating the need for an equinus cast) or not. If you leave an injury of the Achilles

INJURIES OF THE ACHILLES TENDON

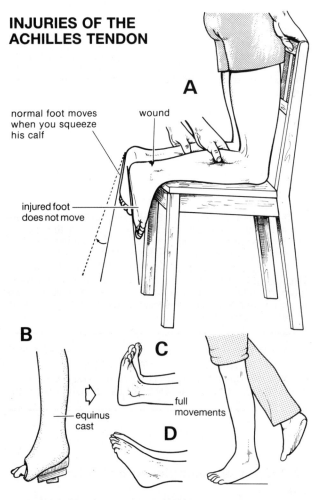

DISPLACEMENT OF THE DISTAL TIBIAL EPIPHYSIS (Type II injury)

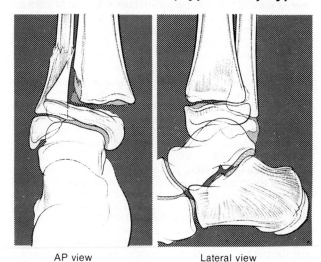

AP view   Lateral view

Fig. 82-12 SEPARATION OF THE DISTAL TIBIAL EPIPHYSIS is a child's equivalent of a malleolar fracture. You can usually manage Salter Harris type II epiphyseal injuries like this one by closed reduction.

Fig. 82-13 ACHILLES TENDON INJURIES. A, testing the integrity of the Achilles tendon. If the patient's foot plantar flexes, his tendon mechanism is intact. B, this patient ruptured his Achilles tendon completely, and has been put in a gravity equinus cast. C, D, and E, after 8 weeks of active walking in his cast he has a normal range of movements and normal lift off.

tendon totally untreated, the patient's calf muscles will pull the proximal end of his tendon upwards, and leave a space that will fill with scar tissue, so that he loses the take off of a normal gait.

ACHILLES TENDON INJURIES

DIAGNOSIS A patient's Achilles tendon mechanism is intact and he needs no special treatment if: (1) He can plantar flex his foot against resistance. Or, (2) his foot plantar flexes when you pinch his calf muscles as he kneels on a chair If it is not intact, his foot will remain still, and he needs treatment as described below.

SPONTANEOUS RUPTURE Keep the patient's foot plantar flexed in a cast in gravity equinus for 8 weeks. This is the amount of equinus which gravity alone produces but no more.

Build up the base of the cast and apply a walking heel as in Fig. 81-3. After 48 hours, encourage him to walk—it will stimulate the repair of his tendon.

At 8 weeks remove the cast. Protect his tendon for a further 8 weeks by raising his heel at least 3 cm (a cobbler should have been doing this during the first 8 weeks). Caution him against running, or any violent excercise for 3 more months.

CUT ACHILLES TENDON Toilet the patient's wound thoroughly, and suture it by the methods in Section 55.11. Leave at least part of it open for delayed primary closure. Or, treat him as above.

If you cannot suture his Achilles tendon, or have decided against suture because his wound is ragged or contaminated, or for any other reason, put him into an equinus cast as described above.

83 The foot

83.1 Conservative treatment for foot injuries

Because feet are usually hidden inside shoes, injuries to them tend to be neglected. You can treat most foot injuries conservatively, and only a few need reduction. Fracture of the body of the calcaneus is the most important one.

CONSERVATIVE TREATMENT FOR FOOT INJURIES Try to diagnose and treat the specific injuries described later. If you have no X-rays, or diagnosis is difficult, proceed as follows:

If there is any obvious displacement of the bones of the patient's foot, correct it, and then apply a short leg walking cast (81.5), taking care to *mould its sole to both the longitudinal and the transverse arches of his foot.* Keep him in bed until his pain subsides and then start him walking in crutches. If you cannot hold the reduction in plaster, fix it with Kirschner wire (70.13).

If he has no obvious displacement, fit him with a short leg walking cast as above.

If his pain is severe and he has only minor injury, or his X-ray is negative, a short leg walking cast will also help him.

**DON'T FORGET TO REDUCE SEVERE
DISPLACEMENT**

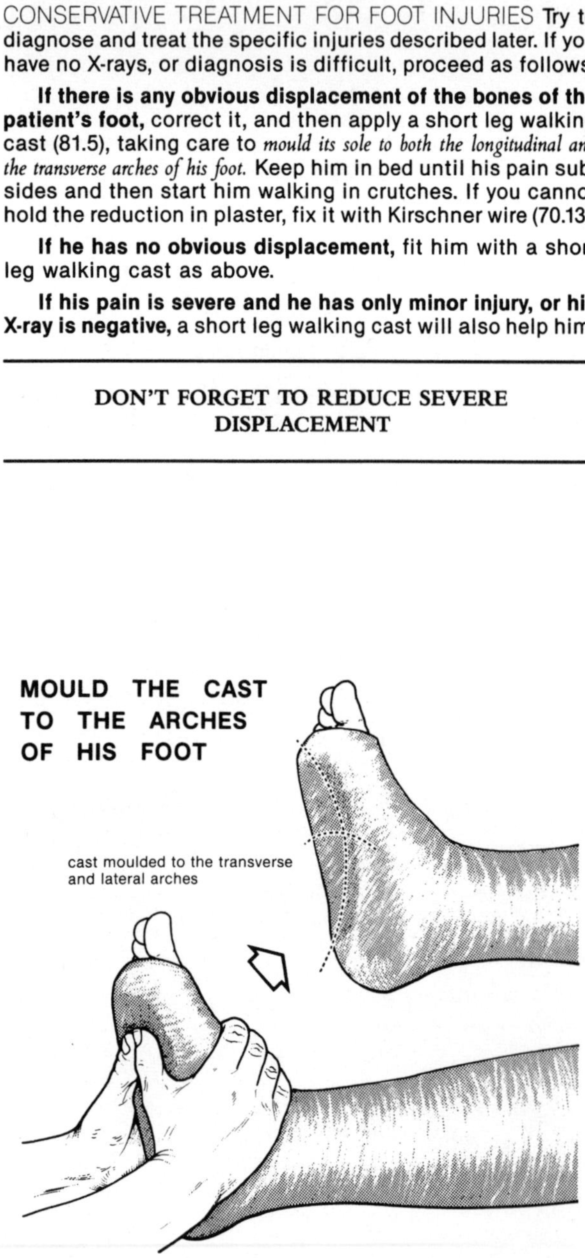

MOULD THE CAST
TO THE ARCHES
OF HIS FOOT

cast moulded to the transverse
and lateral arches

Fig. 83-1 A SHORT LEG WALKING CAST ADAPTED FOR FOOT INJURIES. Make a short leg walking cast as usual (81.5), but be sure you mould it to the arches of the patient's foot. *Kindly contributed by Benjamin Mbindyo.*

83.2 Dislocation of the talonavicular joint

The joint between a patient's talus and his navicular is often strained, and occasionally dislocates, sometimes in association with a dislocation of his forefoot. After some violent injury his foot is turned inwards and displaced under his talus, which remains in its normal place in his ankle joint. The displacement of the front of his foot from around his talus leaves it forming a swelling on the dorsum of his ankle, which presses on the skin and may cause it to necrose rapidly. (A, Fig. 83-2) He is in great pain, and the extreme inversion of his foot makes the diagnosis obvious. Occasionally, his foot is displaced laterally instead of medially. Sometimes, his cuboid and the head of his calcaneus are fractured at the same time. You will see these fractures best after you have reduced his talonavicular dislocation, but even if they are present, they do not alter treatment.

DISLOCATION OF THE TALONAVICULAR JOINT. Reduce the dislocation quickly before the skin over the head of the patient's talus becomes necrotic. If you cannot refer him, anaesthetize him and move his foot back into position. If his foot is unstable, fix it with Kirschner wire (70.13). Splint his ankle, raise it, apply a crepe bandage, and keep him in bed until the swelling is reduced. Then apply a cast with a walking heel, and get him up on crutches. Teach him to walk without a limp, while he is still using crutches. Remove the cast at 3 to 6 weeks. He may need crutches for 6 to 8 weeks.

83.3 Fractures of the dome of the talus

In this injury the patient twists his foot inwards, and shears a small fragment off the upper surface of his talus. An AP X-ray shows a small triangular fragment, like a loose body, at the upper lateral angle of his talus. As his foot returns to its normal position this fragment may turn upside down.

FRACTURE OF THE DOME OF THE TALUS **If the fragment is the right way up,** no treatment is needed.

If the fragment has turned upside down, refer the patient.

If you cannot refer him, remove the fragment by opening his ankle joint. Make an antero–lateral incision just lateral to the long extensors of his foot so as to avoid his superficial peroneal nerve. Fit him with a short leg walking cast for 10 to 14 days. Then remove the cast and encourage him to walk without a limp as soon as he can.

83.4 Fracture of the body of the talus

In this rare injury a patient falls from a height on to his heels and crushes the articular surface of his talus. His ankle is swollen and painful.

FRACTURE OF THE BODY OF THE TALUS If the patient's talus is comminuted, there is no advantage in referring him, so try to mould the comminuted fragments by active movements. As soon as he can move his ankle without too much pain, allow him up on crutches, but don't let him bear weight on it for 3 months. If it becomes too painful, refer him for an arthrodesis.

INJURIES OF THE TALUS

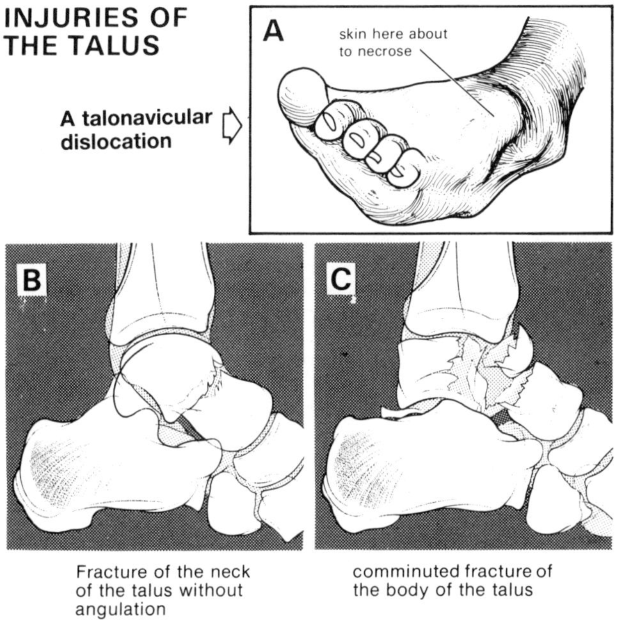

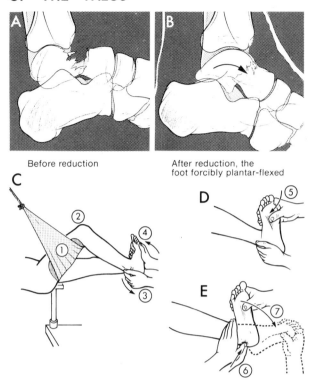

A talonavicular dislocation

skin here about to necrose

Fracture of the neck of the talus without angulation

comminuted fracture of the body of the talus

Fig. 83-2 SOME INJURIES OF THE TALUS. A, the patient's talonavicular joint has dislocated, so that his talus forms a swelling on the dorsum of his ankle. B, an undisplaced fracture of the neck of the talus. C, a comminuted fracture of the body of the talus.

83.5 Fractures of the neck of the talus

These rare fractures are the result of forced dorsiflexion of the patient's foot, and may injure his soft tissues severely. The fracture line runs through the neck of his talus in a coronal plane just in front of the anterior margin of his tibia. There are several varieties: (1) There may be no displacement. (2) The fragments may angulate so that the posterior half of his talus is plantar flexed, while its anterior half is dorsiflexed. You can usually reduce these fractures without too much difficulty by plantar flexing the patient's foot and holding it in a cast. (3) The posterior half of his talus may be displaced posteriorly out of its mortice with his talus leaving the anterior half in place.

FRACTURES OF THE NECK OF THE TALUS

DIAGNOSIS Lateral displacement is easily diagnosed, but you can easily miss an angulation deformity in a lateral X-ray, so examine the posterior half of the patient's subtaloid joint carefully. If its two articular surfaces are not parallel, the fragments have angulated at the fracture line.

TREATING FRACTURES OF THE NECK OF THE TALUS

NO ANGULATION No reduction is needed for a fracture like that in B, Fig. 83-2. Apply a short leg walking cast from below the patient's knee to his toes, with his foot in neutral. Get him up, and teach him to walk bearing weight. Three months later remove the cast.

WITH ANGULATION Internal fixation is sometimes possible.

If his talus is in two parts, refer him for internal fixation.

If you cannot refer him, reduce his fracture by forcibly plantar flexing his foot, as in Fig. 83-3.

Place a canvas sling (1) around the distal end of the patient's thigh, or ask an assistant to hold it.

Flex his knee to 90° (2). Grasp his heel with one hand and his forefoot with the other (3).

REDUCING AN ANGULATED FRACTURE OF THE NECK OF THE TALUS

Before reduction

After reduction, the foot forcibly plantar-flexed

Fig. 83-3 REDUCING AN ANGULATED FRACTURE OF THE NECK OF THE TALUS. A, the fracture before reduction. The body of the patient's talus may also be displaced backwards and rotated. B, the way in which plantar flexion achieves reduction. C, D, and E, the detailed method of reduction. *After de Palma, with kind permission.*

Pull his foot forward into full dorsiflexion (4). While you are pulling forward and maintaining dorsiflexion, strongly evert his foot (5). This will unlock his sustentaculum tali.

While your assistant presses firmly with his thumbs on either side of the patient's Achilles tendon (6), plantar flex his foot (7). A crunching noise shows that reduction is occurring.

Confirm reduction by taking an X-ray. After reduction, apply a cast from just below the patient's knee to his toes, holding his foot in equinus. Keep him in bed, and make him exercise his muscles inside the cast as much as possible.

If you have not been able to reduce his fracture, refer him for open reduction.

If you have been able to reduce his fracture, leave the cast on for 5 to 6 weeks. Then remove it, bring his foot into the neutral position, and apply another cast for 5 to 6 weeks in this neutral postion.

WITH ANTERIOR OR POSTERIOR DISPLACEMENT OF THE FOOT These injuries are rare.

If the patient's foot is displaced forwards, forcibly plantar flex it and push it backwards. Apply a cast with his foot in equinus, and continue as above.

If his foot and with it the posterior half of his talus is pushed backwards, put a Steinmann pin through his calcaneus (70.12). Exert traction so as to open up the space between his calcaneus and his tibia, and push the posterior fragment forwards into his ankle mortice. Apply a cast in equinus as above. If closed reduction fails, refer him.

DIFFICULTIES WITH FRACTURES OF THE NECK OF THE TALUS

If some months later, the patient's FOOT IS STILL PAINFUL and part of his talus looks abnormally dense, aseptic

A SIGN OF A FRACTURED CALCANEUM

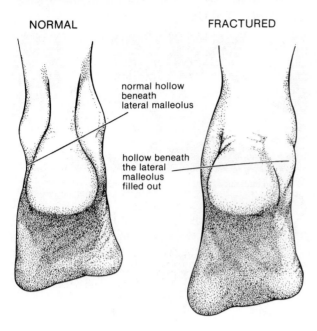

NORMAL   FRACTURED

normal hollow beneath lateral malleolus

hollow beneath the lateral malleolus filled out

Fig. 83-4 A SIGN OF INJURY TO THE CALCANEUS is filling out of the normal hollow under the patient's lateral malleolus. *Kindly contributed by Peter Bewes.*

necrosis has taken place. This is common, especially after a dislocation, so warn him about it. The fragments may unite, even if they look dense on an X-ray. An arthrodesis may eventually be necessary.

83.6 Fracture of the body of the calcaneus

In this common fracture the patient falls on to his feet, usually from only quite a small height. Sometimes, both his calcanei fracture, and his spine too. Always suspect that a patient might have fractured his calcaneus if he complains of pain in his foot after landing on his feet. Although his foot may look fairly normal, you will always find two signs.

(1) His injured calcaneus is widened, so that as you run your finger down the outer side of his leg, it passes over the tip of his lateral malleolus on to his swollen calcaneus *in the same plane.* In a normal foot, your finger sinks into a marked hollow below the lateral malleolus.

(2) The second sign concerns a patient's subtalar joint. Although he can move his ankle through about half its normal range of plantar and dorsiflexion, he cannot invert or evert his heel on his ankle—there is no movement at his subtar joint, either active or passive. Trying to move it is painful.

The fracture lines may not be easy to see on an X-ray, so take a lateral and a special axial view, and look for widening of his calcaneus. Fractures take many forms and vary from small cracks to extensive comminution. Fortunately, an exact diagnosis of the type of fracture is not necessary, because you can treat them all in the same way.

FRACTURE OF THE BODY OF THE CALCANEUS

Don't try to reduce these fractures. Instead, compress the patient's swollen ankle with a crepe bandage to reduce the swelling. Put him to bed for a very short time only (perhaps 3 days), until the pain is bearable and he is able to put his foot to the ground without too much pain.

Then without weight bearing, and with much encourage-

FRACTURE OF THE CALCANEUS

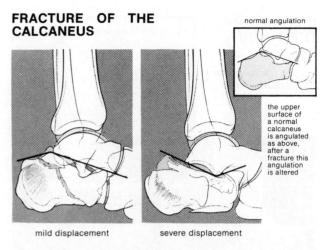

normal angulation

the upper surface of a normal calcaneus is angulated as above, after a fracture this angulation is altered

mild displacement   severe displacement

FIG. 83-5 TWO FRACTURES OF THE BODY OF THE CALCANEUS. A, with mild displacement. B, with severe displacement. C, the upper surface of a normal calcaneus is angulated. A severe fracture destroys this normal angulation. *From Perkins with kind permission.*

ment and careful supervision, encourage active movement of his hip, knee, ankle, and toes for 3 weeks. Follow this by active exercise with partial weight bearing using crutches. Cycling is excellent. All this will be painful, especially early on, so give him plenty of aspirin. Healing takes time, and improvement may continue for 2 years at least. If his fracture is bilateral, early mobilisation will be more difficult and take longer.

CAUTION ! If you have to apply a cast to ease the pain, and make it easier to treat him as an outpatient, leave it on for a few days only, and then get him walking without it.

An occasional patient has enough later disability to need his subtalar joints fused. Don't refer him for 6 months or a year.

83.7 Other fractures of the calcaneus

These are all quite minor injuries. They are not easy to diagnose, but since they can all be treated by active movements, this is fortunately unimportant.

Fracture of the tuberosity of the calcaneus can be diagnosed in a lateral X-ray which may show a fragment prised up from the posterior angle of the bone. Or, an axial X-ray may show a vertical fracture. Treat both these injuries by early active movements.

Fracture of the sustenstaculum tali is difficult to see in an X-ray film, displacement is slight, and no reduction is necessary. Encourage the patient to bear weight immediately.

Fracture of the anterior end of the calcaneus is caused by severe inversion of the patient's foot, or a subtaloid dislocation. A small fragment is pulled off the upper surface of the front end of his calcaneus. Treat it without reduction by active movements as above.

83.8 Fractures of the navicular and cuboid

When a patient's foot is crushed, he may fracture his navicular, or his cuboid; his midtarsal joint may be dislocated, or his metatarsals fractured. These are serious injuries and he may have several of them at the same time.

FRACTURES OF THE NAVICULAR AND THE CUBOID Give the patient a general anaesthetic. Look at his X-rays and carry out any manoeuvre which you think might reduce the fragments, especially if there are signs of a dislocation of his mid–tarsal joint.

If you cannot reduce his injuries, try to refer him.

If you can reduce them, apply a short leg walking cast (81.5) with his foot in neutral. Keep him in bed with his foot raised until the swelling has gone. Then encourage him to walk with crutches, starting with partial weight bearing.

After 3 weeks remove the cast. Check to see if the pain and swelling have subsided enough for him to start walking with crutches and partial weight bearing.

83.9 Fracture subluxation of the tarso–metatarsal joint

This is a difficult fracture to see on an X-ray, but if you look carefully at the bases of all the patient's metatarsals, you will see that he has multiple fractures with minor displacements. This is a severe injury and osteoarthritis often follows, sometimes so severely as to need an arthrodesis.

FRACTURE SUBLUXATION OF THE TARSO–METATARSAL JOINT

If there is severe displacement of the patient's tarso–metatarsal joint, attempt to reduce it as best you can.

If you cannot reduce it with your hands alone, pass a Kirschner wire through the distal ends of his metatarsals, hold this in a tensioner, and use it to help you to manipulate the distal part of his foot. Get this into a good position, and hold it with crossed Kirschner wires. Remove the tensioner and apply a well–padded cast. If you don't have Kirschner wires, try to hold his broken bones with a well moulded cast with his forefoot held in plantar flexion. After a week change this for a short leg walking cast and crutches. Encourage him to walk normally. Four weeks later change this for a shoe.

83.10 Crush fractures of the metatarsals

Any crush injury to a patient's forefoot is serious, and can disable him. His metatarsals usually break through their necks, and he may have an open wound. Diagnosis is difficult without an X-

METATARSAL FRACTURES

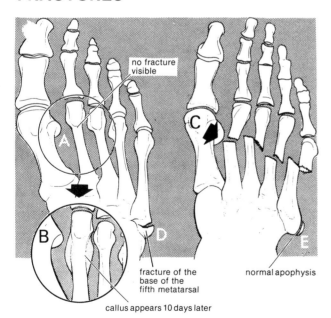

Fig. 83-6 FRACTURES OF THE METATARSALS. In the march fracture A, no injury is visible immediately after the injury, but B, shows callus appearing 10 days later. C, shows several fractured metatarsals. D, shows a fracture of the base of the fifth metatarsal. Compare it with the normal apophysis E.

ray. These fractures are difficult to reduce, but they usually heal without reduction. If they heal in a grossly displaced position, his foot may be painful permanently, so do your best to reduce them. His first metatarsal is a weight bearing bone, so that if it is fractured he is likely to need a cast.

CRUSH FRACTURES OF THE METATARSALS

If there is obvious gross displacement, anaesthetize the patient, reduce his fracture as best you can, apply a below–knee walking cast (81.5), and then elevate his leg (Fig. 81-1). Take care to mould its sole to both the longitudinal and the transverse arches of his feet as in Fig. 83-1. If you fail to correct severe displacement, he will be left with serious disability, so refer him.

If there is no obvious displacement, elevate his leg. As soon as swelling has subsided, and he is comfortable and can walk, give him aspirin and strap his foot in a crepe bandage. If he cannot walk, immobilize his foot in a below–knee walking cast. After 3 weeks in this encourage him to walk in an ordinary shoe.

DIFFICULTIES WITH CRUSH FRACTURES OF THE METATARSALS

If a patient has INTENSE PAIN AND SWELLING, marked stiffness, warm, smooth, glossy skin, bone rarefaction, and in extreme cases, trophic ulcers, he has SUDEK'S ATROPHY which may last several years. It can follow any crush injury of the foot (or hand), even quite a minor one. Keep him walking on his foot as best he can, with weight bearing to tolerance. If he ceases to use it, bone rarefaction will become severe.

83.11 Fatigue (march) fractures

One of the patient's metatarsals, usually his second, fractures spontaneously, without any history of injury. He has localized pain particularly at night, and tenderness over the fracture site. At first the X-ray shows only a fine transverse crack, or nothing at all. But 10 days later a mass of callus appears. Because he may present with pain of gradual onset without a history of injury, and because the fracture may not be visible on an X-ray, you can confuse the callus with a sarcoma, as in the tibia (81.8). Strap the front part of his foot, and advise him to put less stress on the fracture.

83.12 Fracture of the base of the fifth metatarsal

Severe twisting of the front half of the patient's foot tears a fragment bone from the base of his fifth metatarsal. Don't confuse this fracture with an ununited apophysis, which has a characteristic smooth comma shape, and is usually bilateral. If you are in doubt X-ray his other foot.

He will give you a history of having sprained his foot, but his lateral malleolus is not tender, and there is no tenderness over the front of his calcaneus. Instead, there is marked tenderness over and underneath the prominence formed by the base of his fifth metatarsal. This is a painful injury, so fit him with a below–knee walking cast for 2 weeks, or longer if necessary.

83.13 Fractures of the phalanges of the toes

A weight falling on to a patient's toes sometimes breaks them. Reduction is unnecessary, but it may be advisable to evacuate a painful subungual haematoma (75.5). These fractures are not serious and always unite. Splint his injured toe with zinc oxide strapping to the adjacent normal toe. Pad it with a little cotton wool to absorb moisture. As soon as he can get his shoe on, send him back to work. A metal stiffener driven down between the layers of the sole of his shoe will help him to return to work sooner.

INDEX

Note: Section numbers are indicated by a dot (e.g. 55.1) and figures by a dash (e.g. 55-1). D after a section number indicates a difficulty, which is to be found at the end of a particular section.

abdominal cavity
  blood in 66.3
  gas in 66.1, 66-4
abdominal flaps 75.26, 75-35
abdominal girth 66.1, 66-2
abdominal injuries 66.1 to 66-19
  abdominal girth increase 66.1
  abrasion, internal injury with 66.1
  bleeding, into peritoneal cavity 66.1, 66.3, 66.9
    in laparotomy 66.3, 66-7
    in liver injuries 66.7, 66-13
    rectal, after small gut injuries 66.10D
    in ruptured spleen 66.6
  blood loss 53.2, 53-3
  blunt 66.1, 66.3
    incisions for 66.3
    laparotomy 66.3
    viscera injured 66.3
  closed 66.1
  diaphragm, rupture of 66.5
  eviscerated gut 66.4
  examination 66.1
  exploration 66.3, 66-7, 66.8
  fistula formation, see fistula
  further management 66.1
  general methods 66.1
  guarding, rigidity in 66.1, 66.3, 66.19D
  gut, injuries, see gut
  head injuries with 51.5
  history 66.1
  infections in, see infections
  laparotomy in, see laparotomy
  lung collapse in 66.19D
  management 66.1
  organs injured 66-1
  orthostatic hypotension 66.1
  other difficulties 66.19D
  pain in 66.1
  paracentesis 66.1, 66-3
  if patient brought in late 66.19D
  penetrating 66.1, 66.2, 66.9
    conservative treatment 66.2
    of gut 66.9, 66-15, 66-17
    of mesentery 66.10, 66-15
    operative treatment 66.2
  peritoneal lavage in 66.1
  resuscitation 66.3, 66.19D
  severe shock with 66.19D
  small gut injuries 66.9, 66-15
  special methods 66.1
  tenderness 66.1, 66.9, 66.19D
  tests for 66-2
  thoracic injuries with 51.5, 65.3, 65.4, 66.1, 66.19D
    penetrating 66.2, 66-5, 66-6
  in unconscious patient 66.1
  white cell count in 66.1
  X-rays 66.1
  see also individual organs and injuries
abdominal wall injuries 66.2, 66.3
  abscesses 66.14
  bruising 66.9
  rupture 66.4
abscesses
  abdominal wall 66.14
  in burns of ear 58.30
  retroperitoneal 66.17, 66.19D
  subphrenic 66.19D
accidents

accidents (cont.)
  prevention 50.2
  reception area 51-1
  scene of, first aid at 50.3, 51.1
    equipment required at 50.3, 51.1
  severe injuries, see severely injured patient
  trapped patient, extracting of 50-4, 51.1
acetabulum
  in dislocation of hip 77.4, 77.5
  fractures of 76.3
    of floor 76.3, 76-4
    of posterior rim 76.3
Achilles tendon
  cut 82.10
  injuries 82.1, 82.10, 82-13
  rupture 82.10
  in Syme's operation 56.9
acidosis, metabolic 53.2
acromio-clavicular dislocation 71.1, 71-3, 71.6
  slings active movements for 71.2
acromion, injuries 71.7
  examination 71.1
acrylic resins, in mandibular fractures 62.13
adhesions
  around knee 78.6 D
  in emergency splenectomy 66.6
adult respiratory distress syndrome 58.27
agricultural machinery accidents 50.2
air
  draining from pleural cavity 65-2, 65-2, 65.4
    difficulties 65.2D, 65.4D, 65.5D
    see also pneumothorax
  in surgical emphysema 65.10
airway 52.1 to 52.2
  checking, in severely injured patient 51.1
  obstruction, general method for 52.1, 52-1
    diagnosis 52.1, 58.1
    in head injuries 63.1
    prevention 52.1
    in severe burns 58.1
    in thoracic injuries 65.1
    treatment 52.1
  obstruction, laryngotomy, tracheostomy 52.2
  restoration
    in flail chest 65.1, 65.6
    in head injuries 63.1
    in maxillofacial injuries 62.1, 62-2
    in severe burns 58.1
    in severely injured patient 51.1
    in thoracic injuries 65.1
alcohol and trauma 50.2
Allen's test, modified 75.1
alveolus
  comminuted fractures 62.2
  fractures, treatment 62-1, 62.3
  injuries 62.1, 62.2
ambulance
  box, contents of 50.3
  driver, first aid by 50.3
    seriously injured patient 51.1
  minimum requirements 50.3
amputations 50.1, 56.1 to 56.10
  above knee 56.5, 56-11
  anaesthesia 56.1
  below knee 56.1, 56.8, 56-13
  bleeding during 56.1
  in children 56.1
  closing stump 56.1, 56-6
  delayed primary closure 56.1
  difficulties, specific situations 56.1D
  disarticulation

amputations (cont.)
  ankle 56.9
  elbow 56.4
  knee 56.7, 56-12
  wrist 56.5, 56-10
  of elbow 56.4
  equipment 56.1, 56-3
  fat, dealing with 56.1
  fingers, see under finger
  fish mouth flaps 56.1, 56-4, 75.24
  flap
    breakdown 56.1D
    for finger amputation 75.24, 75-30
    in gas gangrene 54.13, 56.1, 56.2
    general methods 56.1
    guillotine 56.2
    of hand, for severe burns 58.29
    immediate suture 56.1
    indications 56.1
    for ischaemic gangrene 56.3
    knife 56.1
    metatarsal 56.10, 56-15
    mid upper arm as site 56.4
    muscle, cutting in 56.1
    nerves, cutting in 56.1
    in paraplegia 64.19
    postoperative care 56.1
    prostheses 56-1, 56.1
    saw 56.1
    scar, position 56.1
    sites 56-2, 56.4
    stumps
      in accidental amputation of finger 75.23, 75-27
      covering whilst sawing 56-5
      painful 75.24D
      perfect, criteria for 56.1
    supracondylar region as site 56.4
    Syme's operation 56.9, 56-14
    through foot, toes 56.10, 56-15, 56-16
    through lower arm, wrist 56.5, 56-9
    through upper arm, elbow 56.4, 56-8
    tourniquet use 56.1
    traumatic 51-5, 75.23
anaemia
  cyanosis not observable in 65.1
  in severe burns 58.1, 58.10
    reasons, treatment 58.10
  skin grafting in 57.4, 57.5
anaerobic infections
  cellulitis 54.13
  gas gangrene 54.13
  streptococcal myositis 54.13
  tetanus 54.12
  see also individual infections
anaesthesia
  in abdominal injuries, for laparotomy 66.3
    in splenectomy 66.6
  for amputations 56.1
  in broad burn contracture release 58.25
  in Colles fractures 74.2
  for fractures of body of mandible 62.10
    for eyelet wiring, arch bars 62.10
  for fractures of vault of skull 63.7
  in hand injuries 75.1
  in hypovolaemic shock 53.2
  in immediate wound toilet 54.1
  in lesser facial wounds 61.1
  local
    for broken ribs 65.3
    in eye injuries 60.1

371

A MASS CASUALTY FORM

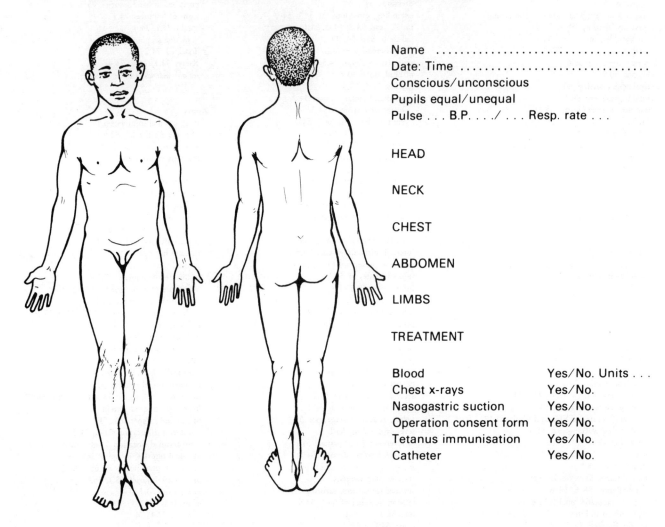

Name ....
Date: Time ....
Conscious/unconscious
Pupils equal/unequal
Pulse . . . B.P. . . ./ . . . Resp. rate . . .

HEAD

NECK

CHEST

ABDOMEN

LIMBS

TREATMENT

Blood   Yes/No. Units . . .
Chest x-rays   Yes/No.
Nasogastric suction   Yes/No.
Operation consent form   Yes/No.
Tetanus immunisation   Yes/No.
Catheter   Yes/No.

A PHYSIOLOGICAL NOMOGRAM

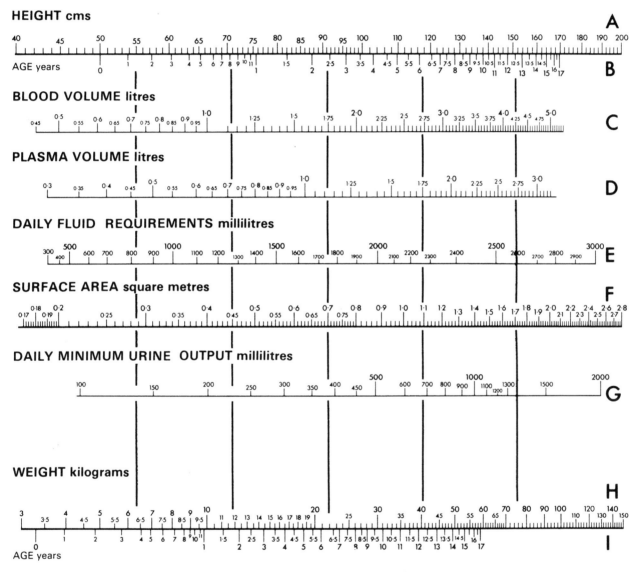

Fig. 58-6 A PHYSIOLOGICAL NOMOGRAM. Don't be defeated by this—it is really quite easy! A patient's blood volume, his plasma volume, his fluid requirements, and his minimum urine output are all proportional to his surface area. This in turn is proportional to his weight and height.

First, align his height and weight with a ruler, this will cross Scale F, at a point which indicates his surface area. Then hold the ruler vertically at this point (hold it parallel to the thick vertical lines) and read off his blood volume etc. For further instructions, see the next figure.

Drawn at the suggestion of Peter Bewes using data from the Ciba–Geigy Scientific Tables.

FLUID AND SODIUM NEEDS
WHEN SHOCK IS OVER

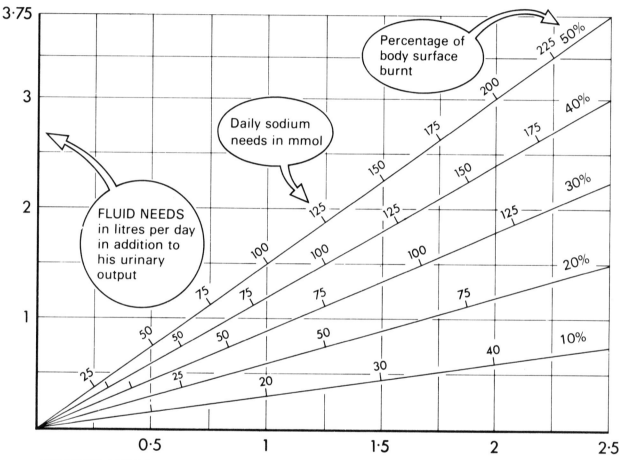

SURFACE AREA in square metres. Read
this off from the previous diagrams

Fig. 58-8 FLUID AND SODIUM NEEDS WHEN SHOCK IS OVER.
Calculate a patient's surface area from Fig. 58-6. Read off his daily
fluid needs. This covers the evaporation from his burn and his respiratory
losses, BUT NOT HIS URINE. Read off the sodium he requires in mmol.

For example, if his surface area is 2 square metres, and he has a 50%
burn and is passing 1500 ml of urine, he will need 3000 ml + 1500 =
4500 ml of fluid a day. He will also need 200 mmol of sodium. *Data
from Cason.*

A BURN CHART

NAME _____ WARD_____ NUMBER _____ DATE _____
AGE _____

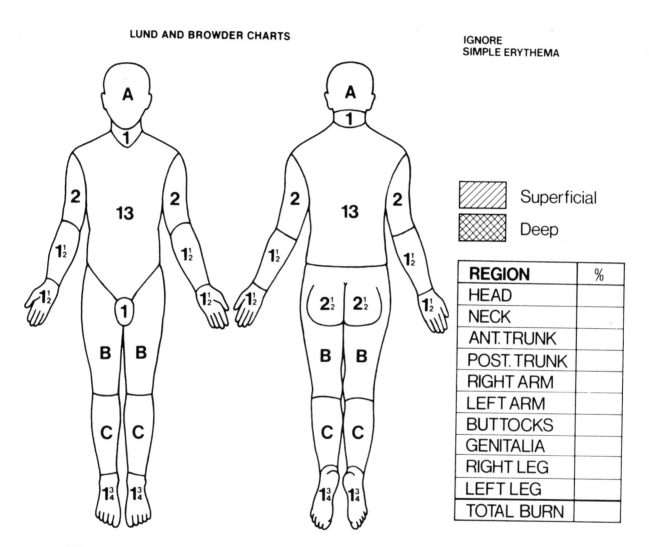

LUND AND BROWDER CHARTS

IGNORE
SIMPLE ERYTHEMA

Superficial

Deep

REGION	%
HEAD	
NECK	
ANT. TRUNK	
POST. TRUNK	
RIGHT ARM	
LEFT ARM	
BUTTOCKS	
GENITALIA	
RIGHT LEG	
LEFT LEG	
TOTAL BURN	

RELATIVE PERCENTAGE OF BODY SURFACE AREA AFFECTED BY GROWTH

AREA	AGE 0	1	5	10	15	ADULT
A = ½ OF HEAD	9½	8½	6½	5½	4½	3½
B = ½ OF ONE THIGH	2¾	3¼	4	4½	4½	4¾
C = ½ OF ONE LEG	2½	2½	2¾	3	3¼	3½

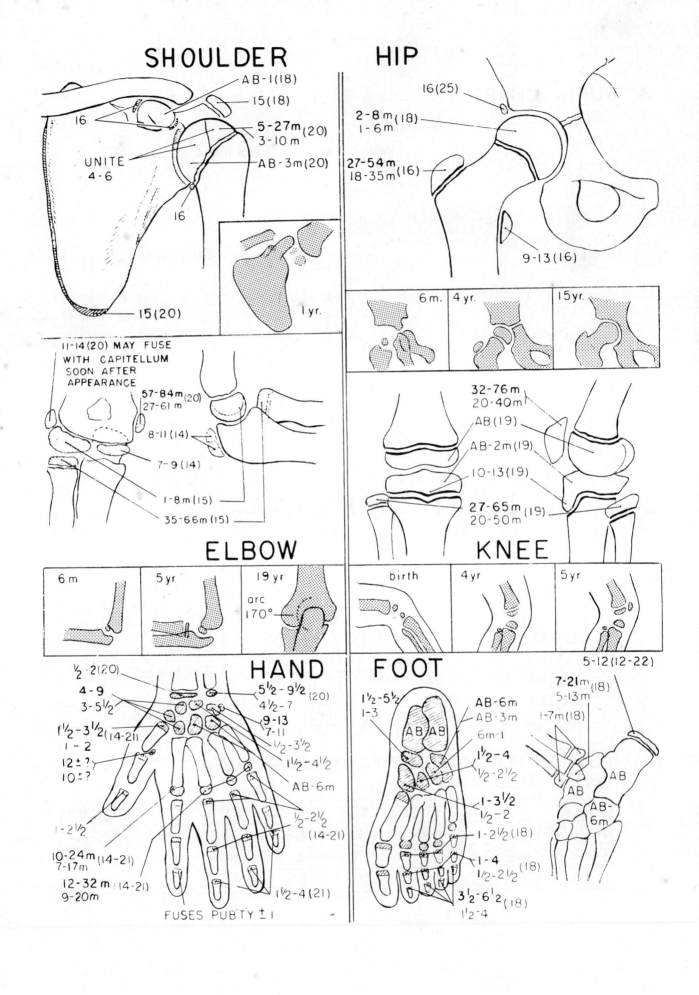

SHOULDER

AB-1(18)
15(18)
16
5-27m (20)
3-10 m
AB-3m(20)
UNITE
4-6
16
15(20)

1 yr.

11-14(20) MAY FUSE
WITH CAPITELLUM
SOON AFTER
APPEARANCE

57-84m(20)
27-61 m

8-11 (14)

7-9 (14)

1-8m(15)
35-66m(15)

ELBOW

| 6 m | 5 yr | 19 yr |

arc
170°

HAND

½-2(20)
4-9
3-5½
1½-3½(14-21)
1-2
12±?
10±?
1-2½
10-24m(14-21)
7-17m
12-32 m (14-21)
9-20m

5½-9½ (20)
4½-7
9-13
7-11
½-3½
1½-4½
AB-6m
½-2½
(14-21)
1½-4(21)

FUSES PUBTY ±1

HIP

16(25)
2-8 m(18)
1-6m
27-54m(16)
18-35m(16)

9-13(16)

| 6 m. | 4 yr. | 15 yr. |

32-76 m
20-40m
AB(19)
AB-2m(19)
10-13(19)
27-65 m (19)
20-50m

KNEE

| birth | 4 yr | 5 yr |

5-12(12-22)

FOOT

1½-5½
1-3
AB-6m
AB-3m
6m-1
1½-4
½-2½
1-3½
½-2
1-2½(18)
1-4
½-2½(18)
3½-6½(18)
1½-4

7-21m(18)
5-13 m
1-7m(18)
AB
AB
AB-
6m